Sanfilippo's Textbook of Pe
and Adolescent Gynecology

Second Edition

Edited by

Joseph S. Sanfilippo MD MBA
Professor, Department of Obstetrics, Gynecology and Reproductive Sciences,
and Academic Division Director, Reproductive Endocrinology and Infertility,
Magee-Womens Hospital of UPMC
University of Pittsburgh Medical Center
Pittsburgh, Philadelphia, USA

Eduardo Lara-Torre MD FACOG
Vice Chair for Academic Affairs and Section Chief,
Academic Specialists in General Obstetrics and Gynecology, Carilion Clinic;
and Professor, Department of Obstetrics and Gynecology and Pediatrics,
Virginia Tech-Carilion School of Medicine, Roanoke, Virginia, USA

Veronica Gomez-Lobo MD
Director of Pediatric and Adolescent Gynecology,
Eunice Kennedy Shriver National Institute of Child Health and
Human Development, Bethesda, Maryland; and MedStar/Children's National;
and Professor of Obstetrics and Gynecology, Georgetown University,
Washington, District of Columbia, USA

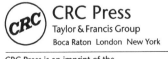

CRC Press
Taylor & Francis Group
Boca Raton London New York

CRC Press is an imprint of the
Taylor & Francis Group, an **informa** business

CRC Press
Taylor & Francis Group
6000 Broken Sound Parkway NW, Suite 300
Boca Raton, FL 33487-2742

First issued in paperback 2021

ISBN 13: 978-1-138-55157-2 (hbk)
ISBN 13: 978-1-03-224004-6 (pbk)

Library of Congress Cataloging-in-Publication Data

Names: Sanfilippo, J. S. (Joseph S.), editor. | Lara-Torre, Eduardo, editor. | Gomez-Lobo, Veronica, editor.
Title: Sanfilippo's textbook of pediatric and adolescent gynecology / edited by Joseph S Sanfilippo, Eduardo Lara-Torre, Veronica Gomez-Lobo.
Other titles: Clinical pediatric and adolescent gynecology. | Textbook of pediatric and adolescent gynecology | Pediatric and adolescent gynecology
Description: Second edition. | Boca Raton, FL : CRC Press, [2019] | Preceded by Clinical pediatric and adolescent gynecology / edited by Joseph S. Sanfilippo ... [et al.]. c2009. | Includes bibliographical references and index.
Identifiers: LCCN 2019006212| ISBN 9781138551572 (hardback) | ISBN 9781315147659 (eBook)
Subjects: | MESH: Genitalia, Female | Genital Diseases, Female | Sexual Development | Child | Adolescent
Classification: LCC RJ478 | NLM WS 320 | DDC 618.92/098--dc23
LC record available at https://lccn.loc.gov/2019006212

Visit the Taylor & Francis Web site at
http://www.taylorandfrancis.com

and the CRC Press Web site at
http://www.crcpress.com

Contents

Preface: We need the tools to get the job done

Where it all began—Prague, September 12, 1940: Rudolf Peter organized the first outpatient clinic for pediatric gynecology. In the United States, Goodrich Shauffler published the first pediatric gynecology (text) book in 1941. However, it was not until 1962 when there was further movement forward with the first faculty position predicated upon pediatric gynecology established at Charles University in Prague under the direction of Peter. Gynecology was now incorporated in pediatric educational curriculums.

In the United States and across the ocean, John Huffman at Northwestern collaborated with Vincent Capraro in Buffalo, New York, and Sir John Dewhurst in England to edit the book, *The Gynecology of Childhood and Adolescence*. Since that time, a number of books by authorities in the field have been published.

A number of us, serving as "Founding Fathers and Founding Mothers," organized the North American Society for Pediatric and Adolescent Gynecology (NASPAG) in 1986. Integral to the society was the *Journal of Pediatric and Adolescent Gynecology*, which I had the privilege of being affiliated with as the editor-in-chief from inception. The first issue included topics we continue to address and are included in this textbook, *viz.*, pubertal neuroendocrine maturation, molecular biology of steroid hydroxylase deficiency, and laparoscopy for chronic pelvic pain in adolescent women, as well as teen-parent programs, uterine and gonadal anomalies, and fertility in individuals with differences in sex development, to mention a few of the topics addressed.

We fast forward and see how expertise has expanded internationally. The Federation Internationale de Gynecologie Infantile et Juvenile (FIGIJ) has established educational forums all over the world (see Figure 0.1).

In this *Textbook of Pediatric and Adolescent Gynecology*, an effort has been made to provide easy access to a number of subjects:

- Establishing a pediatric and adolescent clinical and educational program designed for physicians in training
- Approach to transgender care in adolescents—a modus operandi for adolescents
- Fertility preservation—counseling, preservation of ovarian tissue as well as oocytes
- Obesity—what works and does not work
- Confidentiality in the age of electronic medical records
- Menstrual cycle as a "vital sign"—implications for clinical care
- Congenital anomalies—assessment and management both surgically and nonsurgically
- Common vulvovaginal problems clinicians are likely to manage
- Genital injuries—including acute care
- Dermatology—general and vulvovaginal

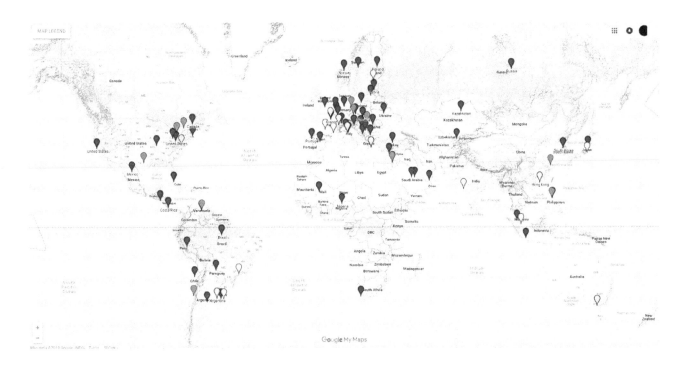

Figure 0.1 Pediatric adolescent gynecology sites across the world. (From http://www.figij.org/members/ with permission from Fédération Internationale de Gynécologie Infantile et Juvénile; accessed January 25, 2019.)

- Breast disorders—staging and assessment
- Polycystic ovarian syndrome—much new information
- Adolescent pregnancy—prevention and early gestation assessment
- Nutrition—designed to change your approach to counseling and follow-up
- Confidentiality—complex and challenging but extremely important
- An additional video section with further common procedures in pediatric and adolescent gynecology

The American Board of Obstetrics and Gynecology (ABOG) has established recognition of Adolescent Gynecology in developing a "Focused Practice" level of certification. Clinicians need to have a venue to be updated with progress in pertinent sectors of medicine germane to their clinical practice. What we have provided in this textbook serves to provide that foundation or complement your current state of knowledge. The education process needs to be ongoing, and thus entities such as the NASPAG, the ABOG, the Society for Adolescent Medicine, the American Society for Reproductive Medicine—Pediatric Adolescent Gynecology Special Interest Group, the American College of Obstetricians and Gynecologists—Committee on Adolescent Health Care, and the American Academy of Pediatricians—Section on Adolescent Health provide such a forum. We hope to meet your every expectation.

Welcome, Bienvenue, Wilkommen, Velkommen, Bem-vindo, Benvenuto, Bienvenido, Witam Cie, Croeso, Bengali, Shagatom, Aloha. Yokodo, Tuloy ka, Welkom, Shalom!

Joseph S. Sanfilippo, MD, MBA

Contributors

Lisa Allen MD FRCSC
Professor
Paediatric & Adolescent Gynaecology
University of Toronto
Toronto, Canada

Amanda Bogart MD
Children's Hospital Colorado
University of Colorado School of Medicine
Aurora, Colorado

Andrea E. Bonny MD
Assistant Professor
Department of Pediatrics
The Ohio State University
Columbus, Ohio

Asma Javed Chattha MD
Assistant Professor of Pediatrics
Mayo Clinic
Rochester, Minnesota

Stephanie Cizek MD
Clinical Fellow, Pediatric and Adolescent Gynecology
Cincinnati Children's Hospital Medical Center
Cincinnati, Ohio

Ellen Lancon Connor MD
Professor of Pediatric Endocrinology
American Family Children's Hospital
University of Wisconsin–Madison
Madison, Wisconsin

Nirupama K. De Silva MD
Professor
Department of Obstetrics and Gynecology
University of Oklahoma School of Community Medicine
Tulsa, Oklahoma

Jennifer E. Dietrich MD, MSC
Professor
Department of Obstetrics and Gynecology and Department
   of Pediatrics
Baylor College of Medicine
Texas Children's Hospital
Houston, Texas

Marcella Donaruma-Kwoh MD FAAP
Public Health and Child Abuse Pediatrics
Baylor College of Medicine
Texas Children's Hospital
Houston, Texas

Shirley M. Dong MD
The Ohio State University
Columbus, Ohio

Maggie Dwiggins MD
Pediatric and Adolescent Gynecology
Medstar Washington Hospital Center
Washington, District of Columbia

Kathleen Ellison MD
Director of Division of Dermatology
Cincinnati Children's Hospital
Cincinnati, Ohio

Susan D. Ernst MD
Associate Professor
Department of Obstetrics and Gynecology
University of Michigan
Ann Arbor, Michigan

Mary E. Fallat MD
Professor of Pediatric Surgery
Division Director of Pediatric Surgery
Department of Surgery
Surgeon-in-Chief, Norton Children's Hospital
University of Louisville
Louisville, Kentucky

Nathalie Fleming MD FRCSC
Professor
Department of Obstetrics and Gynecology
University of Ottawa
Ottawa, Canada

Hanna Goldberg MD MS
Section of Paediatric Gynaecology
Division of Endocrinology
The Hospital for Sick Children
University of Toronto
Toronto, Canada

Veronica Gomez-Lobo MD
Director of Pediatric and Adolescent Gynecology
Eunice Kennedy Shriver National Institute of Child Health
   and Human Development
Bethesda, Maryland

and

MedStar/Children's National

and

Professor of Obstetrics and Gynecology
Georgetown University
Washington, District of Columbia

Monica Henning MD
Assistant Professor
Department of Obstetrics and Gynecology
University of Oklahoma School of Community Medicine
Tulsa, Oklahoma

Geri D. Hewitt MD
Professor of Clinical Obstetrics
Section Chief, Obstetrics and Gynecology
Department of Obstetrics and Gynecology
Nationwide Children's Hospital
The Ohio State University
Columbus, Ohio

Cynthia Holland-Hall MD MPH
Associate Professor of Pediatrics
Section of Adolescent Health
Nationwide Children's Hospital
The Ohio State University College of Medicine
Columbus, Ohio

Emilie K. Johnson MD MPH
Attending Physician
Division of Urology
Ann & Robert H. Lurie Children's Hospital of Chicago
Chicago, Illinois

Paritosh Kaul MD
Children's Hospital Colorado
University of Colorado School of Medicine
Aurora, Colorado

Sari Kives MD FRCSC
Section of Paediatric Gynaecology
Division of Endocrinology
The Hospital for Sick Children
University of Toronto
Toronto, Canada

Eduardo Lara-Torre MD FACOG
Vice Chair for Academic Affairs and Section Chief
Academic Specialists in General Obstetrics
    and Gynecology
Carilion Clinic
and
Department of Obstetrics and Gynecology and
    Pediatrics
Virginia Tech-Carilion School of Medicine
Roanoke, Virginia

Meredith Loveless MD
Department Obstetrics, Gynecology and Pediatrics
Norton Children's Hospital
Gynecology Specialist
Clinical Faculty University of Louisville
Louisville, Kentucky

Veronica Lozano MD
Division of Gynecology
Baylor Scott and White
Temple, Texas

Kalyani Marathe MD MPH
Associate Professor of Dermatology and Pediatrics
Cincinnati Children's Hospital
University of Cincinnati
Cincinnati, Ohio

Tia M. Melton MD
Department of Obstetrics and Gynecology
University Hospitals Cleveland Medical Center
Cleveland, Ohio

Diane F. Merritt MD
Professor, Director of Pediatric and
    Adolescent Gynecology
Department of Obstetrics and Gynecology
Washington University School of Medicine
St. Louis, Missouri

Heather C. Millar MD FRCSC
Department of Obstetrics and Gynaecology
University of Toronto
Toronto, Canada

Lisa Moon MD
Baylor College of Medicine
Houston, Texas

Molly Moravek MD MPH
Assistant Professor
Department of Obstetrics & Gynecology
    and Urology
University of Michigan
Ann Arbor, Michigan

Jasmine Multani MD
Section of Paediatric Gynaecology
Division of Endocrinology
The Hospital for Sick Children
University of Toronto
Toronto, Canada

Anne-Marie Amies Oelschlager MD
Professor of Obstetrics and Gynecology
Department of Obstetrics and Gynecology
Seattle Children's Hospital
University of Washington School of Medicine
Seattle, Washington

Mary A. Ott MD MA
Professor of Pediatrics and Adolescent Medicine
Division of Adolescent Medicine
Indiana University School of Medicine
Indianapolis, Indiana

Bindu N. Patel MD
Pediatric and Adolescent Gynecology
Department of Obstetrics and Gynecology
Washington University School of Medicine
St. Louis, Missouri

Gisselle Perez-Milicua MD
Baylor College of Medicine
Houston, Texas

Elisabeth H. Quint MD
Professor
Department of Obstetrics and Gynecology
Women's Hospital
University of Michigan
Ann Arbor, Michigan

Allison B. Ratto PHD
Assistant Professor
Division of Neuropsychology
Children's National Health System
Washington, District of Columbia

Emily K. Redman MD
Department of Obstetrics and Gynecology
University of Pittsburgh Medical Center
Pittsburgh, Pennsylvania

Ellen S. Rome MD MPH
Professor of Pediatrics
Head, Center for Adolescent Medicine
Cleveland Clinic Children's Hospital
Cleveland, Ohio

Joseph S. Sanfilippo MD MBA
Vice Chairman, Reproductive Sciences
Department of Obstetrics, Gynecology and Reproductive
    Sciences
and
Academic Division Director, Reproductive Endocrinology
    and Infertility
Magee-Womens Hospital of UPMC
University of Pittsburgh Medical Center
Pittsburgh, Philadelphia

Margarett Shnorhavorian MD
Associate Professor of Urology
Division of Pediatric Urology
Seattle Children's DSD Program
University of Washington School of Medicine
Seattle, Washington

Erin H. Sieke MD MS
Cleveland Clinic Lerner College of Medicine at Case
Cleveland, Ohio

Judith Simms-Cendan MD
Professor of Obstetrics and Gynecology
University of Central Florida College of Medicine
Orlando, Florida

Jessica Papillon Smith MD MEd FRCSC
Department of Obstetrics and Gynecology
McGill University Health Centre
Montreal, Canada

Steven R. Smith
Dean Emeritus
California Western School of Law
San Diego, California

Laurel Sofer MD
Resident Physician
Division of Urology
Ann & Robert H. Lurie Children's Hospital of Chicago
Chicago, Illinois

M. Jonathon Solnik MD FACOG FACS
Associate Professor of Obstetrics and Gynaecology
University of Toronto
Toronto, Canada

Joanna Stacey MD
Director, Division of Gynecology
Assistant Professor of Obstetrics and Gynecology
Baylor Scott and White
Temple, Texas

Kathryn Stambough MD
Obstetrics and Gynecology
Pediatric and Adolescent Gynecology
Baylor College of Medicine
Houston, Texas

Julie Strickland MD MPH
Professor
Department of Obstetrics and Gynecology
University of Missouri-Kansas City
Kansas City, Missouri

Julia F. Taylor MD MA
Assistant Professor of Pediatrics
Division of General Pediatrics and Adolescent Medicine
School of Medicine
University of Virginia
Charlottesville, Virginia

Gylynthia Trotman MD MPH
Assistant Professor of Obstetrics and Gynecology
Icahn School of Medicine at Mount Sinai
New York City, New York

Lisa Tuchman MD MPH
Chief, Division of Adolescent and Young Adult Medicine
Children's National Medical Center
Washington, District of Columbia

Nichole Tyson MD
The Kaiser Permanente Medical Group
Roseville, California

Whitney Wellenstein MD
Kaiser Foundation Hospital
Oakland, California

Ariel White MD
Fellow, Division of Adolescent and Adult Medicine
Children's National Medical Center
Washington, District of Columbia

Normal pubertal development and the menstrual cycle as a vital sign*

1

MEREDITH LOVELESS

Puberty consists of a complex interplay of hormonal and physiologic changes that result in sexual maturation and capability for reproduction.[1] This transition is an important phase of development accompanied by physical, social, and behavioral changes. Health-care providers play an important role during this time in monitoring that the process is occurring within normal parameters and providing evaluation if concerns in development arise. In most cases, the process of puberty occurs normally, although there is a broad variation of "normal" that may lead to anxiety in some patients and families. When the pubertal process does not occur within standards of normal, it may represent underlying health concerns and alert the health-care provider of the need for further evaluation and possible interventions. This chapter reviews the stages of normal puberty in females and provides guidance on abnormalities that may require investigation.

TIMING OF PUBERTY

Girls normally begin puberty between 8 and 13 years of age.[2] Thelarche is usually the first sign of puberty followed by pubarche; although 15% of girls will experience pubarche first.[3] Vaginal bleeding before thelarche does not typically represent menarche and should be evaluated. The physiologic mechanism for timing of puberty is not known. There are multiple factors that influence pubertal timing, including genetic, environmental, neuropeptides, energy balance, intrinsic factors, stress, and sleep; however, the key regulatory step for activation of puberty is unknown.[1] Sexual maturation declined rapidly during the first half of the twentieth century attributed to better nutrition as the Western world developed but has remained steady the latter part of the twentieth century. Age of menarche has declined minimally; however, age of thelarche appears to continue to decline.[4] There appears to be a trend toward earlier age to reach Sexual Maturation Rating (SMR) 2 but the age for SMR 3 and age of menarche remains steady.[5] Delayed puberty is defined as lack of pubertal development by an age that is 2–2.5 standard deviations beyond the population mean.[6] In the United States, lack of breast development (SMR 2) by age 13 and menses that has not started within 3 years of thelarche or by age 15 warrant evaluation.[6,7] Precocious puberty is defined as pubertal changes occurring prior to the age of 8 years, although the earlier onset of thelarche makes this age cutoff more controversial. Further discussion on the anomalies of puberty is included in Chapter 5.

It is plausible that the earlier onset of breast development is related to environmental factors. These factors are called *endocrine disruptors* and are environmental chemicals, dietary supplements, and/or medications that interfere with the endocrine system.[8] There is evidence from animal studies that endocrine disruptors affect pubertal timing, but studies in humans have been more difficult and are not currently well understood.[5] More research is needed to understand how medications, environmental agents, and nutritional deficiencies, as well as supplements, can impact pubertal timing. One environmental agent that was found to disrupt puberty in animals and is found in higher levels in children with higher adiposity is biphenol A (BPA). Found in plastic bottles and toys, it has been linked to having an estrogenic effect at low levels and to competing with endogenous estrogen for binding and antiandrogenic properties at higher levels.[9] Chemicals, pesticides, dioxins, polychlorinated biphenyls (PCBs), and flame retardants are present across the ecosystem and have been detected in humans.[9] Exposure to a broad mixture of environmental contaminants makes it challenging to determine if these substances are playing a role in pubertal timing and what that role is; however, growing evidence suggests there is environmental impact on pubertal timing.

Another important factor that may influence pubertal timing is obesity. Multiple studies show a correlation between increased body mass index (BMI) and early puberty.[5] The National Health and Nutrition Examination Survey III (NHANES III) collected pubertal data from 2300 U.S. children ages 8 years and up from 1988 to 1994. This data showed children with a BMI greater than the 85th percentile were strongly associated with earlier age of breast development and menarche, with menarche occurring at a mean age of 12.06 in obese girls compared to 12.57 in nonobese girls.[10] Additional studies suggest that rapid weight gain and early puberty followed by development of obesity, and metabolic syndrome lead to an overall increase in mortality that persists into adulthood.[5] Data have not shown obesity alone as the primary cause of earlier pubertal timing. Some studies suggest leptin, which is related to growth and pubertal development and affects appetite, adiposity, and energy regulation, may be a link associated with this finding.[4] It is also postulated that endocrine disruptors may act on adipocytes, thereby linking early puberty and obesity.[4]

---

* Thanks to Shawn Smith, Kimberley McClanahan, and Hatim Omar for their contributions from the first edition to this chapter.

Early puberty has also been associated with higher rates of depression, anxiety, smoking, delinquent behavior, and early sexual experiences.[5] Chronic stress including a lower socioeconomic status has also been associated with early puberty.[5,10] It is difficult to determine if the consequences of obesity, such as bullying, stress from difficult social situations, or early puberty itself, are related to the link with mood and behavior changes.

HORMONAL CHANGES

Puberty is initiated and controlled by a complex relationship of multiple hormones. The regulatory steps to initiation of puberty are still unknown. The hypothalamus secretes gonadotropin-releasing hormone (GnRH), which signals the gonadotrophs in the pituitary to release gonadotrophins: luteinizing hormone (LH) and follicle-stimulating hormone (FSH). Luteinizing hormone acts on the theca cells in the ovary to produce androgens, and FSH acts on ovarian follicles to produce estradiol, inhibin, and gametes. The interplay is called the hypothalamic-pituitary-gonadal (HPG) axis (Figure 1.1).[3] During the first 3 months of life, under the influence of maternal estrogen exposure in utero, LH and FSH levels are high. By age 6 months, LH levels are almost undetectable. While FSH levels decrease after the first 6 months, they can remain elevated until age 3–4 years.[3] At this point, the HPG axis remains quiescent until activation initiates puberty. The LH level is generally the most useful marker for assessing onset of puberty with elevated levels in childhood indicating central nervous system activity related to onset of puberty.[3] Levels of FSH may be found elevated with thelarche (which can be an isolated event), so they are not a reliable indicator of pubertal onset.[4] Estradiol and testosterone levels are low in prepubertal girls and rise with onset of puberty and should be consistent with laboratory reference levels for age. Leptin does not have a direct role in puberty initiation but likely influences GnRH secretion.[3]

The action of multiple hormones in concerted fashion regulates linear growth in children and adolescents. Growth hormone is the primary growth-stimulating factor during prepubertal growth. Sex hormone augmentations of growth hormone secretion, as well as direct growth-stimulating effects of sex steroids, cause growth acceleration during puberty. Thyroid hormone also plays a key role in growth and development. The concerted actions of both growth hormone and thyroid hormone are largely responsible for skeletal growth. When growth is not occurring on a normal trajectory, evaluation for underlying endocrine etiology should be considered. Failing to appropriately assess a child's growth can often cause a missed or delayed diagnosis of a systemic illness.

GROWTH

The process of normal puberty includes growth, development of secondary sexual characteristics, and onset of menstruation. There is a wide age range in which girls will start the pubertal process. Multiple factors may influence the age at which puberty begins, including family history, environmental factors, underlying health conditions, and nutrition, among others. There are several guidelines to help determine if the child is progressing in a manner that falls within the norm. Growth spurt is typically the first indication of pubertal onset and typically occurs before the onset of secondary sexual characteristics. A longitudinal study reported an increase in both height and foot growth before the onset of secondary sexual characteristics, suggesting change in foot size may be an early marker for puberty.[11] The correct assessment and measurement of growth is an essential component of health supervision. When evaluating a child's growth, it is imperative to determine growth rate, rather than simply relying on a cross-sectional analysis of one measurement in time. Correct monitoring of growth requires careful plotting of data on growth curves. Growth curves are published by the Centers for Disease Control and Prevention and include percentile ranges for girls 2–20 years of age (Figure 1.2).[12] The BMI is an anthropometric index of weight and height combined with age and is a useful index in the evaluation of overall general health (Figure 1.3).[12] The BMI is calculated by dividing weight in kilograms by the square of height in meters. An important difference between using BMI in children and adults is the influence of changing levels of sexual maturity. For example, among patients with similar BMI, the patients with higher sexual maturation will have

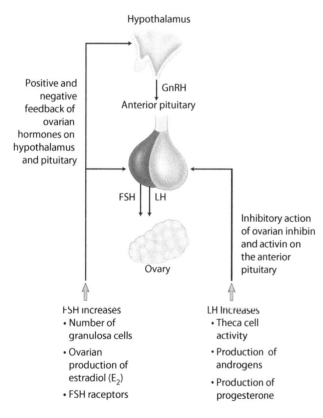

Figure 1.1 Hypothalamic-pituitary-gonadal axis. (With kind permission from Springer Science+Business Media: Normal timing of puberty, 2014, Boswell H. In: Dietrich JE, ed. *Female Puberty: A Comprehensive Guide for Clinicians*, New York, NY, p. 9.)

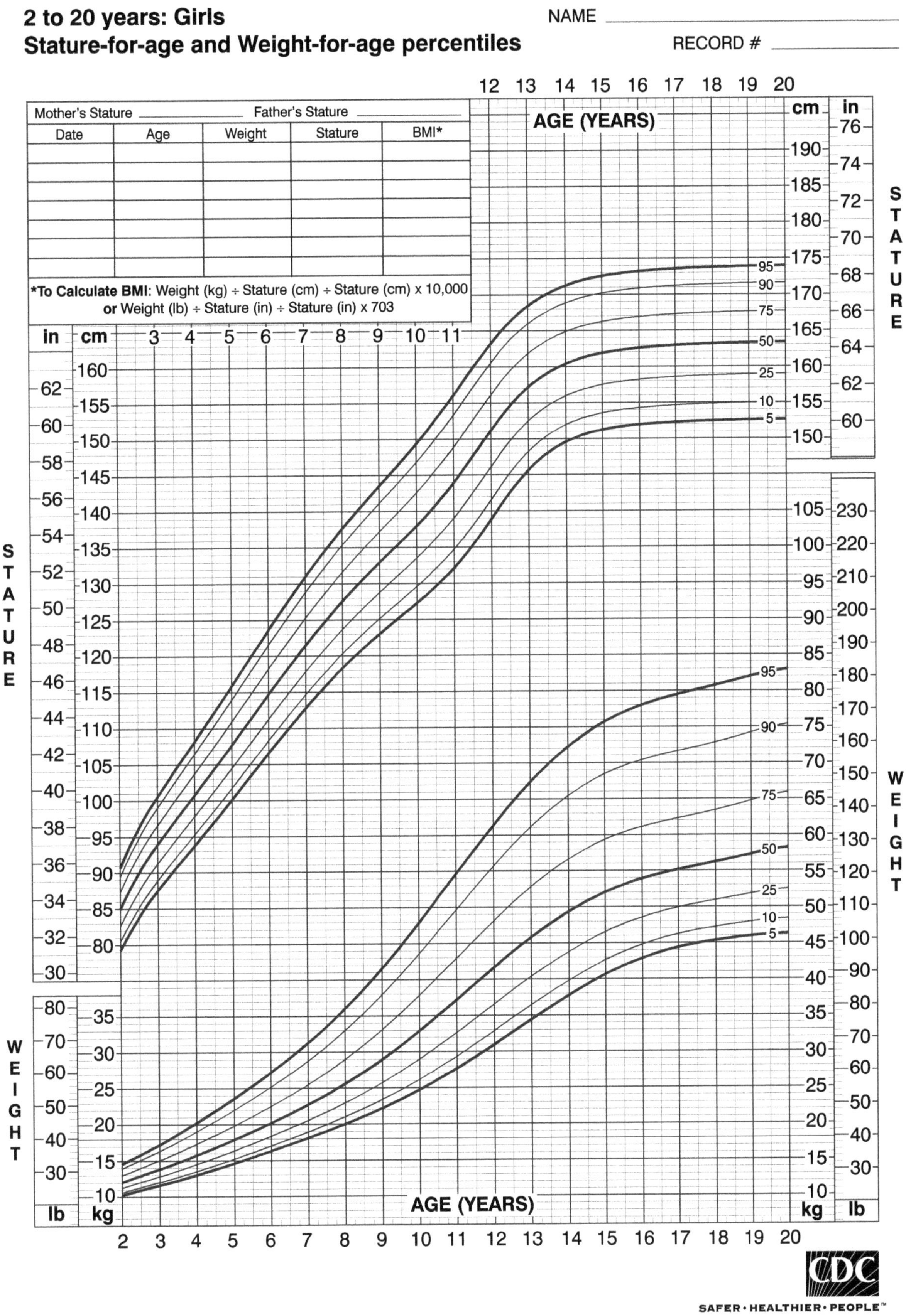
2 to 20 years: Girls
Stature-for-age and Weight-for-age percentiles
NAME
RECORD #
Mother's Stature
Father's Stature
Date
Age
Weight
Stature
BMI*
*To Calculate BMI: Weight (kg) ÷ Stature (cm) ÷ Stature (cm) x 10,000
or Weight (lb) ÷ Stature (in) ÷ Stature (in) x 703
AGE (YEARS)
STATURE
WEIGHT
in
cm
lb
kg
95
90
75
50
25
10
5
SAFER • HEALTHIER • PEOPLE™

Figure 1.2 Growth chart for monitoring of growth in girls aged 2–20 years, developed by the National Center for Health Statistics in collaboration with the National Center for Chronic Disease Prevention and Health Promotion, May 30, 2000 (modified November 21, 2000). (From https://www.cdc.gov/growthcharts/data/set2clinical/cj41c072.pdf.)

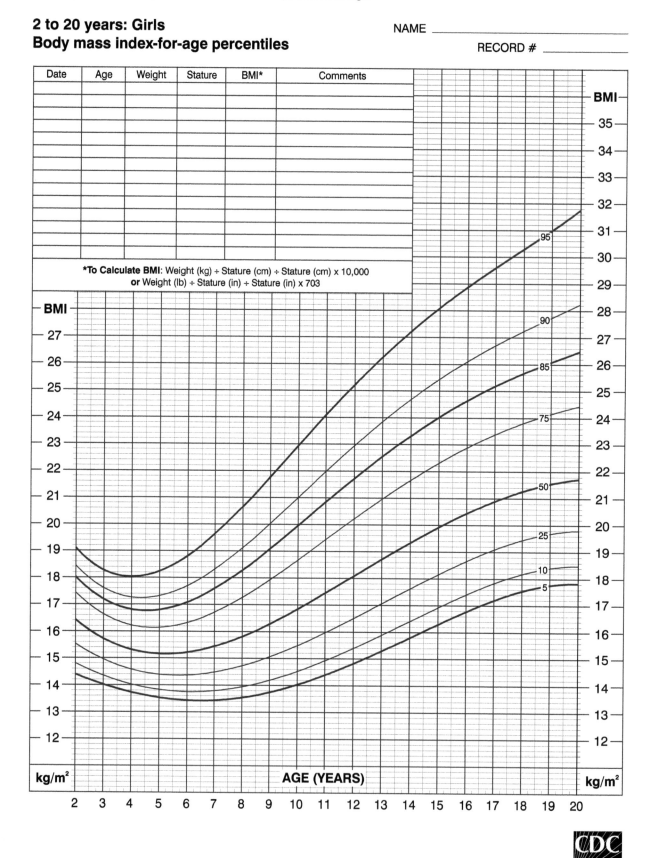

2 to 20 years: Girls
Body mass index-for-age percentiles

NAME _____

RECORD # _____

*To Calculate BMI: Weight (kg) ÷ Stature (cm) ÷ Stature (cm) x 10,000
or Weight (lb) ÷ Stature (in) ÷ Stature (in) x 703

Figure 1.3 Chart for assessing body mass index (BMI) in girls aged 2–20 years, developed by the National Center for Health Statistics in collaboration with the National Center for Chronic Disease Prevention and Health Promotion, May 30, 2000 (modified October 16, 2000). (From https://www.cdc.gov/growthcharts/data/set1clinical/cj41c024.pdf.)

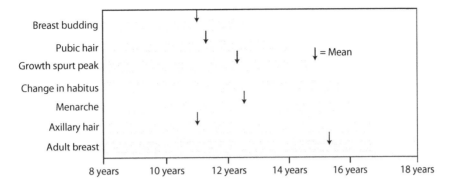

Figure 1.4 Timeline of female pubertal milestones. (Adapted with permission from Fritz MA, Speroff L. *Clinical Gynecologic Endocrinology and Infertility.* 8th ed. Philadelphia, PA: Lippincott Williams & Wilkins; With kind permission from Springer Science+Business Media: Normal timing of puberty, 2014, Boswell H. In: Dietrich JE, ed. *Female Puberty: A Comprehensive Guide for Clinicians*, New York, NY, p. 16.)

a lower percentage of body fat. The importance of including BMI in routine evaluation of growth is to screen for underweight or overweight children and adolescents with respect to age and height. In children and adolescents, a BMI for age greater than 95% is defined as overweight and between 85% and 95% as at increased risk for obesity. Some growth charts have been developed that allow for the variation in growth pattern of a specific medical condition (e.g., Trisomy 21 or gonadal dysgenesis). These charts represent the standard growth for that condition, thereby allowing a child to be compared against standards in his or her own cohort. Many electronic health records will maintain the growth charts within the electronic system, which is a useful tool and allows multiple providers to see growth patterns over time.

PUBERTAL EVENTS

The process of puberty occurs through a series of coordinated events that follow a usually predictable timeline; however, events may overlap or vary slightly in their order (Figure 1.4).

PUBERTAL GROWTH

During puberty, males and females experience the greatest growth velocity, besides that seen during infancy. This growth can be conveniently divided into three stages[13]:

1. The nadir that occurs just before the growth spurt
2. The stage when the adolescent is experiencing the maximum growth velocity
3. The final stage when growth velocity decreases, which occurs before epiphyseal fusion

It is important to remember, especially when examining patients during this period of rapid growth, that although growth is described in centimeters per year, this represents the average growth for that year, and velocity may change throughout this time period. A good marker for following growth of an adolescent through puberty is the peak height velocity (PHV). In girls, PHV ranges from 6 to 10 cm/year, usually coinciding with SMR breast stage

2–3.[3] During puberty, girls will gain an average of 25 cm. For some, this growth velocity is doubled compared with preadolescent rates. The adolescent growth spurt occurs on average 2 years earlier in females compared with males. Thus, for a temporary period, girls may be taller than many boys of the same age.[14–16]

CHANGES IN BODY COMPOSITION

During the rapid growth of puberty, not only is there growth in all tissues, but there are also significant changes in body composition. Girls will experience an increase in percentage of body fat. Body shape changes as the increased body fat is distributed in the lower body to a gynecoid or pear-shaped distribution. The skeleton also undergoes a great amount of growth, not only in length but also in density. Each bone begins with a primary center of ossification and will go through many stages of enlargement and shaping. The adult form is reached when epiphyses ossify and fuse with the main body of the bone. All of these changes are evident on radiographics, as the calcium content of the bone is opaque. The sequence of the changes in bone is the same in all individuals; thus, using radiographs to evaluate skeletal bone age in comparison to chronological age is an excellent clinical tool. The photographic atlas of Greulich and Pyle is the most commonly used resource to compare radiographs of the hand with standards of maturation in a normal population.[17] Growth and puberty are 99% complete by the time bone age reaches 17 years.[3]

BONE DENSITY

Adolescence is an important time for bone density accrual. A longitudinal study demonstrated that during the 4-year adolescent period of peak linear growth, more than 35% of total body bone mineral and 27% of bone mineral at the femoral neck was laid down.[18] This corresponds to as much bone mineral as most adults lose during their remaining life.[1] Many factors can affect the accretion of bone mineral, including genetic factors, ethnicity, body mass, level of physical activity including weight-bearing activity, dietary calcium and vitamin D intake, smoking, and dietary intake of certain products including carbonated beverages. Obtainment of peak bone density requires a high calcium intake, and recommendations for calcium and vitamin intake during this period are 1200 mg calcium and 400 IU vitamin D daily.[19] Estrogen is a key mediator for bone density accrual in females, so disorders that lead to a hypoestrogenic state can negatively impact bone density, such as female athlete triad, anorexia, and conditions resulting in hypothalamic hypogonadism.

SLEEP

Sleep regulation changes during sexual maturation. Teens tend to want to stay up later and sleep in later than younger children. The changes that occur during puberty include a significant decline in non-rapid eye movement (NREM) sleep, melatonin release is later, and circadian rhythm patterns change. Teens and parents often express concern about daytime sleepiness despite adequate overall sleep time, and this may be attributed to the decrease in NREM sleep.[20] The American Academy of Sleep Medicine recommends teenagers 13–18 years of age should sleep 8–10 hours per 24 hours on a regular basis to promote optimal health.[21] The American Academy of Pediatrics published a policy statement in 2014 with recommendations to delay school start times to 8:30 a.m. or later to optimize sleep in students.[22] The report explains that there is a substantial body of research demonstrating that delaying school start times is an effective countermeasure to chronic sleep loss and has a wide range of potential benefits for students regarding physical and mental health, safety, and academic achievement.[22]

BRAIN DEVELOPMENT

Structurally, the brain undergoes changes during puberty that largely affect the frontal and prefrontal cortex. The frontal cortex is responsible for executive function tasks, so teen's tasks involving oculomotor abilities and problem-solving have been shown to improve during adolescence; however, reaction time to assess emotional-related material declines during this time.[1,23,24] Studies have shown the prefrontal cortex is responsible for forward planning and regulatory control of emotional behavior and continues development into the early 20s.[1,25] The definition of adolescence as defined by the World Health Organization (WHO) focuses on ages 13–19 years but has been extended by several organizations into the early 20s in conjunction with timing of brain maturation.[26]

SECONDARY SEXUAL CHARACTERISTICS

Objective measures to evaluate pubertal physical changes allow the clinician to better monitor the normal rate of development. The standard universal system in use today was initially described by Tanner in 1969 and is currently known as the Sexual Maturity Scale (SMS).[3] Activation of the HPG axis leads to production of sex steroids, estrogen and androgens from the ovaries. The effect of estrogen includes breast development, estrogenization of the vagina and growth of female internal reproductive organs, body fat deposition, and linear growth. Androgens secreted by the adrenal gland contribute to body odor and the growth of pubic and axillary hair. Previous studies focused significantly on differences by ethnic background, but now these ages need to be considered carefully, because the pure lines of racial origin are not as clear as in the past.

Thelarche

When evaluating the breast, it is important to include palpation of the breast tissue and visual inspection of the areola, papilla, and breast tissue. Palpation is an important tool to differentiate breast tissue from adipose tissue in overweight females. Age of onset of breast development can be influenced by ethnicity, and mean age of onset is 8.8, 9.3, 9.7, and 9.7 years for African American, Hispanic, white non-Hispanic, and Asians, respectively.[27] In African American and Mexican American girls, breast development may occur up to a year earlier than in other ethnic cohorts and can be normal in the 7th year of age.[4]

SMR is used to describe breast development (Figure 1.5).[28] In SMR stage 1 or the preadolescent stage, there is only elevation of the papilla. Stage 2 progresses to elevation of the breast and papilla as a small mound. Stage 3 represents further enlargement and elevation of breast and areola with no separation of their contours. Projection of the areola and papilla to form a secondary mound above the level of the breast is stage 4. Finally, stage 5 represents the mature stage, which is projection of the areola and papilla due to the recession of the areola to the general contour of the breast. The initial breast tissue in the earlier stage of growth can be unilateral, which may persist for 6–9 months. Knowing this can not only provide reassurance to patients and families, but also may avoid unnecessary diagnostic tests. Historically, menarche occurred 2–2.5 years after thelarche; however, the correlation of age of onset of breast development and menarche has changed in the last decade and therefore is less predictive than it once was.[5,18,29]

Pubarche

Pubarche is the physical findings of growth of pubic and axillary hair. Pubarche is caused by adrenarche, which is the increase in adrenal androgens, principally dehydroepiandrosterone (DHEA) and androstenedione.[1] Mean onset of pubic hair in nonobese girls is 11.57 years and 11.39 years in obese girls. Pubarche begins at a mean age of 10.65 in non-Hispanic black, 11.6 years in non-Hispanic white, and 11.63 in Mexican American girls.[29] As with breast development, SMR is used to describe pubic hair development (Figure 1.6).[28] When examining pubic hair, it is important to make note of the distribution of the hair. For example, from the prepubertal stage 1 to stage 2, pubic hair begins to grow along the labia; as maturity continues, growth occurs over the mons pubis; and finally at stage 5, growth has occurred on the medial thigh. During the progression through the SMR, the hair becomes more pigmented, coarser, and curlier. There is no SMR for axillary hair. However, a gross scale of 1 (no hair) to 3 (adult pattern of hair) is sometimes used. There is an increase in the activity

Tanner stage 1	Preadolescent	Only papilla is elevated
Tanner stage 2	Breast budding	Enlargement and widening of the areola and mound-like elevation of the breast and papilla
Tanner stage 3		Further enlargement of breast and areola with No separation of contours
Tanner stage 4		Projection of the areola and papilla to form secondary mound above the level of the breast and further enlargement
Tanner stage 5	Adult breast	Projection of the papilla only, as the areola recesses to the mature contour of the breast

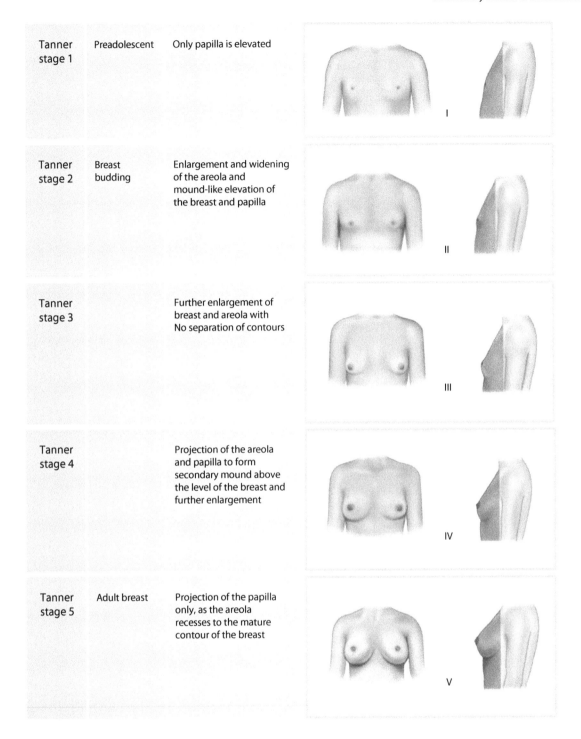

Figure 1.5 SMR staging: female breast development. (With kind permission from Springer Science+Business Media: Normal timing of puberty, 2014, Boswell H. In: Dietrich JE, ed. *Female Puberty: A Comprehensive Guide for Clinicians*, New York, NY, p. 18.)

of glandular tissue, specifically sebaceous glands and merocrine sweat glands. During the initial appearance of pubic and axillary hair, the apocrine glands begin to function.[14]

Premature pubarche is precocious development of axillary and pubic hair caused by premature adrenarche, which is the early increase of adrenal DHEA. Pubarche is considered early or premature when it occurs prior to the age of 8 years in girls. It affects up to 15% of girls and may be considered a normal variant, so the true definition of premature pubarche is not well defined.[2,29] This is more common in girls than in boys, especially in African American girls. Risk for premature adrenarche is increased in small-for-gestational-age infants and has been described as an early marker for development of polycystic ovarian syndrome (PCOS).[30,31] Girls with premature adrenarche have a higher rate of metabolic syndrome, including being overweight, having insulin resistance, and having dyslipidemia.[1,32]

Tanner stage 1	Preadolescent	No discernable difference between vellus hair on the mons and anterior abdominal wall, no pubic hair	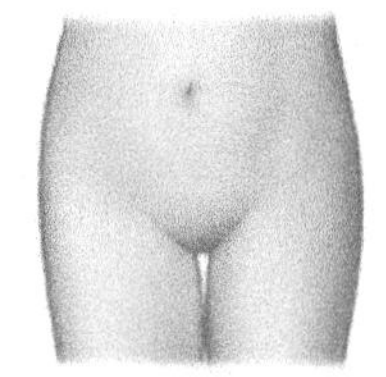
Tanner stage 2		Appearance of few, sparse, lightly pigmented hairs, with minimal curl on the labia	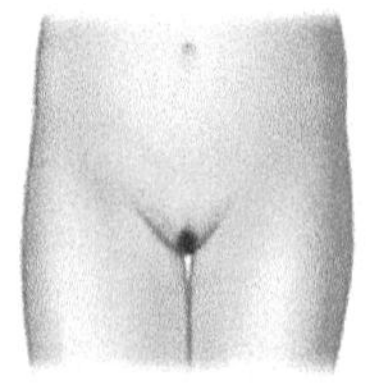
Tanner stage 3		Hair becomes darker, coarser and begins to spread over the junction of the labia	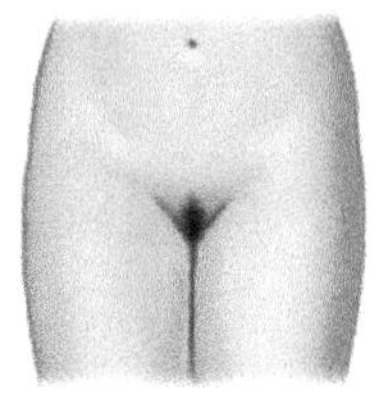
Tanner stage 4		Adult hair type emerges, covers mons pubis, but does not extend to the thighs	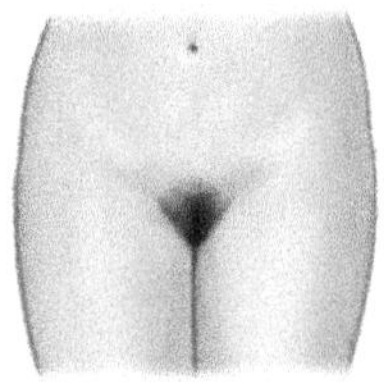
Tanner stage 5	Adult hair pattern	Adult hair type in the classic female pattern	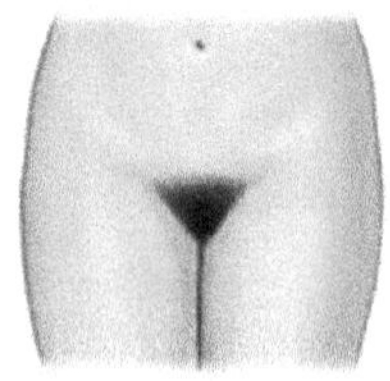

Figure 1.6 SMR female pubic hair development. (With kind permission from Springer Science + Business Media: Normal timing of puberty, 2014, Boswell H. In: Dietrich JE, ed. *Female Puberty: A Comprehensive Guide for Clinicians*, New York, NY, p. 19.)

Menarche

Menarche is often considered the final pubertal milestone. As the HPG axis matures, it leads to the production of estrogen and low levels of androgens from the ovaries, establishing a hormonal feedback loop. Under the influence of estrogen, the uterus will grow, and the endometrial lining will become thickened. When ovulation occurs, there is a surge in progesterone, coupled with a fall in estrogen levels. In the absence of pregnancy, this will trigger the shedding of the endometrial lining and menstrual cycle. Initial menstrual cycles may not all be ovulatory. Menses requires several components, including intact HPG axis, structurally normal end organs (ovaries and uterus), and good overall health. When the body is under stress, the HPG axis does not function normally and results in disruption of menses, making it an excellent marker for overall health. The American College of Obstetricians and Gynecologists (ACOG) Committee on Adolescent Health, endorsed by the American Academy of Pediatrics (AAP), published a committee opinion advocating the use of the menstrual cycle as a vital sign. They encourage asking about last menstrual period and menstrual patterns at each comprehensive or preventive care visit. By including an evaluation of the menstrual cycle as an additional vital sign, clinicians reinforce its importance in assessing overall health status for patients and caregivers.[7]

To use menses as a vital sign, we must understand what normal menstrual function is. The median age of menarche is 12–13 years across well-nourished populations in developed countries.[7] In the past 30 years, there has not been a change in median age of menarche according to NHANES, except among the non-Hispanic black population, which has a 5.5-month earlier median age at menarche than it did 30 years ago.[7,32] Menarche typically follows pubertal onset by 2–2.5 years; however, this historical guide is not always a consistent rule. While the mean age for onset of menarche remains stable, the duration between puberty and menarche varies. Girls starting puberty at age 9 have an average of 2.7 years to menarche, while those starting puberty at age 13 years have an average of 0.7 years to menarche.[1,33] Once menarche has started, the expected interval is every 21–45 days, with a cycle that lasts 7 days or less (see reference[7]). Immaturity of the HPG axis during early years after menarche may result in anovulatory cycles and an irregular pattern; however, 90% of cycles will be within the range of 21–45 days.[33,34] While a long interval due to anovulation is not uncommon in adolescents, it is statistically uncommon for girls to remain amenorrheic for more than 3 months (the 95th percentile for cycle length) and should prompt evaluation.[7] Patients should be encouraged to record their menstrual bleeding to help providers determine if the pattern is within normal limits. This can be made easier with a paper diary or apps that are readily available for this purpose. Adolescent girls may seek medical attention for cycle variations that fall within normal range or be unaware that their bleeding pattern is abnormal and may be attributed to significant underlying medical issues.[7] When the health-care provider inquires as to onset of menses and date of last menstrual period and their bleeding pattern, they have the opportunity to identify patterns that may require evaluation.[7] Providers who care for adult patients may also educate them regarding what is considered normal in adolescents, which may allow them to seek care when menstrual abnormalities are present in their daughters.

Abnormalities in timing of menarche are also a useful marker of overall health. Typically, menarche will occur within 2–3 years after breast budding, characteristically at SMR stages 3–4, and is rare before SMR 3.[35] The process from accelerated growth to menarche is 4.5 years, but the range is between 1.5 and 6 years.[33] Evaluation should occur if menarche has not occurred within 3 years after thelarche, by age 15 with secondary sex characteristics, or by age 14 with signs of hirsutism or evidence for excessive exercise or eating disorder. When abnormalities in the menstrual pattern are found, investigation for underlying causes based on careful history, physical exam, and appropriate imaging and laboratory studies should be undertaken or referral made to a specialist if that is not within the provider's scope of practice.[7]

An abnormal bleeding pattern can also represent underlying health concerns. The typical menstrual flow in adolescents is an interval of 32.2 days with a range of 21–45 days and a flow that lasts 7 days or less requiring 3–6 pads or tampons per day. Menstrual flow requiring a change of sanitary products every 1–2 hours, frequent flooding or soiling, and prolonged bleeding exceeding 7 days are consistent with excessive menstruation (see reference[7]). Teaching adolescents to evaluate the amount of flow using a visual tool such as the pictorial chart may be beneficial. Abnormal uterine bleeding, its causes, and its management are reviewed in Chapter 14.

CONCLUSION

Using the menstrual cycle as a vital sign gives clinicians an important tool to monitor overall health in female youth. Growth, pubertal timing and progression, and the onset of menarche can all provide reassurance of overall health when progressing in a normal fashion but can alert the provider to potential underlying health issues when the process is not proceeding normally. In some cases, abnormality in pubertal development and menses can be the first clue to an underlying health problem, so the practitioner must consider a broad differential, including nongynecological conditions, when abnormalities are encountered. Educating patients and caregivers about normal puberty and menstruation can provide anticipatory guidance so they can seek appropriate evaluation if problems arise. Using the menstrual cycle as a vital sign by checking last menstrual period and menstrual pattern at each visit is a quick and effective diagnostic tool in the care of young women.

REFERENCES

1. Finlayson CA, Styne DM, Jameson, JL. Endocrinology of sexual maturation and puberty. In: Jameson JL, ed. *Endocrinology: Adult and Pediatric*. 7th ed. Philadelphia, PA: Saunders/Elsevier; 2016:2119–29.
2. Herman-Gidden ME, Slora EJ, Wasserman RC et al. Secondary sex characteristics and menses in young girls seen in office practice: A study from the Pediatric Research in Office Settings network. *Pediatrics*. 1997;99(4):505–12.
3. Wolf RM, Long D. Pubertal development. *Peds Rev*. 2016;37(7):292–300.
4. Biro FM, Greenspan, LC, Galvez MP. Puberty in girls of the 21st century. *J Pediatr Adolesc Gynecol*. 2012;25:289–94.
5. Walvoord EC. The timing of puberty: Is it changing? Does it matter? *J Adolesc Health*. 2010;47(5):433–9.
6. Abitol, L, Zborovski, S, Palmaert, M. Evaluation of delayed puberty: What diagnostic tests should be performed in the seemingly otherwise well adolescent? *Arch Dis Child*. 2016;101:767–71.

7. Menstruation in girls and adolescents: Using the menstrual cycle as a vital sign. Committee Opinion No. 651. American College of Obstetricians and Gynecologists. *Obstet Gynecol* 2015;126:e143–6.
8. Gomez-Lobo V. Pharmacological and environmental effects on pubertal development. In: Appelbaum H. (ed.) *Abnormal Female Puberty*. Springer, Cambridge, 2016, pp. 261–70.
9. Greenspan L, Lee Mary M. Endocrine disrupters and pubertal timing. *Curr Opin Endocrinol Diabetes Obes*. 2018;25:49–54.
10. Rosenfield RL, Lipton RB, Drum ML. Thelarche, pubarche and menarche attainment in children with normal and elevated body mass index. *Pediatrics*. 2009;123:84–8.
11. Ford, KR, Khoury, JC, Biro, FM. Early markers of pubertal onset: Height and foot size. *J Adolesc Health*. 2009;44(5):500–1.
12. Centers for Disease Control and Prevention (CDC) Growth Tables. National Center for Health Statistics in collaboration with the National Center for Chronic Disease Prevention and Health Promotion. 2000. https://www.cdc.gov/growthcharts/. Accessed June 5, 2019.
13. Tanner JM, Whitehouse RH, Marubini E, Resele LF. The adolescent growth spurt of boys and girls of the Harpenden growth study. *Ann Hum Biol*. 1976;3:109–26.
14. Marshall WA. Growth and sexual maturation in normal puberty. *Clin Endocrinol Metab*. 1975;4:3–25.
15. Marshall WA, Tanner JM. Variations in the pattern of pubertal changes in boys. *Arch Dis Child*. 1970;45:13–23.
16. Marshall WA, Tanner JM. Variations in pattern of pubertal changes in girls. *Arch Dis Child*. 1969;44:291–303.
17. Greulich WW, Pyle SI. *Radiographic Atlas of Skeletal Development of the Hand and Wrist*. 2nd ed. Palo Alto, CA: Stanford University Press; 1959.
18. Bailey DA. The Saskatchewan Pediatric Bone Mineral Accrual Study: Bone mineral acquisition during the growing years. *Int J Sports Med*. 1997;18(suppl 3):S191–4.
19. American Academy of Pediatrics. *Bright Future*. 3rd ed. (Internet). 2011. https://brightfutures.aap.org/Bright%20Futures%20Documents/BFNutrition3rdEditionSupervision.pdf. Accessed May 24, 2019.
20. Feinberg I, Campbell IG. Sleep EEG changes during adolescence: An index of fundamental brain reorganization. *Brain Cog*. 2010;72:56–65.
21. Paruthi S, Brooks LJ, D'Ambrosio C et al. Recommended amount of sleep for pediatric populations: A consensus statement of the American Academy of Sleep Medicine. *J Clin Sleep Med*. 2016;12(6):785–6.
22. American Academy of Pediatrics Policy Statement. School Start Times for Adolescents. *Pediatrics*. 2014;134:642–9.
23. Blakemore, SJ, Choudury S. Development of the adolescent brain: Implications for executive function and social cognition. *J Child Psychol Psychiatry*. 2006;47:296–313.
24. McGivern RF, Anderson J, Byrd D et al. Cognitive efficiency on match to sample task decreases at the onset of puberty in children. *Brain Cogn*. 2002;50:73–89.
25. Keverne EB. Understanding well-being in the evolutional context of brain development. *Phios Trans R Soc Lond B Biol Sci*. 2004;29:1349–58.
26. World Health Organization (WHO). *Adolescence: A period needing special attention (Internet)*. Geneva, Swizerland: WHO; 2014. http://apps.who.int/adolescent/second-decade/section2/page1/recognizing-adolescence.html. Accessed May 24, 2019.
27. Biro FM, Greenspan LC, Galvez MP et al. Onset of breast development in a longitudinal cohort. *Pediatrics*. 2013;132(6):1019–27.
28. Boswell H. Normal timing of puberty. In: Dietrich JE, ed. *Female Puberty: A Comprehensive Guide for Clinicians*. New York, NY: Springer Science and Business Media; 2014, 22–6.
29. Rosenfield RL. Clinical review: Identifying children at risk for polycystic ovary syndrome. *J Clin Endocrinol Metab*. 2007;92:787–97.
30. Ibanez L, de Zegher F. Puberty and prenatal growth. *Mol Cell Endocrinol*. 2006;254–255:22–5.
31. Utriainen P, Jaaskelainen J, Romppanen J et al. Childhood metabolic syndrome and its components in premature adrenarche. *J Clin Endocrinol Metab*. 2007;92:4282–5.
32. Chumlea WC, Schubert CM, Roche AF et al. Age at menarche and racial comparisons in US girls. *Pediatrics*. 2003;111:110–3.
33. Boswell H. Normal female physiology in females. In: Dietrich JE, ed. *Female Puberty: A Comprehensive Guide for Clinicians*. New York, NY: Springer Science and Business Media; 2014, 7–30.
34. World Health Organization multicentered study on menstrual and ovulatory patterns in the early postmenarcheal period, duration of bleeding episodes and menstrual cycles. World Health Organization Task Force on Adolescent Reproductive Health. *J Adolesc Health Care*. 1986;7:236–44.
35. Biro FM, Huang B, Crawford PB et al. Pubertal correlates in black and white girls. *J Pediatr*. 2006;148:234–40.

Communication strategies with the adolescent patient

2

AMANDA BOGART and PARITOSH KAUL

Effective communication skills with adolescents are important for all health-care providers, both to optimize health outcomes, and to improve patient experiences. These skills are critical in eliciting a history and making a diagnosis. Further, a patient who does not understand the management plan is less likely to follow instructions, or return for recommended follow-up.1 Communication style should be tailored to the patient. Adolescents have unique expectations, communication styles, and lifestyle practices that warrant specific attention. We review the adolescent developmental stages relevant to social behaviors that impact provider-patient communication. In addition, we provide examples of communication styles that could be particularly effective for interactions with this patient population.

Note to Reader: For the purpose of simplification and readability, the authors use she/her pronouns when referring to adolescent gynecology patients. We recognize the importance of honoring the gender identity of all patients, and recommend asking and using the patient's preferred pronouns in daily practice. Details regarding this practice are beyond the scope of this chapter. Recommendations regarding care for transgender and gender nonconforming patients can be found in the American College of Obstetricians and Gynecologists 2011 Committee Opinion[2] and Chapter 7.

STAGES OF ADOLESCENCE

Adolescence is better conceptualized as a continuum of growth, rather than a single phase of development between childhood and adulthood. As a general construct for understanding the psychosocial maturation of young adults, adolescence has been divided into three developmental stages. Adolescents may move through these stages at different times; however, understanding this continuum may assist providers working with this population. It is important to note that physical and cognitive development often occur asynchronously.[3,4,5] For example, a 14-year-old female who has reached adult physical maturity may still struggle emotionally with the concept of consequences of her actions; she may make unhealthy choices like riding in a car with an intoxicated driver.

Early adolescence (age 10–13 years)

This stage is marked by the early establishment of personal identity, concrete thinking, and self-experimentation. Pertinent to the field of gynecology, this stage usually coincides with menarche and early pubertal changes. The role of the adolescent gynecologist in the lives of early adolescent patients focuses on Preventive care, in addition to helping with management of the social impact of menstrual cramps, heavy bleeding, or mood changes. At this age, there is a very strong drive to "fit in" with peer groups and an undeniable desire to be "like everyone else." It can be helpful to normalize developmental changes and use direct, simple language with patients in this stage of development (Table 2.1).

Middle adolescence (age 14–16 years)

During this stage, the adolescent has increasing concerns for outward appearance and the frequently changing platonic and romantic relationships that may dominate daily life. This age coincides with the average age of first sexual experience in the United States.[6] Contraceptive services and confidentiality should be reviewed regularly at visits during middle adolescence, if these have not already been addressed (Table 2.1). This is a time when adolescents engage in high-risk behaviors and are particularly sensitive about their reputation among peers. It is important to communicate openly with your patient about her understanding of romantic relationships, sexuality, and her body. At this age, many adolescents are more focused on instant gratification and living in the moment, which could impact their perception of risk and consequences.

Late adolescence (age 17–21 years)

Adolescents at this stage begin to think more in the abstract (less concrete) and are able to make long-term plans when prompted. There is an increased awareness of the future, interest in goal setting, and an ability to consider options of delayed gratification. An adolescent at this age may have part-time employment and/or be approaching high school graduation. At the same time, she is considering her options for career choices, higher education, and fulfillment as an adult. Adolescents at this age are fast approaching, or have reached, legal adulthood for financial and medical decision-making purposes. While some are eager to acquire this independence, others may still rely on guardians or parents for scheduling appointments and managing their affairs. This is an excellent time to encourage patients to advocate for themselves and "own" their visit, to help foster their sense of independence.

Table 2.1 summarizes adolescent stages, their developmental changes, and examples of effective communication during the different stages of development.

Table 2.1 Adolescent developmental stages and suggested communication strategies.

Adolescent stage (approximate age in years)	Cognitive development	Psychosocial development	Effective communication strategies
Early (10–13)	Concrete thinking	Desire to fit in Timid around health-care providers Parent/guardian often does most of the talking May prefer same-sex friendships	Reassurance and normalization: "Most girls at your age are also going through their first year of periods, and accidents happen to everyone. Let's talk about ways to prevent this from happening at school."
Middle (14–16)	Early abstract thinking May develop early sense of morals, but still engages in high-risk activities Highly susceptible to peer pressure	Preoccupied with improving physical appearance Height of conflict with parent/guardian over independence Average age of first sexual experience	Importance of risk reduction in anticipatory guidance: "I'm glad you came into clinic today for emergency contraception. Have you ever thought of using birth control to help with preventing pregnancy?"
Late (17–21)	Formal operational thinking Personal sense of values and moral compass Future oriented, understands delayed gratification	Less time with peer groups, more intensive personal relationships Often balancing school, family, and job/extracurricular tasks	Anticipatory guidance based on goals/desires of the patient for the future: "You seem to have a lot of personal goals you want to achieve in the next few years. How are you coping with the stress of multitasking?"

CREATING AN ADOLESCENT-FRIENDLY SPACE

Before the visit

Adolescents generally are less likely to access preventive care than other patient age groups, including younger children and adults.[7] Many adolescents seeking gynecological care feel nervous and anxious about their visit. Having friendly office staff including phone operators is important for creating an environment that is welcoming, and not intimidating. Providing reading materials and resources that are appropriate for teens and young adults in the waiting room is a simple way to cater to adolescents in your office space. Adolescents may have preferred names or nicknames, which should be honored when they provide this information. It can be helpful during intake to ask for preferred pronouns (she/her, he/him, they/them, etc.), so that the patient can be identified appropriately.

Many adolescents are accustomed to technology-based communication with peers and may prefer web or text-based communication versus speaking by telephone to arrange medical appointments. When possible, allowing adolescents to schedule appointments and message their providers online can improve their access to health information. In addition, it allows her to feel she has privacy if she is making an appointment for sensitive concerns such as screening for sexually transmitted infections (STIs). Text reminders for appointments are another simple way to communicate easily and increase show rates for appointments. Please see the provider resources at the end of the chapter, which support use of electronic health records (EHRs) to promote adolescent care. We encourage readers

to tailor the use of EHRs to your clinical practice. The use of EHRs as part of adolescent health care is beyond the scope of this chapter.

During the visit: Introductions

The provider should introduce herself/himself to the adolescent first, even when there is a parent/guardian in the room. This simple strategy illustrates to both the adolescent patient and the guardian that the adolescent is the focus of the visit. Adolescent patients should be permitted to remain in their own clothing for the introductions and history-taking parts of the visit. There is an increase in vulnerability placed on the patient who is met and/or interviewed in a gown. With the patient and parent/guardian (if present in the room), ascertain the goals of the visit. The goals of the patient and guardian might be discordant from each other, and this can help you plan the visit accordingly. Setting the agenda should occur at the beginning of the visit. All present for the visit should have a sense of how the visit will go during this introduction. Nonsensitive topics such as medical, surgical, family history, immunization updates, and medications should be addressed with the adult(s) in the room.

Addressing confidentiality

Whether or not the patient can legally consent for treatment, adolescent patients should always be interviewed alone during psychosocial screening. It is recommended to preface the interview by reviewing the limits of confidentiality in the presence of the parent/guardian, before asking any sensitive questions of the adolescent alone. This is to protect her privacy, and also to ensure that you are obtaining the most accurate history your patient is willing to provide. Adults or friends in the room might hinder the ability of the patient to feel she can be honest. Significant others should be requested to leave as well, to allow for open and direct questions pertaining to safety and sensitive history, such as lifetime number of sexual partners and history of domestic violence. Confidentiality is addressed in greater depth in Chapters 27 and 30.

OBTAINING A PSYCHOSOCIAL HISTORY

In addition to information about the patient's menstrual history, vaccination records, and current medical problems and medications, it is imperative that you obtain a confidential psychosocial history from every patient. The major risks for morbidity and mortality can be ascertained during this interview, and endorsed high-risk behaviors can be acted on, using tools discussed later in this chapter. The three leading causes of death in this age group are accidents (including motor vehicle accidents), homicide, and suicide. Unfortunately, feelings of hopelessness or suicidal thinking are prevalent (an estimated 30%–40% of adolescent females).[8] Further, adolescents in the United States represent half of the disease burden of newly diagnosed STIs. Many of the questions asked in a psychosocial screen are personal, and it is very important that providers remain aware of their verbal and nonverbal communication to their patient's responses.

The most commonly used format for this is the HEEADDSS assessment, which has many variations. One example is shown in Table 2.2. The HEEADDSS framework provides an organized approach to adolescent interviewing that starts with nonthreatening topics like home and school, and progresses to more personal questions regarding substance abuse, depression, and sexuality to assist the adolescent in feeling more comfortable in communicating with the health-care provider. The HEEADDSS approach to adolescent interviews was developed in 1972 by Harvey Berman in Seattle, Washington, and was refined and taught by Eric Cohen as a psychosocial risk assessment instrument.[9,10] A HEEADDSS interview addresses home, education, activities, drug use, sexual behavior, and suicidality/depression (Table 2.2). More recently, an additional E for eating and S for safety have been added in response to concerns about obesity, eating disorders, and issues regarding safety and accidents.[11]

When obtaining a sexual history, in particular, the use of presumptive language may result in misleading responses from the adolescent. Table 2.3 gives examples of questions asked differently to the same patient, with the responses these types of questions might elicit. Column A provides questions that are frequently asked and may lead to responses that are less informative than those questions in column B. As noted, asking a female patient if she is straight, lesbian, or bisexual may result in a response of "I identify as a lesbian." A provider could easily make the assumption that a patient who identifies as a lesbian does not have male sexual partners. If there are no further follow-up questions, the provider may miss opportunities to discuss condom use, STI testing, and contraception with that patient who could be at risk of STIs and/or pregnancy.

Asking about frequency of condom use often leads to another pitfall in communication. Adolescents are aware that the "right answer" to this question is, "All of the time." As discussed previously, the average age of first sexual experience occurs during the developmental stage, during which adolescents are still focused on instant gratification and may lack the ability to plan ahead. For more accurate information and discussions about condom use, it can be more helpful to ask about the last time the patient had sex without a condom.

Table 2.2 HEEADDSS assessment.

Home: Who lives at home with you? How many adults and children are in the home? Who in your immediate family lives elsewhere? Do you feel safe when you are at home? How would you describe your relationship with your family?

Education/**E**mployment: What school do you attend, and what grade level are you in? What kind of grades do you make? How are your grades this year compared to last year? Are there struggles at school? Do you work part time or full time? What kind of job do you have?

Eating: How many meals do you eat per day, on average? Has your weight changed significantly in the last year? What do you think about your weight, is it too much, too little, or just right?

Activities: What do you like to do for fun? With whom? Do you have a close group of friends? When was the last time you had fun?

Drug Use: Some people your age may be experimenting with drugs and alcohol. I ask you about this only to provide information to help you make informed decisions for yourself. How often do you smoke cigarettes? How often do you drink alcohol? How often do you use marijuana? Have you used any other drugs like cocaine, ecstasy, amphetamines, IV drugs, or prescription drugs intended for someone else? [If yes, consider using the CRAFFT (car, relax, alone, forget, friends, trouble) screen, and if indicated, refer for treatment.][12]

Depression/Self-Image: Do you like yourself? Does the word "depression" ever apply to you? (Consider using depression screening tools such as the Patient Health Questionnaire [PHQ]-2 and PHQ-9.)

Sexual History: See Table 2.3.

Safety/Suicidality: Has there ever been a time where you did not feel safe with yourself? Have you ever self-harmed with cutting, carving, or scratching? Any history of feeling suicidal? Do you feel safe today? Are there any weapons kept in your home (i.e., guns)?

Table 2.3 Eliciting sexual history in adolescents: Questions and answers.

Column A Common questions	Responses	Column B Suggested alternative questions	Responses
Are you sexually active?	No.	Have you had any form of sexual contact before?	I'm not with anyone right now, but I had oral/anal sex last month.
Are you straight, lesbian, or bisexual?	I identify as a lesbian.	Are you attracted to males, females, or both? Who have your sexual partners been so far? (needs clarification)	I am mostly attracted to women, but I have had sex with men before.
How many boyfriends/ girlfriends have you had in the last year?	None.	How many sexual partners have you had in the last year?	I have never had a boyfriend, but I have had three male sexual partners.
Do you have any children?	No.	Have you ever been pregnant?	Yes, I have had two abortions. I don't have kids.
Have you been tested for STIs before?	Yes, and I don't have herpes or anything.	Have you been tested for Gonorrhea or Chlamydia before, which usually is a urine or swab test? Have you had blood drawn or a cheek swab taken to test for HIV before?	I don't know what I was tested for, but I peed in a cup and they said it was normal.
Have you ever been assaulted or raped?	No.	Have you ever had sex when you didn't want to, or been pressured to have sexual contact with another person?	This one time I was drunk and don't remember what happened. I probably didn't say "No."
How often do you use condoms?	All of the time.	When was the last time you had sex without a condom? What factors determine whether or not you and your partner(s) use a condom?	I usually do, but 4 days ago we didn't have one and had sex anyway. My partner doesn't like condoms.

COMMUNICATION SKILLS FOR PROVIDING ANTICIPATORY GUIDANCE

Motivational interviewing

Motivational interviewing (MI) is a communication style and tool that can be used with adolescents to provide counseling and positive behavior changes. The goal of MI is to work in collaboration with the patient to foster shared decision-making and ultimately strengthen the patient's motivation for change. It has been integrated into primary care settings and is an established practice in psychology and psychiatry. This technique was developed in 1983 by William R. Miller, who worked with patients who struggled with alcohol abuse.[13]

Unlike other counseling techniques in which the provider gives information in a unidirectional flow to the patient, such as "You should stop smoking because it is bad for your health," in MI the provider instead ascertains the patient's motivation to quit smoking first, and provides a safe space for the patient to explore the risks and benefits of making a change to her tobacco use.

The main principles of MI include partnership, acceptance, collaboration, and evocation (PACE). When working with adolescents, it is important to remember that the patient is the most knowledgeable expert on herself. This technique specifically acknowledges the patient's autonomy and encourages collaboration with the provider to improve her health. It relies on the rapport between patient and provider. Adolescents, who are often talked about by adults, rather than talked to, are quite receptive to this approach.

The framework of Ask-Tell-Ask serves as a reminder that the conversation should be patient driven and patient focused. The model is bookended by patient input, with only a middle portion during which the provider is giving information. Begin by asking permission to discuss the behavioral change with the adolescent. This reinforces the patient's autonomy and establishes the provider's respect for the adolescent's opinion as the expert on her life. This is followed by assessing the patient's baseline knowledge about the specific health topic. For example, most adolescents know and are aware that tobacco use is a health hazard associated with and leading to cancer, lung problems, and other health issues. Spending time discussing this is unlikely to be fruitful if the information is not new to the adolescent. She may, however, share with the provider that she has heard that vape pens and electronic tobacco products carry no health risks, which would allow the provider an opportunity to offer new and accurate information. The provider can then ask the patient permission to share appropriate and pertinent information on which the provider might be the expert. Finally, the second Ask refers to checking in with the patient about her thoughts after the exchange of information. It is important to emphasize that the decision to make a change is ultimately the patient's, and not the provider's. The role of the provider is merely to support and provide information to the patient and acknowledge that she has the power to make the change (Table 2.4 demonstrates the use of Ask Tell Ask when interviewing an adolescent about marijuana use.)

Table 2.4 Utilizing Ask-Tell-Ask principles of motivational interviewing (MI): Illustrative example in a 14-year-old with marijuana use.

Dialogue	Principles of MI being utilized
Patient: *I smoke weed every day, but after I get my homework done. I'm still getting As and Bs.*	Patient identifies risky behavior but not a desire to change.
Provider: *I see. It sounds like you don't think marijuana use is impacting your school performance. Would it be all right with you if I share with you what I know about marijuana use in people your age?*	Provider reflects on patient's statement, and **ASK**s permission to provide information.
Patient: *OK, sure. I mean I know you're supposed to tell me not to smoke.*	Patient provides permission.
Provider: *Well, I just want to make sure you can make decisions based on accurate information. Have you thought about why the legal age for marijuana use in states where it is legalized, is 21? It is actually based on brain development. At your age, marijuana use could impact your brain development permanently, because you are still growing and forming connections until at least 21 years of age. The medical profession is concerned that marijuana use at your age could lead to early symptoms of psychosis, stunted brain development, and other irreversible changes, unrelated to your grades in school right now. What do you think about that?*	Provider **TELL**s patient what is known about marijuana use, in objective, nonjudgmental way. Provider **ASK**s patient to reflect on information.
Patient: *I didn't know that about the brain development. So you're saying that smoking now is worse than smoking when I'm older?*	Patient reflects and asks clarifying question.
Provider: *Yes, while experimentation is normal at your age, there are potential harms to you and your brain development that are especially relevant right now because of your age and how often you say you use marijuana. I just want you to have that information so you can weigh the risks and benefits of your marijuana use and decide for yourself what would be best for you.*	Provider normalizes patient behavior and gives additional information.
Patient: *Well, it's not like I need to smoke every day. I'm not addicted. Maybe I will cut back to just special occasions until I'm 21. For my brain development. I still want to be a lawyer when I grow up.*	Patient demonstrates example of change talk.
Provider: *I think that's a great decision. I have resources to help if you find that it is harder to cut back than you think.*	Provider supports patient's change talk and offers resources.

In patient-centered counseling as demonstrated by MI, the provider speaks less than the patient. Reflective listening means the provider sits back and allows the patient to direct the conversation. The provider may ask clarifying questions and provide affirmations, as a demonstration of understanding the patient's feelings on a topic. After reflecting on where the patient stands with respect to the behavioral change, the provider can help elicit Change Talk (CT) by assessing the patient's specific goals and values, and using these as a framework for motivation for change. This interview technique is effective even if the patient is ambivalent or only mildly motivated to make a change.

Example: A 16-year-old female presents for irregular bleeding on her prescribed oral contraceptive pills. Her mother shares that she is forgetting at least three pills per week unless reminded. The patient is on the pills for PCOS.

Patient: I know I'm supposed to take them, but I get busy and forget sometimes. The bleeding is really annoying and is happening two to three times a month. I know I need the pills to help lower the testosterone in my body and stop the extra hair growth and stuff, and to regulate my periods. But sometimes, I think it was easier before when I would go 3 months without a period. I really just forget to take them.

Provider: It sounds like you have a pretty good understanding of how your medication can help you be healthy, and it sounds like being healthy is important to you. You seem to want the bleeding you get from missed pills to go away, which could happen if there was a way to remember to take your pill every day. Can you think of any ways to help you remember to take it?

Patient: I guess I could use my phone to set an alarm? Or take my medicine with dinner instead of with breakfast, since some days I skip breakfast on my way to school?

One tool to assist providers with assessing their patient's motivation for change is the confidence ruler. In this tool, the provider asks the patient to rate the importance of making the change on a scale from 1 to 10. The provider then asks additional questions to prompt the patient to elaborate on her reason for picking the number she did. In a follow-up question, the provider can ask the patient to use the same scale and choose a number to represent her confidence in being able to make the change.

Provider: On a scale of 1–10 with 10 being the highest, how important is it to you to take the pill every day?
Patient: Maybe a 6?
Provider: Six is pretty good. Why didn't you choose 4 or 5?

Patient: Well, I do really want to have regular periods and stay healthy. I also really like that the pills will help with my acne.

Provider: On a scale of 1–10, how confident are you in your ability to take the pill every day?

Patient: Well if I set my phone alarm and schedule it at night that will be easier, so I think a 7/10.

Provider: That's excellent. What do you think could move that to an 8 or 9?

Patient: Maybe if I kept the pill pack near my bathroom since I always brush my teeth after dinner and I would see it there.

Provider: It sounds like you have a pretty good plan for reminders to help you take your pill every day. Is there something you want your mother to do to help you with this?

Example: A 17-year-old high school senior is preparing to go to college. She comes in today and asks for STI testing. You learn that she has a boyfriend of 4 months. You take a comprehensive sexual history and learn that the patient and her sexual partner never use condoms. She is on oral contraceptive pills and is adherent in taking them daily (Table 2.5).

Checking in during the visit

Throughout the visit, it is important to check in with the patient regarding her understanding of what is happening and the next steps of the visit. In the teach-back method, the patient's understanding of what has just been communicated is elicited by the provider. This is a helpful way of making sure that the patient's silence is not the result of confusion or intimidation, and the patient has understanding of the process. An example of this would be,

Table 2.5 Example of motivational interviewing for increased use of barrier contraception.

Dialogue	Comments
Provider: *I am glad you came in today. Tell me about the concern you have for an infection?*	Provider asks open-ended question about patient's concern.
Patient: *Well, we don't use condoms and I just found out that he was with someone else when we broke up, before we got back together. He didn't want to go to the doctor, but I don't want to take chances.*	Patient identifies a concern for risk based on her sexual behavior practices.
Provider: *I see, so it sounds like you want to avoid getting an infection. Is there anything you know of that could help protect you from sexually transmitted infections?*	Provider reflects on patient's response. Provider then assesses patient's knowledge about prevention of STIs.
Patient: *Well yeah, we used to use condoms, but I'm on the pill, and we don't always have condoms, so we stopped.*	
Provider: *On a scale of 1–10, how important to you is it to use a condom right now?*	Provider uses confidence ruler to assess patient's readiness for change.
Patient: *I guess a 3. I know it can help prevent infections, and is a second way to prevent pregnancy, but I think we are OK without it. Neither of us has signs of an infection or anything, and I trust him not to lie to me.*	Patient identifies a somewhat low score for readiness.
Provider: *Would it be OK if I told you a little bit about what I know about sexually transmitted infections?*	Provider **ASK**s permission to share information with patient.
Patient: *Sure.*	Patient provides permission and demonstrates being open to having a conversation about behavioral change.
Provider: *STIs don't always show symptoms, especially in young people. In fact, most infections in young people are asymptomatic. That means a partner could be infected and not know it, and then give the infection to someone else. Using condoms is the only method besides abstinence that helps prevent spreading an infection from one person to another. We actually have free condoms in our clinic for all patients who want them. I know they can be expensive. What do you think about that?*	Provider shares medical information with patient (**TELL**). Provider then **ASK**s patient to reflect on new information.
Patient: *I think part of it is that we get caught up in the moment, and he never buys them in advance. Maybe if we had them, we would use them more. I definitely don't want to take any chances if people with infections don't know they have them.*	Patient identifies indication for behavioral change, or Change Talk (CT).
Provider: *OK, well we can definitely get you tested today, and also give you some free condoms. On a scale of 1–10, how confident are you that you'll be able to use the condoms with your partner, and why?*	Provider uses confidence ruler as a tool to assess readiness for change.
Patient: *I would rate my confidence a 7. I really don't want to get an infection, and I think keeping them in the bedroom will help us remember to use them.*	

"Could you please tell me what you understood from our discussion about how the IUD works?"

Many adolescents are unfamiliar with their own anatomy as a result of never having discussed it with a provider or feeling too uncomfortable to ask another trusted adult. The use of anatomical models and visual aids greatly improves the education of adolescent patients.

The ability to provide strong anticipatory guidance can greatly improve patient care. For example, a 15-year-old patient who is unaware that she may have irregular bleeding on the etonogestrel implant is more likely to be dissatisfied with this method when the bleeding occurs unexpectedly for the next 2 months. If the provider is able to provide information detailing what to expect after a procedure or with a new medication, that will help support the adolescent patient in the event that she forgets or is overwhelmed by information during the visit. Some adolescents may not prefer to have written information, and instead may want to access a web link or online resource with medical information. It is helpful to refer adolescents to age-appropriate and scientifically accurate resources if they have questions or need further information. Please see the list at the end of this chapter of youth-friendly online resources and free applications.

If a clinical practice has access to a patient portal, allowing adolescent patients to directly message a nurse or provider with questions after the visit can be helpful for both patient flow and communication. In addition, releasing lab and test results through this portal can also allow the adolescent to feel knowledgeable about her own health.

INFORMATION SOURCES

Adolescents receive a significant amount of information about their health from the media, their friends, and family members.[14] Sometimes this information is positive (i.e., an adolescent male may learn he could benefit from HPV vaccination from a commercial on television). Sometimes, adolescents do not know where to find the most reliable information and may rely on resources such as YouTube videos or blogs for information about contraception, infections, and general health. This leads to the spread of a lot of scientifically unsupported information.

Adult family members also propagate information that may not be scientifically accurate. A significant portion of adults and adolescents believe that hormone contraception use in adolescents will result in decreased fertility or irreversible changes to the adolescent female's body. Another common concern is that use of contraceptive options, which reduce or stop monthly menses, will result in a build-up of tissue or need for "cleansing" due to the lack of monthly bleeding. Addressing this by discussing with your female patients (and often with their parents present) what the purpose of menstruation is may improve the reception of first-line treatments, like long-acting reversible contraception (LARC). These methods are known to have many health benefits for adolescents but are often declined due to the concern for their impact on menses. Adolescent gynecologists are in a unique position to provide education and promote the empowerment of female adolescents by giving scientifically accurate and reliable information.

WHAT ADOLESCENTS REALLY WANT FROM PROVIDERS

Ultimately, adolescents value communication that is genuine and nonjudgmental.[15,16] Adolescent patients (and their families) come to the health-care provider as the expert on health. By creating a safe space for information sharing and building rapport through open communication, health-care professionals are better able to provide optimal care. Communication skills, like any other skill, require deliberate practice and individual development. It is recommended that every provider develop his or her own unique style of communication that is comfortable and authentic. Using the communication strategies highlighted in this chapter, providers may find that working with adolescents can be both professionally fulfilling and beneficial to their patients and society at large.

REFERENCES

1. Kurtz S, Silverman K, Draper J. *Teaching and Learning Communication Skills in Medicine*. 2nd ed. Oxfordshire, UK: Radcliffe Publishing; 2005.
2. Health care for transgender individuals. Committee Opinion No. 512. American College of Obstetricians and Gynecologists. *Obstet Gynecol*. 2011;118:1454–8.
3. Neinstein L. *Neinstein's Adolescent and Young Adult Health Care: A Practical Guide*. New York, NY: Wolters Kluwer; 2016.
4. Steinberg L. Cognitive and affective development in adolescence. *Trends Cogn Sci*. 2005;9(2):69–74,
5. Hornberger LL. Adolescent psychosocial and development. *JPAG* 2006;19(3):243–6.
6. Finer LB, Philbin JM. Trends in ages at key reproductive transitions in the United States, 1951–2010. *Women's Health Issues*. 2014;24(3):271–9.
7. Klein JD, Wilson KM, McNulty M, Kapphahn C, Collins KS. Access to medical care for adolescents: Results from the 1997 Commonwealth Fund Survey of the Health of Adolescent Girls. *J Adolesc Health*. 1999;25(2):120–30.
8. Kann L, McManus T, Harris WA et al. Youth Risk Behavior Surveillance – United States, 2015. *MMWR Surveill Summ*. 2016;65:1–174.
9. Cohen E, Mackenzie RG, Yates GL. HEADSS, a psychosocial risk assessment instrument: Implications for designing effective intervention programs for runaway youth. *J Adolesc Health*. 1991;12(7):539–44.
10. Goldenring JM, Rosen DS. Getting into adolescent heads: An essential update. *Contemporary Pediatrics*. 2004;21(1):64–90.
11. Klein DA, Goldenring JM, Adelman WP. HEEADSSS 3.0: The psychosocial interview for adolescent updated for a new century fueled by media. *Contemp Pediatr*. 2014;1–16. http://contemporary pediatrics.modernmedicine.com/contemporary-pediatrics/news/probing-scars-how-ask-essential-questions?page=full. Accessed March 1, 2018.

12. Knight K, Sheritt L, Shrier L et al. Validity of the CRAFFT substance abuse screening test among adolescent clinic patients. *Arch Pediatr Adolesc Med.* 2002;156(6):607–14.

13. Miller WR, Rose G. Toward a theory of motivational interviewing. *Am Psychol.* 2009;64(6):527–37.

14. Reznik Y, Tebb K. Where do teens go to get the 411 on Sexual Health? A teen intern in clinical research with teens. *Perm J.* 2008;12(3):47–51.

15. Ambressin A, Bennett K, Patton GC, Sanci LA, Sawyer SM. Assessment of youth-friendly health care: A systematic review of indicators drawn from young people's perspectives. *J Adolesc Health.* 2013;52:670–81.

16. Hoopes A, Benson S, Howard HB, Morrison DM, Ko LK, Shafii T. Adolescent perspectives on patient-provider sexual health communication: A qualitative study. *J Prim Care Community Health.* 2017;8(4):332–7.

ADDITIONAL RESOURCES

Support for adolescent health systems, confidentiality, and EHR use for providers

Achieving quality health services for adolescents. Committee on Adolescence. *Pediatrics.* 2008;121(6):1263–70.

Adolescent confidentiality and electronic health records. Committee Opinion No. 599. American College of Obstetricians and Gynecologists. *Obstet Gynecol.* 2014;123:1148–50.

Beeson T, Mead KH, Wood S. Privacy and confidentiality practices in adolescent family planning care at federally qualified health centers. *Perspect Sex Reprod Health.* 2016;48(1):17–24.

Ford C, English A, Sigman G. Society for Adolescent Medicine. Confidential health care for adolescents: Position paper. *J. Adolesc Health.* 2004;35:160–7.

Lehrer J, Pantell R, Tebb K, Shafer MA. Forgone health care among U.S. adolescents: Associations between risk characteristics and confidentiality concern. *J Adolesc Health.* 2007;40:218–26.

Free resources for adolescent patients on sexual health

https://www.bedsider.org/
  Bedsider Reminders App
  Clue: Period Tracker App
https://www.cdc.gov/healthyyouth
https://youngwomenshealth.org

The physical exam in the pediatric and adolescent patient

3

EDUARDO LARA-TORRE

As we become more familiar with the pathology encountered in the pediatric and adolescent patient with gynecologic disease, knowledge of normal anatomy and proper technique for the performance of the physical exam become an essential part of patient evaluation. During the first visit, it is appropriate to explain to the patient and parents that the examination of the external genitalia, although not always required, is an integral part of the routine physical examination. The pediatric assessment of the internal genitalia is indicated in cases of genitourinary complaints or suspected cases of genitourinary pathology (Table 3.1). Utilizing nontraumatizing techniques during an office examination of a child or adolescent affords the opportunity for the clinician to establish an adequate relationship with his or her patient and allows for the early diagnosis of common conditions found in this age group. Key components of any examination should be covered to the extent allowed by the patient, and in no way should the exam be forced by either the physician or the parent, as it may prevent successful future examinations in these patients and undermines patient agency over her body.

THE PREPUBERTAL FEMALE

Before performing an examination in this age group, one should focus on obtaining the cooperation of the child. Explaining what the exam will entail and allowing the child to have a sense of control (e.g., allowing the child to choose which exam gown to wear) can be ways to enlist cooperation and perform the examination with less difficulty. Preventing multiple examinations in a short period of time may also play a role in the cooperation of the patient.

OVERALL ASSESSMENT OF THE CHILD BEFORE INITIATING THE GENITALIA EXAMINATION

As with any other condition, a physical exam in the prepubertal patient should include a full assessment of other organ systems. Initiating the examination with an overall

Table 3.1 Indications for genital examination in the pediatric patient.

Signs of vaginal bleeding
Presence of vaginal discharge
History of vulvar trauma
Suspicion of solid masses or vulvovaginal cysts
Presence of vulvovaginal ulcerative/inflammatory lesions
Suspected congenital anomalies
Suspected sexual abuse

inspection will afford the opportunity to assess body habitus, hygiene, and the presence of skin disorders, while allowing the young patient to feel more comfortable in the exam room setting. It is also important to evaluate height and weight percentiles, examine the skin, assess breast development, and perform an abdominal and inguinal examination as part of the comprehensive exam. Once the patient is comfortable with the examiner, the genitalia may be examined, and this should probably be done at the end of the examination.

PATIENT POSITIONING FOR THE EXAMINATION

As we attempt to achieve cooperation from our patients for an adequate examination, positioning becomes a key component to a successful pediatric gynecologic assessment. In some situations, more than one position may be required in order to have adequate visualization of the genitalia; the patient's age may also play a role in the exam position. A number of positions have been described to allow adequate visualization of the area, and the most useful will be the one that facilitates the goal at hand. In a child under 2 years of age, the exam can be performed as the parent changes the diaper. The frog-leg position is the most commonly used position in the young prepubertal patient and allows her to have a direct view of the examiner and herself (Figure 3.1). Using stirrups and the lithotomy position may

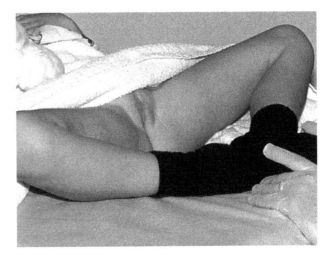

Figure 3.1 A 5-year-old demonstrating the supine "frog-leg" position. (Reproduced with permission from McCann JJ, Kerns DL. Visualization techniques. In: *The Child Abuse Atlas*. Union, MO: Evidentia Learning; 2017. https://www.childabuse-atlas.com.)

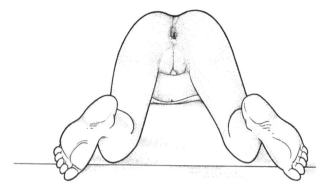

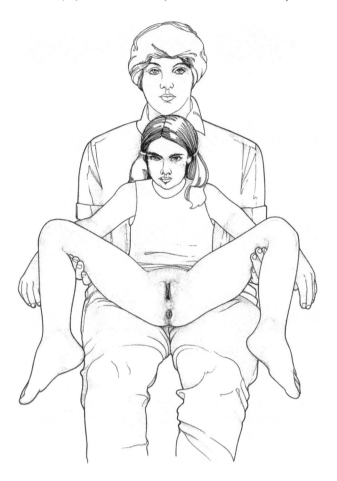

Figure 3.2 Child in lithotomy position while in mother's lap. (Reproduced with permission from Finkel MA, Giardino AP, eds. *Medical Examination of Child Sexual Abuse: A Practical Guide.* 2nd ed. Thousand Oaks, CA: Sage Publications; 2002:46–64.)

assist in better visualization of the perineal area as a child grows older. Asking for mother's assistance with the examination can prove useful, and placing her daughter between her legs may be of assistance (Figure 3.2). Combining the use of low-power magnification as with an otoscope or ophthalmoscope with the knee-chest position, often allows visualization of the lower and upper vagina.[1] This position may be especially helpful in those patients where a vaginal discharge or a suspected foreign body may be a complaint (Figures 3.3 and 3.4). Despite our best efforts, some patients may not cooperate during the exam and an optimal evaluation of the genitalia is not possible. In these patients, it is important to consider the acuity of the complaint and the clinical consequence of the pathology. This will allow a decision regarding a multivisit examination or if an exam under anesthesia is warranted.

Considerations based on age

When evaluating the newborn, attention must be paid to key characteristics of the external genitalia, which are a result of maternal estrogen stimulation. These findings should not be considered abnormal and tend to regress in 6–8 weeks. Becoming familiar with these characteristics is important

Figure 3.3 Child in knee-chest position for genital examination. (Reproduced with permission from Finkel MA, Giardino AP, eds. *Medical Evaluation of Child Sexual Abuse: A Practical Guide.* 2nd ed. Thousand Oaks, CA: Sage Publications; 2002:46–64.)

for the practitioner when called upon to evaluate a newborn. The presence of vulvar edema, vaginal discharge, and breast enlargement are common in this age group; the hymen appears thick and may protrude to the introitus. This particular finding may persist for up to 2 years and may interfere with full visualization of the introitus.[2]

In the prepubertal female, the nonestrogenized nature of the hymeneal and vulvar tissue makes it sensitive to touch and easily torn during an examination. Care should be taken not to cause trauma or pain in the area, as this will promptly make the remainder of the examination difficult to complete. The use of gentle lateral and downward traction improves visualization and does not disrupt the integrity of the normal prepubertal genitalia (Figure 3.5). In young patients, care must be taken to describe the anatomy properly, and not confuse normal findings with signs of abuse. In some patients, the presenting symptom requires an evaluation

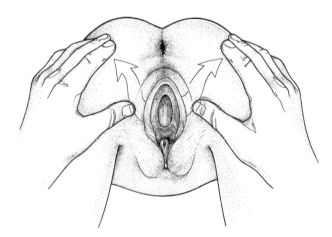

Figure 3.4 Technique for examination of female genitalia in prone knee-chest position. (Reproduced with permission from Finkel MA, Giardino AP, eds. *Medical Evaluation of Child Sexual Abuse: A Practical Guide.* 2nd ed. Thousand Oaks, CA: Sage Publications; 2002:46–64.)

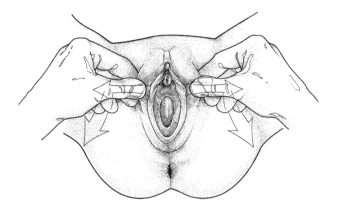

Figure 3.5 Examples of the techniques of labial separation and lateral traction for viewing the hymen of a prepubertal girl. (Reproduced with permission from the North American Society for Pediatric and Adolescent Gynecology. The PediGYN Teaching Slide Set. Elaine E. Yordan, MD, ed.)

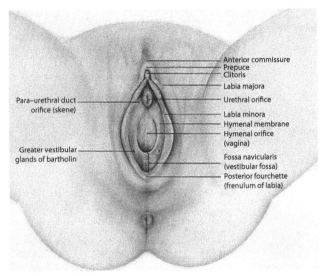

Figure 3.6 Proper nomenclature of the prepubertal external genitalia. (Reproduced with permission from Finkel MA, Giardino AP, eds. *Medical Evaluation of Child Sexual Abuse: A Practical Guide.* 2nd ed. Thousand Oaks, CA: Sage Publications; 2002:46–64.)

of the internal pelvic organs. The use of a recto-abdominal exam may assist in the palpation of the internal organs, as well as possible pelvic masses. This part of the exam is particularly important in cases of suspected vaginal foreign body, abnormal pubertal development, or lower abdominal pain in which the differential diagnosis includes a pelvic mass. This task may prove difficult and should be attempted only in the cooperative patient to prevent trauma. Noninvasive transabdominal ultrasound technology has replaced this type of exam in a large portion of scenarios.

In some instances, the use of radiologic studies is necessary to complete the evaluation of these patients. In order to be able to interpret the findings of such studies, knowledge of the normal appearance of the ovaries and uterus is important and may play a role in the evaluation. Ultrasound is by far the most utilized method of evaluation of the female genitalia and is no different at this age. In 1984, Orsini and coauthors described the normal ultrasonographic appearance of the ovaries and uterus at different ages.[5] Their findings showed that before they reach puberty, most patients will have an ovarian volume of 1 cm³ or less and a uterine volume between 1 and 4 cm³.

DOCUMENTATION

To provide an adequate and consistent description of the examination, proper nomenclature of the female genitalia should be used (Figure 3.6). A systematic approach describing each structure including inspection and palpation characteristics should be included. Components of such an examination include the assessment of pubertal development (Tanner stage), visualization and measurement of the clitoris, and description of the labia majora and minora including any discolorations, ruggae, pigmentations, or lesions. The urethra and the urethral meatus should also be reported. A proper description of the hymen, including type or shape, estrogen status, and abnormalities of configuration, should be detailed. The presence of vaginal notches, ridges, anal erythema, and skin tags is

common and should be thoroughly described. The prepubertal hymen is thin, red, and unestrogenized. At puberty, with estrogenization it thickens, becomes pale pink, and is often more redundant in its configuration. Common normal appearances and variants are shown in Figures 3.7 and 3.8. The location of hymeneal notches and ridges may be important, as those present between the 5 and 7 o'clock positions may be related to prior abuse and may require further questioning.[3] Other findings including presence of hemangiomas or other vulvovaginal lesions should also be described. The presence and appearance of the cervix, if visualized in the knee-chest position, is also important to document.

When documenting genital exams of prepubertal girls, care should be taken to merely describe findings and variations, and not to make diagnostic descriptions in the recording of the exam. Conclusions such as "an interrupted hymen suggestive of sexual abuse is seen," should be placed in the impression and plan portion of the documentation and not in the description of the findings. This will allow for a better interpersonal consistency when a second provider reviews and documents findings. The use of a clock-face method to delineate location of any abnormal findings may be the most helpful way of recording any abnormalities in the exam (Figure 3.9).

SPECIMEN COLLECTION

Certain patients will present with symptoms that require the collection of vaginal secretion samples. When cultures are indicated, moistened small male urethral Dacron swabs may be utilized (Figure 3.10). The hymeneal aperture is small in this age group, and the use of traditional cotton swabs creates discomfort due to their larger size. It may also traumatize the surrounding

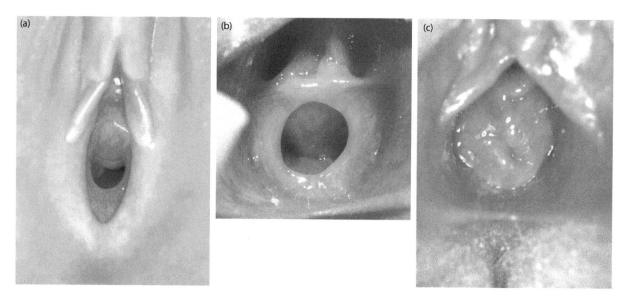

Figure 3.7   Types of hymens: Crescentic (a), annular (b), redundant (c). (Reproduced with permission from Perlman SE et al. *Clinical Protocols in Pediatric and Adolescent Gynecology*. London, UK: Parthenon Publishing Group; 2004.)

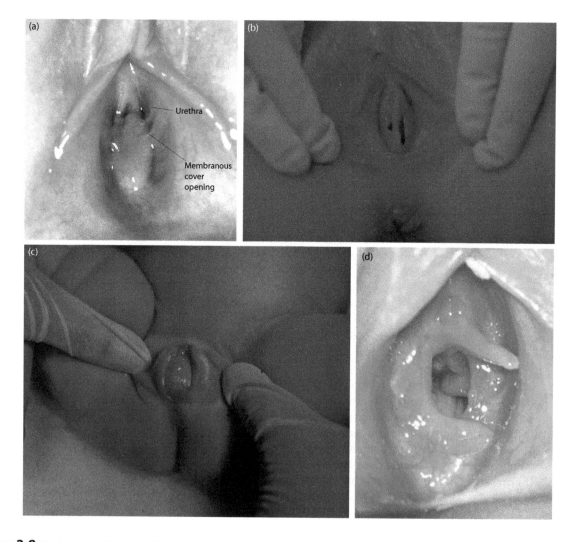

Figure 3.8   Variations in hymens: Microperforate (a), septated (b), imperforate (c), and hymeneal tags (d). (Reproduced with permission from Perlman SE et al. *Clinical Protocols in Pediatric and Adolescent Gynecology*. London, UK: Parthenon Publishing Group; 2004 and McCann JJ, Kerns DL. Visualization techniques. In: *The Child Abuse Atlas*. Union, MO: Evidentia Learning; 2017. https://www.childabuseatlas.com.)

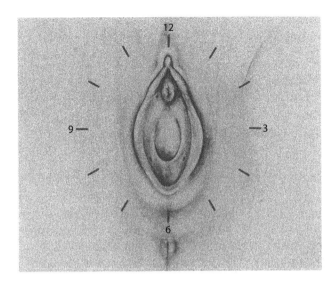

Figure 3.9 Clock-face orientation with patient in frog-leg supine position. (Reproduced with permission from Finkel MA, Giardino AP, eds. *Medical Evaluation of Child Sexual Abuse: A Practical Guide*. 2nd ed. Thousand Oaks, CA: Sage Publications; 2002:46–64.)

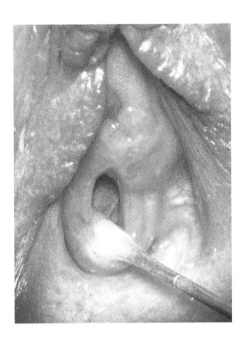

Figure 3.10 Use of small Dacron swabs to obtain vaginal swabs. (Reproduced with permission from McCann JJ, Kerns DL. Visualization techniques. In: *The Child Abuse Atlas*. Union, MO: Evidentia Learning; 2017. https://www.childabuseatlas.com.)

tissue, creating lesions that are not pathologic in nature, but may confuse the examining practitioner. Another helpful method is a catheter-within-a-catheter technique in which a 10-cm intravenous catheter is inserted into the proximal end of a No. 12 red rubber bladder catheter. This is then connected to a syringe with fluid and passed carefully into the vagina. The fluid is then inserted and aspirated multiple times to allow a good mixture of secretions (Figure 3.11).[4]

The presence of a foreign body in the vagina is a common presenting problem encountered in patients with vaginal discharge. The use of a pediatric feeding tube connected to a 20-mL syringe may allow irrigation of the contents of the vagina and determine the nature of the foreign object, negating the use of speculums in these prepubertal patients in whom the small aperture of the hymen will not allow it, and where it would be injured with instrumentation by a speculum. Newer technology with a smaller handheld fiber-optic camera also has allowed for direct visualization of the vagina, and the ability to flush the cavity under direct visualization in the cooperative patient (Figure 3.12, Video 3.1).

Video 3.1 https://youtu.be/_hInvWRVAwI
Endosee (Cooper Surgical, Trumbull, CT) use during a clinical examination of the vagina.

ADOLESCENT GYNECOLOGIC EXAM

Although the peripubertal and adolescent patient may be older and able to understand the specifics of the examination, these patients present another challenge for the examining practitioner. In these patients, self-consciousness about their own body may make the exam even more difficult to perform. The extreme variation in their psychosocial and sexual development contributes to the challenge. Teens develop at varying rates. While some teens have menarche at 10 years, others may just be starting their pubertal development at 13; therefore, careful interviewing and counseling should precede an examination. The use of educational videos and handouts that explain the examination process[6] and the common reasons why this is done may be of benefit when interacting with the patient. Delaying the genital examination, even in a sexually active teen, may prevent the patient from having reservations about her examiner, and allow rapport to be established more easily. While some teens may like to know and see everything that will happen, some would prefer not to look. These preferences

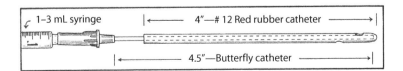

Figure 3.11 Assembled catheter-within-a-catheter aspirator, as used to obtain samples of vaginal secretions from prepubertal patients. (Reproduced with permission from Pokorny SF, Stormer J. *Am J Obstet Gynecol*. 1987;156:581–2.)

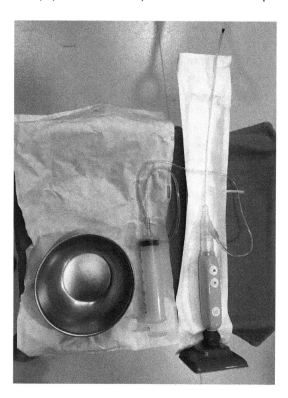

Figure 3.12 Endosee (Cooper Surgical, Trumbull, CT).

Table 3.2 Common indications for pelvic examination in the adolescent.

Delayed puberty
Precocious puberty
Abnormal vaginal bleeding
Abdominal or pelvic pain
History of vaginal intercourse
Pathological vaginal discharge
Suspicion of intra-abdominal pathology

should be taken into account to make the experience as minimally traumatizing as possible.

As in other patients, preventive health care should be a part of the examination in this age group. As recommended by the American College of Obstetricians and Gynecologists (ACOG), the initial visit to the obstetrician gynecologist should occur between the ages of 13 and 15.[7] During this visit, important components of general health, such as immunizations, risk prevention, and screening for tobacco and substance abuse as well as depression and eating disorders should be completed. As we continue to perform "catch-up" vaccinations for human papillomavirus (HPV) in adolescents, opportunities to interact with the adolescent will present during these vaccination visits, which allow the practitioner to improve his or her relationship with the parents and teen as other reproductive needs arise.

As discussed earlier, this examination does not necessarily need to include a pelvic examination. Table 3.2 lists indications for a pelvic examination in the adolescent. After the initial gynecologic visit in sexually active teens, semiannual/annual visits should be scheduled thereafter. Sexually active teens should obtain sexually transmitted infection (STI) screening yearly or with each new sexual partner. With the development of urine and self vaginal swab testing for gonorrhea and chlamydia, STI screening has become easier, without the need for a pelvic exam. In those not sexually active, a visit at each stage of adolescence may be preferred (early adolescence ages 13–15 years, middle adolescence ages 15–17, late adolescence ages 17–19).[7–9]

When a gynecologic exam is indicated, take time to explain the process before you proceed. In all patients,

monitoring of height, weight, blood pressure, and body mass index (BMI) should be performed as components of a preventive visit.[8] Examination of the neck (including a thyroid and lymph node assessment) and evaluation of skin and breast development should precede the pelvic examination. The external genitalia should be visualized, if allowed, in all patients who present for preventive care. This will allow determination of any genital anomalies in this age group, as well as make it the first step toward a pelvic examination. Patients may choose to delay their pelvic examination until cervical cancer screening is indicated (age 21 in most patients), although care should be taken to counsel them about the consequences of nondetection of abnormalities in the female genitalia. Urine screening for gonorrhea and chlamydia should be completed in sexually active teens who choose not to undergo a pelvic examination. In patients who are unable to void or had recent urination and do not meet criteria for urine screening, self vaginal collection is another option to screen. An HIV screening test should be offered as well. A thorough description of the external genitalia should be performed. Those adolescents who do require a pelvic examination should be properly instructed in the methods used. Proper equipment for this age group should be available. A Huffman (half inch wide × 4 inches long) or Pederson speculum (7/8 inch wide × 4 inches long) may be of help in young patients and those who are not sexually active. The use of tampons before their examination and the presence of menses may facilitate the use of a speculum, as they may be more comfortable with vaginal manipulation (Figure 3.13).

The use of a finger applying pressure to the perineal area, away from the introitus, allows for lessening or diffusing of the sensation from the exam ("extinction of stimuli") and may be of benefit in those undergoing their first pelvic examination. Once a finger has been placed in this area, the insertion of a speculum may be easier. Visualization of the external anatomy and confirmation of a vaginal opening would prevent a "blind insertion" in patients with hymeneal and vaginal anomalies. Once access to the cervix is obtained, the collection of vaginal and cervical specimens may be undertaken as indicated. When attempting to palpate the internal organs, the use of a single-digit bimanual examination can be attempted. As with prepubertal patients, the use of transabdominal ultrasound has replaced the use of a rectovaginal exam in most cases to identify internal genitalia pathology.

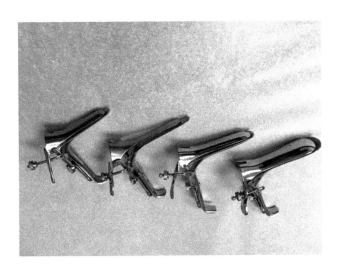

Figure 3.13 Types of specula (from left to right): Infant, Huffman, Pederson, and Graves.

All adolescents should be reassured that the examination, while uncomfortable, is not painful and will not alter their anatomy. This may reassure those who may believe that the exam will alter their "virginity."

After the examination, it is helpful to meet again with the family and the patient together to explain the exam findings and to plan further management. In the sexually active teen, if confidentiality is a concern, first discuss findings with the patient alone while in the exam room. Make a plan together about how to discuss with the parent/guardian before meeting with the family together. Ensure that the adolescent assumes the role of decision-making and help to empower her to take charge of her own health care with her parents and your guidance and assistance. Encourage the patient to allow you to be the liaison between her and the family, stressing the benefits of informing everyone of her health-care needs and the importance of communication; but overall, keep confidentiality consistent with your teen's desire. Further information on adolescent communication and confidentiality is discussed in Chapter 27.

As described in this chapter, the approach to the history and general and genital exam of children and adolescents must include an assessment of their chronological age, physical development, intellectual capacity, risk factors, chief complaint, and emotional maturity. An approach that includes all these characteristics will assure a more thorough assessment of the patient and an evaluation that is nonintimidating and achieves the needs of the patient.

REFERENCES

1. Emans SJ, Golstein DP. The examination of the prepubertal child with vulvovaginitis: Use of the knee-chest position. *Pediatrics.* 1980;65:758.
2. McCann J, Wells R, Simon M et al. Genital findings in prepubertal girls selected for non-abuse: A descriptive study. *Pediatrics.* 1990;86:428.
3. Berenson AB. The prepubertal genital exam: What is normal and abnormal. *Curr Opin Obstet Gynecol.* 1994;6:526.
4. Pokorny SF, Stormer J. Atraumatic removal of secretions from the prepubertal vagina. *Am J Obstet Gynecol.* 1987;156:581–2.
5. Orsini LF, Salardi F, Pilu G et al. Pelvic organs in premenarcheal girls: Real time ultrasonography. *Radiology.* 1984;153:113.
6. https://www.acog.org/Patients/FAQs/Your-First-Gynecologic-Visit-Especially-for-Teens. Accessed September 24, 2018.
7. American College of Obstetricians and Gynecologists. The initial reproductive health visit. Committee Opinion No. 598. American College of Obstetricians and Gynecologists. *Obstet Gynecol.* 2014;123:1143–7.
8. American College of Obstetricians and Gynecologists. Well Women Visit. ACOG Committee Opinion No. 534. *Obstet Gynecol.* 2012;120:421–4.
9. American College of Obstetricians and Gynecologists. *A Guideline for Women's Health Care.* 4th ed. Washington, DC: ACOG; 2014:435–59.
10. McCann JJ, Kerns DL. Visualization techniques. In: *The Child Abuse Atlas.* Union, MO: Evidentia Learning; 2017. https://www.childabuseatlas.com.
11. Finkel MA, Giardino AP, eds. *Medical Examination of Child Sexual Abuse: A Practical Guide.* 2nd ed. Thousand Oaks, CA: Sage Publications; 2002:46–64.
12. The North American Society for Pediatric and Adolescent Gynecology. The PediGYN Teaching Slide Set. Elaine E. Yordan, MD, ed.
13. Perlman SE, Nakajima ST, Hertweck SP. *Clinical Protocols in Pediatric and Adolescent Gynecology.* London, UK: Parthenon Publishing Group; 2004.

Adolescent sexual development and sexuality education

4

JOANNA STACEY and VERONICA LOZANO

INTRODUCTION

Sexuality encompasses sexual knowledge, beliefs, attitudes, values, and behaviors of individuals. Sexual development is a multidimensional process involving the basic human need of being liked and accepted, displaying and receiving affection, feeling valued and attractive, and sharing thoughts and feelings. This development process takes place starting in early childhood and continues throughout adolescence. Children complete a series of tasks, such as developing a body capable of reproducing, learning how to maintain healthy intimate and nonintimate relationships, managing a range of complex emotions, incorporating cultural and moral beliefs into behavior, and learning to think and problem-solve independently. This highly complex interaction of personal and social experiences constitutes the phenomenon known as sexuality.

It is now known that sexuality develops well before adolescence, and it develops alongside the person's overall identity. Sexual self-concept comprises who a person is romantically and sexually attracted to, how that person defines their gender (male, female, both, neither, or someone else), their sexual orientation identity, and their sexual behavior. Although these concepts are closely related, they differ in their definition and are covered extensively in Chapter 23.[1] The person's other identity components, such as gender, ethnic, cultural, occupational, moral, and religious identities, integrate with their sexual identity and form the multidimensional construct of identity.[2,3]

SEXUAL DEVELOPMENT THROUGH THE LIFE CYCLE

There is a dearth of research regarding sexuality in children and young adolescents. These types of studies are difficult to conduct because of requirements for parental permission, restriction about adolescent confidentiality, and society's reluctance to permit sexual studies on adolescents. Current research reflects the complexity of the development of a sexual self and the need for support of sexual development.[4] In utero, genetic, anatomic, and biologic factors begin to shape sexual development. Genetic and biologic factors also influence sexual development by determining the levels of hormones and neurotransmitters that influence sexual response.[5] While children have lower levels of sex hormones than adults or adolescents, the same mechanisms of hormonal influences apply. There is a range of childhood responsiveness, with some children being much more sexually curious and attuned to their bodies than others (Table 4.1).[6-10]

Infants and toddlers

Babies can exhibit sexuality even before birth; males can have erections in utero. Infants often rub their genitals because it gives pleasure, and both genders may experience an orgasm. By age 2 years, children usually will know their own gender and are aware there are differences in the genitals of males and females, and how males and females urinate.[11]

Children ages 3–7 years

Most young children may be curious about other children's genitals. They may imitate adult social and sexual behaviors, such as holding hands or kissing. By age 5 or 6 years, most children become more modest about dressing and bathing. Children of this age are aware of their family's living arrangements and may role-play about being married or having a partner. School-age children may play sexual games with friends of their same sex, and most sex play at this age happens because of curiosity.[11]

Preadolescent and early adolescent, ages 8–14 years

Pubertal growth and development occur in early adolescence (ages 10–14 years). In this stage, adolescents are preoccupied with their own bodies. Adolescents in this age group are likely to ask questions about masturbation, develop crushes on the same or opposite sex based on idealized adults, and may initiate sexual activity as a means of experimentation. Same-gender sexual behavior may be common, but it is usually unrelated to a child's sexual orientation.[6] Menarche typically occurs during this phase and is an important marker of issues between mother and daughter and separation.[11] Masturbation increases during these ages, and it is related to adolescent autonomy. Masturbation is more frequent among boys than girls, and this difference extends into early adulthood.[12,13]

Middle adolescence

In middle adolescence (ages 13–17 years), pubertal changes are reaching an end. Adolescents in this stage are becoming more independent. They may have conflict with parents since they are typically at the peak level of peer conformity. Often, adolescents in this stage make choices even when they do not fully understand the actions or the consequences. This group is most likely to experiment with risk behaviors such as alcohol or substance use, which are known to be associated with increased sexual activity. For this middle adolescent group, romantic involvement is typically characterized by serial monogamy or having several romantic partners in a relatively short period of time.[4]

Table 4.1 Sexual development infancy to puberty.

Age	Behavior and feelings
9–11 months	Sporadic self-stimulation, but may be absent
16–19 months	Pre-Oedipal phase: Turn away from mother to the father for affection; increased genital sensitivity, masturbatory activity, curiosity with own and other's genitalia, awareness of sexual differences in boys and girls
3–4 years	Phallic-Oedipal phase: Increase in masturbation and exhibitionism, preoccupation with own/other's genitalia and may lead to mutual exploration with same- and opposite-sex peers as part of play
5–12 years	Latency Phase: Shift erotic trend from father to mother; begin interest in origin of babies; gradual self-awareness of sexuality and preoccupation with own body

Source: Adapted from Roiphe H. *Psychoanal Study Child*. 1968;23:348–65, with permission.

Late adolescence

In late adolescence (age 18 years and older), the sense of responsibility and capacity for abstract thought are present. They have a more clearly defined body image and gender role. Many older adolescents have accepted some of their parents' values and become less concerned about peer influence. As a result, older adolescents tend to engage in fewer risk behaviors and have a more mature approach to relationships, both romantic and nonromantic.[4] It is expected that at the completion of adolescence, individuals will have achieved characteristics of healthy sexual development (Table 4.2). These include honing critical decision-making skills, being educated about and taking

Table 4.2 Outline of individual characteristics of healthy sexual development.

- Identify and live according to their own values; take responsibility for their own behavior
- Practice effective decision-making; develop critical-thinking skills
- Acknowledge their sexual development, which may or may not include reproduction or sexual experience
- Seek further information about sexuality and reproductive needs, and make informed choices about family options and relationships
- Interact with all genders in respectful and appropriate ways
- Affirm one's own gender identity and sexual orientation, and respect the gender identities and sexual orientations of others
- Appreciate one's body and enjoy one's sexuality throughout life; expresses sexuality in ways that are congruent with one's values
- Express love and intimacy in appropriate ways
- Develop and maintain meaningful relationships, avoiding exploitative or manipulative relationships
- Exhibit skills and communication that enhance personal relationships with family, friends, and romantic partners

Source: Based on data from Breuner CC, Matson G, Committee on Adolescence, Committee on Psychological Aspects of Child and Family Health. *Pediatrics*. 2016;138; and Guidelines for Comprehensive Sexuality Education: Grades K-12. Sexuality Information and Education Council of the United States. https://siecus.org/resources/the-guidelines/ (accessed April 21, 2019).

responsibility for their own sexuality, and expressing love and intimacy in mature and appropriate ways.[14,15]

CULTURAL ASPECTS OF DEVELOPMENT AND EDUCATIONAL PROGRAMS

The way sexuality is experienced and expressed (thoughts, fantasies, desires, beliefs, attitudes, values, behaviors, practices, roles, and relationships) manifests itself not only in biological, physical, and emotional ways, but also in sociocultural ways. This is due to effects of human society and culture, as much as genetics. Human sexuality impacts, and is impacted by, cultural, political, legal, and philosophical aspects of life and can interact with issues of morality, ethics, theology, spirituality, and religion.

A major impact with respect to current adolescent sexuality and development is the increasing time span reported between the onset of reproductive capability and the age of marriage. This span was about two gynecologic years in the 1850s, when the onset of puberty menarche was 16 or 17 years and the average age of marriage was 18 or 19. In 1950, this span was 7–8 gynecologic years. Today the span is 11–14 gynecologic years. This increasing time span from 2 to 11–14 years created a gap of time in which premarital sexual relations are common, and in the 1960s and 1970s a rise in the unwed teen pregnancy rate was seen, and with it, the need for education on contraception and prevention of sexually transmitted infections (STIs).[4]

Interaction between ethnicity and parenting styles affects childhood and adolescent sexual behavior. Differences in beliefs can expose children to multiple and conflicting messages, including those from parents who admonish them about sexual involvement while being proud of and encouraging early romantic nonsexual relationships.[16] Cultures vary considerably in their attitudes toward premarital and adolescent sexuality.

Emerging sexuality outside of North America and Europe can be quite different for adolescents not living in the Western world. In many countries, marriage is the driving factor of adolescent sexual activity. There has been a worldwide emphasis by leading health organizations (the World Health Organization [WHO], for example) on delaying marriage to, or between, young adolescents (those defined as younger than age 15) due to the known health risks of early sexual activity, and this has been successful in many countries.[17] Chapter 28 provides more detail about how various world cultures influence sexuality.

The practice of female circumcision, also known as female genital mutilation, involves the partial or complete removal of the female genitalia. This is done commonly in certain cultures in East and Central Africa, Indonesia, Malaysia, and parts of the Middle East and North Africa as a means of protecting a woman's virginity and honor and can symbolize a girl's passage into adulthood. This practice is criminalized in the United States. Pediatric and adolescent gynecology providers may encounter these complex patients who have migrated to the United States; this aspect is covered in Chapter 9.

Sexuality education

Comprehensive sexuality education should be medically accurate, evidence based, and age appropriate. It should include the benefits of delayed sexual intercourse, while providing the information about reproductive development, contraception, including long-acting reversible contraception to prevent pregnancies, as well as barrier protection to prevent STIs. Sexuality education should begin in early childhood and continue throughout a person's life. Programs should not only focus on reproductive development (including abnormalities in development), but also teach about forms of sexual expression, healthy sexual and non-sexual relationships, gender identity, sexual orientation, and questioning. It should also emphasize communication, recognizing and preventing sexual violence, and consent and decision-making. By incorporating abnormal sexual development into education programs on sexuality, adolescents are given an earlier understanding of the wide variations in development, leading to improved communications and less marginalization of affected children.[18]

How the education is disseminated has much to do with the culture's perspective on sexuality in general. When a culture is highly religious and conservative, sexuality education may be more fear based and focused on abstinence. When adolescents are accepted as sexual beings with a right to information, the education tends to be more comprehensive. This is evident through education programs available in the European Union (EU), which are open to adolescent sexuality and also offer free and convenient access to contraception through a national health service in most countries. Differences in sexuality education in different jurisdictions may be associated with different outcomes; so some countries in the EU with the least extensive sexuality education programs have the highest rates of HIV/AIDS.[19] Policy-driven sexuality education in the United States, occurring at the state and local levels, has been done in the past without referring to data on effectiveness; existing data on the effects of state abstinence policies at best show no change in teen pregnancy and STI rates. Several studies show an association between increasingly strict policies on abstinence teaching (such as abstinence-only taught, not just "stressed") and higher rates of adolescent pregnancy, births, and chlamydia infections.[20]

Further, challenges lie in conservative or developing nations, where resources may be sparse, and treatment of those of different genders and sexual orientations is unequal. Because of the paucity of educational opportunities in some parts of the world, adolescents may lack basic knowledge of sexual and reproductive health, promoting dangerous health myths instead (e.g., that HIV can be spread through a mosquito bite or a woman cannot get pregnant the first time she has sex).[21] A large randomized controlled trial in Kenya found that the national HIV/AIDS school curriculum that is abstinence-only based, without mention of condoms or contraception, did not reduce pregnancy rates or STIs and had the unintended consequence of encouraging early marriage.[22]

Current sexuality education programs in the United States vary widely in the accuracy of content, emphasis, and effectiveness. Evaluations of biological outcomes of sexuality education programs, such as pregnancy rates and STIs in adolescents, are expensive and complex. They can be unreliable due to self-reported behaviors that are difficult to measure. State definitions of "medically accurate" vary widely as well, and most states require school districts to allow parental involvement in sex education programs. Many states have requirements regarding topics that must be included in sex education programs, including abstinence-only education. Evidence has shown that the majority of abstinence-only education programs do not delay sexual intercourse; however, a study of four select abstinence-only education programs reported no increase in the risk of adolescent pregnancy, STIs, or rates of adolescent sexual activity compared with students in a control group who received information on contraception and STI prevention.[23]

Data have shown that not all programs are equally effective for all ages, races and ethnicities, socioeconomic groups, and geographic areas. There is no "one size fits all" program. One key component of an effective program is to encourage community-centered efforts. Innovative, multicomponent, community-wide initiatives that use evidence-based adolescent pregnancy prevention interventions and reproductive health services have dramatically reduced pregnancy rates in certain populations.[23] No studies of comprehensive programs to date have found evidence that providing adolescents with reproductive health information and education results in an increase in sexual risk-taking.[24]

Sexuality education should not marginalize LGBTQ (lesbian, gay, bisexual, transgender, questioning their sexual identity-queer) individuals and those who have variations in sexual development (e.g., primary ovarian insufficiency, Müllerian anomalies). Because there is a link between early sexual debut (sexual intercourse before the age of 13 years) and high-risk sexual behaviors and violence-related behaviors, school-based programs that are inclusive of sexual minority students, encourage the delay in sexual intercourse, and coordinate with substance use and violence-prevention programs can positively impact these negative outcomes.[25] Curricula that emphasize empowerment and gender equality tend to engage learners to question prevailing norms through critical thinking and encourage adolescents to adopt more egalitarian attitudes and relationships, resulting in better sexual and health outcomes.[2]

SEXUAL DEBUT

Antecedents to activity

The antecedents for adolescent initiation of sexual intercourse have been studied.[26] Historically, religion has been the greatest influence on sexual behavior in the United States, but this has been replaced by the media and a child's peers as two of the strongest influences. The primary motivation for adolescent girls aged 12–15 years to initiate sexual intercourse has been associated with their friends' sexual behavior and social processes.[27,28] According to the National Longitudinal Study of Adolescent Health, the most important predictor of sexual experience among participants in grades 7–12 was having been in a romantic relationship during the previous 18 months.[29] Non-sexual romantic relationships in the seventh grade (age 12–13 years) independently contribute to the onset of sexual intercourse by the ninth grade (age 14–15 years) for both males and females. Among females, 12- to 13-year-olds in serious relationships with older teens (2 or more years older) have an increased likelihood of sex at age 14–15 years. It is important to note that both male and female 12- to 13-year-olds who had serious romantic relationships were already different in sixth grade from those who were not: they had peers who were more accepting of sexual activity, had experienced more unwanted sexual advances that could lead to sex (i.e., limited parental monitoring), and the females had undergone earlier menarche.[30] Furthermore, 11- and 12-year-olds whose mothers gave birth to them at young ages, and who have older adolescent friends, are much more likely to have sexual initiation between the ages of 13–14 and 15–16 years. This should be viewed as a "red flag" for early sexual activity and a risk factor for teenage pregnancy.[31] There is some evidence that hormonal levels affect female sexual practice,[32] but there have been no studies that assess whether there are hormonal effects on sexual debut or activity in adolescents.

FACTORS DELAYING THE INITIATION OF ADOLESCENT SEXUAL ACTIVITY

Parental influence

Parental influence is very important. Parents who communicate about sex, are emotionally close to their adolescents, express reasonable values, and are moderately strict have daughters who are less likely to engage in sex before the age of 16 years.[33–35] A longitudinal study of psychosexual adolescent development in girls from an urban adolescent medical clinic confirmed these findings. Girls who described their families as being expressive, having a moral-religious emphasis, providing supervision, having greater maternal education, and who experienced menarche at an older age were older at the time of sexual initiation.[36] Finally, parent and child connectedness and clear communication of disapproval about sexual activity have been associated with a delay in sexual initiation.[37] In contrast, parents with extreme parenting styles, either authoritarian-controlling or permissive styles of parenting, are associated with earlier sexual debut.[38] Growing up in a single-parent household or in households with significant levels of family conflict are also associated with earlier initiation of sexual activity.[39–41] Longitudinal data from community samples of girls followed prospectively from age 5 to 18 years reveal that the absence of a father was strongly associated with early sexual activity as well as adolescent pregnancy.[42]

Religious affiliation and attendance

Attendances at religious services and a person's religious affiliation have little impact on sexual behaviors once intercourse occurs. An evaluation of nationally representative data from the 1995 National Survey of Family Growth suggests that both affiliation and attendance at religious services are associated with age at first sexual occurrence. Multivariant analysis shows that religious affiliation shares few associations with sexual behaviors. However, frequent attendance at religious services at age 14 years continues to have a strong delaying effect on the timing of first intercourse.[43]

Factors associated with early initiation

Girls who are very young at first intercourse (13 years or younger) report that their peers having sex is a greater reason for sexual debut than love or romantic feelings. They are also more likely to report not particularly desiring to have sex or having nonvoluntary sex. If the male partner is 2 or more years older than the girl, intercourse tends to take place earlier in the relationship.[44] Having a greater number of lifetime partners by age 19 years is also associated with initiation of romantic relationships at an early age, and this is indirectly associated with more frequent alcohol use in middle adolescence. The timing of first romantic relationship and alcohol use at age 16 years are associated with complicated paths, including sociability and impulsivity at age 30 months, early physical maturation, physical attractiveness at age 13 years for girls, and higher-quality friendships and increased peer acceptance in early adolescence. This would imply that young people who are sociable, have a more mature appearance, and date early in adolescence would benefit from learning to responsibly manage their relationships in the midst of their emerging sexuality.[42]

Adverse risks of early sexual debut

Early sexual debut (first sexual intercourse before age 13 years) is associated with increased prevalence of sexual risk-taking, among both heterosexual and LGB (lesbian, gay, bisexual) students; these risks include not wearing a condom and four or more partners before graduating high school. Additionally, higher rates of substance abuse and violence-related behavior were associated with early sexual debut among LGB and heterosexual students.[26]

ADOLESCENT SEXUAL BEHAVIOR

Precoital behavior

Most research on sexual behavior in adolescents has been done on penile-vaginal intercourse, STIs, and pregnancy, but girls' sexual lives begin long before first intercourse. Teen sexual behavior includes a range of activity from kissing, petting, and fondling, to oral, anal, and vaginal sex. Many of these other sexual behaviors may serve as a prelude to intercourse or substitute for intercourse for teens wishing to preserve their "virginity."

A small study of girls ages 12–15 years old who were interviewed at baseline and then 1 year later showed changes in attitudes toward sex based on their sexual experiences. Girls with no breast-fondling experience at either time point had stronger abstinence values, peer approval, and sexual self-esteem scores, and lower arousal, compared with girls who initiated breast fondling over the year ("transitioners"). These "transitioners" had similar sexual cognition to girls who had experience at baseline, a finding that suggests changes in sexual cognitions precede actual sexual experience.[45]

Noncoital behavior

Noncoital sexual behavior, which includes mutual masturbation, oral sex, and anal sex, is a common expression of adolescent sexuality. Data from the National Survey of Family Growth (NSFG) does not indicate any increase in the prevalence of oral or anal sex among adolescents and young adults over the past two decades. Compared with oral or vaginal sex, which is common in more than 90% of males and females by age 25 years, anal sex is less common and often initiated later. Noncoital sexual behavior commonly co-occurs with coital behavior. Oral sex and anal sex are much more common in adolescents who have already had vaginal intercourse, compared with those who have not. Likewise, the prevalence of oral sex among adolescents jumps dramatically in the first 6 months after initiation of vaginal intercourse, which suggests that both experiences are often initiated around the same time and with the same partner. Although noncoital sexual behavior carries little or no risk of pregnancy, adolescents who engage in noncoital sexual behavior are at risk of acquiring STIs. There are no guidelines for STI screening in those who report anal and oral sex and are asymptomatic, so careful questioning about sexual practices should occur and guide a clinician in deciding who should be screened.[46]

Adolescent sexual behavior (coitus): National data

Several surveys are available to monitor trends in female and male adolescent sexual behavior. Both the NSFG and the Youth Risk Behavior Survey (YRBS) collect information about adolescent sexual behavior. The NSFG reports detailed information on fertility-related behavior, and YRBS monitors sex categories of health-risk behaviors (such as smoking, alcohol use, and behaviors that contribute to unintended pregnancy and STIs) among high school students, grades 9–12.

Table 4.3 Students by sexual orientation and sexual contacts.

	Heterosexual	Gay or lesbian	Bisexual	Not sure
Identify as…	88%	2.0%	6.0%	3.2%
	Opposite sex only	Same sex only	Both sexes	No sexual contact
Percentage of students, by sex of sexual contacts	48%	1.7%	4.6%	45.7%

Source: Based on data from Youth Risk Behavior Surveillance—United States, 2015. www.cdc.gov/mmwr/volumes/65/ss/ss6509a1. htm?s_cid=ss6509_whats (accessed April 21, 2019).

The most recent NSFG data from 2013 show that 44% of females between ages 15 and 19 years have had intercourse, down from 46% in 2002. YRBS shows 30.1% of all students to have been sexually active in the past 3 months, which is also a decrease from 37.1% in 1991.[47,48]

YRBS data also outline how adolescents identify themselves sexually and who they have sex with. Identification as heterosexual, gay/lesbian/bisexual, or "not sure" is relatively new data and has not been trended until recently (Table 4.3).

Several positive trends are noted: increased use of condoms at last sexual intercourse, decline in teenage unintended pregnancies, and increase in contraception use. Unfortunately, there are still several areas that highlight need for more attention, such as high rates of alcohol and drug use, especially concomitant with sexual activity. There are more risk-taking behaviors noted among gay, lesbian, and bisexual students (such as increased sexual violence, decreased contraceptive and condom use, increased rates of suicide attempts, and increased alcohol and drug use), which shows a demographic group who are more vulnerable to adverse health and social consequences (Figure 4.1).

Emerging adults and noncommitted relationships

More recently, the traditional forms of courting and the pursuit of romantic relationships have shifted to more casual interactions. Dating for courting purposes has decreased, but not disappeared, and sexual behavior outside of traditional committed romantic pair-bonds has become increasingly typical and socially acceptable. These casual "hookups" have emerged from more general social shifts taking place during the last century (rise of novel entertainment venues, automobile usage, and finally the internet culture), and "dating" during this period gave way to a more permissive social-sexual script. Hookups may include any sexual behavior in a seemingly uncommitted context. Nearly all involve kissing (98% of undergraduates responding in one study reported kissing within a hookup), but other behaviors are less ubiquitous. They may involve

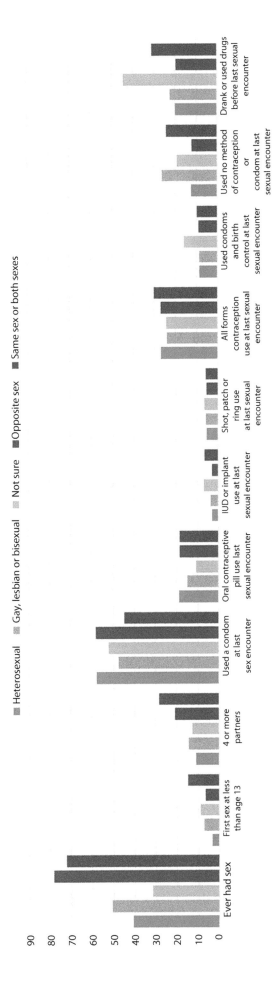

Figure 4.1 Percentage of students engaging in risky versus safer sex encounters, by sexual orientation and sex of sexual contacts. (Based on data from Youth Risk Behavior Surveillance—United States, 2015. www.cdc.gov/mmwr/volumes/65/ss/ss6509a1.htm?s_cid=ss6509_whats (accessed April 21, 2019).

sexual touching above the waist, below the waist, oral sex (giving and receiving), or penetrative intercourse. The term *hookup* focuses more on the uncommitted nature of a sexual encounter rather than on what behaviors "count." Although loving, committed relationships certainly do occur in large percentages in this age group, the uncommitted sexual encounter is becoming an accepted norm; it can even exist within the bounds of a committed relationship as an extra-relationship experience.

Despite the high prevalence of uncommitted sexual behavior, emerging adults often have competing nonsexual interests. One study quotes 63% of college-age men and 83% of college-age women preferred a traditional romantic relationship as opposed to a casual sexual experience. The negative consequences of hookups can include emotional and psychological injury, sexual violence, STIs, and/or unintended pregnancy.[49]

Despite various health risks, nearly half of participants in a college study were unconcerned with contracting STIs. Most students reported not considering their own health risks during hookups, particularly those that occurred within their own community (such as on their college campus). Additionally, there is concern over comorbidity with substance use—men and women who use marijuana or cocaine were more likely than nonusers to have had nonmonogamous sex in the past 12 months.[49]

SOCIAL MEDIA

More than half of all high school students report using the internet as a regular resource for health information. Adolescents can benefit from the use of social media in multiple facets of their lives, including personal, social, and physical aspects. The internet can provide a place of social connection, affording adolescents the opportunity to connect with friends and acquaintances, improve social skills, and foster creativity. Technology can also be a powerful tool for expanding information about sexual health; however, the potential influence of social media on digital health education is unclear. A systematic review of studies looking at the effects of digital media-based interventions on adolescent sexual health showed that such interventions have mixed results. Some studies reveal improved sexual health outcomes for this age group, including improved condom use and improved knowledge about STIs and HIV, contraception, and pregnancy risks. Other studies showed that use of social media increased early onset sexual activity. Other challenges include exposure to incomplete or inaccurate information, pornography, and filters blocking access to legitimate and evidence-based sites.

In addition to the positive effects of accurate health information, there are negative aspects to the internet for children and adolescents. Internet addiction, which is evidenced by uncontrollable use of the internet that results in excess time consumption, can lead to social dysfunction. Internet addiction has been linked to depression, self-injurious behavior, sleep disturbance, increased alcohol and tobacco use, and obesity.

Furthermore, over 70% of children under the age of 18 years report accidental exposure to pornography while using the internet. This can cause significant health implications, because childhood exposure to pornography, even in adolescence, has been linked to a more permissive attitude toward unprotected sex, high-risk sexual behaviors, multiple partners, and use of drugs and alcohol during sex. Pornography also has been shown to have a negative influence on attitudes and ideas toward women, sexuality, and healthy relationships; exposure to violent pornographic material has been linked to sexually aggressive behaviors in boys exposed during early adolescence.

Adolescents also need to be aware of their "digital footprint," the data left behind when a user accesses social media. This record of websites visited, pictures and videos posted, and personal information shared online cannot be removed and can possibly lead to long-term implications if inappropriate information is shared. A trend of sexualized text communication (or "sexting") has emerged. Sending sexually explicit messages or suggestive images can create long-term embarrassment and humiliation, negative effects on future educational and employment opportunities, and potential for physical or emotional harm to the adolescent or others, and can have significant legal consequences. Dissemination of images of a juvenile to another person is prohibited under current child pornography laws; it may be considered a misdemeanor or a felony, depending on the state.[50]

Sexting specifically has been linked to increased odds of sexual activity; although frequent general social media use is not associated with certain risky behaviors per se, sexting is. Sexting as a form of sexual expression increases in frequency with age, and those who sexted had higher odds of engaging in oral, vaginal, and anal sex. This behavior typically occurs within 1 year of sexting.[51]

Internet dating has exploded in popularity among adults as well as adolescents, and many websites have been designed with adolescents in mind. The internet allows users to explore sexual interest with anonymity, perceived safety, and hidden identity. Although these sites usually warn against sharing personal information, this advice is often ignored. Adolescents who have participated in online dating have been shown to have an increased risk of STIs and high-risk sexual behaviors. Dating violence has been associated with internet dating in adolescents.[50]

Studies have shown that only half of parents have discussed privacy settings with their adolescents. Parental interest in their children's online activity is associated with a higher likelihood of an adolescent having a private online profile, but the same discussions with teachers or peers was not found to be as protective. Although formal education and peers might influence social media behavior, this highlights the importance of parental discussions about social media safety to dissuade unsafe online behaviors.[51]

SPECIAL POPULATIONS

Adolescents with disabilities

Like all adolescents, teens with disabilities have the desire for love, friendships, marriage, children, and normal adult sex lives. Adolescents with disabilities should not be considered "asexual" or excluded from sexuality education. Teens with disabilities face the same issues that nondisabled teens face: pubertal development and risk behaviors. Puberty for disabled teens often begins earlier and ends later in males and females, but their knowledge of anatomy, sexuality, contraception, and STI prevention (including HIV) should be on par with their peers.[18] Furthermore, youth with cognitive deficits may be more easily manipulated. Children with disabilities may be more vulnerable to sexual abuse because of their daily dependence on others for intimate care, increased exposure to a large number of caregivers and settings, inappropriate social skills and poor judgment, inability to seek help or report abuse, and a lack of strategies to defend themselves from abuse.[52,53] Expressions of sexuality among adolescents with disabilities are similar to typically developing peers. Age at first intercourse for females does not differ from that of the control population, as noted from data in the U.S. National Longitudinal Study of Adolescent Health.[54] For more guidance in caring for adolescents with disabilities, see Chapter 24.

Sexual minorities (lesbian, gay, bisexual, transgender, and queer)

The YRBS asks youth about their sexual behaviors, and according to the most recent (2015), approximately 2% identify as gay or lesbian, 6% identify as bisexual, and 3.2% report being not sure about their identity or attraction, as referenced in Table 4.3.[47] Sexual behavior alone, however, is not a specific or sensitive predictor of adolescent gender identification, sexual orientation, or sexual identity. Adolescents who are gay, lesbian, transgender, or bisexual or questioning/gender fluid (LGBTQ) have a psychosocial developmental process similar to their heterosexual peers. The majority of clinical research of LGBTQ populations are done with largely white, middle-class, well-educated samples. This demographic limits our understanding of more marginalized subpopulations that are also affected by racism, classism, and other forms of oppression. Queer theory attempts to alter how we define sexual orientation by rejecting the idea of a set outcome and hence the effects of labeling, allowing a more flexible and fluid concept of sexuality.[55]

Adolescents may initially explore heterosexual relationships before homosexual relationships, but uncertainty about sexual orientation decreases with age. Sexual minority students have a higher prevalence of many health-risk behaviors compared with nonsexual minority students. In most of the high-risk behaviors tracked in the YRBS in 2015, students who identified as gay, lesbian, or bisexual engaged in these behaviors in higher percentages than their heterosexual counterparts (Figures 4.2 and 4.3). The rates of some of these high-risk behaviors are even higher in students who report being "not sure" about their sexual identity.[47,56]

HEALTH-CARE PROVIDERS

Although sexuality is a universal component of human development, many providers may miss the opportunity to discuss these topics with adolescents. Barriers to care include clinic accessibility for adolescents, lack of perceived confidentiality, mandatory parental consent laws related to contraception, lack of communication coordination among health programs, biases among providers, stigma associated with various aspects of sexuality including specific sexual behaviors, and financial or practical constraints of the clinic or provider.

Discussions regarding risk-taking behaviors and sex should be routine. Risk assessment for STIs includes inquiring about the gender and sexual behaviors of all partners. The Centers for Disease Control and Prevention (CDC) recommend screening adolescents not involved in high-risk behaviors once per year; however, adolescents with multiple or anonymous partners, those having unprotected intercourse, or those with substance abuse issues should be tested in shorter intervals.[57,58] It is important to ask questions regarding sexual practice, for example, "Are you attracted to boys or girls or both sexes?" Avoid terms such as *boyfriend* or *girlfriend*, but instead ask about *romantic or sexual partners*. Open-ended or gender-neutral questions allow the adolescent to reveal the genders of their partners and begin a conversation about sexual identity and behaviors. It is also important to inquire about vaginal, anal, and/or oral sexual practices as well as screen for early sexual contact such as breast fondling, mutual masturbation, and genital touching. This will allow appropriate counseling for the patient's stage of sexual development. Some adolescents do not consider oral or anal sex "sexually active," and as such may not understand the health risks involved. Questions should include information regarding date of last sexual activity, whether a condom was used, and what type, if any other birth control was used.[58]

Emphasizing confidentiality, showing respect for the teen, listening to the teen's responses, and avoiding medical jargon promote trust between the provider and adolescent. Many adolescents consider their provider to be the most valued and trusted source of advice about issues of health and sexuality. Many youth indicate that they "definitely would not" talk to their parents, citing "embarrassment" as the main reason to avoid discussion. When talking to young people about sexuality and safer sex, an important factor is to help patients make connections between their sexual risk-taking and other aspects of their lives. Teens who engage in sex while under the influence of drugs or alcohol may need to recognize the link and devise a comprehensive risk-reduction strategy. Other "links" include domestic violence, exchanging sex for money or drugs,

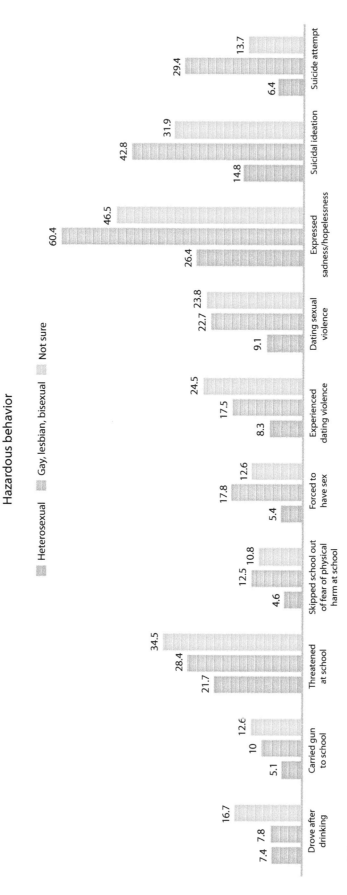

Figure 4.2 Hazardous sexual behavior among those identifying as heterosexual, gay/lesbian/bisexual, or not sure of their sexual orientation. (Based on data from Youth Risk Behavior Surveillance—United States, 2015. www.cdc.gov/mmwr/volumes/65/ss/ss6509a1.htm?s_cid=ss6509_whats (accessed April 21, 2019); MMWR. Sexual identity, sex of sexual contacts, and health-related behaviors among students in grades 9–12—United States and selected sites, 2015. August 12, 2016;65(9). https://www.cdc.gov/mmwr/volumes/65/ss/pdfs/ss6509.pdf. Accessed January 17, 2018.

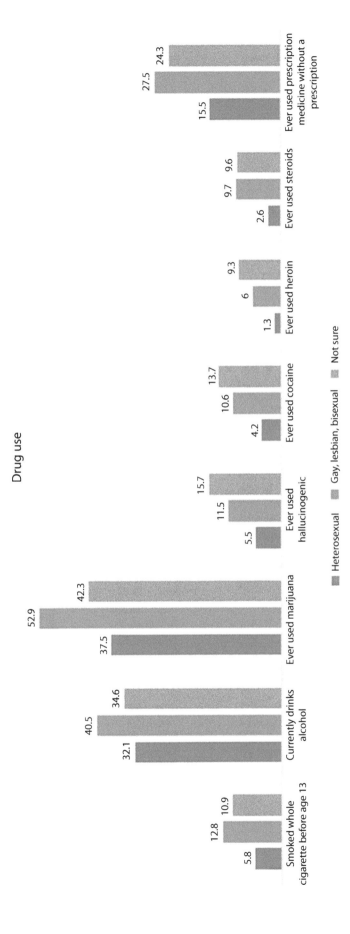

Figure 4.3 Drug use among those identifying as heterosexual, gay/lesbian/bisexual, or not sure of their sexual orientation. (Based on data from Youth Risk Behavior Surveillance—United States, 2015. www.cdc.gov/mmwr/volumes/65/ss/ss6509a1.htm?s_cid=ss6509_whats (accessed April 21, 2019); MMWR. Sexual identity, sex of sexual contacts, and health-related behaviors among students in grades 9–12—United States and selected sites, 2015. August 12, 2016;65(9). https://www.cdc.gov/mmwr/volumes/65/ss/pdfs/ss6509.pdf. Accessed January 17, 2018.

Table 4.4 Provision of care for sexual minority youth.

- Provide time and space for confidential conversations
- Assess and build on the youth's strengths
- Approach sensitive topics respectfully; engage the youth in conversation instead of lecturing
- Aim to foster healthy psychosexual development, integrated identity formation, and adaptive functioning

Make the office welcoming to sexual minority youth (whether or not they have disclosed their orientation). This may encompass:

- Staff who ensure privacy and confidentiality
- Staff who ask patients for their preferred name and gender on intake
- Forms and questions that do not assume heterosexuality and permit nonbinary responses to questions about gender and orientation
- Provision of information and resources for sexual minority youth
- A policy of openness, respect, and value of the individual patient's experience
- Waiting and exam room environments containing health promotion materials and resource information for sexual minority youth

Source: From Society for Adolescent Health and Medicine. *J Adolesc Health*. 2013;52:506, with permission.

and sexual assaults. Each of these risks represents an opportunity for counseling, support, and referral.[2] Sexual minorities routinely report discrimination, bias, and lack of trained providers when attempting to use the healthcare system, leading some to avoid health care altogether. General principles outlined by the American Academy of Pediatrics (AAP), the Society for Adolescent Health and Medicine (SAHM), and the American Academy of Child and Adolescent Psychiatry (AACAP) for the care of sexual minority youth are outlined in Table 4.4.[2,59,60]

REFERENCES

1. Reiter L. Sexual orientation, sexual identity and the quest of choice. *Clin Soc Work J*. 1985;9.
2. Committee on Adolescence. Office-based care for lesbian, gay, bisexual, transgender and questioning youth. *Pediatrics*. 2013;132:198.
3. Luyckx K, Schwartz SJ, Goossens L, Beyers W. Processes of personal identity formation and evaluation. In: Schwartz SJ, Luyckx K, Vignoles VL, eds. *Handbook of Identity Theory and Research*. New York, NY: Springer Science + Business Media; 2011:77–98.
4. Ponton LE, Judice S. Typical adolescent sexual development. *Child Adolesc Psychiatric Clin N Am*. 2004;13:497–511.
5. Hull EM, Lorrain DS. Hormone-neurotransmitter interactions in the control of sexual behavior. *Brain Res*. 1999;105:105–16.
6. Sugar M. Female adolescent sexuality. *J Pediatr Adolesc Gynecol*. 1996;9:175–83.
7. Roiphe H. On an early genital phase: With an addendum on genesis. *Psychoanal Study Child*. 1968; 23:348–65.
8. Galenson E. Development from one to two years: Object relations and psychosexual development. In: Noshspitz JD, ed. *Basic Handbook of Child Psychiatry*. Vol. I. New York, NY: Basic Books; 1979.
9. Roiphe H. A theoretical overview of preoedipal development in the first four years of life. In: Noshspitz JD, ed. *Basic Handbook of Child Psychiatry*. Vol. I. New York, NY: Basic Books; 1979.
10. Whisnant L, Brett E, Zegans L. Adolescent girls and menstruation. *Adolesc Psychiatry*. 1979;7:157–71.
11. *Sexual Development through the Life-Cycle. Adapted from Life Planning Education, a Comprehensive Sex Education Curriculum*. Washington, DC: Advocates for Youth.
12. Smith AM, Rosenthal DA, Reichler H. High schoolers' masturbatory practices: The relationship to sexual intercourse and personal characteristics. *Psychol Rep*. 1996;79:499–509.
13. Leitenberg H, Detzer MJ, Srebnik D. Gender differences in masturbation and the relation of masturbation experiences in preadolescence and/or early adolescence to sexual behavior and sexual adjustment in young adulthood. *Arch Sex Behav*. 1993; 22:87–98.
14. Breuner CC, Matson G, Committee on Adolescence, Committee on Psychological Aspects of Child and Family Health. Sexuality education for children and adolescents. *Pediatrics*. 2016;138.
15. Guidelines for Comprehensive Sexuality Education: Grades K-12. Sexuality Information and Education Council of the United States. https://siecus.org/resources/the-guidelines/ (accessed April 21, 2019).
16. Hotvedt ME. Emerging and submerging adolescent sexuality: Culture and sexual orientation. In: Bancroft J, Reinisch JM, eds. *Adolescence and Puberty*. New York, NY: Oxford University Press; 1990.
17. Kothari MT, Shanxiao W, Head SK, Abderrahim N. 2012. *Trends in Adolescent Reproductive and Sexual Behaviors. DHS Comparative Reports No 29*. Calverton, MD: ICF International.
18. Education S. Comprehensive sexuality education. Committee Opinion No. 678. American College of Obstetricians and Gynecologists. *Obstet Gynecol*. 2016;128:e227–30.
19. Policies for Sexuality Education. https://hivhealth-clearinghouse.unesco.org/library/documents/policies-sexuality-education-european-union-note (accessed April 21, 2019).
20. Santelli J, Kantor L, Grillo S. Abstinence-only until marriage: An updated review of U.S. policies and programs and their impact. *J Adol Health*. 2017;61:273–80.

21. Boonstra H. Advancing sexuality education in developing countries: Evidence and implications. *Guttmacher Policy Review.* 2011;14(3):17–23. https://www.guttmacher.org/gpr/2011/08/advancing-sexuality-education-developing-countries-evidence-and-implications. Accessed January 19, 2018.

22. Duflo E, Dupas P, Kremer M. Education, HIV, and early fertility: Experimental evidence from Kenya. *Am Econ Rev.* 2015;105:2757–97.

23. Trenholm C, Devaney B, Fortson K. Impacts of abstinence education on teen sexual activity, risk of pregnancy and risk of sexually transmitted diseases. *J Policy Anal Manage.* 2008;27:255–76.

24. Lloyd CB, ed. *Growing Up Global: The Changing Transitions to Adulthood in Developing Countries.* Washington, DC: National Academies Press; 2005.

25. Lowry R, Dunville R, Robin L, Kann L. Early sexual debut and associated risk behaviors among sexual minority youth. *Am J of Prev Med.* 2017;52(3):379–84.

26. Kirby D. Antecedents of adolescent initiation of sex, contraceptive use and pregnancy. *Am J Health Behav.* 2002;26:473–85.

27. Smith EA, Udry JR, Morri NM. Pubertal development and friends: A biosocial explanation of adolescent sexual behavior. *J Health Soc Behav.* 1985;26:183–92.

28. Udry JR. Hormonal and social determinants of adolescent sexual behavior. In: Bancroft J, Reinisch JM, eds. *Adolescence and Puberty.* New York, NY: Oxford University Press; 1990.

29. Blum RW, Beuhring T, Rinehart PM. *Protecting teens: Beyond race, income and family structure.* Minneapolis, MN: Center for Adolescent Health, University of Minnesota; 2000.

30. Marin BV, Kirby D, Hudes ES, Coyle KK, Gomez CA. Boyfriends, girlfriends and teenagers' risk of sexual involvement. *Persp Sex Reprod Health.* 2006;38:76–83.

31. Cooksey EC, Mott FL, Neubauer SA. Friendships and early relationships: Links to sexual initiation among American adolescents born to young mothers. *Persp Sex Reprod Health.* 2002;34:118–26.

32. Harvey SM. Female sexual behavior: Fluctuations during the menstrual cycle. *J Psuchosom res.* 1987;31:101–10.

33. Zelnick M, Kahter J, Ford K. *Sex and Pregnancy in Adolescence.* Beverly Hills, CA: Sage; 1981.

34. Furstenberg FF, Brooks-Gunn J, Morgan SP. *Adolescent Mothers in Latter Life.* New York, NY: Cambridge University Press; 1987.

35. Inazu JK, Fox GL. Maternal influences on the sexual behavior of teenage daughters. *J Fam Issues.* 1980;1:81–102.

36. Rosenthal SL, von Ranson KM, Cotton S et al. Sexual initiation: Predictors and developmental trends. *Sex Transm Dis.* 2001;28:527–32.

37. Sieving RE, McNeely CS, Blum RW. Maternal expectations, mother-child connectedness, and adolescent sexual debut. *Arch Pediatr Adolesc Med.* 2000;154:809–16.

38. Thornton A. The courtship process and adolescent sexuality. *J Fam Issues.* 1990;11:239–73.

39. Brewster K. Race differences in sexual activity among adolescent women: The role of neighborhood characteristics. *Am Sociol Rev.* 1994;59:408–24.

40. Crockett L, Bingham D. Family influences on girl's sexual experience and pregnancy risk. *Presented at the Biennial Meeting of the Society for Research on Adolescence*, San Diego, CA, April 1994.

41. McBride CK, Paikoff RL, Holmbeck GN. Individual and familial influences on the onset of sexual intercourse among urban African American adolescents. *J Consult Clin Psychol.* 2003;71:59–67.

42. Ellis BJ, Bates JE, Dodge KA et al. Does father absence place daughters at special risk for early sexual activity and teenage pregnancy? *Child Dev.* 2003;74:801–21.

43. Jones RK, Darroch JE, Singh S. Religious differentials in the sexual and reproductive behaviors of young women in the United States. *J Adolesc Health.* 2005;36:279–88.

44. Abma J, Driscoll A, Moore K. Young womens' degree of control over first intercourse: An exploratory analysis. *Fam Plann Perspective.* 1998;30:12–8.

45. Sullivan LF O, Brooks-Gumm J. The timing of changes in girls' sexual cognitions and behaviors in early adolescence: A prospective, cohort study. *J Adolesc Health.* 2005;37:211–19.

46. Addressing health risks of noncoital sexual activity. Committee Opinion No. 582. American College of Obstetricians and Gynecologists. *Obstet Gynecol.* 2013;122(6):1378–82.

47. Youth Risk Behavior Surveillance—United States, 2015. www.cdc.gov/mmwr/volumes/65/ss/ss6509a1.htm?s_cid=ss6509_whats (accessed April 21, 2019).

48. Data from the National Survey of Family Growth. 2017. https://www.cdc.gov/nchs/nsfg/key_statistics.htm. Accessed January 19, 2018.

49. Garcia JR, Reiber C, Massey SG. Sexual hookup culture: A review. *Rev Gen Psychol.* 2012;16(2):161–76.

50. Concerns regarding social media and health issues in adolescents and young adults. Committee Opinion No. 653. American College of Obstetricians and Gynecologists. *Obstet Gynecol.* 2016;127(2):414.

51. Romo DL, Garnett AP, Younger MS. Social media use and its association with sexual risk and parental monitoring among a primarily Hispanic adolescent population. *J Pediatr Adolesc Gynecol.* 2017;30:466–74.

52. DeLoach CP. Attitudes toward disability impact on sexual development and forging of intimate relationships. *J Appl Rehabil Couns.* 1994;25:18–25.

53. Maclean MJ, Sims S, Bower C. Maltreatment risk among children with disabilities *Pediatrics.* 2017;139(4): e20161817.

54. Cheng MM, Udry JR. Sexual behaviors of physically disabled adolescents in the United States. *J Adolesc Health.* 2002;31:48–58.

55. Human Sexuality and Culture, 2015. https://courses lumenlearning.com/boundless-psychology/chapter/ sexuality/. Accessed January 19, 2018.

56. Kann L, Olsen EO, McManus T et al. Sexual identity, sex of sexual contacts, and health-related behaviors among students in grades 9–12—United States and selected sites, 2015. *MMWR Surveill Summ* 2016;65(No. SS-9):1–202.

57. Workowski KA, Berman SM, Centers for Disease Control and Prevention. Sexually transmitted diseases treatment guidelines, 2010. *MMWR Recomm Rep.* 2010;59(RR-12):1–110.

58. American Academy of Pediatrics Committee on Adolescence. Office-based care for lesbian, gay, bisexual, transgender and questioning youth. *Pediatrics.* 2013;132(1):198–203.

59. Society for Adolescent Health and Medicine. Recommendations for promoting the health and well-being of lesbian, gay, bisexual and transgender adolescents: A position paper of the Society for Adolescent Health and Medicine. *J Adolesc Health.* 2013;52:506.

60. Bell DL, Breland DJ, Ott MA. Adolescent and young adult male health: A review. *Pediatrics.* 2013;132:535.

Pubertal abnormalities

Precocious and delayed

ELLEN LANCON CONNOR

5

Puberty encompasses biochemical, physical, and emotional changes that result in full sexual maturation and adult height and physique.

The biochemical initiation of puberty follows many years of quiescent hypothalamic-pituitary-ovarian function. It is actually the second puberty of postnatal life, occurring after the "mini-puberty of infancy" characterized by gonadotropin-releasing hormone (GnRH) stimulation of the infant pituitary in the first 6 months or more of a baby's life, producing measurable levels of luteinizing hormone (LH) and follicle-stimulating hormone (FSH). LH and FSH stimulate ovarian production of estradiol in early months of infancy, and then fall to prepubertal levels during an interval in which the hypothalamus is particularly sensitive to negative feedback, approximately ages 5–10 years, with LH declining in the first year of life, followed by FSH by age 4 years.[1] Recognizing the timing of the postnatal peaks and troughs of LH and FSH can inform decisions about whether to evaluate children at specific ages using random gonadotropin values. Adolescent puberty is initiated by leptin stimulation of kisspeptin production, resulting in pulsatile GnRH release to stimulate LH and FSH production again. Kisspeptin is produced in the arcuate and anteroventral periventricular nuclei in a pulsatile manner, binding to the kisspeptin receptor and stimulating leptin release. With GnRH pulse amplifications stimulating anterior pituitary gonadotropes, LH and FSH rise and begin to activate the ovary to produce increasing levels of estradiol. Pubertal progression may be altered by genetic variations, congenital or acquired structural defects of the brain, congenital or acquired defects of the ovary or its life span, nutrition, stress, or chronic disease.

Timing of puberty refers specifically to when pubertal events occur, and certain pubertal events mark this timing, namely, thelarche and menarche. *Thelarche* is defined by the appearance of the initial breast bud, noted by the rubbery disc of tissue beneath the areola. In the United States, thelarche is generally normal after age 7 years, occurring slightly earlier on average in African American girls and Hispanic girls, and later in white European American girls.[2] True thelarche corresponds to a bone age of approximately 10 years, regardless of the chronological age of the girl.

While a recent trend toward slightly earlier thelarche has been described in the United States, the average age of menarche has been stable since the 1970s. Factors believed to be affecting thelarche include nutrition, body mass index (BMI), genetics, environmental exposures, and exposures to severe psychological stress. The cross-sectional analysis reported by Herman-Giddens in 1997 (PROS Study) found that 48% of African American (AA) girls and 15% of white girls had thelarche by inspection at age 8 years, while the average age of menarche was 12.2 years for AA girls and 12.9 years for white girls.[2] Chumlea et al. analyzed data from the National Health and Nutrition Examination Survey (NHANES) III (1988–1994) and found ethnic variation for menarche, but all averages were greater than age 12 years.[3] Girls with earlier puberty tend to have a longer duration of puberty, while those with delayed puberty may have a shorter duration of puberty.

The *tempo of puberty* refers to timing of increased estradiol production by the ovaries, most commonly followed by thelarche, adrenarche with increasing dehydroepiandrosterone sulfate (DHEA-S) and androstenedione from the adrenal glands, and finally, menarche, full adult height, and sexual maturation. Normally, the physical signs of thelarche are separated from menarche by at least 2.5 years. A girl may grow 0–5 cm additionally after menarche. Examples of the girl with abnormal tempo of puberty would include a girl with a hypothalamic hamartoma experiencing menarche 6 months after thelarche, as well as a girl with a craniopharyngioma who experienced thelarche at age 10 years but still has not had menarche 6 years later.

Pubertal progression can be an early indicator of underlying health conditions in a child. Evaluating both the *timing* and the *tempo* of puberty permits the practitioner to identify both normal, familial variations in puberty as well as pubertal disorders of precocity or delay. Counseling a child and family about normal variations in pubertal timing and tempo can alleviate significant psychological distress, while identifying true pubertal abnormalities permits identification of and causes for deviation from expected, often permitting intervention to improve physical and psychological health outcomes. Interpretation of history, growth curves, and physical findings, with prudent use of laboratory evaluation and bone age radiographs, will streamline diagnosis to implement appropriate therapeutic interventions (Figures 5.1 and 5.2).

EARLY PUBERTY

Population studies indicate varied incidence of precocious puberty (PP). In the United States, an incidence of 1/5000 to 1/10,000 has been reported. In Denmark, a national patient registry informed an incidence of 1/500 girls.

Thelarche

Premature thelarche is a variant typically seen in young girls ages 1–3 years. It is characterized by unilateral or bilateral breast enlargement without accelerated growth velocity, advancement of bone age, or any other signs of puberty. It does not initiate full pubertal progression, but rather only breast changes. Premature thelarche may be temporary or may continue until the girl is 7–10 years old and begins to show other normal pubertal signs. It should never be treated surgically, as excision would remove all the future breast tissue from that side, necessitating cosmetic repair and preventing lactation on that side. Premature thelarche does not alter reproductive potential.

Adrenarche and pubarche

Adrenarche refers to the process of androgenic maturation, beginning with increasing production of the adrenal hormones, androstenedione and DHEA-S, and culminating with *pubarche*, the appearance of axillary and pubic hair, as well as increased oiliness of the scalp and skin, apocrine body odor, and potential for acne. Pubarche usually but not always occurs after thelarche. In contrast to adrenarche and pubarche, *virilization* describes abnormal androgen production leading to clitoromegaly, muscle enlargement, and hirsutism. Normal female puberty does not include hirsutism, clitoromegaly, deep voice, and/or muscular hypertrophy. A cause for virilization should always be sought, considering exogenous androgen exposure, congenital adrenal hyperplasia, mixed gonadal dysgenesis, other genetic disorders previously unrecognized in the child's life (such as 5-α reductase deficiency) or ovarian, adrenal, or rare hepatic tumors. Virilization can decrease reproductive potential.

Premature adrenarche refers to the premature appearance of acne, apocrine odor, and pubic and axillary hair, and is more common in some ethnicities. Premature adrenarche, especially in girls who were small for gestational

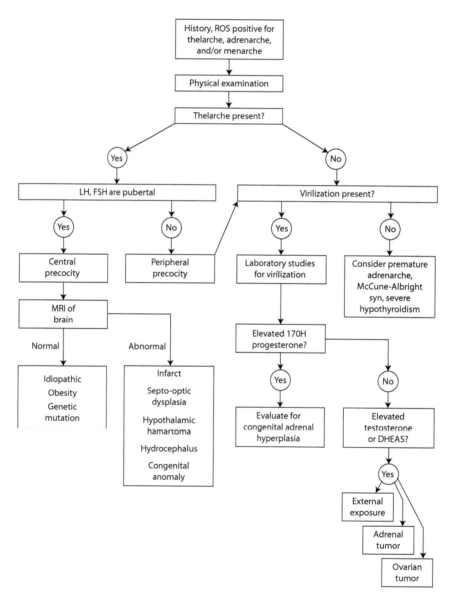

Figure 5.1 Evaluation of precocious puberty.

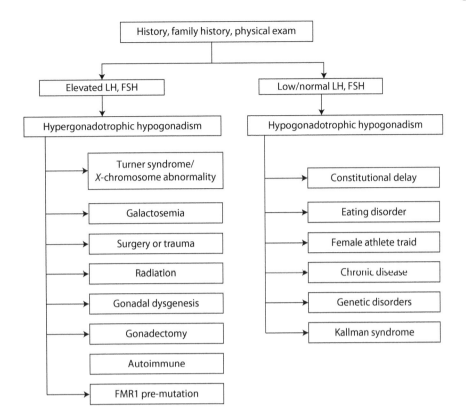

Figure 5.2 Evaluation of delayed puberty.

age, may be a harbinger of insulin resistance and polycystic ovary syndrome (PCOS).[4] After excluding virilizing causes of adrenarche (Table 5.1) or PP, the child should be watched carefully for increasing BMI and, after menses is later established, for signs and symptoms of possible evolving PCOS. PCOS may cause a reduction in reproductive potential. By contrast, some girls with premature adrenarche do not progress to PCOS and will not have altered reproductive potential.

Menarche

A third variant of puberty is *premature menarche*, which must be distinguished from urethral, rectal, perineal, or vaginal introitus bleeding due to structural issues or assault. Ovarian cysts, isolated or as part of severe hypothyroidism (van Wyk-Grumbach syndrome) or McCune-Albright syndrome, may produce unexpected menstrual bleeding, even without thelarche. Van Wyk-Grumbach syndrome does not affect reproductive capability once

Table 5.1 Causes of virilization.

- Exogenous androgen exposure
- Congenital adrenal hyperplasia
- Mixed gonadal dysgenesis
- 5-α reductase deficiency
- Adrenal tumor
- Ovarian tumor
- Hepatic tumor

the hypothyroidism is adequately treated. In contrast, McCune-Albright syndrome may include other endocrinopathies, such as hyperthyroidism, growth hormone excess, or Cushing syndrome, which could impair the ability to conceive or maintain pregnancy.

Precocious puberty

PP describes pubertal changes occurring more than 2.5 standard deviations earlier than the mean. Again, causes can be separated into those resulting from early hypothalamic-pituitary-ovarian axis activation and those resulting from peripheral causes, including ovarian, exogenous, and other (Table 5.2). Those etiologies with central nervous system (CNS) origin are often described as causes of gonadotropin-dependent or central precocious puberty. Peripheral causes are described as gonadotropin independent. In precocious puberty, significant acceleration of linear growth velocity and bone age advancement occur, potentially compromising final adult height. Evidence suggests that height is not significantly impacted if central precocity occurs after age 6 years, although concerns about emotional maturity, final height in small-statured families, and risk-taking behaviors have been reported as reasons for use of therapy to delay puberty. Families must be counseled that although the girl is currently tall for her age, she could lose height potential if bone age advancement is rapid in untreated central PP.

Some children with congenital hydrocephalus, cerebral palsy, septo-optic hypoplasia, or brain injury may develop

Table 5.2 Central and peripheral causes of precocious puberty.

Central	Peripheral
Hypothalamic hamartoma	Exogenous sex steroid exposure
Idiopathic	McCune-Albright syndrome
Central nervous system malignancy	Adrenal tumor
Optic nerve hypoplasia syndrome	Ovarian tumor
Genetic mutations	Hepatic tumor
Familial benign precocity	Endocrine disruptors
Stress	Severe primary hypothyroidism
Hydrocephalus	
Brain injury	
Long-standing peripheral precocity	
Obesity	

central precocious puberty due to loss of GnRH inhibition. Such central PP may occur even in toddlers with these brain lesions. Families may request delay of menarche beyond an age when menarche is typically allowed to occur, due to a desire to avoid the additional hygiene issues, the child's fear of blood, or the risk of unintended pregnancy. In such cases, both short-term and long-term goals regarding therapy must be discussed, as estrogen does benefit bone health, and prolonged use of GnRH agonist or depot-progesterone into the teen years could adversely affect trabecular bone accrual.

Genetic defects leading to central precocity include mutations and single nucleotide polymorphisms (SNPs). Defects have been identified in genes coding for kisspeptin and its receptor, neuropeptide Y, DLK1, POU1F1, and LIN28B. Among the familial cases of central precocity, inactivating mutations in the gene for the makorin ring finger protein 3 (MKRFN3) are most commonly identified, although activating mutations in the genes for KISS1 or KISS1 receptor are also known.[5] Each of these mutations can result in early activation of the GnRH axis. Patients with pituitary hormone deficiencies due to defects in POU1F1 can present with central precocious puberty due to GnRH activation.[6] A defect in the delta-like homolog 1 gene (DLK-1) can also produce central precocity, with a risk for adipose-driven complications involving metabolic syndrome.[7] Peripheral precocity genetic mutations include those in McCune-Albright syndrome.

Approach to precocious puberty

The approach to precocity has been stratified by ethnic and racial groups by the Pediatric Endocrine Society, after careful analysis of the Herman-Giddens and NHANES III data. Their recommendation for otherwise healthy children is that precocity be evaluated in AA girls with pubertal changes before age 6 years and in white girls before age

7 years.[8] Regardless of ethnicity, however, evaluation of girls 6–8 years old is influenced by the severity of growth acceleration, bone age advancement, and family and child concern (Figure 5.1).

Central precocious puberty

Central precocity is characterized by growth acceleration, bone age advancement, thelarche, and adrenarche occurring at earlier than expected ages, with pubertal levels of LH and FSH. Menarche may also occur early. Hypothalamic hamartomas (HHs) may be found, particularly now that magnetic resonance imaging (MRI) is more advanced, though idiopathic causes remain frequent in girls. Among patients with CNS causes, the benign HH is most common. HH may be accompanied by seizures, laughing spells, and other neurologic findings. Concurrent follow-up with a neurosurgeon should be recommended. Genetic or syndromic causes may cause central precocity, as can trauma or surgery, all by interrupting the feedback inhibition of GnRH secretion. Obesity may advance bone age in girls and lead to central pubertal activation. Given that a third of U.S. children are overweight or have obesity, elevated BMI is a frequent cause of referral for early pubertal change. Additionally, one must consider early puberty to have a genetic cause in a girl with obesity if she has had other family members with precocious puberty.

Peripheral precocious puberty

Peripheral precocity will also have growth acceleration and rapid epiphyseal maturation; the order of pubertal changes may be typical or may have predominance of estrogen- or androgen-driven changes, depending on the etiology of precocity. Sources may be exogenous, ovarian, adrenal, or ectopic. LH and FSH levels are usually prepubertal, although long-standing peripheral precocity may lead eventually to activation of central puberty.

One form of precocious peripheral puberty, seen more commonly in girls than in boys, is McCune-Albright syndrome due to a postzygotic activating mutation in *GNAS1*, increasing G-stimulating α protein signaling leading to chronically activated adenyl cyclase and increased cyclic adenosine monophosphate (cAMP). The syndrome is characterized by hyperfunction of multiple endocrine glands, leading to presentations of peripheral precocity, hyperthyroidism, Cushing syndrome, renal phosphate wasting, and/or growth hormone excess. The classic triad in McCune-Albright syndrome (MAS) is that of endocrinopathy, unilateral, irregular bordered café au lait macules, and polyostotic fibrous dysplasia; however, the mutation is postzygotic, and thus affected girls may not demonstrate the entire triad, depending on which tissues contain the mutation. Ultrasonography reveals recurring autonomous ovarian cysts, and premature menarche may be seen. Thelarche may be absent or much less significant than the extent of the menstrual bleeding. Other rare manifestations may include malignancy, cholestasis, and arrhythmia. Both timing and tempo of puberty in these girls may be affected. Treatment may include estrogen receptor modulation with tamoxifen or aromatase inhibitor therapy with the potent long-acting inhibitor letrozole.[9,10]

Severe primary hypothyroidism may produce a syndrome of peripheral precocity known as the van Wyk-Grumbach syndrome. Thelarche and/or early menarche may occur in a girl with poor growth velocity, delayed bone age, and a significantly elevated thyroid-stimulating hormone (TSH) level. The syndrome is believed to be the result of an FSH receptor allele with increased affinity for TSH in some individuals.[11] One should note that significant pubertal changes not associated with a growth spurt or advancing bone age are likely due to hypothyroidism.

Evaluation of precocious puberty

Evaluation of precocious puberty should include a careful history and physical examination, radiograph determination of bone age, and reconstruction of the growth curve. History should include birth weight, history of CNS injury or surgery, timing of pubertal findings, tempo of findings, family history of early puberty, possible exposure to sex steroids, and a review of systems focusing on CNS symptoms as well as abdominal pain.

LH and FSH levels with serum estradiol should be obtained. LH levels are preferable for diagnosis of precocity and should be obtained by immunofluorometric, immunochemiluminometric, or electrochemiluminometric assay. A baseline LH using one of these methods is diagnostic if greater than 0.3–0.5 IU/L. Serum estradiol may be elevated, low, or normal in precocity—very high levels would suggest the presence of a tumor secreting estradiol. Depending on findings from the history, review of systems, and physical exam, obtaining TSH, androstenedione, 17-OH progesterone, total testosterone by liquid chromatography/tandem mass spectrometry, β-HCG, and DHEA-S levels may be needed. GnRH stimulation testing may be needed to establish that the precocity is central if baseline LH is not elevated.

The GnRH stimulation test uses GnRH or one of its analogs to stimulate the pituitary gland. Commonly, a single measurement of LH is obtained 30–45 minutes after administration, with a value greater than 5–8 IU/L being diagnostic.

If confirmed, central precocity should be evaluated with CNS imaging by MRI (Table 5.3). Some authors have advocated for obtaining genetic testing for MKRN3 in patients with a history of familial precocity before considering MRI. Estimates of the frequency of abnormal MRI findings in a cohort of girls with CPP range from 8% to 33%. Only 2% of girls whose precocity was noted after 6 years of age had abnormal MRI findings.

Treatment of precocious puberty

Treatment of precocity varies depending on etiology and degree of severity. For idiopathic central precocity, GnRH analog therapy can provide the benefit of delaying menses until a girl is psychologically ready for puberty and preventing rapid advancement of bone age that would compromise final height. The agonist may be given by injection daily (rarely prescribed), monthly, or every 12 weeks (leuprolide), by nasal spray (Nafarelin) or by intradermal implant (histrelin). The goal is to block GnRH to prevent pulsatile release of FSH and LH in response to GnRH until the provider and family believe the child should undergo pubertal maturation. Girls diagnosed over the age of 8

Table 5.3 Evaluation of suspected precocious or delayed puberty.

Study	Value	Comment
Bone age	Assess effect of diagnosis on growth potential	Radiograph of left hand unless hand is unable to be opened
LH, FSH	Elevation of LH > 0.3 is consistent with puberty; marked elevation of FSH and LH is consistent with ovarian insufficiency Low levels indicate central pubertal delay, peripheral precocity, or suppression by exogenous estrogen	Choose ultrasensitive assay
β-HCG	Elevation can produce changes similar to LH	
17-OH progesterone	Elevated with congenital adrenal hyperplasia	
DHEA-S	Elevated with adrenal causes of precocity	
Testosterone	Elevated with ovarian or adrenal tumor, or exogenous exposure	Use liquid chromatography–tandem mass spectometry
Estradiol	Marked elevation may indicate tumor	Estradiol assay may not separate prepubertal from beginning puberty; LH is preferable for this determination
Androstenedione	Elevated in adrenal and some ovarian tumors	
Gonadotropin-releasing hormone test	Precocity may be diagnosed with pubertal LH response; delayed versus permanent gonadotropin deficiency requires addition of 24-hour post-GnRH measure of LH	

Abbreviations: DHEA-S, dehydroepiandrosterone sulfate; FSH, follicle-stimulating hormone; GnRH, gonadotropin-releasing hormone; HCG, human chorionic gonadotropin; LH, luteinizing hormone.

years will usually not require GnRH analog therapy.[12] Patients undergoing GnRH suppression should have LH monitored 30–120 minutes after administration of a GnRH agonist. LH should be less than 4.5 IU/L during suppression. Patients with suppression by implant should have LH monitored 4 weeks after implantation and again every 6 months after suppression is achieved. Best height outcomes have been reported when GnRH therapy is discontinued by 12–12.5 years. Menarche occurs on average 16 months after leuprolide is discontinued. Because menarche occurring before age 11 years is associated with a higher risk for metabolic syndrome, cardiovascular disease, and cancer, GnRH agonists are generally continued to age 10–11 years.

Peripheral precocity therapy varies depending on the source of the pubertal activation. For van Wyk-Grumbach syndrome, levothyroxine is prescribed, initiating dose based on body weight. For McCune-Albright syndrome, estrogen receptor blockade is desired, and tamoxifen or letrozole may be used to prevent menses and preserve height potential.[25] Congenital adrenal hyperplasia would be addressed with glucocorticoid replacement, initially hydrocortisone every 8 hours at a dose of 10–12 mg/m², a suppressive dose higher than expected replacement therapy. Spironolactone may be added to block androgen effect. Tumor excision, with or without chemotherapy and/or radiation, is indicated for hormone-secreting tumors. Removal of exogenous estrogen and/or androgen exposure in children with exogenous exposure must begin with identification of the source of the exposure and may include creams or gels used by a parent or childcare provider, animal feed products that contain estrogen, estrogen-like compounds, and compounds than enhance skin absorption of estrogen. If peripheral precocity is long standing, a GnRH agonist may also be needed to block the secondary CNS activation. Recent studies suggest that early puberty may be tied to adverse health outcomes, including malignancy and cardiovascular/metabolic disease, findings that could ultimately influence practice regarding when to treat precocity.[13,23,24]

DELAYED PUBERTY

Delayed timing of puberty for girls in the United States refers to thelarche not occurring by 13 years or menarche by 15 years, or to the absence of menarche more than 3 years after thelarche (Figure 5.2). The most common form of delayed puberty in the United States is constitutional delay of growth and puberty (CDGP), also known as self-limited delayed puberty (SLDP). CDGP is characterized by delayed bone age, late pubertal onset timing, and usually a family history of a similar growth pattern. Inheritance may be autosomal dominant or recessive, or X-linked.[14] Girls with CDGP eventually enter puberty with final adult heights commiserate with family genetics. When evaluating delayed puberty, the first and most important question is whether the cause is *central*, that is, originating from the brain, or *peripheral*, related to abnormalities of the genitourinary system (Table 5.4). *Central causes of delayed puberty* are characterized by prepubertal levels of LH and FSH.

Table 5.4 Central and peripheral causes of delayed puberty.

Central	Peripheral
Malnutrition	Ovarian agenesis
Genetic mutations involving GnRH	Autoimmune ovarian failure
Genetic mutations involving kisspeptin	Pelvic radiation
Genetic mutations involving leptin	Galactosemia
Constitutional delay of growth and puberty	Genetic cause of ovarian failure including Turner syndrome, fragile X syndrome, and others
Brain tumor	Surgery or trauma to ovary
Craniopharyngioma or Rathke cleft cyst	
Chronic disease	

Peripheral causes of delayed puberty will usually be characterized by postmenopausal (elevated) levels of LH, FSH, and, if permanent, low or undetectable anti-Müllerian hormone (AMH) due to absence or failure of the ovaries.

Some pubertal delay refers primarily due to the absence of menarche in a girl who has had breast development. Causes can include PCOS or anatomic blockage of menstrual flow. Such etiologies of delayed menarche are accompanied by pubertal LH and FSH levels. By contrast, a girl who presents with normal growth velocity, with thelarche without adrenarche, or with minimal adrenarche, should be evaluated for the possibility of androgen insensitivity syndrome; karyotype would reveal 46XY in this girl with an androgen receptor defect, and pubertal LH and FSH levels would be accompanied by pubertal testosterone levels.

A girl who is found to have genital ambiguity at puberty should be evaluated for mosaicism of gonadal dysgenesis, 5-α reductase deficiency, or partial androgen insensitivity syndrome. Gonadal dysgenesis may be suspected in the setting of ambiguity with inguinal hernia or mass. Girls with 5-α reductase deficiency often virilize when they produce pubertal testosterone levels and are able to convert to dihydrotestosterone. Partial androgen insensitivity can produce more virilization at puberty than what is seen with complete androgen insensitivity syndrome.

Central delayed puberty (hypogonadotropic hypogonadism)

Among the central causes of delayed puberty, malnutrition is most common worldwide, and CDGP and chronic diseases are main causes in the United States. These causes are often described as *reversible hypogonadotropic hypogonadism* or *functional hypogonadotropic hypogonadism*. Malnutrition may be seen due to poverty, eating disorder, relative energy deficit disorder (formerly known as the female athlete triad), withholding of food from a child, or chronic disease. Chronic disease may delay puberty not only through malnutrition, but also by inflammation or hormone excess, such as in hyperprolactinemia or hypercortisolemia. CDGP will be characterized by delayed bone age, prepubertal short stature, late but normal pubertal progression, and ultimately, height commiserate with midparental height.

Hypogonadotropic hypogonadism that is permanent may result from congenital or acquired lesions of the brain that involve the hypothalamus and/or pituitary gland and is characterized by low LH and FSH levels. Congenital lesions may be primarily structural or may involve genetic defects in the production of one or more hypothalamic or pituitary factors. In contrast, hypergonadotropic hypogonadism signals a failure to produce estradiol because of congenital or acquired absence or damage of the ovaries and is characterized by elevated levels of LH snd FSH.

Isolated GnRH deficiency includes the various forms of Kallman syndrome, in addition to idiopathic hypogonadotropic hypogonadism (IHH). Kallman syndrome may involve anosmia or hyposmia, and delayed puberty due to defects in migration of GnRH neurons with the olfactory placode in fetal development.[15] Genes that may be involved in IHH/KS may be X-linked as in *KAL1*, also known as *ANOS1* (rarely affecting females) or autosomal dominant (*CHD7*, *FGFR1*) or recessive (affecting females and males). Some forms of KS may be associated with cleft palate and/or deafness (*CHD7*), dental anomalies or agenesis (*FGFR1*), or synkinesia (*ANOS1*). Some isolated forms of hypogonadotropic hypogonadism involve genes for GnRH (*GNRHR* gene) or kisspeptin or its receptor.[16]

Peripheral delayed puberty (hypergonadotropic hypogonadism)

Among the causes of primary ovarian insufficiency, Turner syndrome is most common, occurring in 2000–2500 live births of female infants. The girl with Turner syndrome may have monosomy of X, a ring chromosome of X, or varying degrees of abnormalities of the X chromosome; she may have mosaicism, with some cell lines involving a Y chromosome or a second X. As a result of the lack of a fully intact second X, ovarian atresia beings in utero and continues postnatally. In some girls, spontaneous puberty or fertility may occur, particularly if mosaicism is present to support ovarian function.[17] As girls with spontaneous puberty in the setting of Turner syndrome have a high likelihood of premature ovarian insufficiency, fertility preservation counseling should be provided.

The girl with Turner syndrome may be diagnosed in utero due to increased nuchal fold lucency, at birth due to lymphedema or congenital heart defect, in early childhood due to growth failure, or in adolescence after primary or secondary amenorrhea occur. Girls may be found to have absent thelarche due to lack of estrogen but normal adrenarche, since the adrenal glands are unaffected. Girls not diagnosed until puberty may have escaped earlier diagnosis because they were not <5th percentile for height, which in fact may reflect that they have tall parents. Taller parents have taller daughters with Turner syndrome. Girls with

Table 5.5 Turner syndrome features.

- Short stature relative to midparental height
- Lymphedema of hands and feet
- Low posterior hairline
- Deep-set eyes, epicanthal folds, ptosis
- Low-set posteriorly rotated ears
- High arched palate, small mandible, dental crowding
- Congenital heart defects
- Nail hypoplasia, hyperconvexity
- Cubitus valgus and increased muscularity of limbs
- Increased venous prominence
- Increased pigmented nevi
- Tendency for keloid formation
- Conductive and sensorineural hearing loss
- Primary or secondary amenorrhea
- Wide-spaced nipples
- Increased autoimmunity
- Intestinal telangiectasia
- Anxiety, difficulties with spatial reasoning, difficulties with nonverbal cues and reading faces

Turner syndrome with a Y component are at increased risk of dysgerminoma or gonadoblastoma. Other features of the syndrome affect multiple organ systems (Table 5.5). Girls with Turner syndrome usually have normal intelligence, although some specific areas of learning challenges may be identified.

Girls who do not have Turner syndrome but have deletions in a portion of the Xq region only may also have premature ovarian insufficiency.[18] Girls with XY gonadal dysgenesis (previously called Swyer syndrome) or mixed gonadal dysgenesis (45X/46XY) will present with ovarian insufficiency but also have risk for dysgerminoma or gonadoblastoma (see Chapter 7). Another group of girls with ovarian insufficiency can be 16% of those with fragile X heterozygote permutation carrier status, particularly if the affected X was of paternal origin. Galactosemia may lead to ovarian failure in 70%–80% of affected girls. Other rare forms of hypergonadotropic hypogonadism, including mutations in the FSH-β subunit or FSH receptor, or type 1 blepharophimosis-ptosis-epicanthus inversus syndrome due to an autosomal mutation in chromosome 3, can also occur.

Other causes of ovarian insufficiency can be iatrogenic due to surgical removal of or damage to ovaries (most often due to chemotherapy and radiation), autoimmune, or idiopathic. Autoimmunity may occur concurrently with Hashimoto thyroiditis, with the autoimmune polyglandular syndromes, or in isolation. Elevation of 21 hydroxylase or 17 hydroxylase antibodies has been described in autoimmune ovarian insufficiency.

Evaluation of delayed puberty

Evaluation of pubertal delay should begin with a careful history and review of systems, reconstruction of the growth height and weight curves, and physical examination looking for signs of chronic disease, genetic abnormalities, eating disorder, and vaginal patency. Bone age should be reviewed to assess whether radiologic evidence of delay is present but does not change the evaluation. More severely delayed bone ages can be seen in severe hypothyroidism, pituitary deficiencies, or long-standing severe chronic disease. A bone age of 12 years or greater is usually present when menarche occurs. Random LH and FSH using an ultrasensitive assay with estradiol, prolactin, free T4, and TSH should be obtained, in addition to sedimentation rate, comprehensive metabolic panel to assess hepatic and renal function, complete blood count, and urinalysis. Karyotype should be included in patients with elevated FSH, if features of Turner syndrome are noted, or if all other causes of delay have been excluded. Anti-Müllerian hormone and inhibin B may also assist in diagnosis if hypergonadotropic hypogonadism is present. Prudent use of GnRH stimulation testing may separate temporary from permanent hypogonadotropic hypogonadism, although some overlap is possible in laboratory results. LH and FSH are measured at baseline, 1 hour, 2 hours, 3 hours, and 24 hours after administration of a GnRH analog. Failure to note a pubertal rise in LH (defined earlier in precocious puberty evaluation) on the first day suggests central etiologies of delayed puberty. Measuring the 24-hour LH sample distinguishes reversible causes (LH is elevated at 24 hours) from permanent causes (LH remains prepubertal).

Radiologic evaluation may be indicated in pubertal delay. MRI of the brain can delineate CNS anatomic lesions causing pubertal delay. Ultrasound or MRI of the pelvis should be performed when hypergonadotropic hypogonadism is diagnosed, or when presence of the vagina and/ or uterus is in question. Additionally, pelvic imaging may sometimes indicate a multicystic ovary in PCOS, although adolescent PCOS does not require ovarian morphology for diagnosis or an ectopic gonad in gonadal dysgenesis.

Treatment of permanent hypogonadism

Treatment of permanent hypogonadism, whether central or peripheral, involves regimens to mimic typical pubertal development, beginning with initiation of low-dose estrogen for 12–24 months, followed by introduction of progesterone therapy to permit menses if a uterus is present. Low-dose estrogen escalation in the form of transdermal estrogen 0.025–0.1 mg daily, oral ethinyl estradiol 0.02–0.2 mg, or conjugated equine estrogen 0.3–1.2 mg may be used. Estrogen therapy alone, in increasing doses every 6 months, is usually indicated for 18 months to 2 years. Micronized progesterone in a daily dose of 100–200 mg is currently recommended for 10 days when menses is desired.[19] Menstruation may be induced to occur monthly or at some other fixed interval.

Genetics of puberty

The previous decade has been significant for advances in understanding how human genetics affects pubertal timing and progression.[20] Furthermore, links between the timing of puberty and subsequent risks for malignancy,

Table 5.6 Genetic contributions to puberty.

Precocious puberty	Delayed puberty
• MKRN3 • DLK1	• IGSF10—GnRH migration • TAC3, TACR3—neurokinin B and its receptor
• Rare gain of function KISS1, KISS1R • POU1Fi mutations	

Thelarche and menarche	Thelarche only
• LIN28B	• FSHR

cardiovascular disease, and diabetes are being uncovered. Elucidation of these links should inform individualized medical decisions for children and adolescents in the future to avoid the severe morbidity and the mortality of chronic diseases. Though much work remains to cogently describe the entire pubertal pathway's genetics, several key findings have recently been described (Table 5.6). Mutations from MKRN3 (located at chromosome 15q11.2) that are maternally imprinted commonly cause familial precocious puberty. Another imprinted gene, DLK1, can also produce precocity. Temple syndrome is the precocity syndrome seen with a deletion of the DLK1 gene. Mutations in the POU1F1 gene present with infantile combined pituitary hormone deficiencies, and later with precocious puberty. Though rare, gain of function mutations of the kisspeptin gene and its receptor have also been described in patients with precocious puberty. Similarly, a single gene mutation of the IGSF10 gene causing delayed puberty has now been described, perhaps causing delay by affecting GnRH neuronal migration. Defects in neurokinin B and its receptor have been identified as another cause of pubertal delay, caused by mutations in the TAC3 and TAC3R genes. Some genes act principally at certain stages of puberty. For example, mutations in the LIN28B gene alter thelarche and menarche timing, while mutations in FSHR, the FSH receptor gene, appear to be primarily manifested to alterations in thelarche timing.

Endocrine disruptors and puberty

Endocrine disruption has been suggested as an etiology of pubertal alterations. Endocrine disruptors can be naturally occurring, such as phytoestrogens, or artificially introduced into an environment. Polybrominated biphenyls (PBBs), for example, were accidentally given more than 40 years ago to more than 4000 Michigan residents through contaminated cattle, with subsequent decrease in menarche age by approximately 1 year in girls with exposure compared to unexposed girls.[21] Earlier thelarche has been observed in girls with higher urine and serum phthalate levels.[22] The effects of environmental exposures on puberty are very difficult to study, as dose of exposure and the confounding effects of obesity and genetics are difficult to quantify. Thus, cause and effect can often not be determined, but endocrine disruptor research may yield further insight into causes for pubertal variation among populations.

CONCLUSION

Careful assessment of the girl referred for precocity or delay of puberty, with history, physical examination, bone age radiograph, and targeted use of laboratory studies based on findings can permit diagnosis, treatment, and counseling of options for pubertal progression and/or reproductive capacity. Genetic studies of puberty offer the promise of earlier and clearer diagnosis, with future opportunities for targeted intervention.

REFERENCES

1. Winter JS, Faiman C, Hobson WC et al. Pituitary-gonadal relations in infancy. I. Patterns of serum gonadotropin concentrations from birth to four years of age in man and chimpanzees. *J Clin Endocrinol Metab*. 1975;40(4):545 51.
2. Herman-Giddens ME, Slora EJ, Wasserman RC et al. Secondary sexual characteristics and menses in young girls seen in office practice: A study from the Pediatric Research in Office Settings Network. *Pediatr*. 1997;99(4):505–12.
3. Chumlea WC, Schubert CM, Roche AF et al. Age at menarche and comparisons in US girls. *Pediatr*. 2003;111(1):110–3.
4. Ibanez L, Potau N, Francois I, de Zegher F. Precocious pubarche, hyperinsulinism, and ovarian hyperandrogenism in girls: Relation to reduced fetal growth. *J Clin Endocrinol Metab*. 2006;91:1275–83.
5. Latronica AC, Brito VN, Carel JC. Causes, diagnosis, and treatment of precocious puberty. *Lancet Diabetes Endocrinol*. 2016;4(3):265–74.
6. Bas F, Abali ZY, Toksoy G et al. Precocious or early puberty in patients with combined pituitary hormone deficiency due to *POU1F1* gene mutation: Case report and review of possible mechanisms. *Hormnoes (Athens)*. November 20, 2018 Eprint.
7. Gomes LG, Curha-Silva M, Crespo RP et al. DLK-1 is a novel link between reproduction and metabolism. *J Clin Endocrinol Metab*. November 19, 2018 Eprint.
8. Kaplowitz PB, Oberfield SE, Drug and Therapeutics and Executive Committees of the Lawson Wilkins Pediatric Endocrine Society. Reexamination of the age limit for defining when puberty is precocious in girls in the United States: Implications for evaluation and treatment. *Pediatr*. 1999;104(4):936–41.
9. Estrada A, Boyce AM, Brillante BA et al. Long-term outcomes of letrozole treatment for peripheral precocity in girls with McCune-Albright syndrome. *Eur J Endocrinol*. 2016;175:477–83.
10. Neyman A, Eugster EA. Treatment of girls and boys with McCune Albright syndrome with precocious puberty—Update 2017. *Pediatr Endocrinol Rev*. 2017;15(2):136–41.
11. Christens A, Sevenants L, Toelen J et al. Van Wyk and Grumbach syndrome: An unusual form of precocious puberty. *Gynecol Endocrinol*. 2014;30(4):272–6.
12. Fuqua JS. Treatment and outcomes of precocious puberty: An update. *J Clin Endocrinol Metab*. 2013;98(6):2198–207.
13. Day FR, Elks CE, Murray A et al. Pubertal timing associated with diabetes, cardiovascular disease and also diverse health outcomes in men and women: The UK Biobank Study. *Sci Rep*. 2015;5:11208.
14. Sedlmeyer IL. Pedigree analysis of constitutional delay of growth and maturation: Determination of familial aggregation and inheritance patterns. *J Clin Endocrinol Metabol*. 2002;87:5581–6.
15. Malone L, Dwyer AA, Francou B et al. Genetics in endocrinology: Genetic counseling for congenital hypogonadotropic hypogonadism and Kallman syndrome: New challenges in the era of oligogenism and next generation sequencing. *Eur J Endocrinol*. 2018;178(3):R55–80.
16. Topaloglu AK. Update on the genetics of idiopathic hypogonadotropic hypogonadism. *J Clin Res Pediatr Endocrinol*. 2017;9(Suppl 2):113–22.
17. Gravholt CH, Andersen NH, Conway GS et al. Clinical practice guidelines for the care of girls and women with Turner syndrome: Proceedings from the 2016 Cincinnati International Turner Syndrome meeting. *Eur J Endocrinol*. 2017;177(3):G1–G70.
18. Toniolo D, Rizzolio F. X chromosome and ovarian failure. *Seminars in Reprod Med*. 2007;25:264–71.
19. Taboada M, Santen R, Lima J et al. Pharmacokinetics and pharmacodynamics of oral and transdermal 17-β estradiol in girls with Turner syndrome. *J Clin Endocrionl Metab*. 2011;96:3502–10.
20. Zhu J, Kusa TO, Chan Y-M. Genetics of pubertal timing. *Curr Opin Pediatr*. 2018;30.
21. Blanck HM, Marcus M, Tolbert PE et al. Age at menarche and Tanner stage in girls exposed in utero and postnatally to polybrominated biphenyl. *Epidemiology*. 2000;11:641–7.
22. Chou YY, Huang PC, Lee CC et al. Phthalate exposure in girls during early puberty. *J Pediatr Endocrinol Metab*. 2009;22:223–33.
23. Prentice P, Viner RM. Pubertal timing and adult obesity and cardiovascular risk in women and men; a systemic review and meta-analysis. *Int J Obes London*. 2013;37:1036–43.
24. Carel JC, Leger J. Clinical practice. Precocious puberty. *N Engl J Med*. 2008;358(22):2366–77.
25. Carel J, Eugster EA, Rogol A et al. Consensus statement on the use of gonadotropin releasing hormone analogues in children. *Pediatrics*. 2009;123:e752–62.

Congenital anomalies of the reproductive tract

MAGGIE DWIGGINS and VERONICA GOMEZ-LOBO

6

INTRODUCTION

Congenital anomalies of the female reproductive tract are varied, either obstructing or nonobstructing, a combination of the two, or they result in complete agenesis. Prevalence ranges from 1:1000 to 1:70,000 depending on the anomaly. These anomalies may present at birth or during childhood; however, the majority of cases are not diagnosed until puberty. Nonobstructing anomalies often are not diagnosed for several years and can present as abnormal uterine bleeding, as pain with use of tampon or during intercourse, during routine ultrasound, or at the time of delivery. In addition to isolated reproductive tract anomalies, extrophy and cloacal anomalies, which may involve the urologic, digestive, and reproductive tracts, are diagnosed either prenatally or immediately after birth, and are associated with high complications, multiple surgeries, and lifelong follow-up. Differences of sexual development (DSDs) can often present in a similar manner. Treatment of each anomaly varies greatly; however, only an experienced surgeon with knowledge of embryologic development and pelvic anatomy should attempt surgical repair, as improper management can lead to devastating stricture formation, pelvic pain, and sexual dysfunction. Furthermore, it is important to note that many of the surgeries described in this chapter have not been submitted to rigorous study.

EMBRYOGENESIS

When discussing congenital Müllerian anomalies, it is important to have a basic understanding of the embryology of the reproductive tract. Development of the reproductive tract begins at approximately 6 weeks of gestational age and is complete by 14 weeks.[1] The Müllerian structures derive from the primitive mesoderm, as do the heart, lungs, and urogenital system.[2] These will give rise to the fallopian tubes, uterus, cervix, and upper two-thirds of the vagina. The ovaries, however, arise from the endoderm and develop independently of other female structures.[1] The external genitalia and lower third of the vagina develop from the urogenital sinus, derived from primordial ectoderm, also giving rise to the bladder, excluding the trigone and the urethra. Internally, female reproductive development is driven by the absence of the *SRY* gene and possibly an unidentified female determining factor.[3] The Müllerian ducts develop in close proximity to the Wolffian ducts, which eventually form the urinary tract. The two Müllerian ducts begin to migrate medially then fuse and descend into the pelvis around 6 weeks of gestational age.[1] Fusion is generally complete by 14 weeks of gestational age, at which time the structures canalize. During this time, the urogenital sinus invaginates and differentiates into the sinovaginal bulb.[4] At approximately 12 weeks gestation, the sinovaginal bulb grows cephalad and fuses with the most caudal portion of the Müllerian ducts. This then becomes the vaginal plate, which also canalizes by 14 weeks gestation. The hymen is the embryologic septum between the urogenital sinus and the sinovaginal bulb; it perforates during embryogenesis and represents the most caudal aspect of the vaginal plate.[5]

Congenital anomalies can occur when there is failure of any step in development, including fusion of paired Müllerian ducts, fusion of Müllerian ducts with the sinovaginal bulb, canalization of the Müllerian ducts or vaginal plate, or atresia of one or more structures.[3] Also, the female reproductive tract develops in close association with many other organ systems; therefore, when presented with these anomalies, there is a high likelihood of other concomitant anomalies. Due to the proximity of development, the most common associated anomaly occurs in the renal system. However, other structures deriving from the mesoderm may also be affected.

CLASSIFICATION

Classifying Müllerian anomalies has been challenging, but determining the anatomy leads to correct surgical repair and counseling on long-term outcomes. The first and most widely accepted system for characterization is the American Fertility Society (AFS)/American Society for Reproductive Medicine (ASRM) classification from 1988.[6] Under this system, uterine anatomy could be grouped into six different categories based on impact on reproductive potential, and this categorization was accompanied by a scoring system designed to help formulate a prognosis.[7] This classification, however, only included those structures that could impact fertility; thus, the AFS/ASRM classification system is lacking as a diagnostic tool for the pediatric and adolescent gynecology provider (Table 6.1).

In order to address the other common Müllerian anomalies, Oppelt et al. developed the Vagina Cervix Uterus Adnexa-Associated Malformation (VCUAM) classification system for genital malformations.[8] This system is also based on anatomy, including all the structures of the female reproductive tract and outside malformations, mirroring the tumor-node-metastases (TNM) scheme in oncology. The comprehensive subcategories allow for detailed description of reproductive tract anomalies while also acknowledging malformations of other systems; however, the system is not simple and is, therefore, not as widely accepted among providers (Table 6.2).

Table 6.1 American Fertility Society (AFS)/American Society for Reproductive Medicine (ASRM) classification.

Class	Subclass
I. Müllerian agenesis or hypoplasia	A. Vaginal B. Cervical C. Fundal D. Tubal E. Combined (any)
II. Unicornuate uterus	A1. With endometrial cavity 　　a. Communicating rudimentary horn 　　b. Noncommunicating horn A2. No endometrial cavity in horn B. No horn
III. Uterus didelphys, complete	
IV. Uterus bicornuate	A. Complete (to internal os) B. Partial
V. Arcuate uterus	
VI. Septate uterus	A. Complete (to internal os) B. Partial
VII. Diethylstilbestrol (DES) anomalies	

Source: Used with permission from Buttram V, Gibbons W. *Fertil Steril.* 1979;32(1):40–6.

While both systems describe differences in Müllerian structures, they fail to detail the associated anomalies. Acien et al. created a third classification system based on embryology that would be comprehensive, always including the renal system, to be used as a guide for diagnosis and treatment.[3] This system describes five groups of malformations among four locations of embryologic origin, again with many subcategories in each group (Table 6.3).

Most recently, the European Society of Human Reproduction and Embryology (ESHRE) and the European Society for Gynaecological Endoscopy (ESGE) developed a new system based on scientific research and consensus measurements among experts and the scientific community.[9] This group analyzed all published works regarding Müllerian anomalies and created a system primarily based on anatomy with a secondary inclusion of embryologic origin to detail anomalies of the uterus, cervix, and vagina, in a way that was both comprehensive and simple.[10] With this system, nearly every case of Müllerian anomalies can be categorized and diagnosed, at the expense of including associated anomalies (Table 6.4).

Correct and comprehensive classification of Müllerian anomalies in a way that is easy for the practitioner to use continues to be elusive. No matter the classification system, one must always keep in mind the embryology and anatomy to ensure a complete workup and appropriate treatment.

APPROACH TO THE PATIENT

If an infant presents with concern for a reproductive tract anomaly in the absence of a DSD, extrophy, or cloacal anomaly, an external exam may be difficult due to the enlarged external genitalia from estrogen exposure *in utero*. Ultrasound imaging, however, may be instructive in the first few months of life due to uterine enlargement secondary to maternal hormones and the neonatal "mini-puberty." Prior to puberty, isolated reproductive tract anomalies do not require any intervention unless there is associated hydronephrosis, ectopic ureter, bladder outlet obstruction, or infection.

When presented with a young girl or adolescent in whom a congenital anomaly is suspected, it is imperative that careful clinical assessment be performed so that correct diagnosis is made. Any patient who presents with primary amenorrhea, which is absence of menses by age 15 years in the presence of secondary sexual characteristics or lack of menarche within 2–3 years of initial breast development, warrants further examination.[11] If the patient also presents with cyclic or chronic pelvic pain, evidence of a pelvic mass, or disruption of normal bladder and bowel function, an obstructive anomaly should be considered. Obstruction should also be ruled out in patients with worsening dysmenorrhea, or for those who do not respond to medications. Physical exam should include palpation of the abdomen as well as visual inspection of the external genitalia. When hymenal or vaginal patency is in question, or if length of vagina needs to be determined, a moist swab can be gently inserted into the introitus. If vaginal opening is difficult to determine visually, one must first ensure the location of the urethra to avoid probing it, as it may be caudally positioned in cases of vaginal agenesis. A rectal exam can also be performed when assessing for pelvic mass or determining distance of obstruction from introitus. It is important to remember that when a vaginal mass is noted, simple needle drainage without ensuring continued track patency should never be performed, as this could lead to ascending infection, pyometra, and reaccumulation of menses.

Imaging is another important aspect of diagnosing congenital anomalies. Transabdominal ultrasound is a useful initial exam, as it is readily available at most institutions and can show the presence of obstruction. Magnetic resonance imaging (MRI) remains the gold standard assessing for the presence of Müllerian structures, such as uterus or vagina, determining the length of the vagina, thickness of the septum, and presence of fluid collection within the vagina, uterus, and fallopian tubes.[12] Depending on the anomaly, other imaging may be indicated and will be discussed.

OBSTRUCTIVE ANOMALIES

Obstructing anomalies can present with or without menses, with increasing dysmenorrhea, pelvic pain, and/or with pelvic masses. It is thought that increased retrograde menstruation results in endometriosis, which generally improves once the obstruction is relieved.[13] Thus, pelvic masses associated with obstructive anomalies often represent endometriomas, which should be managed medically or through relief of the obstruction

Table 6.2 Vagina Cervix Uterus Adnexa-Associated Malformation (VCUAM) classification system.

Anatomic location	Class	Subclass
Vagina (V)	0: Normal	
	1: Hymenal atresia	a. Partial
		b. Complete
	2: Septate	a. Incomplete (<50%)
		b. Complete
	3: Stenosis of the introitus	
	4: Hypoplasia	
	5: Atresia	a. Unilateral
		b. Complete
	S: Sinus urogenitalis	1. Deep confluence
		2. Middle confluence
		3. High confluence
	C: Cloaca	
	+: Other	
	#: Unknown	
Cervix (C)	0: Normal	
	1: Duplex cervix	
	2: Atresia/aplasia	a. Unilateral
		b. Bilateral
	+: Other	
	#: Unknown	
Uterus (U)	0: Normal	
	1:	a. Arcuate
		b. Septate <50% of cavity
		c. Septate >50% of cavity
	2: Bicornate	
	3: Hypoplastic	
	4: Rudimentary or aplastic	a. Unilateral
		b. Bilateral
	+: Other	
	#: Unknown	
Adnexa (A)	0: Normal	
	1: Tubal malformation, ovaries normal	a. Unilateral
		b. Bilateral
	2: Hypoplasia/gonadal streak	a. Unilateral
		b. Bilateral
	3: Aplasia	a. Unilateral
		b. Bilateral
	+: Other	
	#: Unknown	
Associated malformation (M)	0: None	
	R: Renal system	
	S: Skeleton	
	C: Cardiac	
	N: Neurologic	
	+: Other	
	#: Unknown	

Source: Used with permission from Oppelt P et al. *Fertil Steril.* 2005;84(5):1493–7.

rather than by resection in order to preserve ovarian function. The mainstay in treatment for obstruction is surgical correction. Furthermore, it is important to note that some obstructions require postoperative dilation in order to avoid stricture and resulting reaccumulation of blood or pyometra. Many young adolescents are not able to carry out this postoperative management, and thus, they are best managed through menstrual suppression and delay of surgery until they can perform postoperative dilation.

Table 6.3 Embryological and clinical classification.

Embryology	Pathogenic anomaly	Anatomic findings
i. Agenesis or hypoplasia of entire urogenital ridge	a. Bilateral Müllerian agenesis b. Unicornuate uterus	a. MRKH with unilateral renal agenesis b. Contralateral renal agenesis
ii. Mesonephric anomalies, absence of Wolffian duct opening in urogenital sinus, absence of ureteral bud sprouting	a. Blind hemivagina b. Gartner's pseudocyst c. Longitudinal vaginal septum d. Complete unilateral vaginal or cervicovaginal agenesis	a. OHVIRA b. Ipsilateral renal agenesis c. Partial reabsorption, noted along entire length or isolated near cervix d. With/without communicating uterine horn, ipsilateral renal agenesis
iii. Isolated Müllerian anomalies	a. Paramesonephric or Müllerian ducts (per AFS) b. Müllerian tubercle c. Both Müllerian tubercle and ducts; MRKH syndrome d. Fusion and reabsorption of superior and inferior uterine segments	1. Agenesis and uterine hypoplasia 2. Unicornuate uterus 3. Didelphys uterus 4. Bicornuate uterus 5. Septate uterus 6. Arcuate uterus 7. Anomalies related to DES 1. Complete vaginal or cervicovaginal agenesis/atresia 2. Transverse vaginal septum and segmental atresia
iv. Gubernaculum dysfunction	Accessory or cavitated rudimentary uterine horn	
v. Anomalies of the urogenital sinus	Imperforate hymen, congenital vesicovaginal fistulas, cloacal anomalies	
vi. Malformative combinations	Cloacal anomaly with bladder exstrophy, renal anomaly with contralateral Müllerian anomaly, etc.	

Source: Used with permission from Acién P, Acién M. *Hum Reprod Update*. 2011;17(5):693–705.

Abbreviations: AFS, American Fertility Society; DES, diethylstilbestrol; MRKH, Mayer-Rokitansky-Küster-Hauser; OHVIRA, obstructed hemivagina with ipsilateral renal agenesis.

OBSTRUCTIVE ANOMALIES WITHOUT MENSES

Imperforate hymen

As previously mentioned, the hymen is the embryologic septum between the urogenital sinus and sinovaginal bulb and is the distal boundary of the vaginal plate. The incidence of imperforate hymen is 0.1% (1:1000), making this the most common congenital anomaly.[5] These can be diagnosed in the newborn by the presence of bulging mucocolpos; however, the majority present in adolescents.[14] Patients will often present with primary amenorrhea 2–3 years after initial breast development. They may also present with cyclic abdominal pain, urinary retention, or constipation.[12,15] On exam, a bluish bulge of the hymenal membrane at the vaginal introitus can be seen.[14] Physical exam alone can generally elicit a diagnosis; however, transperineal or transabdominal ultrasound can provide confirmation. If a bulge is not easily seen, the patient can be asked to Valsalva or pressure can be applied to the abdomen, and if the bulge is still not visible, transverse vaginal septum or lower vaginal agenesis should be suspected.

Timing of surgery is controversial and can be performed during the newborn period or after the patient undergoes puberty when the hymen is well estrogenized, thus avoiding stricture.[14] Surgery is performed under general anesthesia. A Foley catheter can be placed to further delineate the anatomy. A cruciate or U-shaped incision is then made in the hymenal membrane, and the hematocolpos is allowed to drain (Figure 6.1). The hymenal tissue is then resected with careful attention being paid to avoid the vaginal wall, as this could cause more bleeding or pain.[12] If thick, the exposed edges are then suture ligated to prevent scar formation (Video 6.1). The risk of stenosis is very low, and postoperative vaginal dilation is not routinely recommended.

Video 6.1   https://youtu.be/eBxk8fAInns

Thick imperforate hymen. (Courtesy of Drs. Mary Ann Jamieson and Amanda Black.)

Table 6.4 European Society of Human Reproduction and Embryology (ESHRE)/European Society for Gynaecological Endoscopy (ESGE) classification.

Class	Anatomic findings
U0: Normal uterus	Normal uterine cavity
U1: Dysmorphic uterus	a. T-shaped
	b. Infantilis
	c. Other
U2: Septate uterus	a. Partial
	b. Complete
U3: Bicorporeal uterus	a. Partial
	b. Complete
	c. Bicorporeal septate
U4: Hemi-uterus	a. With rudimentary cavity
	b. Without rudimentary cavity
U5: Aplastic uterus	a. With rudimentary cavity
	b. Without rudimentary cavity
C0	Normal cervix
C1	Septate cervix
C2	Double normal cervix
C3	Unilateral cervical aplasia
C4	Cervical aplasia
V0	Normal vagina
V1	Longitudinal nonobstructing vaginal septum
V2	Longitudinal obstructing vaginal septum
V3	Transverse vaginal septum and/or imperforate hymen
V4	Vaginal aplasia

Source: Under Creative Commons Attribution License. Grimbizis G et al. *Gynecol Surg.* 2013;10:199–212.

Transverse vaginal septum

The upper vagina is derived entirely from the Müllerian ducts, and incomplete canalization or abnormality of the vaginal plate may result in a septum.[4] Another cause may be when the sinovaginal bulb fails to meet the Müllerian ducts, thus resulting in a septum in the middle or upper vagina.[4] Like other anomalies, the pathology is often multifactorial; therefore, the finding of a septum should prompt the provider to evaluate for other Müllerian anomalies.[16] The incidence of vaginal septum is 1:70,000, making this the rarest of all congenital anomalies.[5] The septum may be perforate or imperforate. Perforate septums allow for menstrual outflow, and patients may only present with difficulty inserting a tampon or with intercourse, as well as during routine obstetric or gynecologic examination.[14] Imperforate septum may present similarly to an imperforate hymen, either without a visible bulge, or in cases of thin low septums, with hymenal tissue visible in front of a bulge.

MRI is the imaging modality of choice when evaluating a septum for preoperative planning.[17] Knowing both the thickness and the location is essential for determining the approach to surgery and in preparing for long-term complications. The location is determined by measuring the distance between the vaginal introitus and the distal end of the septum and is classified as low (<3 cm), mid (3–6 cm), or high (>6 cm).[4] The septum is described as thin if it is <1 cm, or thick when ≥1 cm.[17]

Low or thin septums can be resected without significant struggle from the vaginal approach. Mid to high or thick septums are associated with more complex surgeries and may require a combined abdominal and vaginal approach. During surgery, needle aspiration under ultrasound guidance or a sound placed through the upper vagina abdominally may assist in ascertaining where to incise the septum in order to avoid injury to other organs (Figure 6.2). These surgeries are associated with a high rate of reobstruction requiring repeat surgery, and in extreme cases, hysterectomy. Several strategies have been made in an effort to simplify these surgeries. Often, preoperative dilation is utilized to increase the length of the distal vagina and thin the septum.[18] Also, insertion of a guidewire through the septum with placement of a balloon can be done in an effort to thin the septum and bring the proximal vagina to the distal portion without

(a)

(b)

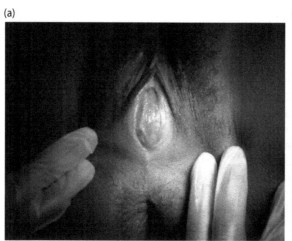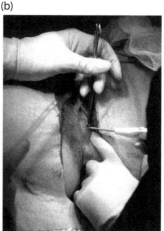

Figure 6.1 (a) Imperforate hymen. (b) Incision and drainage.

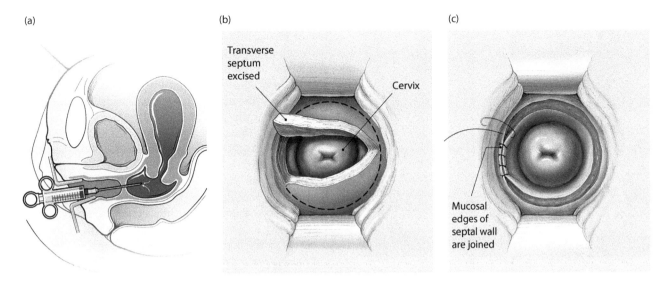

Figure 6.2 Septoplasty for transverse vaginal septum and vaginal agenesis. (a) Sagittal view of a transverse vaginal septum with accompanying hematocolpos, spinal needle inserted into space with aspiration of material to provide for clear evaluation of the anatomy. (b) A horizontal incision is made and carried down through the entire thickness of the septum, revealing the cervix and proximal vagina. The anterior and posterior leaflets are then cut circumferentially, flush with the vaginal wall. (c) The raw edges are then reapproximated with interrupted sutures.

tension.[19] In addition, thick septums may require a tissue graft or Z-plasty procedure in order to cover the large gap in epithelium that may result from removal of the septum[20,21] (Figure 6.3). For thick septums where the need for an interposition graft or injury to bowel or bladder is high, a team approach with urology, plastic surgery, and/ or colorectal surgery may be warranted.[22]

Pregnancy following vaginal septum excision is not well documented in the literature. One review suggested a mid to high septum was directly correlated with infertility, possibly due to increased risk of prolonged

obstruction and damage caused by hematosalpinx or endometriosis.[4] However, several other studies have shown a 100% pregnancy rate in those who attempted pregnancy, suggesting there is no detrimental impact on fertility.[4,17] There is no suggested mode of delivery, with roughly 50% of patients undergoing cesarean section and 50% vaginal delivery.[16,17]

Partial vaginal agenesis

Incomplete atresia of the Müllerian ducts may result in partial vaginal agenesis (Figure 6.4). As with other

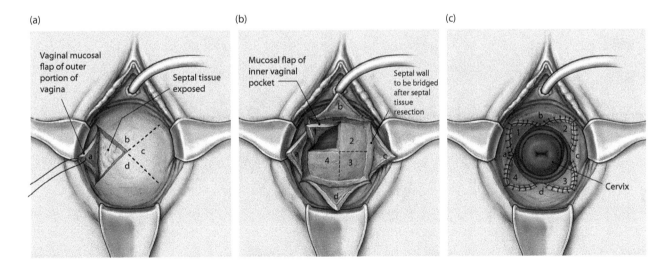

Figure 6.3 Z-plasty. (a) Vaginal view of thick septum. The distal septal mucosa is incised with an "X" to create four triangular leaflets (a–d). These leaflets are then retracted to expose the underlying connective tissue. (b) The thick connective tissue is then bluntly and sharply dissected to the proximal septal mucosa. The proximal mucosa is then incised with a "+" to create four additional distinct leaflets (1–4). (c) The four proximal (a–d) and four distal (1–4) leaflets are then intercalated and sutured together to bridge the thickness of the resected septum. The cervix and proximal vagina are revealed.

(a)   (b)

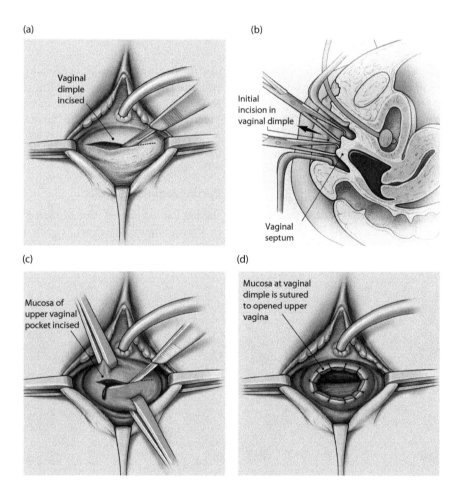

Figure 6.4 Vaginal atresia. (a) Vaginal atresia. (b) After pull-through. (From Dr. Marta C. Mendez and NASPAG PediGyn Teaching Slide Set CD-ROM, NASPAG 2001, with permission.)

vaginal anomalies, the incidence is approximately 1:4000 female births.[23] They often present with increasing cyclic pain and a hematocolpos without bulging at the introitus. Surgical repair can be accomplished by vaginal pull-through procedures. The introitus is dissected below the urethra, and the areolar space between the urethra and rectum is bluntly dissected until the bulging vagina is encountered. The vagina is then grasped, dissected from the surrounding tissues, and "pulled through" to the introitus.[24,25] The bulge is then entered and sutured to the mucosa at the initial incision (Figure 6.5). It is important to ascertain the distance from the hematocolpos to the introitus, as a distance of greater than 3 cm is associated with greater stricture rate.[15] When the distance from the introitus to the hematocolpos is significant (>4 cm), tissues such as skin, buccal mucosa, or bowel have been used to bridge this gap.[22] Postoperative stricture is again common, and follow-up for pain and reobstruction should be performed regularly.[24]

(a)

Vaginal
dimple
incised

(b)

Initial
incision in
vaginal dimple

Vaginal
septum

(c)

Mucosa of
upper vaginal
pocket incised

(d)

Mucosa at vaginal
dimple is sutured
to opened upper
vagina

Figure 6.5 Vaginal pull-through. (a) Vaginal view of vaginal agenesis or thick lower vaginal septum. Distal mucosa at the vaginal dimple is noted and incised horizontally with a scalpel. (b) Sagittal view, the incised mucosa is grasped anteriorly and posteriorly with Allis forceps and retracted toward the operator. Thick connective tissue is then dissected both sharply and bluntly to the level of the proximal mucosa. (c) Vaginal view, the distal vaginal mucosa has been grasped both anteriorly and posteriorly and the connective tissue dissected to reveal the proximal mucosa. This mucosa is then incised horizontally and hematocolpos evacuated. (d) The proximal mucosa is then brought down to the distal mucosa, the new vaginal introitus, and raw edges reapproximated with interrupted sutures.

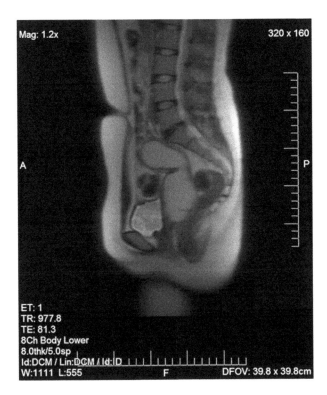

ET: 1
TR: 977.8
TE: 81.3
8Ch Body Lower
8.0thk/5.0sp

Figure 6.6 Cervical agenesis.

Cervical agenesis

Cervical agenesis occurs when the cervix fails to develop with an otherwise normal reproductive tract (Figure 6.6).[26] Cervical agenesis can encompass isolated agenesis of the cervix or agenesis of the cervix and vagina. Several types of cervical agenesis have been described (Figure 6.7). This anomaly is rare with true incidence unknown but estimated to be 1:80,000, and the classical treatment has been by total hysterectomy[27]; while this does definitely relieve symptoms of obstruction, it renders the patient irreversibly infertile.

Uterovaginal anastomosis has been described. The procedure is accomplished by laparotomy, dissection of the anterior space, followed by modified vaginal pull-through, and finally, catheterization of the uterine cavity and attachment of the neovagina to the uterine body.[27] When anastomosis is performed, resection of abnormal cervical tissue must be performed, and then the graft or vagina is attached to the uterine corpus. This procedure, however, is associated with significant morbidity, including stenosis and severe infection.[28]

However, recent advances in surgical technique have improved overall outcomes and lead to continued relief of menstrual obstruction and successful pregnancies. When the remaining cervical stroma is at least 2 cm in

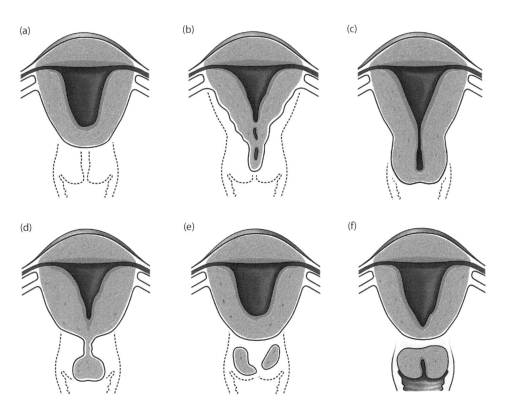

Figure 6.7 Congenital cervical agenesis. (a) Complete agenesis of the cervix, corpus of the uterus noted. (b) The cervix is composed of fibrous bands that may contain endocervical glands. (c) Intact cervix with obstruction at the external os. (d) Stricture of the midportion of the cervix, which is noted to be hypoplastic with a bulbous distal end. No active endocervical glands are present. (e) Hypoplastic cervix is noted with fibrous fragments not connecting to the uterine corpus. (f) Noncommunicating cervix is present with complete stricture at the level of the internal os causing obstruction of the uterine corpus. Normal appearing external cervix with endocervical glands can be seen vaginally.

diameter, an effective neocanal can be created.[28] To promote long-term patency, a 14-French Foley catheter can be placed inside the uterine cavity and extend into the vagina, anchored to a T-shaped intrauterine device, until epithelialization is complete.[29] Successful pregnancy has been reported in these patients who have adequate cervix remaining, both with and without the use of a permanent cervical cerclage.[23,26,28,29] The use of transmyometrial embryo transfer in those who have had unsuccessful cervical canalization is controversial. To date, four pregnancies have been reported, and all have delivered preterm via cesarean section.[30–33] The question of how to manage first- or second-trimester loss in these patients continues to be difficult; therefore, this method of achieving pregnancy is not widely practiced.

If there is vaginal agenesis associated with cervical agenesis, the vagina can be lengthened preoperatively through dilation. Vaginal reconstruction can also be performed with skin, buccal, or bowel graft, as in the case of thick transverse septum or agenesis.[22] Often, a stent such as a Foley catheter needs to be placed in order to avoid stricture.

OBSTRUCTIVE ANOMALIES WITH MENSES

Patients with obstructive anomalies with menses generally present with dysmenorrhea or worsening pelvic pain following menarche. Although they may be seen in the office, many patients will present with severe pain and an acute abdomen in the emergency department. Due to the presence of menses, diagnosis is often delayed by 3–5 months; however, cases of delay of up to 20 years have been described.[34–37] Some patients may have a small communication or fistula between the obstructed and patent vagina or uterus. These cases often present later as pain is periodically relieved, and are accompanied by a history of irregular menses, chronic brown and malodorous vaginal discharge, or with pyocolpos or pyometra.[38–40]

Rudimentary uterine horn with functional endometrium

Rudimentary uterine horns occur due to failure of fusion of the paired Müllerian ducts.[3] The incidence is extremely rare, occurring in 1:100,000 to 140,000 female deliveries.[41] When a rudimentary uterine horn contains functional endometrium, it will also have cyclic proliferation and shedding. When the horn is not communicating, it may become distended with menstrual products, causing severe abdominal pain.[42] Rudimentary horns may also have small communications with the functional unicornuate uterus, allowing menstrual blood to efflux. While a noncommunicating horn generally presents early due to abdominal pain, a communicating horn may take several years to diagnose.[42] Pregnancy can occur in a rudimentary uterine horn, and it generally presents as a surgical emergency as the rate of uterine rupture is high if a pregnancy progresses past the first trimester.[41] MRI is the gold standard to diagnose a uterine horn, allowing for detection of endometrium. When a single obstructed horn

is diagnosed, immediate surgical resection, including removal of ipsilateral tube, should be performed to avoid pain, severe endometriosis, pregnancy, or other complications.[14] If communication is present, oversewing the remaining uterus may be necessary to prevent laxity of the uterine wall and subsequent rupture[15] (Video 6.2).

Video 6.2 https://youtu.be/k7ol1jxUPE4

Rudimentary uterine horn removal. (Courtesy of Drs. Ted Lee, Richard Guido, and Michael Haggerty.)

Obstructed Hemivagina Ipsilateral Renal Agenesis

Purslow first documented a patient with a duplicated reproductive system and obstructed hemivagina in 1922.[43] Since that time, many cases of obstructed hemivagina ipsilateral renal agenesis (OHVIRA) have been described, especially under the name Herlyn-Werner-Wunderlich Syndrome (HWWS) or obstructing longitudinal vaginal septum with corresponding uterine anomalies.[5] The incidence is unknown, as this traditionally has been under-reported in the literature. This anomaly is thought to be a result of abnormal development of the caudal portion of the Wolffian duct, resulting in ipsilateral renal agenesis.[34] Complete ipsilateral renal agenesis is the most common associated anomaly found in at least 74% of patients, while the remainder may have ipsilateral renal anomaly such as duplicated ureter, dysplastic or polycystic kidneys, or ectopic ureter inserting into obstructed hemivagina.[13,44] Much like other anomalies, OHVIRA does not appear to have a have a clear genetic etiology.[45]

On physical exam, a bulge in the lateral vaginal sidewall may be appreciated, and in cases of prolonged obstruction, a tender abdominal mass can be felt. While ultrasound is acceptable to make the diagnosis, MRI remains the gold standard for imaging.[13]

Management

In the past, laparoscopy and two-stage procedures were advocated in the management of OHVIRA (Video 6.3). However, with MRI, laparoscopy is no longer needed to diagnose these anomalies.[34,45] Long-term studies have now shown that surgery by a single-stage resection of the vaginal septum through a vaginal approach results in complete resolution in symptoms for more than 90% of patients, and a two-stage procedure with both vaginal and abdominal approaches should be reserved for complex cases.[13] Septum excision is accomplished in a manner similar to those described before, with care to identify the borders of the obstructed vagina to ensure complete septum excision. The vaginal defect is then closed by suturing the mucosal surfaces together. If a communication is observed, a Foley catheter may be inserted into the obstructed hemivagina and used as a guide for resection. When the anatomy is not clear, a spinal needle can be inserted under ultrasound guidance to identify the correct hemivaginal space

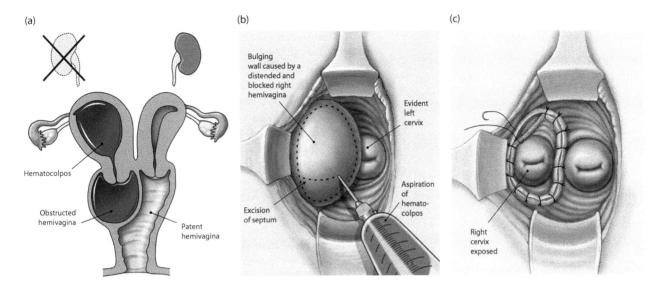

Figure 6.8 OHVIRA and surgical management. (a) Right obstructed hemivagina ipsilateral renal agenesis with accompanying right hematometrocolpos due to obstruction of menses. (b) Vaginal view with distended right vaginal side wall due to obstructed hemivagina, left cervix noted. Obstructed vagina can be drained with a spinal needle to allow for clear visualization of the anatomy. A horizontal incision is then made along the obstructed vaginal sidewall, and septum excision is carried out circumferentially (dotted line). (c) After complete excision of the septum has been performed, the raw edges are then reapproximated using interrupted sutures. Two cervixes are clearly noted and right hemivagina obstruction completely resolved.

(Figure 6.8; Video 6.4). Some experts endorse placing a vaginal mold or stent postoperatively; however, this is not universally practiced.

Video 6.3   https://youtu.be/WIGbyQVq6eQ
Uterus didelphys with obstructed hemivagina. (Courtesy of Dr. Diane Merritt.)

Video 6.4   https://youtu.be/GDsvbPI5YDk
Obstructed hemivagina. (Courtesy of Drs. Mary Ann Jamieson and Amanda Black.)

Due to prolonged menstrual obstruction, patients with OHVIRA have been noted to have endometriosis at a rate of up to 23%.[34–37,45] However, improvement of endometriosis symptoms usually occurs spontaneously after obstruction is relieved and does not need surgical treatment at the time of septum excision.[13,46] As mentioned before, when a communication between the obstructed and unobstructed vagina is present, vaginal bacteria is able to ascend into the vagina, uterus, and fallopian tubes, causing infection and pelvic inflammatory disease. In the literature, cases of severe infection and sepsis have been documented, disastrously resulting in hemi- or total hysterectomy.[34–37] Otherwise, in most cases, every effort should be made to preserve the obstructed uterus and vagina.

Long-term prognosis

Complete resolution of pain symptoms, endometriosis, and obstruction can be expected after vaginal septum excision. Pregnancy rates are fair, and infertility has been noted in 5%–15% of these patients, consistent with the general population.[34–37] Pregnancies in both ipsilateral and contralateral uterus have been recorded. Delivery method has been largely based on provider preference, but overall, half of deliveries are accomplished vaginally and half by cesarean section. Histologically, the obstructed vaginal mucosa approaches mature squamous epithelium; however, it continues to remain abnormal even after several years.[13,47] Rare cases of adenosis have been reported, suggesting a possible need for increased surveillance in these patients.[13]

Prepubertal diagnosis

Although the vast majority present after puberty due to pain and irregular menses, increased prenatal ultrasound screening has led to increased diagnosis of renal anomalies prenatally, and in roughly 2% of patients, diagnosis of OHVIRA shortly after birth.[48] The obstructed hemivagina may have accumulated menstrual blood or mucus secondary to mini-puberty or urine due to vaginal insertion of ectopic ureter. About 13% of patients will require surgery for urinary obstruction to alleviate renal impact.[48] The rate of resolution of vaginal distention is only about 30% before 1 year of age, and in these cases, a vaginal approach to septum resection may be accomplished in collaboration with urology.[37] These children will require close surveillance around the time of puberty to ensure obstruction has not recurred.

NONOBSTRUCTIVE ANOMALIES

Longitudinal vaginal septum

Longitudinal vaginal septum results from a defect in canalization of any region of the vagina, but more commonly in the upper vagina near the cervix.[36] This is a more common anomaly, with an incidence of about 1:1000. Patients who present with nonobstructive longitudinal vaginal septums often have presenting symptoms that may be complaints of difficulty placing a tampon or pain with intercourse; however, some may present during the course of a routine pelvic exam. Many such septums are asymptomatic and do not require treatment. It is important when there is a complete duplication that Pap smears of both cervixes be collected. When the septum is associated with discomfort, these can be resected in the operating room with Bovie cautery or the LigaSure device.[42] Care must be taken to avoid deep incisions or burns in order to prevent bladder and bowel injury. Once the septum is resected, the mucosa can be approximated with absorbable suture. This surgery does not require postoperative dilation.

Other nonobstructing anomalies

Many other uterine anomalies have been categorized and described by the AFS/ASRM, VCUAM, Acien, and ESHRE-ESGE and include bicornuate or septate uterus and uterine didelphys, and have an incidence of 4.3% in the general population.[3,6,8,9] These anomalies, while important to be cognizant of, often do not need treatment from the pediatric and adolescent gynecologist. Diagnosis is usually made by hysteroscopy or hysterosalpingogram in the adult patient, often due to infertility. A uterine septum may cause implantation failure or recurrent miscarriage, and in these cases, septoplasty by operative hysteroscopy is indicated.[6] Pregnancy rates are unchanged in patients with bicornuate or didelphic uterus, patients have increased rates of abnormal fetal lie, and preterm deliveries have been described.[7] The arcuate uterus does not have any implications related to pregnancy and does not need treatment. Rarely, a Thompkins or Jones metroplasty may be indicated for complex intrauterine anomalies; however, these are difficult surgeries to perform and are associated with increased risk of uterine rupture.

MAYER-ROKITANSKY-KÜSTER-HAUSER SYNDROME

Background

Congenital absence of the vagina and uterus has long been described in the literature. Mayer described the first patient in 1829, and the syndrome was later defined more precisely by von Rokitansky, Küster, and Hauser from 1910 to 1961. The prevalence of Mayer-Rokitansky-Küster-Hauser (MRKH) syndrome is 1:4000–5000 and is the second most common cause of primary amenorrhea, behind gonadal dysgenesis.[49] Patients with MRKH tend to present in adolescence about 2–3 years after normal development of other secondary sex characteristics with absence of menarche. The differential diagnosis includes low

transverse vaginal septum, androgen insensitivity syndrome, or 17α-hydroxylase deficiency.[49] The syndrome is a result of a failure of the Müllerian ducts to fuse, resulting in vaginal agenesis as well as complete or partial uterine agenesis in patients with a 46,XX karyotype and typical female hormone profile.[50] The Müllerian system is embryologically derived from the mesoderm; therefore, other organ systems also derived from mesoderm, such as heart, lungs, or urogenital, may also be involved.[2] The ovaries, arising from the endoderm, are not typically abnormal in MRKH.[1] Due to their proximity to the Wolffian ducts, MRKH is often associated with renal anomalies. Although MRKH is not considered a heritable mutation, other gene mutations can be noted in individuals, especially those involved in midline or limb development, such as WNT or HOX.[2,50] Therefore, an array of other congenital anomalies may be found in patients with MRKH, including skeletal anomalies, inguinal hernias, deafness, and many others (Table 6.5).

Evaluation

Some experts believe that there are two types of MRKH, each carrying different prognosis and implications. The most common form is isolated absence of the vagina and uterus, Type 1, or the typical form. The less common types, Type 2 as well as Müllerian, renal, cervicothoracic, somite abnormalities (MURCS), are associated with at least one other concomitant congenital anomaly and are considered atypical forms.[1] In order to differentiate

Table 6.5 Associated anomalies in Mayer-Rokitansky-Küster-Hauser (MRKH) syndrome.

Anomaly	Prevalence (%)
Any other anomaly	44.4–54.4
No associated anomaly	45.6–54.9
Uterine	100
• Rudimentary	• 83.5–88.8
• Hypoplastic with endometrium	• 0.7–11.2
• Absent	• 16.5
• Other	• 5.6
Renal	28.8–57.6
• Unilateral agenesis	• 31–52.8
• Pelvic kidney	• 2–9.3
• Horseshoe kidney	• 1.1–4.5
• Duplicated system	• 2.4–12.3
Skeletal	7.7–44.4
• Scoliosis	• 5.5–54.9
• Hip dysplasia	• 0.8–15.5
• Caudal fusion of vertebrae	• 4.2–4.8
• Klippel-Feil syndrome	• 1.5–3.1
Cardiac	0.7–14.6
Inguinal hernia	1.8–15.6

Source: Adapted from data in Oppelt P et al. *Reprod Biol Endocrinol.* 2012;10:57; Rall K et al. *Pediatr Adolesc Gynecol.* 2015;28:362–8; Kapczuk K et al. *Eur J Obstet Gynecol Reprod Biol.* 2016;207: 45–9; Creatsas G. *Fertil Steril.* 2010;94(5):1848–52.

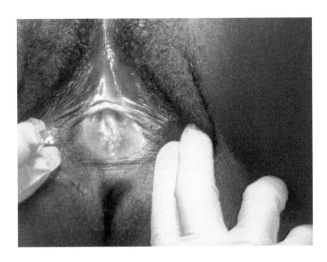

Figure 6.9 MRKH on physical exam.

these types, a careful history and physical exam should be conducted and proper imaging obtained (Figure 6.9; Video 6.5). A study was conducted by Oppelt et al. to determine the best diagnostic modalities for concomitant anomalies.[1] They determined that physical exam for vaginal and cervical malformations was most sensitive. Both MRI and ultrasound were sufficient in determining presence or absence of uterus, endometrium, and renal abnormalities. Laparoscopy is no longer recommended for initial diagnosis. Skeletal anomalies are also found up to 20% of the time, so complete spinal x-ray can also be considered.[50] Other imaging can also be obtained as needed; however, diagnosis of cardiac malformation or inguinal hernia often has occurred prior to the diagnosis of MRKH.

Video 6.5 https://youtu.be/Z2e_I8EOlUw

Vaginal agenesis. (Courtesy of Drs. Mary Ann Jamieson and Amanda Black.)

After complete absence of the uterus and cervix, bilateral rudimentary or aplastic uterine horns are the most commonly associated anomaly, occurring in upward of 85% of patients.[1] It is important to determine if these uterine structures have functioning endometrium prior to recommending a treatment strategy. Often, surgery is not necessary, as the remnants are composed mainly of fibrous tissue. However, if active endometrium is noted, there is a high likelihood of menstrual obstruction and pain. The uterine remnants are still incapable of supporting a pregnancy. In these cases, menstrual suppression should be offered, as well as removal of these dysplastic horns.[49] Such surgery can be easily accomplished through laparoscopic hemihysterectomy.

Management

A diagnosis of MRKH is often unexpected, and patients experience a period of understanding and grieving.[51]

These women are abruptly confronted with perceived loss of sexual function, as well as infertility, and each person becomes ready to discuss or pursue treatment at different times. It has been our practice to see patients multiple times over the course of 3 months from diagnosis in order to offer support and answer questions as patients are ready. Several case reviews have also shown that women have more successful outcomes in terms of vaginal creation and satisfying sexual function when they have regular access to physicians, nurses, psychosexual support, and physical therapy by trained professionals.[52,53] Following vaginal creation, after passive perineal dilation or surgery, women continue to indicate dissatisfaction with their genitals and overall body image.[51] This was found at higher rates with the surgical group. Difficulties with continued sexual function are also higher among the surgery group, with almost half of these women indicating pain and inability to produce adequate lubrication.[51] We therefore recommend a team approach to management, including gynecologist, nursing support, pelvic floor physical therapist, and experienced counselor or therapist.

Neovagina creation

Several approaches to creating a neovagina in patients with MRKH have been described, including nonsurgical dilation, as well as multiple surgical options. Complications after these surgeries are high, and include vaginal and introital stenosis, disfiguring scar formation, fistula, chronic pain, vaginal prolapse, and copious, malodorous discharge. In comparison, passive perineal dilation has been shown to be highly effective in creating a normal vaginal length, resulting in good sexual function, with very few complications (Table 6.6).

Primary perineal dilation

Primary or progressive vaginal dilation was first described by Frank in 1938.[54] He suggested progressive dilation using hard dilators placed at the vaginal dimple for 10–20 minutes, three times per day (Figure 6.10). Patients and providers found this method to be difficult, because it was time consuming, required a private space and dedicated time, and could lead to muscle fatigue. In 1981, Ingram proposed an alternative form of dilation, involving progressive dilators on a bicycle seat.[55,56] With this method, patients could sit upright and perform other activities while dilating. Since then, it has been concluded that dilation should occur when a patient is mentally and emotionally ready, in a fashion that she is comfortable with and has support for during its course. In one study of a single center with 245 patients with MRKH, they found that patients younger than age 16 were significantly less likely to succeed at primary perineal dilation (PPD) than older counterparts.[57] A review of the literature suggests that among all patients, the success rate of creating a functional vagina that allowed for satisfying sexual function was at least 96%.[51-53,57-59] A recent report reveals that in North America the education of physicians caring for

Table 6.6 Techniques for creation of neovagina in Mayer-Rokitansky-Küster-Hauser (MRKH) syndrome.

Procedure	Advantages	Disadvantages	Complications
Progressive perineal dilation	• Lower complication rate • Good long-term functionality • Noninvasive • Epithelium histologically converts to vaginal tissue • 96% functional success	• Patient fatigue • Time consuming	• Recurrent urinary tract infection • Stress urinary incontinence
Split-thickness graft (McIndoe, autologous membrane graft)	• Vaginal approach to surgery • Lower rate of prolapse • 89.5% functional success (improved with use of autologous graft to 93%)	• Large scar from donor site (28% found disfiguring) • Mold left in situ for 3 months	• 14% overall rate • Injury to bladder or rectum • Fistula • Vaginal stenosis (9.3%) • Recurrent infection • Graft shrinkage • Lack of lubrication • Vaginal hair growth • Rejection of graft (9.3%) • Risk of malignancy
Peritoneal vaginoplasty (Davydov)	• No donor site scar • 93% functional success	• Need for special training	• Bladder/bowel injury (7%) • Vesicovaginal fistula (3.6%) • Vaginal stenosis (14.3%) • Ascending infection
Labial skin flap (Williams, Creatsas)	• Can be performed after previous vaginoplasty • Noninvasive vaginal approach • 95% functional success	• Angle of repair not anatomic, creates awkward angle for intercourse	• Wound dehiscence • Hematoma from trauma • Vaginal hair growth
Active perineal dilation (Vecchietti)	• Preserves vaginal tissue • Lower risk of stenosis • 96% functional success	• Not approved by U.S. Food and Drug Administration • Associated with pain and need for long inpatient admission	• Perforation of vital organs • Stress urinary incontinence • Vaginal prolapse
Bowel vaginoplasty	• Achieve vaginal length 9–12 cm • Grows with patient • Produces lubrication • Dilating postoperative not required • 90% functional success	• Major abdominal surgery • Copious foul-smelling mucous discharge	• 16%–26% overall rate • Organ prolapse (3.5%–8.3%) • Introital stenosis (14%) • Increased risk of HIV • Risk of malignancy or colitis

Source: Compiled from data in Callens N et al. *J Sex Med.* 2012;9:1842–51; Gargollo PC et al. *J Urol.* 2009;182:1882–91; Frank RT. *Am J Obstet Gynecol.* 1938;35:1053; Ingram. *Am J Obstet Gynecol.* 1981;140(8):867–73; Williams JK et al. *J Obstet Gynecol Neonatal Nurs.* 1985;14(2):147–50; Callens N et al. *Hum Reprod.* 2014;20(5):775–801; Callens N et al. *Am J Obstet Gynecol.* 2014;211:228.e1–12; Oelschlager AA et al. *Curr Opin Obstet Gynecol.* 2016;28:345–9; McIndoe AH, Banister JB. *J Obstet Gynaecol Br Emp.* 1938;45:490–4; Strickland J et al. *Adolesc Pediatr Gynecol.* 1993;6:135–7; Vecchietti G. *Attual Ostet Ginecol.* 1965;11(2):131–47; Burruto F et al. *Int J Gynaecol Obstet.* 1999;64(2):1530158; Burruto. *Clin Exp Obstet Gynecol.* 1992;19(4):273–4; Veronikis D et al. *Obstet Gynecol.* 1997;90(2):301–4; Davydov SN. *Akush Ginekol (Mosk).* 1969;45(12):55–7; Williams EA. *J Obstet Gynaecolo Br Commonw.* 1964;71:511–2; Laufer MR. *Curr Opin Obstet Gynecol.* 2002;14:441–4; Allen LM et al. *Fertil Steril.* 2010;94(6):2272–6; Willemsen WN, Kluivers KB. *Fertil Steril.* 2015;103(1):e1; Giannesi A et al. *Hum Reprod.* 2005;20(1):2954–7; Nahas S et al. *J Minim Invasive Gynecol.* 2013;20(5):553; Dong X et al. *Zhonghua Fu Chan Ke Za Zhi.* 2015;50(4):278–82; Pator Z et al. *Sex Med.* 2017;5(2): e106–13; Kisku S et al. *Int Urogynecol J.* 2015;26(10):1441–8; Karateke A et al. *Fertil Steril.* 2010;94(6):2312–5; Creatsas G. *Fertil Steril.* 2010;94(5):1848–52.

women with MRKH is often lacking in hands-on experience with dilation teaching and may explain the lack of success with dilation in many practices.[60] We find that engagement with an experienced pelvic floor physical therapist not only increases success with dilation, but may also prevent resultant pain and pelvic floor sensitivity. It is important to note that many women achieve adequate vaginal length through dilation with attempted intercourse.

Typically patients can elongate a vagina within 2–18 months. It was also a long-held belief that successful dilation depended on a longer starting length of the vaginal pouch, of at least 2–3 cm.[57] However, starting length does not correlate to final vaginal length, and those with just a vaginal dimple are still able to create a vagina at least 6 cm in length, or within two standard deviations of the mean of 9.6 cm.[51,52,57–59,61] The suggested treatment regimen is dilation for 10–20 minutes one to three times a day

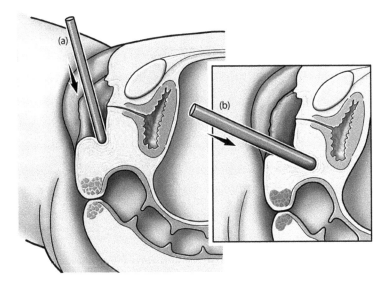

Figure 6.10   Vaginal dilation. (a) Sagittal view of complete Müllerian agenesis, vaginal dilator introduced into the vaginal dimple at a 45° angle. In this way, accidental dilation of the urethra can be avoided. (b) After initial insertion, the dilator is then dropped to a nearly horizontal angle, and gentle inward pressure is applied.

until successful vaginal creation has been completed, but there is great variability in dilators and schedules recommended by gynecologists involved in such care.[53,60,62] Of note, functional success (usually thought as the ability to have satisfying sexual relations) was not associated with the number of episodes of dilation per day; however, those who dilated more often were able to achieve longer vaginal length.[61]

After therapy has concluded, it is recommended to either dilate or have penetrative intercourse twice per week for continued vaginal patency.[61] Complications following dilation are very few, with recurrent urinary tract infection and urethral dilation being the most common.[53,58,59,61] Therefore, every patient who has indicated readiness for vaginal creation should be offered dilation first, no matter what her starting vaginal length is, and be supported throughout the process.

Surgical neovagina creation

As previously discussed, rates of complications are higher with surgical management, and most procedures require postoperative dilation. Thus, most experts in the field agree that nonsurgical vaginal dilation should be first-line treatment for neovaginal creation.[49] At times, with shared decision-making, the patient and her physician may choose surgical management for neovagina creation. It is important to note that although many procedures have been performed, none has been noted to have superior outcomes, and each has unique risks and benefits (Table 6.6).[52–59,61–81]

Perineal approach: McIndoe (split thickness, full-thickness skin, buccal mucosa grafts) and shears procedure

Gynecologists have traditionally performed McIndoe procedures, and there are many variations of this procedure. McIndoe first described this procedure in 1938 as

a noninvasive surgical approach to correction of vaginal agenesis.[63] Essentially, with a Foley in place, an incision is made in the perineum below the urethra. The areolar space between the urethra and the rectum is bluntly dissected, and the vaginal space is thus created and hemostasis achieved (Figure 6.11). In the classic McIndoe procedure, a split-thickness graft was obtained from the thigh or buttocks and sutured with the dermis facing around a soft mold (Mentor stent or one created by filling a condom or glove with foam) (Figure 6.12). This stent is placed within the vaginal space, and the external tissue edge is sutured to the incision at the introitus. Patients have traditionally been maintained in-house on bedrest with a suprapubic tube, constipating agents, and venous thromboembolism prophylaxis to avoid disturbance of the graft. After 7 days, the stent was removed, and the patient was instructed to place a dilator at least two to three times per week.[64]

This same procedure has been performed with full-thickness grafts, often from the lower abdominal wall, as this avoids the large graft scar and leaves one that can have the appearance of a large Pfannenstiel incision.[22] Full-thickness skin may be more difficult to graft into the space. Buccal mucosa has also been used. Given the smaller surface area that can be removed, multiple small slits are placed in the tissue in order to expand it over the mold. These spaces then epithelize later.

Other nonautologous tissues such as amnion and artificial material have been used, but the Shears procedure relies on the body's ability to epithelialize the vaginal space over time. The space is created as previously described, and a mold is kept in place for 3 months until the vagina is fully covered with epithelium.

Active perineal dilation: Vecchietti procedure

The Vecchietti procedure was first described in 1965 as another noninvasive method of vaginal creation.[65]

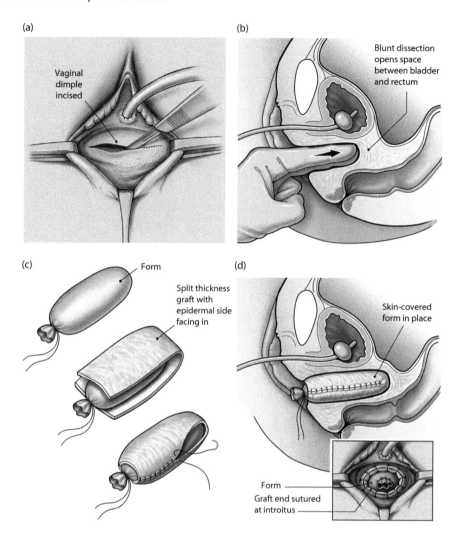

Figure 6.11 McIndoe vaginoplasty. (a) Vaginal view of vaginal agenesis. Distal mucosa at the vaginal dimple is noted and incised horizontally with a scalpel. (b) Sagittal view, blunt dissection is then carried out between the bladder and rectum to create a canal for the neovagina. (c) A vaginal graft is then made by covering a created mold with tissue (in this case, split thickness skin graft with epidermal side facing in), and suturing the tissue around mold. (d) The mold is then placed in the newly created vaginal canal, and graft tissue sutured circumferentially along the mucosa of the vaginal dimple (inset).

This procedure entails the placement of an "olive" at the perineum, which is attached to sutures.[66,67] These sutures are advanced through the vaginal space into the abdominal cavity. Though originally described as an open approach, now currently laparoscopic, these sutures are advanced laterally anteriorly behind the peritoneum and finally through the abdominal wall. These sutures are then attached to a metal device that allows increasing tension in order to actively dilate the vagina.[68] This procedure, similar to the McIndoe procedure, often requires prolonged hospitalization and analgesia with an epidural for about 7 days.

Autologous/membranous graft: Davydov procedure

The Davydov or peritoneal advancement procedure was first described in 1933.[69] Neovagina creation is approached both laparoscopically and from the perineum. The vaginal space is created as described in the McIndoe until the vaginal peritoneum is encountered, grasped, and pulled

through to the introitus. Laparoscopically, the peritoneum is sutured closed with a purse-string suture with or without release of the peritoneum laterally (Video 6.6).

Video 6.6 https://youtu.be/09Xh5knKI7o
Davydov vaginoplasty. (Courtesy of Drs. S. Paige Hertweck and Sari Kives.)

Labial skin flap: Williams/Creatsas

The Williams procedure was created in 1964 as the most noninvasive and simple form of vaginal creation.[70] The Williams procedure is rarely performed but may be useful in cases of severe scarring from previous procedures or radiation. Essentially, this procedure creates a pouch by incising the labia majora and perineal epithelium in a U-shape. The labia majora are then closed, creating a

(a)   (b)

(c)   (d)

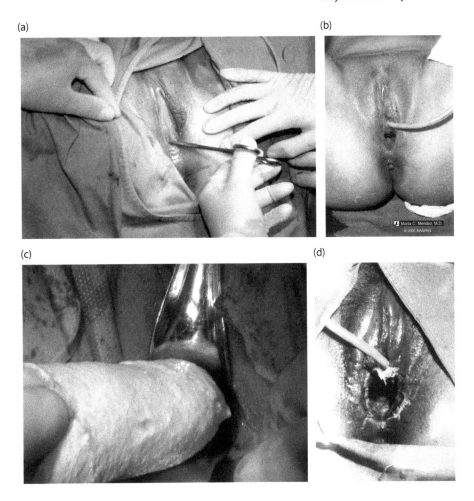

Figure 6.12   Graft placement following McIndoe procedure. (a) Dissection of space. (b) Open space. (c) Graft placement. (d) Healed neovagina. (From [a,b,d] Dr. Marta C. Mendez and NASPAG PediGyn Teaching Slide Set CD-ROM, NASPAG 2001, with permission.)

pouch inferior to the urethra (Figure 6.13). This procedure can be easily reversed if needed.

Bowel vaginoplasty

Bowel vaginoplasty was first described as early as 1892 by Sneguireff and made popular in the United States by Beck and Baldwin in the early 1900s.[71] It has been the preferred procedure performed by pediatric surgeons and urologists for neovagina creation in infancy and childhood. Both small bowel and colon have been utilized for these procedures.[71] The mainstay of such procedures is mobilization of the bowel without disturbing the blood supply. Though bowel vaginas can develop introital stenosis or complete stenosis if the blood supply is injured, these usually do not require immediate postoperative dilation.[72] They can be associated with large quantities of malodorous discharge that may require daily irrigations. These can also be associated with neovaginal polyps, adenomas, and cancer and should be monitored with inspection.[61]

Long-term care

While many patients and providers strive to achieve a functional vagina able to support satisfying sexual intercourse, the provider must not forget to encourage routine gynecologic care.[49] This includes regular pelvic exams, recommending barrier protection to prevent against transmission of disease, and offering routine screening for sexually transmitted infections (STIs).[49,61] A speculum exam continues to be indicated in this group for evaluation of symptoms due to the risk of malignancies, colitis, ulceration, or other pathologic conditions. Vaginal cytologic testing is not routinely recommended.[49] Although evidence is insufficient regarding the human papillomavirus (HPV) vaccination, these patients continue to be at risk for vaginal and vulvar HPV infection and intraepithelial neoplasia as is the general female population, and vaccination should be recommended.[61]

Fertility

Although great advances in assisted reproductive technology (ART) have been made since the 1970s, absolute uterine factor infertility due to congenital absence of the uterus, prior surgical removal, or severe adhesive disease remains a significant challenge. Pregnancy options for patients with MRKH in the United States who desire a genetic child include gestational surrogacy or uterine transplant.[82] While *in vitro* fertilization (IVF) and embryo transfer (ET) has become more successful, IVF using

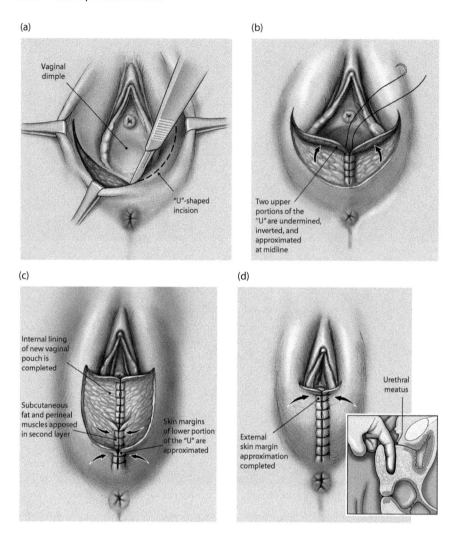

Figure 6.13 Williams vaginoplasty. (a) Perineal view, a "U"-shaped incision is made in the labia major and carried across the perineum to the contralateral labia majora. The hymenal tissue and vaginal dimple remain intact. (b) Beginning in the midline, the anterior flap is then sutured cranially, with the bilateral labia apices meeting in the midline, to create the internal mucosal wall. (c) After the internal mucosal wall has been approximated, a second layer of subcutaneous fat and perineal muscles are approximated at the midline for support. Finally, the posterior skin margins of the lower portion of the "U" are approximated at the midline in a similar manner, forming the external skin of the new pouch. (d) After the external skin has been approximated, the new pouch is complete. Inset shows a sagittal view of the length and orientation of the neovagina.

embryos from patients with MRKH typically results in fewer clinical pregnancies and live births.[83] When transferring good-quality embryos created using oocytes retrieved from MRKH patients, the rate of clinical pregnancy is only 17%, with live birth rate of 12% versus the national average over 40% in similar age groups.[83] At this time, no explanation can be provided for the lower than expected live birth rates in this population.

Uterine transplant is still considered highly experimental and can only be obtained at hospitals enrolled in a clinical trial. The first uterine transplant was performed in Saudi Arabia in 2002, and the first successful pregnancy was in 2014 in Sweden for a 35-year-old with MRKH who received a living donor graft.[84] As of 2017, 17 uterine transplants have been documented in the literature, 14 in patients with MRKH, with a total of 9 live births (Table 6.7).[84–93]

OTHER MALFORMATIONS
Anorectal malformations

Anorectal malformations (ARMs) are complex disorders of the lower genitourinary tract that require a multidisciplinary team approach and occur in 1:5000 live births.[94] The most common ARM in females is the imperforate anus with rectovestibular fistula, followed by imperforate anus with rectoperineal fistula, and then the most complex, the cloacal anomaly.[95] These require surgical repair during infancy with a multidisciplinary team of colorectal surgery, urology, and gynecology. These patients have high rates of concomitant Müllerian anomalies and require close follow-up with an adolescent gynecologist as they enter puberty. Since ovarian function is normal, patients can expect to undergo puberty as expected. Menstrual obstruction requiring additional procedures has been

Table 6.7 Uterine transplant and pregnancy outcome.

	Country	Year	Age	Diagnosis	Donor	Outcome	Pregnancy	Live birth
Fageeh et al.	Saudi Arabia	2002	26	Hysterectomy	Live	Thrombosis/necrosis after 99 days	No	No
Akar	Turkey	2011	21	MRKH	Deceased	Menstruating	One clinical unconfirmed pregnancy with loss, one 8 week spontaneous abortion	No
Brannstrom	Sweden	2013	35	MRKH	Live	Menstruating	Yes	Yes, 31.5, pre-E
Brannstrom	Sweden	2014	28	MRKH	Live	Hysterectomy 3 months postpartum	Yes	Yes, 34.4 Cholestasis
Johannesson	Sweden	2016		Cervical CA	Live	Menstruating	Yes	?
				MRKH	Live	Thrombosis/hysterectomy	No	No
				MRKH	Live	Menstruating	No	No
				MRKH	Live	Menstruating	Yes	Yes
				MRKH	Live	Menstruating	Yes	Yes
				MRKH	Live	Menstruating	Yes	Yes
Flyckt	Cleveland	2016		MRKH	Deceased	Infection/hysterectormy postoperative day 12	No	No
Testa	Houston	2016	32	MRKH	Live	Hysterectomy postoperative day 14	No	No
			33	MRKH	Live	Hysterectomy postoperative day 12	No	No
			34	MRKH	Live	Hysterectomy postoperative day 6	No	No
			28	MRKH	Live	Menstruating	Yes	Yes
			28	MRKH	Live	Menstruating	No	No

Source: Compiled from data in Brännström M et al. *The Lancet.* 2015;385(9968):607–16; Johannesson L, Järvholm S. *Int J Womens Health.* 2016:43–51; Park M. Baby is first to be born in US after uterus transplant, hospital says. CNN: Health. 2017, December 4. Accessed from https://www.cnn.com/2017/12/04/health/uterus-transplant-us-baby-birth/index.html; Fageeh W et al. *Int J Gynaecol Obstet.* 2002;76(3):245–51; Ozkan O et al. *Fertil Steril.* 2013;99(2):470–6.e5; Erman Akar M et al. *Fertil Steril.* 2013;100(5):1358–63; Brännström M et al. *Fertil Steril.* 2016;106(2):261–6; Johannesson L et al. *Fertil Steril.* 2015;103(1):199–204; Flyckt R et al. *J Obstet Gynaecol Can.* 2013;40(1):86-93; Testa G et al. *Am J Transplant.* 2017;17(11):2901–10.

noted in up to 36%–41% of affected individuals.[96] Thus, ultrasound imaging of the reproductive structures should be initiated within 6–9 months after initial breast development and continue every 6–9 months until menarche.

Physical exam should be performed when the patient is ready after puberty to evaluate for scar tissue, introital stenosis, and adequacy of the vagina for sexual intercourse.[96] Some studies suggest that only 20% of adults who had repair during infancy have a vagina of an appropriate caliber to allow for comfortable intercourse.[97] These women should attempt vaginal dilation as a first-line therapy; however, surgical revision or introitoplasty may be warranted.[96]

Pregnancy in patients with ARMs is possible. Preconception evaluation is recommended to assess for uterine anomalies and provide appropriate counseling.[95] Those women with a history of imperforate anus or perineal fistula may be candidates for vaginal delivery. Due to the complexity of surgical repair, women with a history of cloacal anomaly should deliver via cesarean section to avoid disruption of the vascular supply to repairs.

Bladder exstrophy

Another uncommon but complex anomaly is bladder exstrophy, with an incidence of 3.3:100,000 births.[98] In these girls, the bladder is everted on the lower abdomen, the urethra is completely unroofed, the clitoris is bifid, and the vagina is abnormally positioned.[98] Repair of the external genitalia consists of enlarging and relocating the vaginal introitus and typically reapproximating the bifid clitoris. In general, repair leads to good vaginal function and satisfying sexual intercourse.

Vaginal cysts

Vaginal (Gartner's duct) cysts form as a result of incompletely obliterated Wolffian ducts and subsequent accumulation of fluid.[99] Cysts may also be accompanied by other Wolffian duct anomalies, including ectopic ureter, unilateral renal dysgenesis, and renal hypoplasia.[100] These cysts can become quite large, up to 8 cm in diameter, and resemble obstructed vaginal anomalies. However, careful exam will reveal these ducts originating in the lateral vaginal wall with patent vagina. Surgical management can successfully resolve the cysts by excision and marsupialization.[101] However, in asymptomatic patients, conservative treatment with observation may also be a safe and effective management strategy.[100]

CONCLUSION

There is great variation in possible congenital anomalies of the female reproductive system. Pediatric gynecologists need to be aware of the underlying embryology, as well as the most common anomalies and their possible anatomic variations, in order to provide the best care to their patients. In most cases, excellent anatomic evaluation with MRI is necessary for counseling and surgical planning. Surgical treatment should be performed by providers with expertise in such care, taking into account the risks, benefits, patient readiness, and desires. Patients and families

should be counseled about the anatomic condition and impact on future fertility by using simple explanations and maintaining sensitivity of the emotional aspects of such diagnoses.

REFERENCES

1. Oppelt P, Lermann J, Stick R et al. Malformations in a cohort of 284 women with Mayer-Rokitansky-Kuster-Hauser syndrome (MRKH). *Reprod Biol Endocrinol*. 2012;10:57.
2. Rall K, Eisenbeis S, Henninger V, Henes M, Wallwiener D, Bonin M, Brucker S. Typical and atypical associated findings in a group of 346 patients with Mayer-Rokitansky-Kuster-Hauser Syndrome. *J Pediatr Adolesc Gynecol*. 2015;28:362–8.
3. Acién P, Acién M. The history of female genital tract malformation classifications and proposal of an updated system. *Hum Reprod Update*. 2011;17(5):693–705.
4. Rock J, Zacur H, Dlugi A. Pregnancy success following surgical correction of imperforate hymen and complete transverse vaginal septum. *Obstet Gynecol*. 1982;59:448–51.
5. Joki-Erkkila M, Heinonen P. Presenting and long-term clinical implications in fecundity in females with obstructive vaginal malformations. *J Pediatr Adolesc Gynaecol*. 2003;16:307–12.
6. The American Fertility Society. The American Fertility Society classifications of adnexal adhesions, distal tubal occlusion, tubal occlusion secondary to tubal ligation, tubal pregnancies, Müllerian anomalies and intrauterine adhesions. *Fertil Steril*. 1988;49(6):944–55.
7. Buttram V, Gibbons W. Müllerian anomalies: A proposed classification (and analysis of 144 cases). *Fertil Steril*. 1979;32(1):40–6.
8. Oppelt P, Renner S, Brucker S et al. The VCUAM (vagina cervix uterus adnex-associated malformation) classification: A new classification for genital malformations. *Fertil Steril*. 2005;84(5):1493–7.
9. Grimbizis G, Gordts S, Sardo A et al. The ESHRE-ESGE consensus on the classification of female genital tract congenital anomalies. *Gynecol Surg*. 2013;10:199–212.
10. Di Spiezio Sardo A, Campo R, Gordts S et al. The comprehensiveness of the ESHRE/ESGE classification of female genital tract congenital anomalies: A systematic review of cases not classified by the AFS system. *Hum Reprod*. 2015;30(5):1046–58.
11. Menstruation in girls and adolescents: Using the menstrual cycle as a vital sign. Committee Opinion No. 651. American College of Obstetricians and Gynecologists. *Obstet Gynecol*. 2015;126:e143–6.
12. Dubinskaya A, Gomez-Lobo V. Obstructive anomalies of the reproductive tract. *Postgrad Obstet Gynecol*. 2015;35(24):e1–8.
13. Smith N, Laufer M. Obstructed hemivagina and ipsilateral renal anomaly (OHVIRA) syndrome: Management and follow-up. *Fertil Steril*. 2007;87(4):918–22.

14. Patel V, Gomez-Lobo V. Obstructive anomalies of the gynecologic tract. *Curr Opin Obstet Gynecol.* 2016;28(5):339–44.

15. Dietrich J, Millar D, Quint E. Obstructive reproductive tract anomalies. Committee Opinion NASPAG 2014. *J Pediatr Adolesc Gynecol.* 2014;27:396–401.

16. Haddad B, Louis-Sylvestre C, Poitout P, Paniel BJ. Longitudinal vaginal septum: A retrospective study of 202 cases. *Eur J Obstet Gynecol Reprod Biol.* 1997;74:197–9.

17. Williams CE, Nakhal RS, Hall-Craggs MA, Wood D, Cutner A, Pattison SH, Creighton SM. Transverse vaginal septae: Management and long-term outcomes. *BJOG.* 2014;121:1653–8.

18. Kashimura T, Takahashi S, Nakazawa H. Successful management of a thick transverse vaginal septum with a vesicovaginal fistula by vaginal expansion and surgery. *Int Urogynecol J.* 2012;23:797–9.

19. Layman L, McDonough P. Management of transverse vaginal septum using the Olbert balloon catheter to mobilize the proximal vaginal mucosa and facilitate low anastomosis. *Fertil Steril.* 2010;94(6):2316–8.

20. Garcia R. Z-plasty for correction of congenital transverse vaginal septum. *Am J Obstet Gynecol.* 1967;99(8):1164–5.

21. Wierrani F, Bodner K, Spangler B, Grunberger W. "Z"-plasty of the transverse vaginal septum using Garcias procedure and the Grunberger modification. *Fertil Steril.* 2003;79(3):608–12.

22. Miller RJ, Breech LL. Surgical correction of vaginal anomalies. *Clin Obstet Gynecol.* 2008;51:223.

23. Grimbizis G, Tsalikis T, Mikos T, Papadopoulos N, Tarlatzis B, Bontis J. Successful end-to-end cervico-cervical anastomosis in a patient with congenital cervical fragmentation: Case Report. *Hum Reprod.* 2004;19(5):1204–10.

24. Mansouri R, Dietrich J. Postoperative course and complications after pull-through vaginoplasty for distal vaginal atresia. *J Pediatr Adolesc Gynecol.* 2015; 28:433–6.

25. Van Bijsterveldt C, Willemsen W. Treatment of patients with a congenital transversal vaginal septum or a partial aplasia of the vagina. The vaginal pull-through versus the push-through technique. *J Pediatr Adolesc Gynecol.* 2009;22:157–61.

26. Acién P, Acién MI, Quereda F, Santoyo T. Cervicovaginal agenesis: Spontaneous gestation at term after previous reimplantation of the uterine corpus in a neovagina: Case report. *Hum Reprod.* 2008;23(3):548–53.

27. Deffarges JV, Haddad B, Musset R, Paniel BJ. Utero-vaginal anastomosis in women with uterine cervix atresia: Long-term follow-up and reproductive performance. A study of 18 cases. *Hum Reprod.* 2001; 16(8):1722–5.

28. Rock JA, Roberts CP, Jones HW. Congenital anomalies of the uterine cervix: Lessons from 30 cases managed clinically by a common protocol. *Fertil Stertil.* 2010;94(5):1858–63.

29. Shen F, Zhang X, Yin, C, Ding J, Hua K. Comparison of small intestinal submucosa graft with split-thickness skin graft for cervicovaginal reconstruction of congenital vaginal and cervical aplasia. *Hum Reprod.* 2016;31(11):2499–505.

30. Al-Jaroudi D, Saleh A, Al-Obaid S, Agdi M, Salih A, Khan F. Pregnancy with cervical dysgenesis. *Fertil Steril.* 2011;96(6):1355–6.

31. Anttila L, Penttla TA, Suikkari AM. Successful pregnancy after in-vitro fertilization and transmyometrial embryo transfer in patient with congenital atresia of cervix. *Hum Reprod.* 1999;14:164–9.

32. Lai TH, Wu MH, Hung KH, Cheng YC, Chang FM. Successful pregnancy by transmyometrial and transtubal embryo transfer after IVF in a patient with congenital cervical atresia who underwent utero vaginal canalization during Caesarean section: Case report. *Hum Reprod.* 2001;16:268–71.

33. Thijssen RF, Hollanders JM, Willemsen WN, vander Heyden PM, van Dongen PW, Rolland R. Successful pregnancy after ZIFT in a patient with congenital cervical atresia. *Obstet Gynecol.* 1990;76:902–4.

34. Candiani G, Fedele L, Candiani M. Double uterus, blind hemivagina, and ipsilateral renal agenesis: 36 cases and long-term follow-up. *Obstet Gynecol.* 1997; 90(1):26–32.

35. Tong J, Zhu L, Lang J. Clinical characteristics of 70 patients with Herlyn-Werner-Wunderlich syndrome. *Int J Gynecol Obstetr.* 2013;121(2):173–5.

36. Haddad B, Barranger E, Paniel B. Blind hemivagina: Long-term follow-up and reproductive performance in 42 cases. *Hum Reprod.* 1999;14(8):1962–4.

37. Capito C, Echaieb A, Lortat-Jacob S, Thibaud E, Sarnacki S, Nihoul-Fekete C. Pitfalls in the diagnosis and management of obstructive uterovaginal duplication: A series of 32 cases. *Pediatrics.* 2008;122(4):e891–7.

38. Kapczuk K, Friebe Z, Iwaniec K, Kędzia W. Obstructive Müllerian anomalies in menstruating adolescent girls: A report of 22 cases. *J Pediatr Adolesc Gynecol.* 2018;31(3):252–7.

39. Reis M, Vicente A, Cominho J, Gomes A, Martins L, Nunes F. Pyometra and pregnancy with Herlyn-Werner-Wunderlich syndrome. *Rev Bras Ginecol Obstet.* 2016;38(12):623–8.

40. Jung E, Cho M, Kim D et al. Herlyn-Werner-Wunderlich syndrome: An unusual presentation with pyocolpos. *Obstet Gynecol Sci.* 2017;60(4):374.

41. Jain R, Gami N, Puri M, Trivedi S. A rare case of intact rudimentary horn pregnancy presenting as hemoperitoneum. *J Hum Reprod Sci.* 2010;3(2):113–5.

42. Dietrich J, Millar D, Quint E. Non-obstructive Müllerian anomalies. *J Pediatr Adolesc Gynecol.* 2014;27(6):386–95.

43. Purslow C. A case of unilateral haematokolpos, haematometra and haematosalpinx. *BJOG.* 1922;29(4):643.

44. Fedele L, Motta F, Frontino G, Restelli E, Bianchi S. Double uterus with obstructed hemivagina and ipsilateral renal agenesis: Pelvic anatomic variants in 87 cases. *Hum Reprod.* 2013;28(6):1580–3.

45. Santos X, Dietrich J. Obstructed hemivagina with ipsilateral renal anomaly. *J Pediatr Adolesc Gynecol.* 2016;29(1):7–10.

46. Gholoum S, Puligandla P, Hui T, Su W, Quiros E, Laberge J. Management and outcome of patients with combined vaginal septum, bifid uterus, and ipsilateral renal agenesis (Herlyn-Werner-Wunderlich syndrome). *J Pediatr Surg.* 2006;41(5):987–92.

47. Rock J, Jones H. The double uterus associated with an obstructed hemivagina and ipsilateral renal agenesis. *Am J Obstet Gynecol.* 1980;138(3):339–42.

48. Han JH, Lee YS, Im YJ, Kim SW, Lee MJ, Han SW. Clinical implications of obstructed hemivagina and ipsilateral renal anomaly (OHVIRA) syndrome in the prepubertal age group. *PLOS ONE.* 2016;11(11):e1–3.

49. Müllerian agenesis: Diagnosis, management, and treatment. ACOG Committee Opinion No. 728. American College of Obstetricians and Gynecologists. *Obstet Gynecol.* 2018;131(1):e35–42.

50. Kapczuk K, Iwaniec K, Friebe Z, Kedzia W. Congenital malformations and other comorbidities in 125 women with Mayer-Rokitansky-Kuster-Hauser syndrome. *Eur J Obstet Gynecol Reprod Biol.* 2016;207:45–9.

51. Callens N, De Cuypere G, Wolffenbuttel KP et al. Long-term psychosexual and anatomical outcome after vaginal dilation or vaginoplast: A comparative study. International Society for Sexual Medicine. *J Sex Med.* 2012;9:1842–51.

52. Gargollo PC, Cannon GM, Diamond DA, Thomas P, Burke V, Laufer MR. Should progressive perineal dilation be considered first line therapy for vaginal agenesis? *J Urol.* 2009;182:1882–91.

53. Edmonds DK, Rose GL, Lipton MG, Quek J. Mayer-Rokitansky-Kuster-Hauser syndrome: A review of 245 consecutive cases managed by a multidisciplinary approach with vaginal dilators. *Fertil Steril.* 2012;97(3):686–90.

54. Frank RT. The formation of an artificial vagina without operation. *Am J Obstet Gynecol.* 1938;35:1053.

55. Ingram JM. The bicycle seat stool in the treatment of vaginal agenesis and stenosis: A preliminary report. *Am J Obstet Gynecol.* 1981;140(8):867–73.

56. Williams JK, Lake M, Ingram JM. The bicycle seat stool in the treatment of vaginal agenesis and stenosis. *J Obstet Gynecol Neonatal Nurs.* 1985;14(2):147–50.

57. Roberts CP, Haber MJ, Rock JA. Vaginal creation for Müllerian agenesis. *Am J Obstet Gynecol.* 2000;185:1349–53.

58. Callens N, De Cuypere G, De Sutter P, Monstrey S, Weyers S, Hoebeke P, Cools M. An update on surgical and non-surgical treatments for vaginal hypoplasia. *Hum Reprod.* 2014;20(5):775–801.

59. Callens N, Weyers S, Monstrey S, Stockman S, van Hoorde B, van Hoecke E, De Cuyypee G, Hoebeke P, Cools M. Vaginal dilation treatment in women with vaginal hypoplasia: A prospective one-year follow-up study. *Am J Obstet Gynecol.* 2014;211:228.e1–12.

60. Patel V, Hakin J, Gomez-Lobo V, Oelschlager AA. Providers' experiences with vaginal dilator training for patients with vaginal agenesis. *J Pediatr Adolesc Gynecol.* 2018;31(1):45–7.

61. Oelschlager AA, Debiec K, Appelbaum H. Primary vaginal dilation for vaginal agenesis: Strategies to anticipate challenges and optimize outcomes. *Curr Opin Obstet Gynecol.* 2016;28:345–9.

62. Adeyemi-Fowode OA, Dietrich JE. Assessing the experience of vaginal dilator use and potential barriers to ongoing use among a focus group of women with Mayer-Rokitansky-Kuster-Hauser syndrome. *J Pediatr Adoles Gynecol.* 2017;30:491–4.

63. McIndoe AH, Banister JB. An operation for the cure of congenital absence of the vagina. *J Obstet Gynaecol Br Emp* 1938;45:490–4.

64. Strickland J, Cameron W, Krantz K. Long-term satisfaction of adults undergoing McIndoe vaginoplasty as adolescents. *Adolesc Pediatr Gynecol.* 1993;6:135–7.

65. Vecchietti G. Creation of an artificial vagina in Rokitansky-Kuster-Hauser syndrome. *Attual Ostet Ginecol.* 1965;11(2):131–47.

66. Burruto F, Chasen ST, Chervenak FA, Fedele L. The Vecchietti procedure for surgical treatment of vaginal agenesis: Comparison of laparoscopy and laparotomy. *Int J Gynaecol Obstet.* 1999;64(2):1530158.

67. Burruto F. Mayer-Rokitansky-Kuster syndrome: Vecchietti's personal series. *Clin Exp Obstet Gynecol.* 1992;19(4):273–4.

68. Veronikis D, McClure GB, Nichols DH. The Vecchietti operation for constructing a neovagina: Indications, instrumentation, and techniques. *Obstet Gynecol.* 1997;90(2):301–4.

69. Davydov SN. Colpopoeisis from the peritoneum of the uterorectal space. *Akush Ginekol (Mosk).* 1969;45(12):55–7.

70. Williams EA. Congenital absence of the vagina, a simple operation for its relief. *J Obstet Gynaecolo Br Commonw* 1964;71:511–2.

71. Baldwin JF. The formation of an artificial vagina by intestinal transplantation. *Ann Surg.* 1904;40(3):398–403.

72. Laufer MR. Congenital absence of the vagina: In search of the perfect solution. When, and by what technique, should a vagina be created? *Curr Opin Obstet Gynecol.* 2002;14:441–4.

73. Allen LM, Lucco KL, Brown CM, Spitzer RF, Kives S. Psychosexual and functional outcomes after creation of a neovagina with laparoscopic Davydov in patients with vaginal agenesis. *Fertil Steril.* 2010;94(6):2272–6.

74. Willemsen WN, Kluivers KB. Long-term results of vaginal construction with the use of Frank dilation and a peritoneal graft (Davydov procedure) in patients with Mayer-Rokitansky-Kuster syndrome. *Fertil Steril.* 2015;103(1):e1.

75. Giannesi A, Marchiole P, Benchaib M, Chevret-Measson M, Mathevet P, Dargent D. Sexuality

after laparoscopic Davydov in patients affected by congenital complete vaginal agenesis associated with uterine agenesis or hypoplasia. *Hum Reprod.* 2005;20(1):2954–7.

76. Nahas S, Yi J, Magrina J. Mayo Clinic experience with modified Vecchietti procedure for vaginal agenesis: It is easy, safe, and effective. *J Minim Invasive Gynecol.* 2013;20(5):553.

77. Dong X, Xie Z, Jin H. Comparison study between Vecchietti's and Davydov's laparoscopic vaginoplasty in Mayer-Rokitansky-Kuster-Hauser syndrome. *Zhonghua Fu Chan Ke Za Zhi.* 2015;50(4): 278–82.

78. Pator Z, Fronek J, Novackova M, Chmel R. Sexual life of women with Mayer-Rokitansky-Kuster-Hauser syndrome after laparoscopic Vecchietti vaginoplasty. *Sex Med.* 2017;5(2):e106–13.

79. Kisku S, Varghese L, Kekre A, Sen S, Karl S, Mathai J, Thomas RJ, Kishore R. Bowel vaginoplasty in children and young women: And institutional experience with 55 patients. *Int Urogynecol J.* 2015;26(10): 1441–8.

80. Karateke A, Haliloglu B, Parlak O, Cam C, Coksuer H. Intestinal vaginoplasty: Seven years' experience of a tertiary center. *Fertil Steril.* 2010;94(6):2312–5.

81. Creatsas G. Creation of a neovagina after Creatsas modification of Williams vaginoplasty for the treatment of 200 patients with Mayer-Rokitansky-Kuster-Hauser syndrome. *Fertil Steril.* 2010;94(5):1848–52.

82. Beski S, Gorgy A, Venkat G, Craft I, Edmonds K. Gestational surrogacy: A feasible option for patients with Rokitansky syndrome. *Hum Reprod.* 2000;15(11):2326–8.

83. Raziel A, Friedler S, Gidoni Y, Ben Ami I, Strassburger D, Ron-El R. Surrogate in vitro fertilization outcome in typical and atypical forms of Mayer-Rokitansky-Kuster-Hauser syndrome. *Hum Reprod.* 2011;27(1):126–30.

84. Brännström M, Johannesson L, Bokström H et al. Livebirth after uterus transplantation. *The Lancet.* 2015;385(9968):607–16.

85. Johannesson L, Järvholm S. Uterus transplantation: Current progress and future prospects. *Int J Womens Health.* 2016;8:43–51.

86. Park M. *Baby is first to be born in US after uterus transplant, hospital says.* CNN: Health. 2017, December 4. Accessed from https://www.cnn.com/2017/12/04/health/uterus-transplant-us-baby-birth/index.html

87. Fageeh W, Raffa H, Jabbad H, Marzouki A. Transplantation of the human uterus. *Int J Gynaecol Obstet.* 2002;76(3):245–51.

88. Ozkan O, Akar M, Ozkan O et al. Preliminary results of the first human uterus transplantation from a multiorgan donor. *Fertil Steril.* 2013;99(2):470–6.e5.

89. Erman Akar M, Ozkan O, Aydinuraz B et al. Clinical pregnancy after uterus transplantation. *Fertil Steril.* 2013;100(5):1358–63.

90. Brännström M, Bokström H, Dahm-Kähler P et al. One uterus bridging three generations: First live birth after mother-to-daughter uterus transplantation. *Fertil Steril.* 2016;106(2):261–6.

91. Johannesson L, Kvarnström N, Mölne J et al. Uterus transplantation trial: 1-year outcome. *Fertil Steril.* 2015;103(1):199–204.

92. Flyckt R, Davis A, Farrell R, Zimberg S, Tzakis A, Falcone T. Uterine transplantation: Surgical innovation in the treatment of uterine factor infertility. *J Obstet Gynaecol Can.* 2018;40(1):86–93.

93. Testa G, Koon E, Johannesson L et al. Living donor uterus transplantation: A single center's observations and lessons learned from early setbacks to technical success. *Am J Transplant.* 2017;17(11):2901–10.

94. Wood R, Levitt M. Anorectal malformations. *Clin Colon Rectal Surg.* 2018;31(2):61–70.

95. Breech L. Gynecologic concerns in patients with anorectal malformations. *Semin Pediatr Surg.* 2010;19: 139–45.

96. Breech L. Gynecologic concerns in patients with cloacal anomaly. *Semin Pediatri Surg.* 2016;25:90–5.

97. Warne SA, Wilcox DT, Creighton S, Ransley PG. Long-term gynecological outcome of patients with persistent cloaca. *J Urol.* 2003;170:1493–6.

98. Jones HW. An anomaly of the external genitalia in female patients with exstrophy of the bladder. *Am J Obstet Gynecol.* 1973;117(6):748–56.

99. Blackwell WJ, McElin TW. Vaginal cysts of mesonephric duct origin (Gartner's duct cysts). Report of 22 cases. *Q Bull Northwest Unive Med Sch.* 1955;29(2):94–7.

100. Rios SS, Pereira LCR, Santos CB, Chen ACR, Chen JR, de Fatima M. Conservative treatment and follow-up of vaginal Gartner's duct cysts: A case series. *J Med Case Rep.* 2016;10:147–50.

101. Cope AG, Laughlin-Tommaso SK, Famuyide AO, Gebhart JB, Hopkins MR, Breitkopf DM. Clinical manifestations and outcomes in surgically managed Gartner duct cysts. *J Minim Invasive Gynecol.* 2017;24(3):473–7.

APPENDIX: ADDITIONAL ONLINE RESOURCES

Miklos JR, Moore RD. Laparoscopic Neovagina: Minimally Invasive Pelvic Reconstruction (Atlanta, Georgia, 2010). (Accessed May 23, 2019.) Available online at: https://www.youtube.com/watch?v=SctFnQ63nzo

Neomedic International. Technique mini-invasive de Vecchietti [Vecchietti's surgical technique for vaginal agenesia with Agers, the less invasive treatment for the Rokitansky Syndrome]. (Madrid, Spain, 2012). (Accessed May 23, 2019.) Available online at: https://www.youtube.com/watch?v=EgLRn0Qky6o

Ramesh B, Prasanna G, Chandana A, Gupta P. Veichetti's laparoscopic vaginoplasty procedure (Bangaloru, India, 2015). (Accessed May 23, 2019.) Available online at: https://www.youtube.com/watch?v=uOzouV9qIHE

Variation of sex differentiation

7

ANNE-MARIE AMIES OELSCHLAGER and MARGARETT SHNORHAVORIAN

INTRODUCTION

The first question that is usually asked after the delivery of a newborn is "Is it a boy or a girl?" However, if the genitalia is ambiguous and the infant has a difference of sex development, this question cannot be answered immediately. Differences of sex development (DSDs) include a heterogeneous group of conditions where the chromosomal, gonadal, or anatomic sex is considered atypical. The incidence ranges between 1:200 and 1:5000 births.[1] These conditions may be identified antenatally, through prenatal genetic testing with atypical sex chromosomes, by physical examination of ambiguous external genitalia at birth, during evaluation for a hernia in childhood, through evaluation of aberrant pubertal development, or during evaluation for infertility. Understanding the typical embryologic development of the fetus is essential to understanding the causes of variations in sex development.

EMBRYOLOGY OF SEX DIFFERENTIATION

The process of sex development follows three stages: the *chromosomal sex* is established at fertilization, which guides the differentiation of *gonadal sex* into a testis or an ovary, and then the hormonal production of the gonad causes internal reproductive structure and external genital differentiation, or *anatomic sex*.[2,3]

Chromosomal sex and the genetics of sex differentiation

Chromosomal sex occurs when the sperm, carrying an X or a Y sex chromosome, fertilizes the ovum, which carries an X. Typically, the XX zygote will become a phenotypic female, and the XY zygote will become a phenotypic male. There are multiple critical genes involved in the differentiation of the bipotential gonad, which then determine the gonadal sex (Table 7.1). It is important to note that the scientific knowledge of the genetics of sex differentiation is rapidly evolving.

Gonadal sex

Internally, the bipotential gonad develops from somatic and germ cells. The somatic cells arise from the mesonephric cells and the coelomic epithelium and develop into the Sertoli cells of the testes and the granulosa cells of the ovary. The germ cells migrate to the genital ridge, medial to the mesonephros, by 6 weeks' gestation, at which point they are surrounded by the somatic cells, which regulate differentiation. Thus, gonadal sex is determined by about 7 weeks' gestation.[3]

At this point, the Sertoli cells of the testis begin producing anti-Müllerian hormone (AMH), also known as Müllerian inhibiting substance (MIS). The fetal pituitary, under the influence of human chorionic gonadotropin (HCG) produced by the placenta, produces luteinizing hormone (LH), which prompts the fetal Leydig cells of the testes to secrete testosterone around week 9 or 10 of gestation.

Anatomic sex

Internal reproductive structure development

In the first trimester, the prototypes for both the internal male (wolffian) and female (Müllerian) ducts are present. The wolffian, or mesonephric, ducts connect the capillaries of the mesonephros to the urogenital sinus. The Müllerian, or paramesonephric, ducts are adjacent and connect distally at the urogenital sinus. The distal portion of the urogenital sinus is influenced by external genital development. The internal urogenital sinus will develop into the bladder, trigone, and posterior urethra[4] (Figure 7.1).

The development or regression of the internal reproductive structures is dictated by the differentiation of the gonad. If a testis develops, the Müllerian (or paramesonephric) ducts regress due to production of AMH from the Sertoli cells. The wolffian duct will differentiate into the epididymis, vas deferens, seminal vesicles, and the ejaculatory ducts under the influence of testosterone produced by the fetal Leydig cells. The embryologic remnant of the distal Müllerian duct is the prostatic utricle and the appendix testis cephalically. Distally, the urogenital sinus differentiates into the urethra and the prostate glands in the male.

Although differentiation into female was considered the "default" pathway previously, it is now clear that internal Müllerian development occurs due to the presence of multiple genes. In the typical female, the Müllerian (or paramesonephric) ducts, which originate from the coelemic epithelium, will elongate, invaginate, and migrate medially and form the fallopian tubes, uterus, cervix, and upper one-third of the vagina. The wolffian ducts involute in the absence of high levels of testosterone; the distal embryologic remnant is the Gartner duct. The two uterine horns will then join together and will fuse. The transverse and longitudinal vaginal septae will then resorb through the second trimester. The distal urogenital sinus separates into the urethra and distal one-third of the vagina in the female in the process of external genital development.

External genital development

In the early first trimester, the external genitalia are undifferentiated. The protogenitalia of the clitorophallus, labioscrotal folds, and the urogenital sinus will begin to differentiate around week 8, and this process continues through the second trimester.

External male genital development: Dihydrotestosterone (DHT) is produced from testosterone by the 5α-reductase

Table 7.1 Genes critical for sex differentiation.

Gene	Locus	Function	Associations
DAX1	Xp22	Necessary for testis differentiation. Involved in upregulation of *SOX9*.	Duplication of *DAX1* in 46,XY individuals results in a female phenotype and gonadal dysgenesis.
SRY (Sex-determining Region of the Y chromosome) *TDF* (Testis-Determining Factor)	Yp11.2	Expression of *SRY* makes sex-determining region Y protein, a transcription factor that controls genes associated with testicular development. Protein directs medullary region of undifferentiated gonad to develop Sertoli cells, testicular cords, and seminiferous tubules.	
WT1 (Wilms Tumor Gene 1)	11p13	WT1 protein is a transcription factor necessary for the development of kidneys, ovaries, and testes. WT1 protein promotes cell growth, cell differentiation, and apoptosis in the gonads and kidneys.	Denys-Drash syndrome. Frasier syndrome, *WAGR* (Wilms tumor, aniridia, genitourinary anomalies, intellectual disability). Associated with leukemia, lung, prostate, breast, and ovarian cancer.
SF1 (Steroidogenic Factor 1) *NR5A1* (nuclear receptor subfamily 5 group A, member 1)	9q33.3	*SF1* regulates activity of genes for gonad and adrenal gland development. *SF1* interacts with β-catenin to express *DAX-1/NROB1* genes. Regulates steroid hormone encoding. Promotes anti-Müllerian hormone (AMH) production by Sertoli cells of the testes, which causes Müllerian duct regression.	Adrenal failure
SOX9	17q24.3	SOX9 protein is a transcription factor critical for skeletal development and sex differentiation.	Camptomelic dysplasia and testicular dysgenesis in 75% of XY individuals.
WNT4	1p35	Causes the Müllerian ducts to form. Prevents the Leydig cells from developing in the testes.	Mutation associated with virilization of the 46,XX individual and Müllerian duct regression. *WNT4* duplication associated with increased *DAX1* expression and 46,XY DSD with female phenotype.
DMRT1	9p24.3	Controls testis development and spermatogonia meiosis.	
FOXL2	3q23	Essential for ovarian development, fertility, and maintenance of ovarian function.	Deletions are associated with blepharophimosis-ptosis-epicanthus inversus syndrome.
GATA4	8p23.1	Transcription factor involved in genital ridge formation, gonadal differentiation, and fertility. Works in synergy with *SRY*, *SOX9*, and *NR5A1* to promote AMH.	Mutations associated with testicular and congenital cardiac anomalies.

type 2 enzyme in genital tissues. DHT is a more potent androgen that causes the protophallus to enlarge to form the penis, the labioscrotal folds to fuse in the midline to form scrotum, and the urethra to migrate distally to the tip of the penis. Additionally, the scrotal skin will darken and rugate. This process begins at 8 weeks of gestation and continues through into the second trimester. The testes begin their abdominal descent in the first trimester and descend into the inguinal and then scrotal region between 25 and 35 weeks. The testes may continue to descend postnatally.

External female genital development: Without high levels of DHT, the protophallus remains small as the clitoris and the labioscrotal folds remain separated and develop into the labia majora. The urethra remains in the perineal location, and the distal vagina and hymen separate from the urogenital sinus. The labia minora remain separated below the dorsal hood of the clitoris. Distally, the distal urogenital sinus separates into the urethra and distal one-third of the vagina.

CAUSES OF DIFFERENCE OF SEXUAL DEVELOPMENT CONDITIONS

Classification of DSD conditions is based on underlying karyotype, including 46,XX DSD; 46,XY DSD; and sex chromosome DSD. In general, ambiguous genitalia

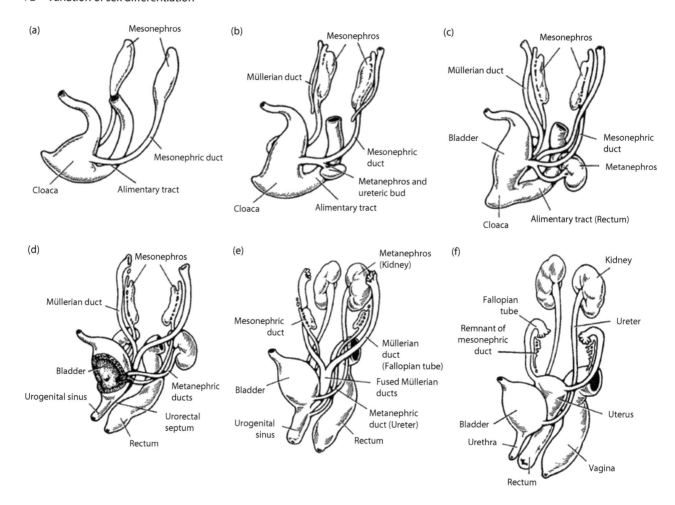

Figure 7.1 Embryonic differentiation of the female genitourinary tract. (a) The mesonephric ducts connect the mesonephric kidneys to the cloaca. (b) The ureteric buds develop from the mesonephric duct and induce differentiation of the metanephros, which will later develop into the functional kidneys. (c) The Müllerian ducts develop adjacent to the mesonephric ducts. (d) The rectum and the urogenital sinus separate. (e) The distal Müllerian ducts fuse to the urogenital sinus. (f) The vaginal plate canalizes, and the distal vagina and urethra separate. (Reprinted with permission from Markam S, Waterhouse T. *Curr Opin Obstet Gynecol.* 1992;4;867–73.)

in infancy with 46,XX DSD conditions are due to excess virilization, and 46,XY DSD conditions are due to under-virilization. Sex chromosome disorders include gonadal dysgenesis; Turner syndrome (45,X); mixed gonadal dysgenesis (45,X/46,XY); Klinefelter's syndrome and variants (47,XXY); and ovotesticular DSD (45,X/46,XY or 46,XX/46,XY). Additional genetic etiologies include mosaicism and chimerism. The causes of DSD can be broadly categorized as sex steroid excess or deficiency due to a central or peripheral etiology, hormonal receptor deficiencies, or atypical or slowed migration of the Müllerian or wolffian ducts (Tables 7.2 and 7.3).

46,XX difference of sexual development conditions

Congenital adrenal hyperplasia

The pathway of conversion of cholesterol into sex steroids is complex and involves multiple enzymes. If an enzymatic process is compromised, then there will be a reduction in the product. Due to decreased downstream by-products, there may be upregulation of the precursors, which may

result in congenital adrenal hyperplasia (CAH) and higher or lower levels of testosterone, dihydrotestosterone, and estrogen (Figure 7.2).

21-Hydroxylase deficiency is an autosomal recessive condition involving the *CYP21A2* gene. The worldwide incidence of homozygous CAH is close to 1:15,000 and for heterozygous CAH is 1:60. The Alaskan Yupik Eskimo population has the highest incidence of CAH of 1:131. The carrier rate for mutations in the *CYP21A2* gene for the Yupik population may be as high as 1:10 to 1:25.[5,6]

21-Hydroxylase deficiency results in an underproduction of cortisol and aldosterone, which increases adreno-corticotropic hormone (ACTH). Increased ACTH induces adrenal hyperplasia and overproduction of 17-hydroxy-progesterone (17-OHP) and testosterone. The impact of elevated testosterone is not externally evident in the 46,XY newborn; however, the 46,XX newborn will demonstrate virilization of the external genitalia. Due to life-threatening hypoglycemia and hyponatremia associated with classic salt-wasting CAH, universal screening is performed in

Table 7.2 46,XX causes of difference of sex development (DSD) conditions.

Disorders of gonadal development	Testicular DSD (*SRY* positive)
	Ovotesticular DSD
	Gonadal dysgenesis
Disorders in androgen synthesis or action	**Excess androgen effect**
	Congenital adrenal hyperplasia
	21-Hydroxylase deficiency
	11-Hydroxylase deficiency
	3β-Hydroxysteroid dehydrogenase deficiency
	Fetoplacental
	Aromatase deficiency
	Maternal etiology
	Maternal adrenal, ovarian tumors, or luteoma
	Maternal congenital adrenal hyperplasia
	Exogenous exposure
	Ingestion of progestins and androgens
	Testosterone creams
Central hormone deficiencies	Panhypopituitarism
	Growth hormone
	Adrenocorticotropic hormone deficiencies
	Kallmann syndrome
Field effects	Cloacal anomalies
	Epispadias
	Mayer-Rokitansky-Küster-Hauser
	Vaginal atresia

Table 7.3 46,XY Causes of difference of sex development (DSD) conditions.

Disorders of gonadal development	Gonadal dysgenesis (Swyer: complete, partial)
	Gonadal regression (vanishing testes)
	Ovotesticular DSD
	Testicular DSD (*SRY* positive, duplicate *SOX9*)
Disorders in androgen synthesis or action	**Decreased androgen effect**
	Androgen insensitivity syndrome (partial or complete)
	Testosterone biosynthesis defect
	17β-Hydroxysteroid hydrogenase type 3 deficiency
	3β-Hydroxysteroid Dehydrogenase deficiency
	17α-Hydroxylase or 17.20 lyase deficiency
	Congenital lipoid adrenal hyperplasia
	5α-Reductase deficiency
	Receptor defects
	Androgen receptor: Complete or partial androgen insensitivity
	Luteinizing-hormone receptor Leydig cell hypoplasia or aplasia
	Anti-Müllerian hormone deficiency or receptor defect: persistent Müllerian duct syndrome
	Maternal exposures
	Progestins, spironolactone, phenytoin, cimetidine
Central hormone deficiencies	Panhypopituitarism
	Growth hormone deficiency
	Adrenocorticotropic hormone deficiency
	Kallmann syndrome
Field effects	Cloacal anomalies
	Hypospadias

the United States and results in many infants being diagnosed at birth.

Medical treatment includes administration of cortisol and mineralocorticoid to prevent salt wasting, adrenal insufficiency, precocious puberty, and progressive virilization. Infants and children are treated with hydrocortisone to replete cortisol and with fludrocortisone to replete mineralocorticoids. Stress-dose steroids are given to prevent adrenal crisis during infection, trauma, and surgery. Longer-acting steroid repletion may include prednisone or dexamethasone after adult height is achieved. After puberty, females may also use antiandrogens and combination estrogen and progestin contraceptives to decrease hyperandrogenism.[7] Consultation with a reproductive endocrinologist to adjust medication to improve ovulation may increase fertility for those women with CAH who desire pregnancy.[8,9] Given the urogenital sinus and consequent vaginal narrowing, women with CAH do have higher rates of cesarean delivery.[10]

11β-Hydroxylase deficiency is caused by a mutation in the *CYP11B1* gene, which results in increased 11-deoxycortisol and mild elevation in 17-OHP. Presenting 46,XX infants may have mild virilization and later may develop hypertension and hypokalemia.

3β-Hydroxysteroid dehydrogenase deficiency type 2 is caused by a deleterious *HSD3B2* gene. This results in low cortisol and aldosterone and, consequently, salt wasting with adrenal insufficiency. The 46,XX infants may have mild clitoromegaly.

P450 oxidoreductase deficiency, also known as *POR*, results in virilization of the 46,XX individual as well as possible salt wasting and adrenal crisis. Serum levels of 17-OHP and 17-hydroxypregnenolone may be elevated, and dehydroepiandrosterone (DHEA) and androstenedione levels may be low.

Exogenous intrauterine exposure

Excess androgen exposure resulting in virilization of the genitalia of a 46,XX patient may be a result of antenatal androgen exposure only during gestation. This may be related to the production of androgen from a maternal ovarian luteoma or tumor in pregnancy or may be related to environmental exposures, including inadvertent exposure to testosterone gels or creams. The mother should be asked about any medications used in pregnancy, including teratogens (i.e., phenytoin), as well as endocrine medications (i.e., danazol and progestins).

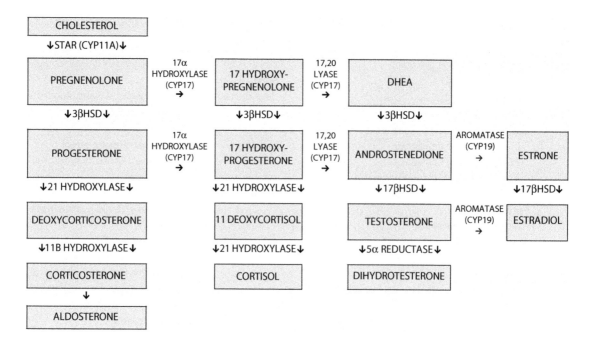

Figure 7.2 Sex steroid biosynthesis pathway.

Central hormone deficiencies

Central hormone deficiencies include decreased gonadotropin-releasing hormone or LH production. This may result in decreased gonadal hormonal production *in utero*, resulting in ambiguous external genitalia at birth or pubertal delay. The etiologies include panhypopituitarism or more isolated deficiencies in growth hormone, ACTH, or gonadotropin-releasing hormone (Kallmann syndrome). Often patients with Kallmann syndrome will present with pubertal delay. Associated findings include midline congenital anomalies (i.e., cleft palate) and anosmia.

Placental aromatase deficiency

Aromatase converts testosterone to estradiol and androstenedione to estrone. Aromatase deficiency is an autosomal recessive condition and results in virilization of the 46,XX infant due to reduced placental ability to convert precursors to estrogens, with high levels of placental testosterone and androstenedione. Adolescents may present with hypergonadotropic hypogonadism and progressive virilization.[11] Additionally, the mother may experience virilization during pregnancy.

Field effects

Cell migration during fetal development may be impaired and result in differences in the development of the external genitalia or internal reproductive structures. These conditions are also associated with multiple other anomalies.[12] For example, genitourinary anomalies are common with VACTERL or VATER association, which represents vertebral anomalies, anorectal malformation, cardiovascular anomalies, tracheoesophageal fistula, esophageal atresia, renal anomalies, and limb anomalies. In 46,XX individuals, Mayer-Rokitansky-Küster-Hauser syndrome, which

occurs in 1:4000–1:5000 females, is associated with renal, spine, and ear anomalies.[13] Cloacal anomalies, including cloacal exstrophy or bladder exstrophy, are less common. Typically, these patients will have normal ovarian function but often have underdevelopment or anomalies of the clitorophallus, labia, vagina, or uteri.[14]

Other

SRY translocation, *SOX9* duplication, and ovotesticular DSD are rare causes of 46,XX DSD with virilization. Each is associated with testicular hormone production, which can be measured by assessment of serum AMH, inhibin B, and testosterone levels, the latter which may be elevated after a HCG stimulation test.

46,XY difference of sexual development conditions

The 46,XY DSD conditions are characterized by the lack of virilization of the external genitalia.

Receptor deficiencies

Androgen insensitivity syndrome: Androgen receptor dysfunction is caused by mutations in the androgen receptor (*AR*) gene with an incidence of 1:20,000 to 1:64,000 births. Androgen insensitivity syndrome may present as female phenotype in complete androgen insensitivity (CAIS), ambiguous genitalia in partial androgen insensitivity (PAIS), and hypospadias or mild undervirilization in males. Due to AMH production by the testes, the uterus and upper vagina are absent. Given the lack of testosterone effect on the external genitalia, individuals may have typical external female genitalia with CAIS or clitoromegaly and urogenital sinus present with PAIS. Although women with CAIS have testes and levels of testosterone that are higher than the typical male range, they have systemic estrogen through peripheral aromatization of testosterone. Adolescents with CAIS often present with primary amenorrhea. Physical exam reveals typical breast development, vulvar appearance, and fat distribution, but individuals have little to no pubic hair or other signs of adrenarche.[15]

The *AR* gene is located on the X chromosomes (Xq11–12). Many adults have received the clinical diagnosis of CAIS or PAIS without genetic testing; confirmatory testing should be encouraged to exclude other causes of 46,XY DSDs.[16]

AMH receptor defect: Persistent Müllerian duct syndrome is associated with an AMH receptor defect. Usually this is not associated with ambiguous external genitalia but is discovered when Müllerian structures are identified in evaluation for a hernia or undescended testis. This condition is autosomal recessive due to a mutation in the *AMH* gene, location 19p13.3, or the receptor gene, *AMHR2*, location 12q13.13.

Luteinizing hormone receptor defect: HCG stimulates the Leydig cells to produce testosterone. Leydig cell hypoplasia is notable for absent or low levels of Leydig cells with high levels of LH and follicle-stimulating hormone (FSH), and low levels of testosterone. This has been associated with a LH receptor defect. The Sertoli cells will produce AMH; therefore, affected individuals do not have internal Müllerian structures. Clitorophallic enlargement will occur with testosterone supplementation.[17]

Decreased androgen synthesis

To convert cholesterol to testosterone and dihydrotestosterone, multiple enzymes are essential, and enzymatic dysfunction may result in undervirilization (Figure 7.1). DSD conditions associated with abnormal androgen production include 5α-reductase type 2 deficiency (5αRDS), 17β-hydroxysteroid dehydrogenase type 3 deficiency (17βHSD), 3β-hydroxysteroid dehydrogenase deficiency II (3βHSD), and 17α-hydroxylase/17,20 lyase deficiency.

5α-Reductase Type 2 Deficiency (5αRDS) is an autosomal recessive condition that prevents conversion of testosterone to the more potent dihydrotestosterone. Dihydrotestosterone drives the virilization of the external genitalia. Therefore, 46,XY patients with 5αRDS may present with ambiguous genitalia at birth, often with the testes in the inguinal canals or labioscrotal folds. Alternately, patients may present at puberty with the onset of virilization from elevated testosterone. Due to AMH production by the testes, the Müllerian structures will be absent, and the wolffian-derived structures are typically well developed. There is a wide spectrum of prepubertal external phenotype of 5αRDS from typical female external genitalia to male phenotype with hypospadias.[18] At puberty, there is progressive masculine pubertal changes, including deepening of the voice, increased muscle mass, and male pattern hair growth. Gender assignment for 5αRDS is challenging, as there are reports of adolescents raised female identifying as male in adolescence.[19,20]

Testing for 5αRDS includes assessment of the testosterone-to-dihydrotestosterone ratio. The normal ratio in the newborn is 4:1; infants with this disorder may have ratios closer to 14:1.[3] Mutations in the *SRD5A2* gene, located on 2p23.1, have been identified. This condition is more common in communities in the Dominican Republic, Papua New Guinea, Turkey, and Egypt. Although uncommon, there may be potential for fertility in some individuals.[21,22]

17β-Hydroxysteroid dehydrogenase type 3 deficiency (17βHSD) reduces the enzymatic conversion of androstenedione to testosterone (Figure 7.1). It is an autosomal recessive condition that may present at birth with typical female genitalia or ambiguous genitalia, or in childhood with inguinal hernia. At puberty, there is progressive virilization with enlargement of the clitorophallus and labioscrotal tissue, deepening of the voice, increased muscle mass, and male pattern hair growth. Hormonal testing in mini-puberty or in adolescence will reveal elevated androstenedione levels and low testosterone levels. Androstenedione levels prepubertally may be normal, however. Genetic testing for the *17βHSD3* gene, located at 9p22.32, may confirm the diagnosis.

46,XY 3β-Hydroxysteroid dehydrogenase type 2 deficiency (3βHSD). The 3β-hydroxysteroid dehydrogenase converts pregnenolone to progesterone, 17-hydroxypregnenolone to 17-hydroxyprogesterone, and DHEA to androstenedione. The *3βHSD* results in decreased aldosterone, cortisol, androgens, and estrogen. This enzymatic deficiency may occur on a spectrum in 46,XY individuals with phenotype variation from typical female genitalia to ambiguous genitalia to typical male genitalia. Regardless of appearance, there is a risk of salt-wasting crisis with this condition. Testing for a mutation of *HSD3B2* gene, located on 1p12, may confirm the diagnosis.

17α-Hydroxylase/17.20 lyase deficiency is caused by a mutation in the cytochrome P450c17 gene (*CYP17A1*). The gene is located at 10q24.32. The CYP17A1 enzyme converts pregnenolone to 17-hydroxypregnenolone and progesterone to 17-hydroxyprogesterone by hydroxylation. Also, 17,20 lyase activity converts 17-hydroxypregnenolone to DHEA (Figure 7.1). A genetic mutation may result in deficiency in hydroxylation and/or lyase reactions. This results in low androgen and estrogen levels. Affected 46,XY individuals appear phenotypically female with absent Müllerian structures and typical external female genitalia. Individuals not identified at birth may present with pubertal delay. Cortisol synthesis is blocked, but due to elevated ACTH, there is an increase in aldosterone with resultant hypokalemia and hypertension. Glucocorticoid treatment addresses the ACTH overproduction and, therefore, suppresses corticosterone overproduction. Sex steroid hormonal induction and maintenance are necessary at puberty.

P450 oxidoreductase deficiency, also known as POR, may lead to salt wasting and adrenal crisis. Serum levels of 17-OHP and 17-hydroxypregnenolone may be elevated, and DHEA and androstenedione levels may be low. Testosterone levels will be low in 46,XY individuals, resulting in undervirilization and delayed puberty.

Gonadal dysgenesis

The clinical diagnosis of gonadal dysgenesis includes either the complete failure of the gonads to differentiate into a functional ovary or testes, or partial differentiation with premature cessation of hormonal function. The cessation may occur in utero or prior to puberty; although some individuals may partially progress through puberty, they have early onset gonadal insufficiency.

Complete gonadal dysgenesis with a 46,XY karyotype is the result of failure of the gonadal tissues to develop into functioning testicular tissue. As a result, there is no Sertoli production of AMH and no Leydig cell production of testosterone. Müllerian structures develop, and external genitalia appear typical for a female. This clinical condition is named *Swyer syndrome*. Often these individuals are identified with pubertal delay and elevated gonadotropins or when they present with a gonadoblastoma. *SRY* gene mutations have been identified in 15% of individuals with Swyer syndrome. Additional mutations associated with 46,XY complete gonadal dysgenesis have been identified in the *MAP3K1, DHH,* and *NR5A1* genes (Table 7.1).

Partial gonadal dysgenesis: The 46,XY partial gonadal dysgenesis and testicular regression syndrome usually present with genital ambiguity in the newborn period. Given the presence of some testicular function early in embryologic development, there may be regression of the Müllerian structures. If this occurs late in utero, the condition has been named testicular regression or vanishing testes syndrome.

Central hormone deficiencies

Central hormone deficiencies include congenital hypogonadotropic hypogonadism. Similar to the 46,XX individual, the 46,XY individual will have decreased gonadal hormonal production in utero. This may present with cryptorchidism and microphallus or with pubertal delay. The etiologies include panhypopituitarism or more isolated deficiencies in growth hormone, ACTH, or gonadotropin-releasing hormone (Kallmann syndrome). Mutations in the Kallmann syndrome genes have been associated with 46,XY DSDs, including isolated hypospadias.[23]

Field effects

46,XY individuals may have an absent or underdeveloped clitorophallus or scrotum. Hypospadias, the most common external genital anomaly, is included in this category. It is important to note that if a hypospadias is proximal or associated with undescended testes, additional investigation for a genetic etiology should be pursued, particularly for partial androgen insensitivity syndrome and 5α-reductase deficiency. 46,XY cloacal exstrophy may be associated with complete absence of the phallus and scrotum. It is important to note that although the external genitalia are underdeveloped, the testes have typical function.

Sex chromosome disorders

Turner syndrome

The most common etiology for patients presenting with primary amenorrhea with pubertal delay is Turner syndrome.[24] Turner syndrome affects 1:2500 live-born female infants and is diagnosed with physical findings combined with complete or partial absence of a sex chromosome.[25] These chromosome abnormalities may be detected prenatally by fetal karyotype; however, diagnosis must be confirmed postnatally with physical findings including nuchal folds, edema, cardiac or renal anomalies, and short stature. It is the most common etiology for primary amenorrhea for adolescents age 16 years and older.[26,27] Some individuals with Turner syndrome will be able to enter puberty spontaneously and even menstruate; therefore, they may not be diagnosed until they experience early ovarian insufficiency or recurrent pregnancy loss.

The most common chromosomal anomaly associated with Turner syndrome is monosomy X (45,X), but 7%–10% of patients may have Y chromatin present. Additional testing for mosaicism with a Y chromosome should be considered, particularly when there is a marker present (a fragment of a sex chromosome of uncertain X or Y origin) or if there is virilization noted on physical exam. The presence of Y chromatin is associated with an increased risk of gonadoblastoma and is an indication for gonadectomy.[28,29]

Early identification of Turner syndrome can allow time for growth hormone therapy, which may increase adult height by 0–11 cm (on average 7 cm) over untreated controls.[30,31] Although 30% of girls will experience spontaneous puberty, most experience early gonadal failure; therefore, induction of puberty with low-dose estradiol treatment is typically required until menarche. After menarche, combination estrogen and progestin therapy can prevent osteoporosis.[32,33] Pregnancies with donor egg are possible for patients with Turner syndrome; however, there is a risk of aortic dissection. Cardiac evaluation is essential prior to any pregnancy.[26,34–37]

Ovotesticular DSD

Ovotesticular DSD is diagnosed by the presence of ovarian and testicular tissue, either in the same or opposite gonads. 46,XX/46,XY chimerism may result in ovotesticular DSD, although the most common karyotype is 46,XX followed by 46,XX/46,XY chimerism, and 46,XY karyotype. Although a range from typical male to typical female phenotypes has been described, most individuals are identified with genital ambiguity at birth. The labioscrotal folds may be asymmetric, and a uterus and vagina are often present.

CLINICAL EVALUATION OF THE PATIENT WITH DIFFERENCE OF SEXUAL DEVELOPMENT

History

Family history: A detailed family history is critical in the assessment of an infant with ambiguous genitalia or an adolescent with atypical pubertal development. Specific questions include whether there is a history of known congenital anomalies, including renal and gynecologic anomalies, male or female infertility, primary amenorrhea or pubertal delay, or gonadal tumors. Additionally, parents should be asked about any history of DSD or early neonatal death. For example, 46,XY individuals with congenital adrenal hyperplasia do not appear with ambiguous genitalia; therefore, the infant may have died prior to diagnosis. Additionally, a family history of polycystic ovarian syndrome (PCOS) is important, as often symptoms of PCOS are seen with nonclassic CAH.[6]

The history should include questions regarding consanguinity and region of origin associated with a high incidence of autosomal recessive genes. For example, Yupik Alaska has a high rate of CAH, the Dominican Republican has a high rate of 5αRDS, and the Gaza strip has a high rate of 17 βHSD deficiency.[5]

Prenatal history: Virilization may occur from a maternal source, including a luteoma, an androgen-secreting tumor, or another virilizing condition. The mother should be asked about any noteworthy virilization during pregnancy, including excessive acne, hirsutism, deepening of the voice, or clitoromegaly. A detailed history should include exogenous exposures to hormones in pregnancy, which may include use of synthetic progestins or spironolactone, or contact with a family member using testosterone cream. The parents should be asked about assisted reproductive technology and medications. Endocrine disrupters have also been implicated in reproductive tract anomalies; therefore, asking about environmental exposures is essential. Finally, a detailed history of any complications of pregnancy that may increase the risks of fetal malformations is warranted, as some field effects have been associated with maternal diabetes, pregnancy-induced hypertension, abnormal placentation, and multiple gestation. Additionally, preterm birth and low birth weight are both risk factors for cryptorchidism.[38]

Medical history: A careful history of other anomalies is important to assess for syndromes associated with DSD conditions. Although a unified genetic etiology has not been identified for VATER and VACTERL association, the association often includes anomalies of the external genitalia, vagina, and Müllerian structures. Additionally, any history of neonatal hypoglycemia or jaundice may indicate hypopituitarism or growth hormone deficiencies.

Pubertal history: For the adolescent patient, careful questioning of the progress of puberty is critical. Patients should be asked about the onset of thelarche and pubarche. Symptoms of progressive androgenization include enlargement of the clitoris, erections of clitoral tissue, deepening of the voice, male pattern adrenarche, and acne. The patient should be asked about any history of pain or swelling in the labia or the inguinal region, which can indicate a hernia and an inguinal or labial gonad. Finally, symptoms of recurrent urinary incontinence or recurrent urinary tract infections may indicate vaginal reflux of urine with a urogenital sinus. Privately, the adolescent should be asked about difficulty with placing tampons or penetrative intercourse, which may be related to an anatomic etiology.

Surgical history: Patients should be asked about any prior history of genital surgery or any history of herniorrhaphy. Although the incidence of androgen insensitivity syndrome is 1:20,000 in the general population, for girls who have had an inguinal herniorrhaphy, the rate may be as high as 2.4%.[39]

Physical examination

Any hormonal excess in a 46,XX individual may cause external virilization, or any deficiency of hormonal function in a 46,XY may cause undervirilization. It is very important to note that any of these changes appear on a spectrum, and therefore, findings may be very subtle. A careful physical examination can provide clear information about the possible etiology of the DSD condition.

Vital signs: Head circumference, weight, and length in the newborn may reflect growth restriction. In the older child, the height measurement may reveal short stature (associated with Turner syndrome) or an early growth spurt (associated with CAH with early onset puberty). Blood pressure may be elevated with steroidogenic enzyme deficiencies.

General physical examination: A complete head-to-toe examination with attention to any other associated anomalies, including dysmorphic features, eye or ear anomalies, cleft lip or palate, cardiac murmur, and limb anomalies, can help to determine whether the patient has an underlying syndrome or VACTERL association. In the child or adolescent, skin examination may reveal acne or hirsutism (associated with CAH) or may reveal minimal or absent pubarche or adrenarche (associated with androgen insensitivity).

Sexual maturity (Tanner) staging: In the adolescent, careful staging is necessary to assess for presence and degree of thelarche, adrenarche, and pubarche. The presence of adrenarche indicates that the androgen receptor is at least partially sensitive to androgens, and the presence of thelarche typically indicates gonadal hormonal production, either estrogen from the ovary or from aromatization of testosterone produced by the testes into estrogen.

Genital examination: Genital examinations for patients with DSD conditions may be embarrassing and stressful. Adolescent and adult patients have reported humiliation associated with photography, multiple examiners, or repeated examinations. Care should be taken to minimize the trauma that may be associated with genital examinations. A clear explanation of the reason to perform the examination should be given and only with parental and/or patient agreement. After diagnosis, further examinations should be performed only when necessary and when there is clear patient benefit. The number of examiners should be limited, and care should be taken so that the examination is performed with the least amount of discomfort and embarrassment for the patient.

Given the complexity and variation of sex differentiation, it is not surprising that there is significant overlap in

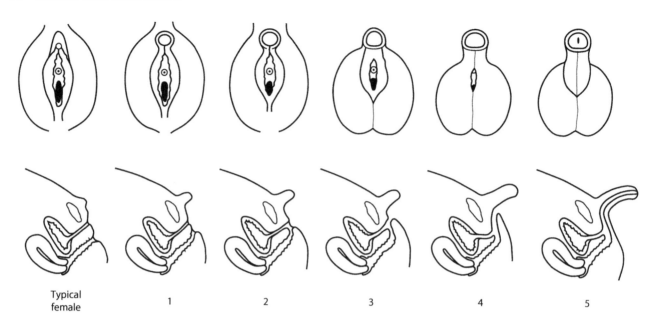

Figure 7.3 Prader staging of degree of virilization of the 46,XX individual. (Adapted from Allen L. *Obstet Gynecol Clin N Amer.* 2009;36:25–45.)

genital examination findings between different etiologies. A careful and detailed examination may provide many clues to the type of disorder as well as the timing of *in utero* androgen exposure. There are two standardized methods for reporting the extent of virilization or under-virilization: Prader staging (Figure 7.3) and the external masculinization score (EMS) (Table 7.4).[40,41] In general, Prader staging is useful to communicate the extent of virilization of the 46,XX patient, and the EMS is useful to classify the degree of undervirilization of the 46,XY patient. The genital examination provides essential clues to the underlying etiology and includes multiple critical components.

Table 7.4 External masculinization score (EMS) used to describe the degree of genital virilization.

Feature		Points
Scrotal fusion	Yes	3
	No	0
Micropenis	Yes	0
	No	3
Urethral meatus	Normal	3
	Glandular	2
	Penile	1
	Perineal	0
Right and left gonad score (score for each)	Scrotal	1.5
	Inguinal	1
	Abdominal	0.5
	Absent	0

Source: See Ahmed S et al. *BJU Int.* 2000;85:120–4.

Note: An EMS score of 12 is considered typical male virilization, 7–11 indicates mild undervirilization, and less than 7 is reflective of ambiguous genitalia.

Assessment of the clitorophallus: It is important to note that palpation of the corporal tissue is the most accurate method for assessing width and length of the corporal tissue. In the newborn, swelling of the labia and the clitoral hood may be misleading; therefore, care must be taken to retract the clitoral hood if the tissue is edematous to assess for true clitoromegaly. For the most accurate measurement, the clitorophallus should be stretched and measured from the pubic ramus to the tip of the glans (stretched length). The width should be measured in the midshaft. The tethering of the clitorophallus on the ventral side by residual urethral tissue is called a *chordee*, and this may prevent stretching to assess the length. If stretching the tissue is not possible, palpating the corporal tissue is an option. For a term male infant, a typical stretched phallic length is >2.5 cm and width is >0.9 mm. Stretched length less than 2 cm is considered a microphallus. For a term female infant, clitoromegaly is defined as width greater than 6 mm and length greater than 9 mm. It is important to note that this is impacted by gestational age, gestational size (large or small for gestational age), and twinning.[42]

Presence and degree of posterior fusion of the labioscrotal tissue: With early androgen exposure *in utero* in the first trimester, the labioscrotal folds may fuse from the posterior to anterior direction. The degree of fusion may range from mild posterior fusion of the labia majora to complete fusion, which mimics a scrotal appearance. Additionally, high androgen exposure may result in hyperpigmentation and rugation of the labioscrotal folds, which may suggest CAH. If the phallus is below the labioscrotal folds, this is called penoscrotal transposition. The labia minora may fuse over the glans of the clitorophallus.

Location of the urethra and vagina: Determining the location of the urethra and vagina with particular attention to the degree of separation of the structures is most important. A persistent urogenital sinus occurs when the urethra and vagina do not separate distally. There may be the presence of a normal upper vagina and cervix, which is typical for 46,XX patients with CAH, or there may be a blind ending vagina. In the male, hypospadias is the presence of a urethral opening below the tip of the glans, which may range from a mild glandular hypospadias to a perineal hypospadias. The length of the urogenital sinus prior to separation into the urethra and the vagina is important for surgical planning to achieve a separate vaginal opening. Measurement of this length often requires an endoscopic examination or genitourethrogram.

Location of the gonads: All patients being evaluated for a DSD condition should have careful palpation of both inguinal regions and labia for the presence or absence of gonadal tissue. If there are palpable gonads in the labia, this is highly suggestive of a 46,XY karyotype, although hernias with ovaries and uterine structures are also found in 46,XX individuals.

Position of the anus in relation to the anal muscle complex: This is important to assess for anorectal malformations. Additionally, the anogenital distance can be measured from the center of the anus to the junction of smooth perineal skin and rugated skin of the posterior convergence of the fourchette. The average length is 1 cm in newborn females and 2 cm in newborn males.[43]

Sexual maturity (Tanner) staging: In the adolescent, careful staging is necessary to assess for presence and degree of thelarche, adrenarche, and pubarche. The presence of adrenarche indicates that the androgen receptor is at least partially sensitive to androgens, and the presence of thelarche typically indicates gonadal hormonal production, either estrogen from the ovary or from aromatization of testosterone produced by the testes into estrogen.

Imaging

Ultrasound: A pelvic ultrasound to assess for the presence of the uterus is more sensitive in the newborn given the maternal stimulation of the endometrium and relative enlargement of the uterus. After the maternal estrogenization recedes, the uterus shrinks prior to puberty and can be difficult to image with ultrasound. It is important to note that the inability to image the uterus prior to puberty is not diagnostic for Müllerian agenesis.[44] Ultrasound may be able to identify the location of testes, but this may not be accurate. Additionally, ultrasound is important to assess for renal anomalies, which can be associated with Müllerian anomalies and with Turner syndrome.

Genitourethrogram: The genitourethrogram is a fluoroscopic study where dye is injected into the perineal opening to assess the presence of the vagina or prostatic utricle and to assess the length of the urogenital sinus.[45]

Magnetic resonance imaging: Magnetic resonance imaging (MRI) is particularly useful for the adolescent with primary amenorrhea and 46,XX karyotype, where Müllerian agenesis is suspected and ultrasound is unable to visualize a uterus. The MRI can assess for rudimentary uterine structures and whether there is functional endometrium

present.[46,47] Given that MRI requires sedation for infants and young children, ultrasound is seen as the preferential initial screening tool.

Laboratory testing

Karyotype evaluation

In an infant with ambiguous genitalia, on day of life one, a stat karyotype should be sent immediately with fluorescence in situ hybridization (FISH) for the *SRY* gene. Typically, the preliminary karyotype will be available in 48 hours, and this can guide additional hormonal testing. FISH may also allow detection of mosaicism or *SRY* translocation to an *X* gene. Although rapid and useful, it is essential that FISH be confirmed with complete karyotype.

Hormonal testing

On day of life one, testosterone and dihydrotestosterone levels can be sent, as these levels will fall quickly after birth. If CAH is suspected, then on day of life two or three, a 17-hydroxyprogesterone, 17-hydroxypregnenolone, DHEA, androstenedione, and plasma renin activity can be drawn. Additionally, testing for sodium and potassium daily to assess for salt-wasting crisis is essential.[3]

To assess the etiology for undervirilization in a 46,XY individual, gonadal dysgenesis may be assessed by testing the FSH level. Gonadotropins are typically suppressed immediately at birth; therefore, FSH and LH are best assessed after the first week of life. Between weeks 2 and 8, typical males have a physiologic testosterone surge. This mini-puberty is a window of opportunity to assess gonadal function and for 5α-reductase deficiency, androgen insensitivity, or a LH receptor defect. The AMH level can assess for Sertoli cell function. To assess for a testosterone biosynthesis defect, a HCG stimulation test can be administered. HCG binds the LH receptor and should increase serum testosterone produced by the Leydig cells.[48] There also may be an increase in clitorophallic size with this test. To assess for 5α-reductase deficiency, a testosterone-to-dihydrotestosterone ratio may be measured. A normal ratio is less than 8:1; however, it is important to note that the testosterone level must be high enough for this to be accurately interpreted. See Table 7.5 to review the optimal timing of laboratory assessment of the infant. After hormonal testing, specific genetic testing aimed at the suspected underlying etiology can confirm the diagnosis.

The combination of karyotype, physical exam, imaging, and hormonal assessment allows the narrowing of the differential diagnoses. Refer to Figure 7.4 for the approach to the newborn with ambiguous genitalia, Figure 7.5 for the approach for the patient with pubertal delay, and Figure 7.6 for the approach to the patient with primary amenorrhea.

GENERAL APPROACH TO THE CARE OF A PATIENT WITH A DSD CONDITION

The first question that is usually asked after the delivery of a newborn is "Is it a boy or a girl?" However, if the genitalia is ambiguous, the answer should not be a guess. The first step is to avoid making any assumptions without

Table 7.5 Ideal time frame for testing for infants identified with genital ambiguity.

Time	Test	Why	Notes
Newborn	• Stat karyotype • FISH for SRY	FISH may also allow detection of mosaicism and SRY translocation to an X gene.	Essential that FISH be confirmed with complete karyotype.
Day of life 1	• Testosterone • Dihydrotestosterone		Unstimulated androgen levels may be useful for evaluation of CAH; however, maternal hormones may prevent accurate interpretation. Use liquid chromatography-mass spectrometry to avoid maternal steroid interaction. Follow testing is warranted.
Day of life 2–4	• 17 hydroxyprogesterone • 17-hydroxypregnenolone, Dehydroepiandrosterone (DHEA) • Androsteinedione • Plasma renin activity • Sodium and potassium daily to assess for a salt wasting crisis	Assessment for CAH	
Week 1–2	• Follicle stimulating hormone • Luteinizing hormone	Gonadotropins are typically suppressed immediately at birth	
Weeks 2–12	• Anti-Müllerian hormone level to assess Sertoli cell function • HCG stimulation test to assess testosterone to dihydrotestosterone ratio	The physiologic testosterone surge, alternately called the mini-puberty, occurs from 1–6 months. The mini- puberty is a window of opportunity to assess for gonadal insufficiency, a LH receptor defect, 5 alpha reductase deficiency, and androgen insensitivity.	HCG binds the LH receptor, which stimulates Leydig cells to produce testosterone. There may be an increase in phallic size with the HCG stimulation test. A normal T:DHT ratio is usually 4:1, however it is important to note that the testosterone level must be high enough for this to be accurately interpreted. Infants with 5 alpha reductase deficiency typically have a T:DHT ratio over 10:1.

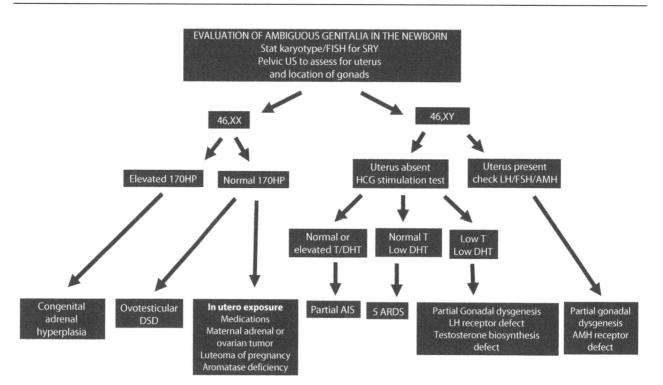

Figure 7.4 Evaluation of ambiguous genitalia in the newborn.

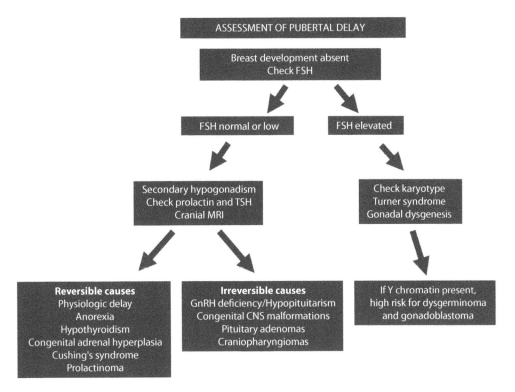

Figure 7.5 Assessment of pubertal delay.

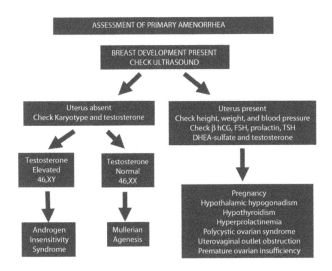

Figure 7.6 Assessment of primary amenorrhea.

further information. Sex assignment should be delayed until the baby has been evaluated by an experienced multidisciplinary team.

Excellent and compassionate communication

The provider should share with the family that there are differences in the appearance of the genitalia and that additional testing is necessary to determine the etiology. All team members should coordinate their discussions to minimize confusion and harmful terms that may anger or scare the family. Flippant statements or guessing about the sex of rearing should be avoided, as these statements can be harmful, misleading, and contribute to confusion.

Given the stress of the uncertainty of undetermined sex of rearing as well as concerns that parents have regarding the health of their baby, emphasize positive statements, including "You have a healthy baby" or "Your baby is healthy and has genital differences. This is not an uncommon finding. Often there are medical explanations for the genital differences."

Terms such as "hermaphrodite" or calling the baby "it" should be avoided. Confusing and controversial terms, including true hermaphrodite, pseudohermaphrodite, XX male, sex reversal, testicular feminization, and undermasculinization, have been replaced with categorization by karyotype and include 46,XY DSD; 46,XX DSD; and sex chromosome DSD. Initially, the term DSD was "disorders of sex development," but more currently, DSD is used to signify "differences of sex development," Some patients and parents will prefer the term "intersex" to "DSD." Refer to Table 7.6 for current terminology describing DSD conditions.[49]

The next step is to reach out to a multidisciplinary DSD team to discuss initial appropriate tests and plan for further evaluation. A stat karyotype with FISH for SRY is particularly helpful to begin narrowing the differential. Testing for congenital adrenal hyperplasia, which is the most common cause of ambiguous genitalia, is particularly important to provide appropriate early treatment to avoid a salt-wasting crisis. Additionally, a pelvic ultrasound in the newborn may be more sensitive for the presence of the uterus given the stimulation of the uterus from maternal hormones.

Involvement of the multidisciplinary team

The family should be scheduled to see a multidisciplinary team, which ideally should include pediatric and

Table 7.6 Current terminology used to describe difference of sexual development (DSD) conditions.

Current terminology	Old terminology
46,XY DSD	Male pseudohermaphrodite
	Undervirilized/undermasculinized male
46,XX DSD	Female pseudohermaphrodite
	Virilized/masculinized female
Ovotesticular DSD	True hermaphrodite
46,XY complete gonadal dysgenesis	XY female
46,XX testicular DSD	XX male
	XX sex reversal
Androgen insensitivity syndrome	Testicular feminization

Source: See further Lee P et al. *Pediatrics.* 2006;118;e488–500.

Note: Terms including hermaphrodite and testicular feminization have been replaced.

adolescent gynecology, pediatric endocrinology, pediatric urology, genetics and genetic counselors, psychology/psychiatry, nursing, social work, ethics, and legal advisors.[50] Key members of the team should meet with the family to obtain a detailed history and to examine the child. The team should review all the tests, discuss the results and the physical examination findings together, and be able to come to a consensus with the family on sex of rearing as soon as possible. If the sex of rearing cannot be recommended at this initial visit, then close follow-up with the family is essential.[51]

Early involvement of psychosocial support

Early involvement of mental health support is critical, ideally from a psychologist or psychiatrist with experience caring for families impacted by DSD conditions. Parents of children with ambiguous genitalia report increased levels of stress, anxiety, and depression, and later report post-traumatic stress disorder.[52] Early referral to peer support networks may be especially helpful to help families to understand that they are not alone. Close follow-up with parents is essential to increase their knowledge and acceptance of their child's condition, as well as to provide ample support so they can best nurture and support their child.[53]

Education of patient and family

Age-appropriate discussions with ongoing education are necessary and required for children and adolescents to understand their condition.[54,55] As patients age and their ability to comprehend biology increases, more precise explanation of their condition should be revisited. Patients with DSD conditions require ongoing support throughout their lives.[56]

Understanding gender identity

Assigning sex of rearing is a complex decision-making process that is evolving with more precise diagnoses of DSD conditions.[57] Gender identity is not expressed until the patient is older. Although most individuals identify with their sex of rearing, gender dysphoria is more common in patients with DSD conditions, particularly 17βHSD, 5αRDS, partial androgen insensitivity syndrome, and congenital adrenal hyperplasia.[55,58–60] Gender identity should not be assumed, even with conditions associated with low rates of gender dysphoria, such as complete androgen insensitivity syndrome.[61] As the patients age, they will begin to express their gender identity and voice their own opinions. The provider should ask patients what pronouns they prefer and follow their guidance. Each individual with a DSD condition is unique and should be supported in their identity.[62]

MANAGEMENT
Goals of therapy

In general, the goal of medical and surgical treatment should be to minimize physical and psychosocial risk for the child, preserve potential for fertility, and preserve or increase the capacity for a satisfying sex life. Providers should understand that the child will grow to express their gender identity and should also consider and respect the cultural background, beliefs, and wishes of the family.[63,64]

Given the heterogeneity of DSD conditions and the limited long-term outcomes research of surgery, clear consensus about the best timing for surgical intervention has not been established.[65] Surgeons with expertise in the care of children and specific training in the surgery of DSDs should perform these procedures. The goal of surgery should focus on functional outcome rather than strictly cosmesis. All procedures involve risk of complications and may require additional surgical intervention later. Given that gender identity may not be clear until a patient is older, some have advocated for delaying surgery until gender identity has been established and the patient can be involved in the surgical decision-making process. Any discussion about surgical intervention should include a clear discussion of expected benefits, known short- and long-term risks, and the pros and cons of delaying surgery until the patient is older.

Surgical and nonsurgical options

Urogenital sinus surgery: For patients with a urogenital sinus, there is a solitary opening for the urethra and the vagina. The two structures remain joined distally through the confluence where the two structures separate. In general, the higher the Prader stage externally, the longer is the urogenital sinus. The urogenital sinus results in hydrocolpos in some individuals due to reflux of urine and may also result in subsequent leaking of urine. A persistent urogenital sinus impedes tampon usage and penetrative vaginal intercourse. To achieve a separate vaginal and urethral opening, the most common procedures include flap vaginoplasty and urogenital sinus mobilization.

Flap vaginoplasty is used for a shorter urogenital sinus. A wide, omega-shaped perineal flap is mobilized, and the

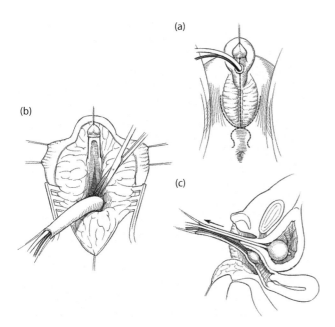

Figure 7.7 The partial urogenital sinus mobilization. (a) Catheters are placed into the bladder and proximal vagina through the urogenital sinus. (b) The urogenital sinus is mobilized. (c) The vagina and urethra are mobilized distally to provide two separate openings at the perineum. (Reproduced with permission from Rink R et al. *J Pediatr Urol.* 2006;2:351–6.)

posterior wall of the urogenital sinus is then dissected. The flap is advanced to the level of the proximal posterior vagina.[66] This procedure is commonly performed with Y-V advancement labiaplasty, which separates the fused labia majora and advances them distally to separate the labia and widen the vaginal introitus.

The urogenital sinus mobilization involves dissecting anteriorly to the urethra and posteriorly to the vagina, and moving the urogenital sinus *en bloc* distally to the perineum. This brings the confluence distally (Figure 7.7).[67–69]

Clitoral surgery: Surgical techniques used to decrease the size of an enlarged clitoris have included total clitorectomy, clitoral recession, and clitoroplasty.[70] Due to concerns about loss of sensation with clitoral surgery, current techniques aim to preserve the glans and preserve the neurovascular bundle while decreasing the corporal tissue.[71–73]

Vaginal dilation and surgery: Most patients with a well-developed distal vagina, for example, patients with CAIS and Mayer-Rokitansky-Küster-Hauser syndrome, are able to elongate the vagina without surgery through primary vaginal dilation with dilators or coital activity.[74] With proper coaching and support, 86%–95% of patients will achieve adequate vaginal length with primary vaginal dilation alone.[75] Compared to vaginoplasty, there is no significant difference in sexual desire, arousal, and satisfaction, but dilation is more cost effective than surgical intervention ($796 versus $18,520) and has much lower risk of complications.[76] The process of vaginal dilation

should be delayed until after puberty and when the patient herself is ready and committed to the process.

Vaginoplasty has been used for patients who have not been able to achieve adequate vaginal length for comfortable sexual activity with dilation alone or for patients where a vaginal dimple or distal vagina is not present. Refer to Chapter 6 regarding vaginoplasty techniques.

Gonadal surgery: The purposes of gonadectomy include treating or preventing a gonadal tumor, or decreasing virilization in a patient who identifies female with testes.[77] For patients with Y chromatin present, there may be an increased risk of gonadal tumor development. The risk of gonadal malignancy is based on the underlying etiology, with dysgenetic gonadal tissue conferring the greatest risk (Table 7.7). The highest risk of tumor development is in dysgenetic gonadal tissue; therefore when there is no potential for fertility or hormonal function, gonadectomy is recommended.[78] For patients with a low risk of tumor, including androgen insensitivity syndrome, retaining the testes will allow spontaneous pubertal progression with a low risk of tumor development through adolescence.[79] Given the low risk of tumor with CAIS, current recommendation is that gonadectomy should be delayed until the patient can consent to the procedure.

The best method for monitoring for tumor development with in situ testes is unclear. Orchiopexy may be an option to permit self-examination. Alternatively, surveillance by imaging and biopsies may be reasonable, although there

Table 7.7 Risk of gonadoblastoma can vary based on the underlying etiology.

Risk	Type of disorder of sexual development (DSD)	Prevalence of tumor (%)
High	Gonadal dysgenesis	15%–35%
	intra-abdominal	50%[a]
	PAIS nonscrotal	60%
	Fraiser	40%
	Denys-Drash	30%
	46,XY GD	15%–40%
Intermediate	45,X/46,XY GD	12%
	PAIS scrotal gonad	Unknown[a]
	17βHSD	28%
Low	CAIS	2%[a]
	Ovotesticular DSD	3%
	45X (no Y chromatin)	1%
Unknown	5α-Reductase deficiency	0%
	Leydig cell hypoplasia	0%

Source: See further Lee P et al. *Pediatrics.* 2006;118;e488–500.
Abbreviations: 17βHSD, 17β-hydroxysteroid dehydrogenase type 3 deficiency; CAIS, complete androgen insensitivity; DSD, difference of sexual development; GD, gonadal dysgenesis; PAIS, partial androgen insensitivity.
[a] Note that these estimates are based on historical clinical diagnoses. For example, individuals with CAIS and PAIS may not have had androgen receptor sequencing; therefore, these estimates may not reflect the true risk of developing gonadoblastoma for specific conditions.

are no evidence-based guidelines for monitoring intra-abdominal testes.[80] Finally, for a patient where gender identity is not clear, but virilization at puberty is possible, the patient and family may be offered pubertal suppression until the patient is ready to be involved in the decision-making process regarding retaining or removing functional gonadal tissue.

Any discussion of gonadectomy should include a discussion on hormone replacement therapy. The risks of osteoporosis with gonadal dysgenesis and with gonadectomy are high; therefore, adequate hormone therapy is necessary to prevent bone mineral loss and osteoporosis.[81,82]

FUTURE DIRECTIONS

With advances in genetic testing, individuals with DSD conditions can now receive more specific diagnoses than were previously available. Therefore, much of our long-term outcomes research involves patients with clinical diagnoses that oversimplify a heterogeneous group of diagnoses. Additionally, natural history data, particularly involving risk of gonadal tumors, is lacking given that many individuals underwent gonadectomy early in life. Given the shame and secrecy surrounding some of these conditions, most outcomes research has been based off small, single-institution studies. Future research is needed to assess long-term outcomes for patients with DSD conditions, with the aim to improve physical and psychological health throughout life.

CONCLUSION

Caring for patients with DSDs requires multidisciplinary expertise and an understanding of the complexity, both medically and psychologically, of living with a DSD condition. Goals of medical and surgical treatment should be to maximize health, minimize physical and psychosocial risk, and optimize fertility and sexual health.

REFERENCES

1. Lee PA, Nordenstrom A, Houk C et al. Global disorders of sex development update since 2006: Perceptions, approach and care. *Horm Res Paediatr.* 2016;85:158–80.
2. Jost A, Proce D, Edwards R. Hormonal factors in the sex differentiation of the mammalian fetus. *Biol Sci.* 1970;259:119–31.
3. Shnorhavorian M, Fechner P. Disorders of sex differentiation. In: Gleason C, Juul S, eds. *Avery's Diseases of the Newborn.* 10th ed. New York, NY: Elsevier; 2017:Chapter 97.
4. Markam S, Waterhouse T. Structural anomalies of the reproductive tract. *Curr Opin Obstet Gynecol.* 1992;4;867–73.
5. Pang S, Wallace M, Hofman L et al. Worldwide experience in newborn screening for classical congenital adrenal hyperplasia due to 21-hydroxylase deficiency. *Pediatrics.* 1988;81:866–74.
6. Speiser P, Dupont B, Rubinstein P et al. High frequency of nonclassical steroid 21-hydroxylase deficiency. *Am J Hum Genet.* 1985;37:650–7.
7. Speiser P, Azziz R, Baskin L et al. Congenital adrenal hyperplasia due to steroid 21-hydroxylase deficiency: An Endocrine Society clinical practice guideline. *J Clin Endocrinol Metab.* 2010;95:4133–60.
8. Casteras A, De Silva P, Rumsby G, Conway GS. Reassessing fecundity in women with classical congenital adrenal hyperplasia (CAH): Normal pregnancy rate but reduced fertility rate. *Clin Endocrinol.* 2009;70:833–7.
9. Bidet M, Bellanne-Chantelot C, Galand-Portier M et al. Fertility in women with nonclassical congenital adrenal hyperplasia due to 21-hydroxylase deficiency. *J Clin Endocrinol Metab.* 2010;95:1189–90.
10. Hoepffner W, Schulze E, Bennek J, Keller E. Pregnancies in patients with congenital adrenal hyperplasia with complete or almost complete impairment of 21-hydroxylase activity. *Fertil Steril.* 2004;81:1314–21.
11. Conte F, Grumbach M, Ito Y et al. A syndrome of female pseudohermaphrodism, hypergonadotropic hypogonadism, and multicystic ovaries associated with missense mutations in the gene encoding aromatase (P450arom). *J Clinic Endocrinolo Metab.* 1994;78:1287–92.
12. Oppelt P, Renner SP, Kellermann A et al. Clinical aspects of Mayer-Rokitansky-Kuster-Hauser syndrome: Recommendations for clinical diagnosis and staging. *Hum Reprod.* 2006;21:792–7.
13. American College of Obstetricians and Gynecologists Committee on Adolescent Health. Mullerian agenesis: Diagnosis, management and treatment. Committee Opinion 562. *Obstet Gynecol.* 2018;131:e35–42.
14. Breech L. Gynecologic concerns in patients with anorectal malformations. *Semin Pediatr Surg.* 2010;19:139–45.
15. Ahmed S, Cheng A, Dovey L et al. Phenotypic features, androgen receptor binding, and mutational analysis in 278 clinical cases reported as androgen insensitivity syndrome. *J Clin Endocrinol Metab.* 2000;85:658–65.
16. Mongan N, Tadokoro-Cuccaro R, Bunch T, Hughes I. Androgen insensitivity syndrome. *Best Pract Res Clin Endocrinol Metab.* 2015;29:569–80.
17. Latronico A, Anhold I. Inactivating mutations of the human luteinizing hormone receptor in both sexes. *Semin Reprod Med.* 2012;30:382–6.
18. Maimoun L, Philibert P, Cammas B et al. Phenotypical, biological, and molecular heterogeneity of 5α-reductase deficiency: An extensive international experience of 55 patients. *J Clin Endocrinol Metab.* 2011;96(2):296–307.
19. Houk C, Damiani D, Lee P. Choice of gender in 5α-reductase deficiency: A moving target. *J Pediatr Endocrinol Metab.* 2005;18:339–45.
20. Herdt G, Davidson J. The Sambia "turnim-man": Sociocultural and clinical aspects of gender formation in male pseudohermaphrodites with 5α-reductase deficiency in Papua New Guinea. *Arch Sex Behav.* 1988;17:33–56.

21. Kang H, Imperato-McGinley J, Zhu Y, Rosenwaks Z. The effect of 5α-reductase-2 deficiency on human fertility. *Fertil Steril.* 2014;101:310–6.

22. Nordenskjöld A, Ivarsson S. Molecular characterization of 5α-reductase type 2 deficiency and fertility in a Swedish family. *J Clin Endocrinol Metab.* 1998;83:3236–8.

23. Eggers S, Sadedin S, van der Bergen J et al. Disorders of sex development: Insights from targeted gene sequencing of a large international patient cohort. *Genome Biol.* 2016;17:243.

24. Reindollar R, Byrd J, McDonough P. Delayed sexual development: A study of 252 patients. *Am J Obstet Gynecol.* 1981;140:371–80.

25. Sybert V, McCauley E. Turner's syndrome. *New Engl J Med.* 2004;351:1227–38.

26. Boissonnas C, Davy C, Bornes M et al. Careful cardiovascular screening and follow-up of women with Turner syndrome before and during pregnancy is necessary to prevent maternal mortality. *Fertil Steril.* 2009;91:929.

27. Gunther D, Eugster E, Zagar A et al. Ascertainment bias in Turner syndrome: New insights from girls who were diagnosed incidentally in prenatal life. *Pediatrics.* 2004;114:640–4.

28. Gravholt C, Fedder J, Naeraa R, Muller J. Occurrence of gonadoblastoma in females with Turner syndrome and Y chromosome material: A population study. *J Clin Endocrinol Metab.* 2000;85:3199–202.

29. Brant W, Rajimwale A, Lovell M et al. Gonadoblastoma and Turner syndrome. *J Urol.* 2006;175:1858–60.

30. Baxter L, Bryant J, Cave C, Milne R. Recombinant growth hormone for children and adolescents with Turner syndrome. *Cochrane Database Syst Rev.* 2007;24:CD003887.

31. Bondy C. Turner Syndrome Consensus Study Group. Care of girls and women with Turner syndrome: A guideline of the Turner syndrome study group. *J Clin Endocrinol.* 2007;92:10–25.

32. Pasquino A, Passeri F, Pucarelli I et al. Spontaneous pubertal development in Turner's syndrome. Italian Study Group for Turner's Syndrome. *J Clin Endocrinol Metab.* 1997;82:1810–3.

33. Tanaka T, Igarashi Y, Ozono K et al. Frequencies of spontaneous breast development and spontaneous menarche in Turner syndrome in Japan. *Clin Pediatr Endocrinol.* 2015;24:167–73.

34. Hadnott T, Gould H, Gharib A, Bondy C. Outcomes of spontaneous and assisted pregnancies in Turner syndrome: The U.S. National Institutes of Health experience. *Fertil Steril.* 2011;95:2251–6.

35. Karnis M, Zimon A, Lalwani S et al. Risk of death in pregnancy achieved through oocyte donation in patients with Turner syndrome: A national survey. *Fertil Steril.* 2003;80:498–501.

36. Chevalier N, Letur H, Lelannou D et al. Materno-fetal cardiovascular complications in Turner syndrome after oocyte donation: Insufficient prepregnancy screening and pregnancy follow-up are associated with poor outcome. *J Clin Endocrinol Metab.* 2011;96:260–7.

37. Practice Committee of the American Society for Reproductive Medicine. Increased maternal cardiovascular mortality associated with pregnancy in women with Turner syndrome. *Fertil Steril.* 2012;97:282–4.

38. Viranen H, Toppari J. Epidemiology and pathogenesis of cryptorchidism. *Hum Reprod Update.* 2008;14:49–58.

39. Sarpel U, Palmer S, Dolgin S. The incidence of complete androgen insensitivity in girls with inguinal hernias and assessment of screening by vaginal length measurement. *Horm Res Paediatr.* 2016;85:158–80.

40. Allen L. Disorders of sexual development. *Obstet Gynecol Clin N Amer.* 2009;36:25–45.

41. Ahmed S, Khwaja O, Hughes I. The role of a clinical score in the assessment of ambiguous genitalia. *BJU Int.* 2000;85:120–4.

42. Feldman K, Smith D. Fetal phallic growth and penile standards for newborn male infants. *J Pediatr.* 1975;86:395–8.

43. Thankamony A, Ong K, Dunger D et al. Anogenital distance from birth to two years: A population study. *Environ Health Perspect.* 2009;117:1786–90.

44. Michala L, Aslam N, Conway G, Creighton S. The clandestine uterus: Or how the uterus escapes detection prior to puberty. *BJOG.* 2010;117:212–5.

45. Vanderbrink B, Rink R, Cain M et al. Does preoperative genitography in congenital adrenal hyperplasia cases affect surgical feminizing genitoplasty? *J Urol.* 2010;184:1793–7.

46. Preibsch H, Rall K, Wietek BM et al. Clinical value of magnetic resonance imaging in patients with Mayer-Rokitansky-Kuster-Hauser (MRKH) syndrome: Diagnosis of associated malformations, uterine rudiments and intrauterine endometrium. *Eur Radiol.* 2014;24:1621–7.

47. Chauvin N, Epelman M, Victoria T, Johnson AM. Complex genitourinary abnormalities on fetal MRI: Imaging findings and approach to diagnosis. *AJR.* 2012;199:222.

48. Douglas G, Axelrad M, Brandt M et al. Consensus in guidelines for evaluation of DSD by the Texas Children's Hospital multidisciplinary gender medicine team. *Int J Pediatr Endocrinol.* 2010;2010:919707.

49. Lee P, Houk C, Ahmed S, Hughes A. Consensus statement on management of intersex disorders. *Pediatrics.* 2006;118:e488–500.

50. Auchus R, Witchel S, Leight K et al. Guidelines for the development of comprehensive care centers for congenital adrenal hyperplasia: Guidance from the CARES foundation initiative. *Int J Pediatr Endocrinol.* 2010;2010:275213.

51. Lee P, Nordenstrom A, Houk C et al. Global disorders of sex development update since 2006: Perceptions, approach, and care. *Horm Res Paediatr.* 2016;85:158–80.

52. Suorsa K, Mullins A, Tackett A et al. Characterizing early psychosocial functioning of parents of children

with moderate to severe genital ambiguity due to disorders of sex development. *J Urol.* 2015;194:1737–42.

53. Sandberg D, Gardner M, Cohen-Kettenis P. Psychological aspects of the treatment of patients with disorders of sex development. *Semin Reprod Med.* 2012;30:443–52.

54. Liao L, Green H, Creighton S et al. Service users' experiences of obtaining and giving information about disorders of sex development. *BJOG.* 2010;117:193–9.

55. Dessens A, Slijper F, Drop S. Gender dysphoria and gender change in chromosomal females with congenital adrenal hyperplasia. *Arch Sex Behav.* 2005;34:389–97.

56. Poland M, Evans T. Psychologic aspects of vaginal agenesis. *J Reprod Med.* 1985;30:340–4.

57. Kolesinska Z, Ahmed S, Niedziela M et al. Changes over time in sex assignment for disorders of sex development. *Pediatrics.* 2014;134:710–5.

58. Frisen L, Nordenstrom A, Falhammar H et al. Gender role behavior, sexuality, and psychosocial adaptation in women with congenital adrenal hyperplasia due to CYP21A2 deficiency. *J Clin Endo Metab.* 2009;94:3432–9.

59. Diamond M, Sigmundson K. Sex reassignment at birth: Long-term review and clinical implications. *Arch Pediatr Adolesc Med.* 1997;151:298–304.

60. Cohen-Kettenis P. Gender change in 46,XY persons with 5α-reductase-2 deficiency and 17β-hydroxysteroid dehydrogenase-3 deficiency. *Arch Sex Behav.* 2005;34:399–410.

61. T'Sjoen G, De Cuypere G, Monstrey S et al. Male gender identity in complete androgen insensitivity. *Arch Sex Behav.* 2011;40:635–8.

62. Fisher A, Ristori J, Fanni E et al. Gender identity, gender assignment and reassignment in individuals with disorders of sex development; a major dilemma. *J Endocrinol Invest.* 2016;39:1207–24.

63. Hughes I, Houk C, Ahmed S, Lee P. Lawson Wilkins Pediatric Endocrine Society/European Society for Paediatric Endocrinology Consensus Group. Consensus statement on management of intersex disorders. *J Pediatr Urol.* 2006;2:148–62.

64. Wiesemann C, Ude-Koeller S, Sinnecker G, Thyen U. Ethical principles and recommendations for the medical management of differences of sex development (DSD)/intersex in children and adolescents. *Eur J Pediatr.* 2010;169:671–9.

65. Mouriquand P, Gorduza D, Gay C et al. Surgery in disorders of sex development (DSD) with a gender issue: If (why), when, and how? *J Pediatr Urol.* 2016;12:139–49.

66. Freitas Filho L, Carnevale J, Melo C et al. A posterior-based omega-shaped flap vaginoplasty in girls with congenital adrenal hyperplasia caused by 21-hydroxylase deficiency. *BJU Int.* 2003;91:263–7.

67. Pena A. Total urogenital mobilization: An easier way to repair cloacas. *J Pediatr Surg.* 1997;32:263–7.

68. Leslie J, Cain M, Rink R. Feminizing genital reconstruction in congenital adrenal hyperplasia. *Indian J Urol.* 2009;25:17–26.

69. Rink R, Metcalfe P, Kaefer M et al. Partial urogenital mobilization: A limited proximal dissection. *J Pediatr Urol.* 2006;2:351–6.

70. Gross RE, Randolph J, Crigler JF Jr. Clitorectomy for sexual abnormalities: Indications and technique. *Surgery.* 1966;59:300–8.

71. Crouch N, Liao L, Woodhouse C et al. Sexual function and genital sensitivity following feminizing genitoplasty for congenital adrenal hyperplasia. *J Urol.* 2008;179:634–8.

72. Minto C, Liao L, Woodhouse C et al. The effect of clitoral surgery on sexual outcome in individuals who have intersex conditions with ambiguous genitalia: A cross sectional study. *Lancet.* 2003;361:1252–7.

73. Schober J, Meyer-Bahlburg H, Ransley P. Self-assessment of genital anatomy, sexual sensitivity and function in women: Implications for genitoplasty. *BJU Int.* 2004;94:589–94.

74. Frank R. The formation of an artificial vagina without operation. *Am J Obstet Gynecol.* 1938;35:1053–5.

75. Edmonds D, Rose G, Lipton M, Quek J. Mayer-Rokitansky-Kuster-Hauser syndrome: A review of 245 consecutive cases managed by a multidisciplinary approach with vaginal dilators. *Fertil Steril.* 2012;97:686–90.

76. Routh J, Laufer M, Cannon G et al. Management strategies for Mayer-Rokitansky-Kuster-Hauser related vaginal agenesis; a cost-effectiveness analysis. *J Urol.* 2010;184:2116–21.

77. Cools M, Drop S, Wolffenbuttel K et al. Germ cell tumors in the intersex gonad: Old paths, new directions, moving frontiers. *Endocr Rev.* 2006;27:468–84.

78. Kanakatti Shankar R, Inge T, Gutmark-Little I, Backelijauw P. Oophorectomy versus salpingo-oophorectomy in Turner syndrome patients with Y-chromosome material: Clinical experience and current practice patterns assessment. *J Pediatr Surg.* 2014;49:1585–8.

79. Patel V, Casey R, Gomez-Lobo V. Timing of gonadectomy in patients with complete androgen insensitivity syndrome: Current recommendations and future directions. *J Pediatr Adolesc Gynecol.* 2016;29:320–5.

80. Wunsch L, Holterhus P, Wessel L, Hiort O. Patients with disorders of sex development (DSD) at risk of gonadal tumour development: Management based on laparoscopic biopsy and molecular diagnosis. *BJU Int.* 2012;110:958–65.

81. Danilovic D, Correa P, Costa E et al. Height and bone mineral density in androgen insensitivity syndrome with mutations in the androgen receptor gene. *Osteoporos Int.* 2007;18:369–74.

82. Hans T, Goswani D, Trikudanathan S et al. Comparison of bone mineral density and body proportions between women with complete androgen insensitivity syndrome and women with gonadal dysgenesis. *Eur J Endocrinol.* 2008;159:179–85.

Common vulvar and vaginal complaints

8

JUDITH SIMMS-CENDAN

INTRODUCTION

Vulvovaginal concerns are the most common reason prepubertal girls present for gynecologic care. While dermatologic disorders of the vulva are covered in a separate chapter, this chapter addresses vulvovaginal disorders resulting from anatomic/structural differences, as well as vulvovaginal disorders presenting as vaginal discharge and prepubertal vaginal bleeding.

LABIAL ADHESIONS

Labial adhesion, also known as labial agglutination and labial synechiae, refers to fusion of the labia minora in the midline. The appearance can generate concern in parents and providers for urinary obstruction, or even reproductive tract anomaly, leading patients to present for evaluation and treatment even in the absence of symptoms.

Girls usually develop labial adhesions while still in diapers, with an estimated peak incidence of 3.3% in girls 13–23 months of age.[1] The adhesions arise from the perfect storm of a prepubertal hypoestrogenic vulva and an inflammatory inciting event occurring in a girl predisposed to developing adhesions. Even with meticulous hygiene practices, some girls with very sensitive skin may be predisposed to inflammation from the presence of urine or feces in the diaper. The variable hygiene habits of toilet-training toddlers may exacerbate the problem. As the adhesions progressively close the labia minor over the vestibule, urine can become trapped in the vagina during voiding, then with slow release the perineum becomes wet and irritated, further increasing adhesion formation. Triggers of labial adhesions include vaginal infections and inflammatory skin conditions such as lichen sclerosus (see Chapter 10), and trauma to the perineum from straddle injury or sexual abuse. In areas where female genital mutilation is endemic, labial adhesions are unfortunately an intended outcome of this practice.

Labial adhesions most often are asymptomatic, detected by providers at the time of well-child examination, or by caretakers at the time of diaper changes. They can also present with symptoms of vulvar irritation and vaginitis. Patients with dribbling urine from behind the adhesions after voiding may report feeling wet, and caregivers or teachers may notice staining or odor of underwear. Less commonly, labial adhesions can present with urinary tract infections, urinary frequency, or urinary retention.[2] Diagnosis is based on clinical examination of the labia minora. Most commonly, the adhesions develop posteriorly with the superior aspect of the labia minora spared. A thin median raphe can be seen at the junction of the labia minora in the midline. The adhesions may cover the vaginal opening but should be distinguished from imperforate hymen. The provider should look as well for signs of infection, inflammation, and trauma, which could induce adhesion development (Figure 8.1).

The decision on whether to treat labial adhesions depends on the presence of symptoms. Often the condition is self-limiting and resolves spontaneously with normal wiping after voiding or at the onset of pubertal estrogen production.[2] In the absence of symptoms, current recommendations are to monitor conservatively. Vulvar hygiene should be optimized. When treatment is indicated in the setting of urinary tract infections or vulvar irritation due to dribbling of urine, medical management is preferred over surgical management. The treatment of labial adhesions has been directed either at treating the hypoestrogenic state through use of topical estrogen cream, or treating the inflammation through use of topical steroids, most often betamethasone ointment (Table 8.1). With use of either medication, gentle traction or pressure over the adhesion on the labia at the time of application has been shown to increase efficacy. A randomized trial comparing emollient cream to Estrace showed improvement in both groups, supporting the importance of application technique. A trend to better resolution was observed with Estrace, although

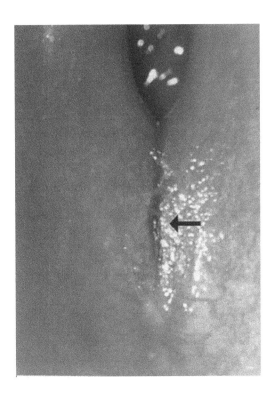

Figure 8.1 Labial adhesions. (From NASPAG PediGyn Teaching Slide Set CD-ROM, NASPAG 2001, with permission.)

Table 8.1 Medical management of labial adhesions.

Therapy	Medication	Application	Duration	Side effects	Success rates
Topical estrogen	Conjugated estrogen cream *or* Estradiol 0.01% vaginal cream	Pea-size amount applied by fingertip or cotton applicator, once or twice daily	2–6 weeks	Transient irritation, redness, and hyperpigmentation of the vulva, breast budding, rarely vaginal bleeding	50%–89%
Topical steroid	Betamethasone 0.05% cream	Twice-daily application	4–6 weeks	Erythema, pruritus, folliculitis, skin atrophy, fine pubic hair growth	68%–79%

Source: Adapted from data in Bacon J et al. *J Pediatr Adolesc Gynecol.* 2015;28(5):405–9.

results were not statistically significant.[34] It is important to teach this to the parents who may be afraid to touch their child's genitalia. Older cooperative prepubertal girls can be shown how to do this and may be more willing to gently separate the labia themselves.

Surgical management of labial adhesions should be limited to symptomatic patients failing medical therapy. Adequate topical anesthesia with lidocaine ointment or topical prilocaine/lidocaine cream and, if necessary, sedation should be provided to prevent pain and undue anxiety prior to any separation. Because the adhesions occur related to inflammation, surgical procedures should minimize trauma to the surrounding tissue. Gentle use of a lubricated cotton-tipped applicator is usually successful. A scalpel can be used for particularly dense adhesions.

Recurrences of labial adhesions can occur after medical or surgical management. The recurrence rate in one study of 151 girls was 35% after estrogen cream, 15.8% after steroid cream, and 26% after surgical management.[3] Decision to retreat should again depend on symptoms, and not simply the presence of adhesions.

LABIAL HYPERTROPHY

Puberty is a time of rapid growth of the genitalia. At times growth occurs asymmetrically, or the labia minora become more prominent than the labia majora, especially in the absence of significant body fat. Adolescent girls, sometimes prompted by their mothers, other times through their own concerns, are presenting with increasing frequency for evaluation of labial hypertrophy. Whether because of increased internet availability of idealized genital images, including in pornography or exposure through marketing for genital aesthetic procedures, there has been a marked increase in girls seeking labioplasty, or surgical reduction of the labia minora. Labial hypertrophy, referring to the excessive growth or elongation of the labia minora, yet lacks a uniform definition, as the "normal" appearance of the labia minora varies widely. There have been no large anatomic surveys documenting labia minora size in adolescent girls, and studies in adults can demonstrate a range of normal from 3 to 50 mm.[4]

Girls may present for evaluation of labial hypertrophy due to symptoms of swelling and pain with sports activities, hygiene difficulty with menstruation, or concern about visibility in tight-fitting clothes such as leggings and

bathing suits. Other girls may have significant psychological distress with the appearance of the genitalia and can develop body dysmorphic disorder.

Evaluation should include a detailed external genital examination, ideally with the patient as an active participant, holding a mirror if necessary for visibility. Labia should be assessed for evidence of edema, excoriation, infection, or inflammation. Labia minora can be measured from the cusp of the labia minora to the apex.

Management of labia minora enlargement begins with thoughtful education on the variations of normal, aided by resources such as the *Petals* book by Nick Karras or the Labia Library online resource.[5,6] For girls with vulvar irritation with sports, silicon-based emollients can be helpful. Use of a peribottle or increasingly available, inexpensive toilet bidets can help with hygiene. Reduction of use of tight-fitting clothing, especially for daily use, can be helpful as well.

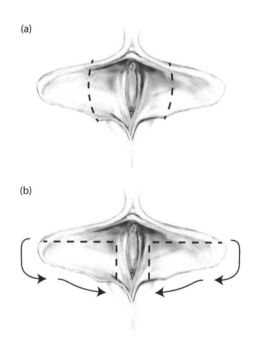

Figure 8.2 Labioplasty: (a) edge excision and (b) wedge excision. (With kind permission from Springer Science+ Business Media: Case of a girl with vulvar swelling, Simms-Cendan J, Santos X. *Adolescent Gynecology: A Clinical Casebook.* 2018. pp. 35–40. New York, New York.)

Labioplasty is recommended for adolescents under the age of 18 only if they have a significant congenital malformation or persistent physical symptoms directly related to the labial anatomy. The labia minora are highly innervated along the edge, and excision of excess labia minora tissue may affect future sexual function.[7] Procedures should be delayed until full development is completed, especially in the setting of asymmetry, as this may resolve spontaneously. Many states have laws criminalizing adolescent labioplasty as a kind to female genital mutilation, and practitioners should be aware of their own states' laws.[8] The decision to perform labioplasty on a girl with significant body dysmorphic disorder related exclusively to the labia presents an ethical quandary and should be made in partnership with her mental health provider.[9] Labioplasty techniques include the edge excision, involving excision of the excess labial tissue from the edge, and the wedge excision, involving excision from the lower labial edge, and modifications involving both procedures (Figure 8.2).

HYMENAL VARIANTS

The configuration of the hymen varies substantially, and certain developmental configurations may produce symptoms prompting patients to seek care. Imperforate hymen and assessment of hymenal anatomy for determination of sexual abuse are outside the coverage of this chapter. The most common configurations of the hymen can be seen in Figure 8.3. The prepubertal hymen is very thin, often with fine vascularity noted, whereas the postpubertal estrogenized hymen becomes thickened and opaque. The microperforate hymenal shape can cause retention of vaginal secretions or collection of urine after voiding, resulting in dribbling after voiding. Both the microperforate and cribriform shape can

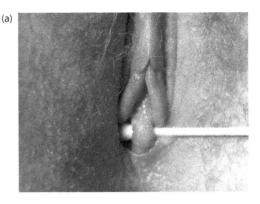
(a)

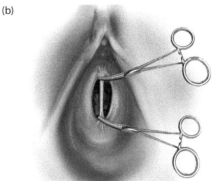
(b)

Figure 8.4 Hymenal septum, diagnosis and excision. (a) The hymenal septum is demonstrated, distinguished from a vaginal septum by visualizing the cotton applicator on both sides of the septum. (b) The placement of hemostats for septum excision. ([a] Courtesy of Veronica Gomez-Lobo.)

preclude tampon insertion, whereas a hymenal septum is more often noticed as difficulty with tampon extraction. Diagnosis of the hymenal septum can be made by passing a plastic cervical os finder, small dilator, or cotton-tipped applicator behind the septum, visualizing it on either side of the septum.

In general, for nonobstructing hymenal variants, performing surgical procedures on the hymen after onset of menarche is preferable to optimize healing in the presence of estrogenization. Depending on the patient tolerance for office procedures, as well as the thickness of the septum, hymenal septum excision can take place in the office or the operating room. Local anesthetic at the superior and inferior margins of the septum, followed by clamping with a hemostat for 2 minutes, then excision of the intervening septum often allow excellent hemostasis and avoidance of sutures (Figure 8.4). Care should be taken to avoid clamping too close to the urethra.

VULVOVAGINITIS

Vulvovaginal irritation and vaginal discharge, hallmark symptoms of vulvovaginitis, are among the most common presenting complaints in pediatric adolescent gynecology. When present, especially in the prepubertal patient, they can create significant anxiety for parents and caregivers. Most often the symptoms have a benign etiology, with approximately 5% of patients referred with suspected

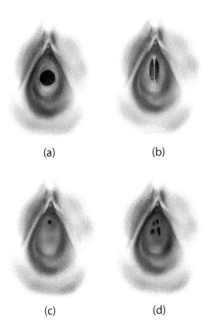
(a)   (b)

(c)   (d)

Figure 8.3 Hymenal configurations: (a) annular, (b) septate, (c) microperforate, and (d) cribriform.

sexual abuse.[10] The pathophysiology, differential diagnoses, treatment, and management of vulvovaginitis depend on the pubertal status of the child; it is related to estrogen exposure and can be correlated to Tanner staging of the breast.[11] Prepubertal girls are physiologically predisposed to vulvovaginitis related to hygiene habits and hematogenously spread infections, whereas postpubertal girls have a clinical picture more like adult women, where *Candida* infections, bacterial vaginosis, and sexually transmitted disease are more common.

Prepubertal vulvovaginitis

Both physiology and young psychosocial development stage conspire to increase risk of vulvovaginitis in young girls. The diminutive labia minora, small hymenal orifice, less prominent labia majora, and absence of pubic hair of the unestrogenized vulva increase collection and trapping of sweat, urine, dirt, and stool in the vagina. The lower levels of lactobacilli produce a more alkaline pH, facilitating the overgrowth of bacteria. Meanwhile, development of good hygiene practices often does not coincide with toilet training, leading to poor handwashing and inadequate wiping after defecation. Common childhood bubble baths can cause skin irritation, and certain living conditions may expose girls to pinworms. Some girls void with their knees pressed together, trapping urine in the vagina, or lack patience for complete voiding, resulting in dribbling of urine, which leaves the vulva wet and irritated.[12] Girls occasionally place foreign objects, most commonly rolled up bits of toilet paper, but also coins, batteries, and a variety of small objects, in the vagina, all of which create a vaginal discharge that can be bloody and associated with a foul odor.

An important consideration for girls presenting with persistent discharge is the presence of an ectopic ureter with vaginal insertion. Although present since birth, it is usually not noticed until after toilet training, and presentation may be further delayed until changes in the anatomy of the vagina with growth may trigger leakage of urine from the vagina. Girls complain of feeling wet all the time, and yellow "discharge" is noticed in the underwear. The moisture leads to vulvovaginal irritation. Diagnosis requires a high index of suspicion and is made by magnetic resonance urography imaging of the pelvis.

Vulvovaginitis in young girls caused by hygiene issues is called nonspecific vaginitis. Nonspecific vaginitis accounts for up to 75% of cases of vulvovaginitis in this population, and vaginal cultures usually demonstrate "normal flora."[13] Studies done to define the normal flora of the prepubertal vagina identify aerobic bacteria, such as *Staphylococcus epidermitis*, enterococci, *Escherichia coli*, lactobacilli, *Streptococcus viridans*, and anaerobic bacteria, such as *Peptococcus* and *Bacteroides*, with significant overlap between symptomatic and asymptomatic girls.[12]

Prepubertal girls may develop specific bacterial vaginitis through direct contamination or hematogenous spread. The most common isolates involve respiratory pathogens, such as group A β-hemolyic streptococcus (*S. pyogenes*), *Haemophilus influenza*, *Neisseria meningitides*, *S. aureus*,

Branhamella catarrhalis, and *S. pneumoniae*. Just as group A streptococcal (GAS) infections produce significant exudate and pain in the pharynx, the vagina and vulva become significantly tender and erythematous, producing symptoms of itching, burning, and dysuria. One study found that 95% of patients with perineal GAS also had a positive pharyngeal culture. The infections appeared to be seasonal, occurring October through March.[14] A significant enteric pathogen that can cause vaginitis is *Shigella*, most often *Shigella flexneri*, which may present with bloody vaginal discharge, and at times, diarrhea. *Yersinia* has also been reported to cause vaginitis.[12]

Another surprisingly common cause of vulvovaginitis in prepubertal girls is pinworm, *Enterobius vermicularis*. It has been identified in some studies in up to 22%–32% of prepubertal girls presenting with vulvovaginitis. The high incidence was associated with crowded living conditions, poor hygiene, and low socioeconomic level.[13] If the patient has been traveling outside the country to endemic areas, other parasitic infections to be considered include *Giardia* and *Schistosomiasis*.

An important point about prepubertal vaginitis is that *Candida* infections are uncommon in this age group, unless precipitated by recent antibiotics, immunosuppression such as chemotherapy, or uncontrolled diabetes.[10,12]

Sexually transmitted infections (STIs), such as gonorrhea, chlamydia, trichomonas, and herpes simplex, can occur in the setting of sexual abuse, but the absence of these infections of course does not rule out abuse, as the rate of STIs in sexually abused children has been found to be 3%–8%. An Argentine study found an incidence of STIs of 4.1% in 1034 girls referred for evaluation of sexual abuse, and nonspecific findings of abuse on exam were still associated with STIs.[15]

The significance of finding genital mycoplasma infection such as *Mycoplasma hominis* and *Ureaplasma* in a prepubertal girl presenting with vulvovaginitis is unclear. Mycoplasma colonization is found in 60%–80% in sexually active women, and vertical transmission is known to occur, yet usually colonization decreases after birth and is not found after 2 years of age. The presence of *Ureaplasma* and *Mycoplasma* on vaginal culture in prepubertal girls has been shown to be significantly correlated with a higher incidence of sexual abuse compared to controls but at this time cannot be considered diagnostic for abuse.[16]

The diagnosis of vulvovaginitis in the prepubertal girl depends on a detailed history, including assessment of hygiene and voiding habits, recent upper respiratory infection, and recent antibiotic use. A screen for history of sexual abuse should be done. Details about the discharge, including quantity, duration, color, and odor, are important.

Physical examination of prepubertal girls should include documentation of Tanner staging, and a head and neck exam to asses for pharyngitis. Examination of the external genitalia can be done in frog-legged or knee-chest position. Nonspecific vaginitis often reveals mild erythema at the introitus and the presence of a small amount of discharge. Poor hygiene can be noted by the presence of

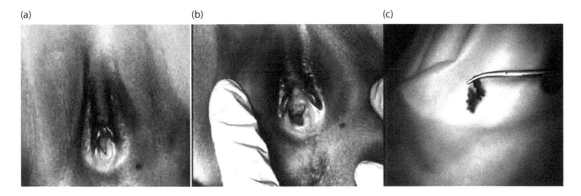

Figure 8.5 Foreign body: 6-year-old patient presenting with malodorous vaginal discharge. (a) Normal external examination. (b) Visualization of foreign body. (c) Stuffing from toy removed.

excessive smegma or soiling from stool. Gentle downward traction of the labia majora can help visualize the lower vagina and may help reveal the presence of a foreign body. Small CalgiSwabs can be used to obtain a vaginal culture. Vaginal irrigation with use of a small pediatric Foley or feeding tube and a syringe with saline can be used to flush out small bits of toilet paper, the foreign body most often found. If the patient cannot tolerate an examination in the office, or if foreign body is suspected, examination under sedation, and vaginoscopy using a small hysteroscope or cystoscope are indicated.[12] Figure 8.5 demonstrates the presence of foreign body, in this case, stuffing from a toy bear, in a 6-year-old girl presenting with a 6-month history of malodorous vaginal discharge.

Treatment of vulvovaginitis in the prepubertal child depends on the etiology. Correction of poor hygiene is important, and educating parents and children may be accomplished with tools including the American Girl Series: *The Care and Keeping of You*, which discusses good hygiene. For teaching girls with special needs, the Vanderbilt Kennedy Center Healthy Bodies Toolkit available online is especially helpful. Symptoms of vulvar irritation can be relieved by use of bland emollients such as petroleum jelly or coconut oil. Sitting in a bathtub of lukewarm water can also relieve symptoms. A low-potency topical steroid, such as 2.5% hydrocortisone cream, may relieve irritation as well. Table 8.2 details the treatment recommendations for specific vaginitis in the prepubertal patient. The penicillin family of antibiotics is effective for most infections and should be considered first line, for all except *E. coli* infection. Pharyngeal *H. influenza* has been found to have significant β-lactam resistance, but vaginal *H. influenza* appears to be more susceptible.[17] Diagnosis and treatment of STIs is covered in Chapter 17.

Vulvovaginitis in adolescent girls

With the onset of puberty, the vaginal flora shifts to resemble that of the adult woman. The glycogen content of the vaginal walls increases, as do the number of lactobacilli, leading to a decrease in vaginal pH to a more acidic environment. Estrogenization substantially increases the normal physiologic discharge prior to the onset of menarche,

prompting some patients to present for evaluation. Onset of ovulatory cycles, which occurs after menarche, is accompanied by increased mid-cycle vaginal discharge due to increased cervical mucus production.

Nonspecific vaginitis remains common in adolescents and can be triggered by poor hygiene in early adolescence, or overzealous hygiene and shaving in older adolescence. Vaginal odor is a very frequent concern of adolescent girls, and in fact is one of the most frequently searched genital concerns by all women.[18] The wearing of tight clothes and excessive sweating associated with exercise and warm climates all can produce normal vaginal odor. Education is critical to reducing worry. Use of panty liners or underwear that are designed to absorb menstrual flow or discharge (e.g., THINX) can improve symptoms. Girls should be taught to avoid douching or use of scented soaps and encouraged to wash with water or rinse very well after any perineal soap use. Retained foreign bodies, including tampons or condoms, are less common in adolescent girls but do occur.

Friction injury during intercourse, associated with vaginal dryness and condom use is a common noninfectious cause of vaginal irritation and discharge in sexually active adolescents. Girls may present with complaints of white vaginal discharge and burning with urination as the stream contacts traumatized vulvar tissue. Sexual dysfunction is not often addressed with adolescents, who may be told to simply abstain, and therefore be hesitant to come forward with complaints. History of sexual abuse, intimate partner violence, inadequate foreplay and arousal, and use of hormonal contraceptives may all lead to vaginal dryness. Embarrassed girls may be reticent to make the association with painful intercourse unless asked directly, and may have been treated multiple times for urinary tract infections and yeast infections. The sexual dysfunction affects self-esteem and can perpetuate symptoms. Careful history, sensitive counseling, and encouraging use of water-based and silicon-based lubricants are key to symptom improvement.

With an increase in the use of progesterone-only long-acting reversible contraception, depo-medroxyprogesterone acetate injections, and continuous oral contraceptives, breakthrough bleeding has become a common complaint of adolescent girls. When the bleeding is very light, it often

Table 8.2 Treatment of specific vaginitis in the prepubertal girl.

Pathogen	Bacteria	Antibiotics	Special considerations
Skin flora	Streptococcus pyogenes, Staphylococcus epidermidis, S. viridans	Ampicillin: 25 mg/kg every 6 hours or 500 mg every 6 hours if over 20 kg for 5–10 days Amoxicillin: 20 mg/kg every 12 hours for 5–10 days Azithromycin 10 mg/kg day 1, then 5 mg/kg for 4 days Cephalaxin 25–50 mg/kg every 6–8 hours or 500 mg twice a day in adolescents	Treat if symptomatic and no response to improved hygiene
	S. aureus	Cephalexin Trimethoprim/sulfamethoxazole (TM/SMX) 5 mg/kg every 12 hours for 5–10 days Amoxicillin clavulanate 25–45 mg/kg every 12 hours for 5–10 days	Consider clindamycin if suspected methicillin resistance
Respiratory pathogens	Group A β-hemolytic streptococcus, S. pneumoniae	Amoxicillin, cephalexin, azithromycin	Guttate psoriasis can occur after treatment
	Haemophilus influenzae	Amoxicillin clavulanate, Cefuroxime 20 mg/kg/day divided every 12 hours for 10 days, TM/SMX	β-lactamase production increasing
Gastrointestinal pathogens	Escherichia coli	Azithromycin	Treat if symptoms do not respond to improvement in hygiene
	Shigella	TM/SMX, ampicillin, azithromycin	40% resistance to TM/SMX, 80% resistance to ampicillin
Helminths	Enterobiasis vermicularis	Mebendazole 100 mg × 1, repeat in 2 weeks Pyrantel pamoate 11 mg/kg × 1, repeat in 2 weeks Albendazole 400 mg × 1, repeat in 2 weeks	Pinworms can be treated empirically if anal itching present

presents as a yellowish vaginal discharge that can be mistaken for infection. Wet mount often reveals red blood cells in various states of degeneration. Treatment in this case would be directed toward management of the breakthrough bleeding. Similarly, girls who have a partially obstructed Müllerian anomaly may present with discharge associated with odor. An ectopic ureter can present in adolescence and should be considered in girls with Müllerian anomalies, especially OHVIRA (obstructed hemivagina with ipsilateral renal agenesis), as the symptomatic drainage may present after septum excision.

Specific vaginal infections in adolescents are correlated with change in flora as well as change in risk factors and behavior. Figure 8.6 shows the shift in causes of specific vaginitis in a cohort of girls based on Tanner staging, with a rise in *Gardnerella, Trichomonas, Ureaplasma*, and *Chlamydia* as girls progressed through puberty.

The three most common causes for specific vaginal infections in adolescent girls are vulvovaginal candidiasis (VVC), bacterial vaginosis, and trichomoniasis. Risk factors for VVC include recent broad-spectrum antibiotic use and immune-compromised status, such as HIV infection, immunosuppressive therapy for organ transplant recipients and rheumatologic disorders, and chemotherapy. Obesity, tight-fitting clothing, and warm climates increase vulvar sweating, moisture, and temperature, leading to an environment that supports fungal infections. Poorly controlled diabetes, unfortunately common in adolescents

with type 1 diabetes, leads to a higher incidence of VVC. The pathophysiology is probably due to decreased immune function in poorly controlled diabetes, as well as increased *Candida* adherence to vaginal epithelium receptors expressed in the setting of elevated glucose levels.[19] The most common cause of VVC is *Candida albicans*, but *Candida glabrata* and *Candida tropicalis* also cause VVC and may be more difficult to treat with standard therapy. Patients with VVC usually present with symptoms of intense pruritus and thick-curd-like vaginal discharge.

Bacterial vaginosis (BV) occurs when an overgrowth of amine-producing bacteria leads to a malodorous discharge that can negatively impact self-esteem, sexual relationships, and quality of life.[20] As the field of biome study has evolved from culture-based assays to gene sequencing, a clearer picture of the normal vaginal flora and the flora leading to symptoms is coming into focus. *Lactobacillus* species, including *Lactobacillus crispatus*, *L. gasseri*, *L. iners*, and *L. jensenii*, dominate the normal vaginal flora of reproductive-age women. *L. crispatus* is the most efficient producer of lactic acid, whereas *L. iners* produces lower levels.[21] Studies have shown higher levels of *L. crispatus* in Caucasian women compared to African American women. Bacterial vaginosis is associated with a reduction in peroxidase, producing lactobacillus colonies, and a rise in *Gardnerella vaginalis*, a facultative anaerobic gram-variable rod. Infection also involves other bacteria, including *Atobium, Ureaplasma, Mycoplasma,*

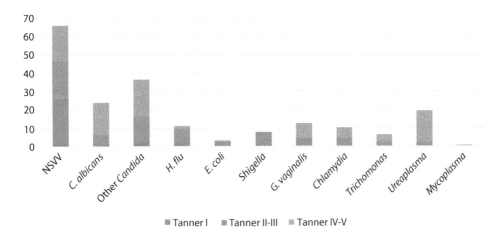

Figure 8.6 Percentage of patients presenting with vulvovaginitis with positive culture, in relation to Tanner staging. (Based on selected data of 229 girls presenting with vulvovaginitis. Ocampo D et al. *Arch Argent Pediatr.* 2014;112[1]:65–74.)

Mobiluncus, Fusobacterium, Megasphera, Sneathia, and *Letptrichia.*[22] While not considered a sexually transmitted disease, BV is diagnosed more often with new onset of sexual activity, with an increased number of male or female sex partners, and lack of condom use with penile-vaginal intercourse.[12] A prospective vaginal microbiota study evaluating vaginal swabs self-collected by university students every 3 months found that sexual activity increased colonization by *L. iners* and *G. vaginalis*; women with BV were also more likely to be sexually active.[21] Screening for sexual activity is, of course, part of standard adolescent care, and although not diagnostic for sexual activity, the presence of BV should prompt careful confidential inquiry about sexual practices.

Trichomoniasis, caused by the *Trichomonas vaginalis* protozoa, is the most prevalent and curable STI, found in 3.1% of reproductive-age women. Non-Hispanic black women have a 10-fold rate of infection (13.3% versus 1.3% of non-Hispanic white women).[23] An 18-month longitudinal study of African American adolescents found a baseline prevalence of 11.7% and a 20% incidence of new infections during the study.[24] Patients with trichomoniasis present with vaginal discharge, vaginal irritation, dysuria, and vaginal malodor.

Coinfection of BV and trichomoniasis is very common, and both infections increase the risk of acquiring other STIs, including chlamydia, gonorrhea, and HIV. Tissue changes in the genital tract caused by *G vaginalis* and *A vaginae* create a biofilm allowing more pathogenic bacteria to adhere. Trichomoniasis creates an inflammatory state with punctate hemorrhagic lesions and influx of leukocytes with CD4 receptors, an environment conducive to HIV spread.[12,20,24]

Diagnosis of vaginitis historically has relied on history, physical examination, and wet mount microscopy with saline and 10% potassium hydroxide (KOH). Physical examination of adolescents with VVC may demonstrate vulvovaginal erythema, excoriation from scratching, and a thick, adherent white vaginal discharge. Patients with bacterial vaginosis may demonstrate a white-gray, frothy vaginal discharge, but they usually do not have vulvovaginal erythema. *Trichomonas* infections classically presents with a frothy vaginal discharge that may be yellow due to light bleeding from punctate hemorrhages found on the cervix. The vaginal pH is normal in patients with VVC, and elevated (>4.5) in patients with BV and trichomonas. Wet mounts showing hyphae and budding yeast for VVC, clue cells for BV, and motile flagellates for trichomoniasis, are convenient and cost effective, yet newer diagnostic methods, including DNA probe assays and nucleic acid amplification testing (NAAT) have demonstrated improved sensitivity and specificity, especially for trichomoniasis. NAAT is now the gold standard for *Trichomonas* testing, as it is three to five times more sensitive than wet mount microscopy and can be done on vaginal, endocervical, and urine specimens.[12] Commercial assays that simultaneously check for *Candida* species, bacterial vaginosis, and *Trichomonas*, along with gonorrhea and chlamydia, are being used more often, especially in clinics where microscopy is not available. These tests also facilitate simultaneous screening for STIs. Point-of-care assays, including self-collection of swabs, are rapidly emerging to improve timely diagnosis.

Treatment of vulvovaginitis in adolescent girls means tailoring therapy to the patient as well as the infection. Adolescent girls may be more comfortable with oral versus topical therapy. Trichomoniasis, VVC, and BV all have significant rates of recurrence or reinfection. Recurrent VVC is defined as four or more symptomatic infections in 1 year. These infections, often due to *C. glabrata* and other nonalbicans species can be more difficult to treat. Table 8.3 includes the current diagnostic strategies and treatments as recommended by the Centers for Disease Control and Prevention (CDC).[25] Note that at the time of publication, there was no molecular test for yeast approved by the U.S. Food and Drug Administration; therefore, these are not included in the table. Although an STI, currently there are no CDC recommendations for expedited partner therapy for trichomoniasis.

Table 8.3 Diagnosis and treatment of vulvovaginitis in adolescent girls.

Etiology	Diagnosis	Selected CDC Recommended Treatments

Vulvovaginal candidiasis	Wet mount with KOH to visualize yeast, hyphae, or pseudohyphae	Uncomplicated VVC:
		OTC:
		  Clotrimazole 2% cream 5 g pv for 3 days
		  Miconazole 4% cream 5 g pv for 3 days
		  Miconazole 1200 mg suppository pv for 1 day

	Candida culture (gold standard)	Prescription intravaginal:
		  Terconazole 0.8% cream pv for 3 days
		  Terconazole 80 mg suppository pv for 3 days
		  Butoconazole 2% cream 5 gm pv for 1 day
		Prescription oral:
		  Fluconazole 150 mg orally single dose
		Recurrent VVC:
		  Fluconazole 150–200 mg orally every 2 days for three doses
		  Fluconazole 150 mg orally weekly for 6 months
		  Boric acid 600 mg gelatin capsule pv daily for 2 weeks

Bacterial vaginosis	Amsel criteria (three of the four must be present):
	 • White thin discharge that coats vaginal walls
	 • Clue cells on wet mount
	 • pH > 4.5
	 • Fishy odor before or after KOH
	  Affirm VP III *G. vaginalis* DNA Hybridization Probe
	OSOM BV Blue test for vaginal sialidase
	Gram stain (gold standard)
		Oral:
		  Metronidazole 500 mg bid for 7 days
		  Tinidazole 2 g orally for 2 days
		  Clindamycin 300 mg bid for 7 days
		Vaginal:
		  Metronidazole gel 0.75% 5 g pv for 5 days
		  Clindamycin cream 2% 5 g pv for 7 days
		  Clindamycin ovules 100 mg pv for 3 days
		Note: Clindamycin ovules have a base that can weaken latex condoms

Trichomonas	NAAT testing Aptima *Trichomonas vaginalis* Assay OSOM *Trichomonas* rapid test Affirm VP III	Metronidazole 2 g orally single dose Tinidazole 2 g oral single dose Alternative: Metronidazole 500 mg twice daily for 7 days[a]

Source: Data from Centers for Disease Control and Prevention (https://www.cdc.gov).

Abbreviations: KOH, 10% potassium hydroxide; NAAT, nucleic acid amplification testing; OTC, over the counter; PCR, polymerase chain reaction; pv, per vagina.

[a] *Caution:* To reduce the possibility of a disulfiram-like reaction, abstinence from alcohol use should continue for 24 hours after completion of metronidazole or 72 hours after completion of tinidazole.

VULVAR ULCERS

Most providers are trained to associate vulvar ulcers with herpes or syphilis infections, yet prepubertal and adolescent girls who are not sexually active most commonly present with vulvar ulcerations that are not related to sexual abuse or sexual activity. A 2012 review of acute genital ulceration (AGU) in girls who are not sexually active found the most common etiology to be idiopathic aphthosis (70%), with no assays positive for genital HSV or syphilis.[26] Idiopathic vulvar aphthosis is also known as Lipschütz ulcers, named after the physician who in 1913 reported vulvar ulcers in adolescent girls who had not been sexually active.[27] Interestingly, the mean age of presentation of AGU is 12.2 years of age, corresponding to the onset of menarche, and the mean age of onset of Behçet disease.[28] The role of hormones in development of vulvar ulcerations has not been studied. Vulvar ulcerations have many similar characteristics and risk factors as oral aphthous ulcers, also known as

canker sores. It appears that for some girls, infection with influenza, Epstein–Barr virus (EBV) or cytomegalovirus (CMV), and other acute viral illnesses triggers ulcers; for most, however, serology for these infections is negative. Oral aphthous ulcers are triggered by vitamin deficiencies, stress, trauma, infection, hormonal changes, and nonsteroidal anti-inflammatory drug (NSAID) use, and it appears AGU may have these same triggers.[26]

A detailed acute and past medical history is important for accurate evaluation of vulvar ulcers. Up to 71% of girls report systemic prodromal symptoms such as fever or myalgias, upper respiratory disease, and gastrointestinal symptoms prior to onset of the ulcers, which occur even in the absence of detectable infection.[26] While it is important to document a history of trauma, abuse, or sexual activity, it is important not to frame the questions with an accusatory tone, as these are not as likely as many presume. History of recurrent oral ulcers should prompt concern for

Behçet disease. Gastrointestinal symptoms should trigger concern for possible Crohn disease.

Vulvar aphthosis is generally exceptionally painful, and the examination needs to be approached very gently, with limitation of ulcer contact as much as possible. As opposed to superficial erosions, vulvar ulcers associated with aphthosis extend into the underlying dermis, are 1–2 cm with irregular borders, and usually are necrotic at the base with a yellow exudate or black eschar present. They occur most commonly in the medial aspect of the labia minora, and often present as "kissing lesions," appearing on bilateral labia minora. The surrounding tissue is often tender and erythematous due to inflammation, not necessarily associated cellulitis (Figure 8.7). The ulcers can appear quite frightening to patients and their caregivers. In contrast to vulvar aphthosis, herpes simplex appears most often as grouped vesicles on an erythematous base. The lesions of Crohn disease are classically "slit" or "knife-like" lesions occurring in genitourinary folds or creases. The presence of perianal fistulae is strongly associated with Crohn disease.[27]

Laboratory testing should be based on exposure risk. It is reasonable to test for HSV with polymerase chain reaction (PCR) assay, and to rule out syphilis and HIV infection. Testing for influenza, EBV, and CMV is controversial, as it usually does not influence treatment, and is costly. Referral to rheumatology for evaluation of Behçet is indicated for recurrent vulvar ulcers occurring in the setting of recurrent oral aphthous ulcers, ocular complaints, or erythema nodosum lesions. Symptoms suggestive of inflammatory bowel disease should prompt referral to gastroenterology.

Most importantly, management of vulvar aphthous ulcers should not await definitive diagnosis or HSV results (Table 8.4). Supportive care with reassurance that aphthae are not contagious, nor sexually transmitted, can produce great relief in the parents and patients. Topical lidocaine gel (2%) or ointment (5%) can relieve pain locally. Sitz baths, use of a peribottle during voiding, and barrier emollients with 40% zinc oxide can be used to manage dysuria, but if pain is severe, a hospitalization with Foley catheter placement

Table 8.4 Management of acute genital ulcers.

History	• Prodromal symptoms
	• Sexual activity or abuse
	• Oral aphthous ulcers
	• Ocular symptoms
	• Gastrointestinal symptoms
	• Arthralgia
	• Lymphadenopathy
Diagnostic tests	• Herpes simplex PCR or culture
	• Syphilis and HIV testing if sexually active or suspect abuse
	• EBV, CMV, influenza serology if signs of systemic infectious process
	• Bacterial culture if suspicious for secondary infection
Treatment for idiopathic aphthosis	• Pain relief: topical lidocaine ointment (5%) or gel (2%)
	• High-potency topical steroid (clobetasol 0.05% ointment)
	• Barrier emollients (zinc oxide 40% ointment, petroleum jelly)
	• Peribottle, sitz baths, ± whirlpool for debridement
	• Foley catheter and systemic pain relief if severe symptoms
Treatment of initial genital HSV (only if strongly suspected by history and/or exam, or positive HSV PCR)	• Acyclovir 400 mg three times per day for 7–10 days or
	• Valacyclovir 1 g twice daily for 7–10 days
	• Age <11 years, acyclovir 40–80 mg/kg/day po divided every 6–8 hours for 5–10 days
Referral	• To rheumatology if vulvar and oral ulcers are recurrent, or if ocular symptoms, arthralgias, erythema nodosum are present
	• To GI if symptoms of inflammatory bowel disease

Abbreviations: CMV, cytomegalovirus; EBV, Epstein–Barr virus; HSV, herpes simplex virus; PCR, polymerase chain reaction.

and wound care may be needed. Although clinical trials are lacking in vulvar ulcer treatment, topical high-potency steroids, such as clobetasol 0.05% ointment, are used successfully in oral aphthous ulcer treatment and are prescribed by many caring for vulvar ulcers. Experience in use of systemic steroids is limited but also recommended in severe cases. In general, the prognosis for full recovery is excellent, with the event being isolated in two-thirds of patients.[26,27]

VULVOVAGINAL LESIONS PRESENTING AS VAGINAL BLEEDING

Abnormal vaginal bleeding, especially in the prepubertal girl, requires careful assessment. Prepubertal vaginal

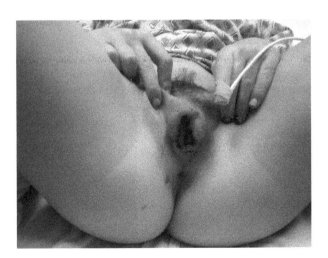

Figure 8.7 Acute genitourinary ulcers. (Courtesy of Veronica Gomez-Lobo.)

Table 8.5 Differential diagnosis of prepubertal vaginal bleeding.

Nonhormonal causes	Trauma
	Vulvovaginitis
	Urethral prolapse
	Genital/vaginal tumor, including rhabdomyosarcoma
	Sexual abuse
	Foreign body
	Lichen sclerosus
Hormonal causes	Precocious puberty
	Hormonal withdrawal bleeding
	Ovarian tumor
	Isolated precocious menarche

bleeding is uncommon, and the frequency of underlying etiology varies based on study author. Table 8.5 includes a differential diagnosis of the most common causes. As can be seen in the table, many of these have a structural origin, versus a hormonal cause seen in postmenarchal adolescent patients; evaluation depends on a careful physical examination, which may include exam under anesthesia and vaginoscopy. In approximately 25% of prepubertal girls, the etiology of the vaginal bleeding is unknown, even after careful investigation.[29] Bleeding associated with hormonal causes may be accompanied by other signs of puberty, including a growth spurt or breast development. Foreign body and vulvovaginitis are covered earlier in this chapter, while lichen sclerosus, trauma, sexual abuse, and precocious puberty are covered elsewhere. Two important causes of prepubertal vaginal bleeding, urethral prolapse and genital rhabdomyosarcoma, deserve mention here.

Urethral prolapse

Urethral prolapse is the protrusion of the distal urethra through the external meatus. The tissue appears as a friable, often donut-shaped mass superior to the hymen. Patients report painless, bright red bleeding, especially with wiping.[30] The volume of bleeding is minimal and is usually noted on tissue or underwear. The frequency of urethral prolapse as a cause of vaginal bleeding depends on the population studied. It has been reported to be more common in African American girls (as well as postmenopausal Caucasian women), and a Swedish case series of 86 prepubertal vaginal bleeding identified no cases related to

urethral prolapse.[29] A series of 89 Chinese girls presenting to a single institution with urethral prolapse over 16 years was published in 2017, prompting reconsideration of risk based on race. In contrast to earlier studies, most of these girls had a body mass index of less than the 50th percentile, challenging obesity as a contributing cause.[31] Predisposing factors can be those that decrease tissue integrity, such as malnutrition, neuromuscular disorders, steroid use, or the hypoestrogenic state, or those that increase intraabdominal pressure, such as chronic cough or constipation. Diagnosis is made based on vulvar examination. The mass may appear red and friable, but if strangulation of vascular supply has occurred with prolapse, the mass may appear dark, necrotic, and malodorous. Management of urethral prolapse depends on the severity of presentation and is covered in more detail in Chapter 11. Conservative management of nonnecrotic urethral prolapse includes correcting underlying constipation, sitz baths, and topical estrogen cream for 2–6 weeks.[30] Recurrent or larger lesions may require surgical resection.

GENITAL RHABDOMYOSARCOMA

Because of its aggressive nature, the diagnosis of genital rhabdomyosarcoma (RMS) should be excluded in girls presenting with unexplained vaginal bleeding. It arises from primitive mesenchymal cells and has four histologic subtypes: embryonic, pleomorphic, spindle cell, and alveolar, with embryonal or mixed type being the most common in girls with genitourinary RMS; sarcoma botryoides is a variant embryonal RMS. Genital RMS may present in prepubertal and adolescent girls. Most cases are sporadic, but there are reports of increased risk of RMS in patients with Li-Fraumeni syndrome, neurofibromatosis I, basal cell nevus syndrome, Costello syndrome, Noonan syndrome, and multiple endocrine neoplasia type 2A.[32] Depending on the study, the incidence ranges from 1.8% to 20% of girls presenting with prepubertal bleeding.[29] In 2017, Nasiuodis et al. published an analysis of 40 years of genital RMS cases from the National Cancer Institute's Surveillance Epidemiology and End Results database.[33] See Table 8.6 for a comparison of prepubertal and adolescent girls presenting with genital RMS. RMS in prepubertal girls is most often vulvovaginal, where in adolescent girls, RMS arises from the cervix.[33] The tumors are rapidly growing and present with a median size at presentation of 6 cm in prepubertal girls, and 8 cm in adolescent girls. Diagnosis of RMS depends on physical exam and vaginoscopy, with biopsy for tissue diagnosis.

Table 8.6 Genital rhabdomyosarcoma in prepubertal and adolescent girls.

Characteristic	Prepubertal	Adolescent
Location	Vulvovaginal 89%; cervical 11%	Vulvovaginal 27%; cervical 72%
Size (median) at presentation	6 cm	8 cm
Presence of regional lymph node metastases	12.5%	54.5%
Presence of distant metastases	5%	9%
Overall 5-year survival	85.6%	77.2%

Source: Data from Nasioudis D et al. *Arch Gynecol Obstet.* 2017;296:327–34.

RMS is sensitive to chemotherapy. Most treatment involves wide local resection and chemotherapy. Neoadjuvant chemotherapy reduces tumor burden and can allow resection with better preservation of reproductive function. The tumors are very responsive to VAC (vincristine, dactinomycin, plus cyclophosphamide). The use of radiation therapy did not improve survival in the SEER data analysis, but its use may have been limited to high-risk patients. While it may be useful to treat tumors difficult to resect, radiation therapy also carries long-term risks of vaginal stenosis, ovarian insufficiency, and increased risk of primary tumors. Long-term follow-up of girls treated for genital RMS is important, as both disease recurrence and second primary tumors can occur.[33]

REFERENCES

1. Leung A, Robson W, Tay-Uyboco J. The incidence of labial fusion in children. *J Pediatr Child Health*. 1993;29(3):235–6.
2. Bacon J, Romano M, Quint E. Clinical recommendation: Labial adhesions. *J Pediatr Adolesc Gynecol*. 2015;28(5):405–9.
3. Mayoglou L, Dulabon L, Marin-Alguacil N, Pfaff D, Schober J. Success of treatment modalities for labial fusion: A retrospective evaluation of topical and surgical treatments. *J Pediatr Adolesc Gynecol*. 2009;22(4):247–50.
4. Runacres S, Wood P. Cosmetic labioplasty in an adolescent population. *J Ped Adol Gynecol*. 2016;29(3):218–22.
5. Women's Health Victoria. The Labia Library. http://www.labialibrary.org.au/. Accessed December 11, 2017.
6. Karras N. *Petals*. San Diego, CA: Crystal River Publishing; 2003.
7. Schober J, Cooney T, Pfaff D, Mayoglou L, Martin-Alguacil N. Innervation of the labia minora of prepubertal girls. *J Pediatr Adolesc Gynecol*. 2010;23(6):352–7.
8. Breast and labial surgery in adolescents. Committee Opinion No. 686. American College of Obstetricians and Gynecologists. *Obstet Gynecol*. 2017;129:e17–9.
9. Spriggs M, Gillam L. Body dysmorphic disorder: Contraindication or ethical justification for female genital cosmetic surgery in adolescents. *Bioethics*. 2016;30(9):706–13.
10. McGreal S, Wood P. Recurrent vaginal discharge in children. *J Pediatr Adolesc Gynecol*. 2013;26(4):205–8.
11. Ocampo D, Rahman G, Giugno S et al. Vulvovaginitis in a pediatric population: Relationship among etiologic agents, age and Tanner staging of breast development. *Arch Argent Pediatr*. 2014;112(1):65–74.
12. Zuckerman A, Romano M. Clinical recommendation: Vulvovaginitis. *J Pediatr Adolesc Gynecol*. 2016;29(6):673–9.
13. Cemek F, Odabas D, Senel U, Tuba Kocaman A. Personal hygiene and vulvovaginitis in prepubertal children. *J Pediatr Adolesc Gynecol*. 2016;29:223–7.
14. Clegg H, Giftos P, Anderson W et al. Clinical perineal streptococcal infection in children: Epidemiologic features, low symptomatic recurrence rate after treatment, and risk factors for recurrence. *J Pediatr*. 2015;167(3):687–93.
15. Rahman G, Ocampo D, Rubinstein A, Risso P. Prevalence of vulvovaginitis and relation to physical findings in girls assessed for suspected child sexual abuse. *Arch Argent Pediatr*. 2015;113(5):390–6.
16. Romero P, Munoz M, Martinez M et al. Ureaplasmas and mycoplasmas in vaginal samples from prepubertal girls and the reasons for gynecological consultation. *J Pediatr Adolesc Gynecol*. 2014;27(1):10–3.
17. Li JP, Hua CZ, Sun LY et al. Epidemiological features and antibiotic resistance patterns of *Haemophilus influenzae* originating from respiratory tract and vaginal specimens in pediatric patients. *J Pediatr Adolesc Gynecol*. 2017;30(6):626–31.
18. Stephens-Davidowitz S. Searching for sex. *The New York Times*. January 24, 2015.
19. Mikamo H, Yamagishi Y, Sugiyama H et al. High glucose-mediated overexpression of ICAM-1 in human vaginal epithelial cells increases adhesion of *Candida albicans*. *J Obstet Gynecol*. 2018;38(2):226–30.
20. Bradshaw C, Sobel J. Current treatment of bacterial vaginosis—Limitations and need for innovation. *J Infect Dis*. 2016;214(Suppl 1):S14–20.
21. Vodstrcil L, Twin J, Garland S et al. The influence of sexual activity on the vaginal microbiota and *Gardnerella vaginalis* clade diversity in young women. *PLOS ONE*. 2017;12(2):e0171856.
22. Fettweis J, Brooks P, Serrano M et al. Differences in vaginal microbiome in African American women versus women of European ancestry. *Microbiology*. 2014;160(Pt 10):2272–82.
23. Sutton M, Sternberg M, Koumans E et al. The prevalence of *Trichomonas vaginalis* infection among reproductive-age women in the United States, 2001–2004. *Clin Infect Dis*. 2007;45(10):1319–26.
24. Swartzendruber A, Sales J, Brown J et al. Correlates of incident *Trichomonas vaginalis* infections among African American female adolescents. *Sex Transm Dis*. 2014;41(4):240–5.
25. Centers for Disease Control and Prevention. CDC website. https://www.cdc.gov/std/tg2015/default.htm. Accessed January 7, 2018.
26. Rosman I, Berk D, Baylis S et al. Acute genital ulcers in nonsexually active young girls: Case series, review of the literature, and evaluation and management recommendations. *Ped Derm*. 2012;29(2):147–53.
27. Bandow G. Diagnosis and management of vulvar ulcers. *Dermatol Clin*. 2010;28:753–63.
28. Chiaroni-Clarke R, Munro J, Ellis J. Sex bias in paediatric autoimmune disease – Not just about sex hormones? *J Autoimmun*. 2016;69:12–23.
29. Soderstrom H, Carlsson A, Borjesson A, Elfving M. Vaginal bleeding in prepubertal girls: Etiology

and clinical management. *J Pediatr Adolesc Gynecol* 2016;29(3):280–5.

30. Dwiggins M, Gomez-Lobo V. Current review of pre-pubertal vaginal bleeding. *Curr Opin Obstet Gynecol.* 2017;29(5):322–7.

31. Wei Y, Wu Sd, Lin T et al. Diagnosis and treatment of urethral prolapse in children: 16 years' experience with 89 Chinese girls. *Arab J Urol.* 2017;15:248–53.

32. Harel M, Ferrer F, Shapiro L, Makari J. Future directions in risk stratification and therapy for advanced pediatric genitourinary rhabdomyosarcoma. *Urol Oncol.* 2016;34(2):103–15.

33. Nasioudis D, Alevizakos M, Chapman-Davis E et al. Rhabdomyosarcoma of the lower female genital tract: An analysis of 144 cases. *Arch Gynecol Obstet.* 2017;296:327–34.

34. Dowlut-McElroy T, Higgins J, Williams KB, Strickland JL. Treatment of prepubertal labial adhesions: A double blinded randomized controlled trial comparing topical emollient versus topical estrogen. *J Pediatr Adolesc Gynecol* 2017;30:268.

35. NASPAG PediGyn Teaching Slide Set CD-ROM, NASPAG 2001.

36. Simms-Cendan J, Santos X. Case of a girl with vulvar swelling. *Adolescent Gynecology: A Clinical Casebook.* New York, New York: Springer, 2018:35–40.

eRESOURCES

NASPAG Clinical Recommendations: Labial Adhesions, Vulvovaginitis. http://www.naspag.org/?page=clinicalrecommend

NASPAG Patient Handouts: Labial Adhesions, Labial Hypertrophy, Vaginal Discharge, Urethral Prolapse. http://www.naspag.org/?page=patienttools

ACOG Committee Opinion 686 2017: Breast and Labial Surgery in Adolescents. https://www.acog.org/Clinical-Guidance-and-Publications/Committee-Opinions-List

The Healthy Bodies Toolkit, Vanderbilt Kennedy Center. http://vkc.mc.vanderbilt.edu/healthybodies/

CDC.gov Sexually Transmitted Diseases (STDs) guidelines. https://www.cdc.gov/std/default.htm

Genital injuries in children and adolescents

9

BINDU N. PATEL and DIANE F. MERRITT

INTRODUCTION

Gynecologic emergencies often induce anxiety in the patient, her parents, and a medical provider who has not developed an organized protocol for assessing and managing these clinical problems. A common gynecologic complaint in the emergency pediatric and adolescent setting is genital trauma. This includes both accidental and non-accidental trauma. Potential causes of genital trauma are discussed later in this chapter, followed by basic management guidelines.

Straddle injuries

Straddle injuries (Figure 9.1) occur when the soft tissues of the vulva are compressed between an object and the bones of the pelvis, the pubic symphysis, and pubic rami. This trauma may result in ecchymosis, abrasions, and linear lacerations. Extravasation of blood into the loose areolar tissue in the labia or along the vagina, the mons, or clitoral area may cause hematoma formation. Accidental straddle injuries commonly occur as a result of falling onto a bicycle frame, playground equipment, or piece of furniture.

Accidental penetrating injuries

Penetrating injuries (Figure 9.2) occur if the victim falls on a sharp or pointed object and impales herself. Common household objects that can cause impalement include in-lawn sprinkling systems, pipes, fence posts, and furniture (e.g., chair-tops, bedposts, legs of stools). The vulva may display signs of injury, but the vagina, urethra, bladder,

anus, rectum, and peritoneal cavity can also be pierced by sharp or pointed objects.

Vaginal injuries related to sexual intercourse

Consensual intercourse or sexual assault should be considered whenever an adolescent presents with vaginal trauma. The patient may be too embarrassed or distressed to explain her injuries, so the medical history may not give a full account of how the injury occurred. Superficial minor lacerations of the introitus and lower vagina often occur with initial coitus. Adolescents who sustain deep vaginal lacerations from coitus may present with intense vaginal pain, profuse or prolonged vaginal bleeding, and shock.

Insufflation injuries

Insufflation injuries can occur when females fall off of personal watercraft or water skis, slide down water chutes, and come in direct contact with pool or spa jets.[1] As pressurized water enters the vagina, the walls may over-distend and tear. Significant blood loss can occur if branches of the anterior division of the internal iliac artery, which

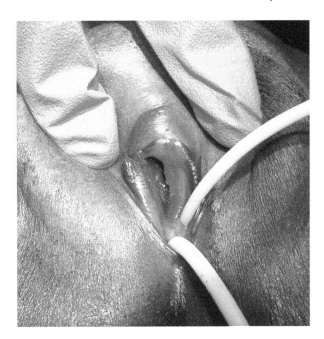

Figure 9.2 This child fell onto a broken metal bed frame and sustained this laceration. Initially, a source of bleeding could not be identified. A Foley catheter was placed in the vagina as a landmark; a second catheter was placed in the bladder. The repair proceeded safely with knowledge of the location of the urethra. (Courtesy of Dr. DF Merritt, MD.)

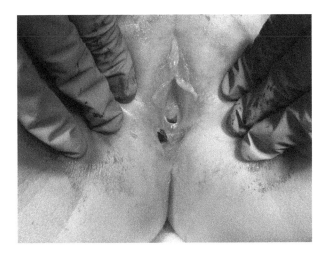

Figure 9.1 Straddle injury. (Courtesy of Dr. DF Merritt, MD.)

(a)   (b)

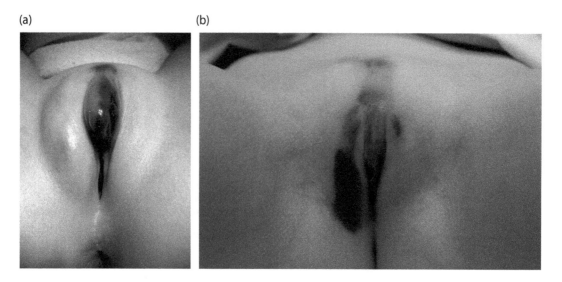

Figure 9.3 This patient was climbing over a chair when she fell, sustaining a periclitoral hematoma (a). The follow-up photo (b) was taken 6 days later. Once it was determined that her hematoma was not expanding, this patient was managed conservatively. Tracking of blood along the tissue planes can be seen as well as documentation of changes in her clinical examination with the passage of time. (Courtesy of Dr. DF Merritt, MD.)

supply the vagina, are avulsed. Such injuries may produce no sign of external genital trauma, and only careful vaginal examination (often under anesthesia) will reveal the source of bleeding and true extent of injury.

Vulvar hematoma

Vulvar hematomas (usually sustained as a result of a straddle injury) and the resulting pain and swelling may prevent a child or adolescent from urinating. If the hematoma is not large, if the perineal anatomy is not distorted, and if the patient has no difficulty urinating, the patient can be managed conservatively with immediate application of ice packs and bedrest (Figure 9.3). As the hematoma resolves, the blood will track along the fascial planes. The ecchymosis discoloration may take weeks to resolve.

Animal and human bites

Animal bites are a rare cause of potentially severe genital trauma, and children are the most common victims.[2] Human bites tend to occur in children as a result of playing or fighting.

Thermal and chemical burns

Accidental immersion burns caused by a child falling into a tub of hot water typically have irregular borders and nonuniform depth because the patient struggled to escape the hot liquid. Accidental burns are rarely full thickness, as they typically involve short contact time. The perineum and buttocks are infrequently involved in accidental burns, and burns in this area are often inflicted.[3] Well-demarcated and simultaneous scald burns to buttocks, feet, and perineum are highly suspicious for physical abuse and warrant a thorough investigation.

Batteries placed in the vagina may cause chemical burns and significant scarring.[4] Additionally, genital burns can occur from use of medications intended to treat genital warts, such as imiquimod, podophyllin, or trichloroacetic acid.

Female genital mutilation

Female genital cutting or mutilation (FGM), often referred to as female circumcision, refers to all procedures involving partial or total removal or injury of the external female genitalia for cultural, religious, or other nontherapeutic reasons. The World Health Organization (WHO) has classified FGM into four types (Table 9.1, Figure 9.4).

Table 9.1 Female genital mutilation types as classified by the World Health Organization.

Type	Description
Type I	Partial or total removal of the clitoris (clitoridectomy) and/or the prepuce
Type II	Partial or total removal of the clitoris and the labia minora, with or without excision of the labia majora (excision)
Type III	Narrowing of the vaginal orifice with the creation of a covering seal by cutting and appositioning the labia minora and/or the labia majora, with or without excision of the clitoris (infibulation)
Type IV	All other harmful procedures to the female genitalia for nonmedical purposes, for example, pricking, pulling, piercing, incising, scraping, and cauterization

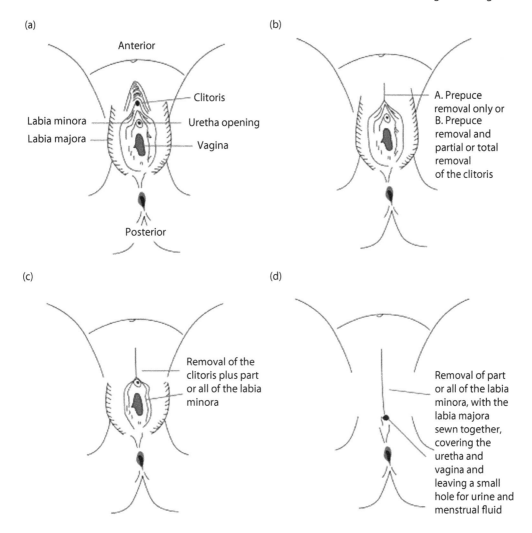

Figure 9.4 (a) Normal female external anatomy. (b) Type I FGM. (c) Type II FGM. (d) Type III FGM. (Courtesy of Wikimedia Commons.)

It is estimated that 200 million girls and women in the world have undergone some form of FGM, and 3 million girls are at risk from the practice each year.[5] Most of these women live in Africa, the Middle East, and Asia. However, as women emigrate from countries where FGM is practiced, medical care providers all over the world are caring for these women.

The WHO, the International Council of Nurses, the International Confederation of Midwives, and the International Federation of Gynecology and Obstetrics have openly condemned this practice of willful damage to healthy organs for nontherapeutic reasons. FGM is considered a form of violence against girls and women. The immediate health consequences of FGM include severe pain, shock, hemorrhage, urinary retention, ulceration of the genital region, and injury to adjacent tissue. Long-term complications include cysts and abscesses, keloid scar formation, damage to the urethra resulting in urinary incontinence, dyspareunia, sexual dysfunction, and difficulties with childbirth.

Increased awareness of the harmful effects of FGM and greater access to health-care services have resulted in requests to "medicalize" FGM and have the operation performed by health-care professionals in clinical settings. The WHO policy prohibits performing this procedure in a medical setting.

MANAGEMENT OF GENITAL TRAUMA
Lacerations, penetrating injuries, and vaginal rupture

When examining patients with genital trauma, the importance of proper positioning and lighting to allow good visualization cannot be overstated. An apparently bloody injury may be superficial or minor. With the patient on an examination table, gently rinse or wipe away blood. Place the patient on a bedpan, and pour warm water over the perineum to find the source of the bleeding. Direct inspection of a laceration will then allow the examiner to determine whether bleeding is active or has stopped.

If the injury is superficial and no longer bleeding, application of a topical ointment and good hygiene are all that is needed. Topical estrogen, an antibiotic ointment, petroleum jelly, or another barrier cream may be used depending on the situation. Whenever there is an injury to the mucosal genital surfaces, application of topical estrogen cream can benefit the healing process and decrease scarring. At our institution, a pea-sized amount is massaged into the tissues once or twice a day until resolution of the injury. Barrier ointments can be applied to prevent irritation from rubbing or pain at the laceration site while urinating. If minor cellulitis is associated with the laceration, an antibiotic ointment should be used. A small sanitary pad can be worn in the underwear as the dressing.

Vaginal lacerations that are not bleeding but are deeper than a few millimeters should be considered for repair with sutures rather than allowed to heal by secondary intent, as the latter process can take several weeks. A deep laceration should be sutured.

Superficial vaginal lacerations that are oozing but not heavily bleeding may be managed with compression. As an initial first aid measure, a clean dressing (washcloth, sanitary pad, or towel) can be held in place over the vulva by the patient or caregiver. By compressing the soft tissues against the underlying pelvic bones, an expanding hematoma can be prevented, and blood loss can be minimized. If the oozing is from a vaginal laceration, the vagina can be packed using tampons or sterile gauze to slow blood loss. The packing should be moistened with estrogen cream or saline to allow for easier removal.

Actively or briskly bleeding vaginal lacerations should always be evaluated by someone with expertise in genital anatomy in this age group. The urethra, bladder, and rectum should be assessed for injury. In a child or young adolescent, who has a small-caliber vagina, begin repair of lacerations with the deepest (most distal from the introitus) vaginal injuries first, and end the repair with introital lacerations to allow for maximum working space and visualization. Again, we have found that application of topical estrogen to the repaired lesion may hasten the healing process, decrease formation of granulation tissue, and promote healing without stricture. Minor lacerations can be repaired under local anesthesia or with conscious sedation.

Patients who have suffered from major trauma or have extensive lacerations may require examination and repair of their injuries under general anesthesia (Table 9.2). General anesthesia is especially needed to thoroughly evaluate the extent of penetrating injuries or if the vaginal injury extends above the hymen such that the true extent of the injury cannot be determined or repaired under local anesthesia.

Table 9.2 Indications for general anesthesia in gynecologic trauma.

- Young or uncooperative patient
- Transection of the hymen with inability to see the full extent of an injury
- Vaginal hemorrhage
- Expanding vulvar or vaginal hematoma
- Concomitant injuries which require examination under anesthesia

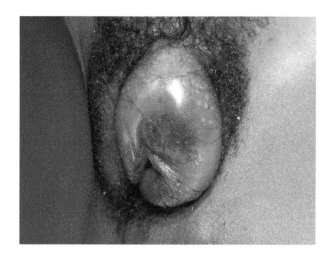

Figure 9.5 This large distorting hematoma needs to be treated with incision and drainage to hasten the patient's recovery. The incision is made in the medial mucosal surface near the vaginal orifice. (Courtesy of Dr. DF Merritt, MD.)

Blunt forceful penetrating vaginal injuries can include lateral vaginal wall and posterior fornix lacerations, and a tear may extend along the vagina and enter the peritoneal cavity, avulsing the cervix from its attachment to the vagina. This is called vaginal rupture, or colporrhexis, and while it is rare, examples have been described.[6] In such cases, the bowel, omentum, or fallopian tubes may eviscerate through the laceration (Figure 9.6). These patients present with vaginal bleeding and may be at risk of morbidity or death from exsanguination if not properly diagnosed and managed. If it is necessary to inspect the vagina of a trauma victim and a standard speculum is too large for a prepubertal child or young adolescent, vaginoscopy may be done. In this case, it is important to monitor the fluid deficit to avoid filling the abdomen or peritoneal cavity with saline through an unseen laceration extension. Perforations into the rectum or peritoneal cavity mandate an exploratory laparotomy or laparoscopy to determine whether other structures, such as the bowel or blood vessels, have been injured. Rectal injuries above the sphincter may mandate need for a diverting colostomy, and consultation with a pediatric surgeon is warranted.

Hematomas

If the patient has a large vulvar hematoma and is unable to urinate, place an indwelling urinary catheter and continue bladder drainage until the swelling resolves. Large vulvar hematomas may dissect into the loose areolar tissue along the vaginal wall and along the fascial planes overlying the symphysis pubis and lower abdominal wall. Pressure from an expanding hematoma can cause necrosis of the overlying skin (Figure 9.5). Evacuating the hematoma will reduce pain, hasten recovery, and prevent necrosis, tissue loss, and secondary infection. When incising large vulvar hematomas, care should be taken

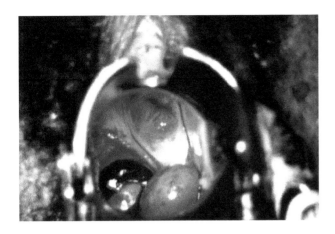

Figure 9.6 This adolescent was forcibly raped, and her cervix was avulsed from the vagina, resulting in evisceration of the small bowel and clot into the vagina. This injury should be repaired under general anesthesia. Consideration should be given to performing a diagnostic laparoscopy or exploratory laparotomy to determine the extent of intraabdominal injuries.(Courtesy of Dr. DF Merritt, MD.)

to start at the medial mucosal surface near the vaginal orifice. Note that the periclitoral area has a rich blood supply, so it is important to achieve complete hemostasis when operating in this area. If adequate hemostasis is not attained, the patient will be at risk for bleeding and reaccumulation of her hematoma. When the bed of the hematoma has been debrided of clot and devascularized tissue, and hemostasis has been attained, place a closed system drain (i.e., Jackson-Pratt) to prevent reaccumulation of blood, reduce pain, and reduce the risk of bacterial growth. Allow the drain to exit the skin in a dependent position, and close the skin primarily. In most cases, the drain can be removed in 24 hours.

Animal and human bites

Initial management of all types of bite injuries involves extensive irrigation and debridement. Whether to repair a wound with primary closure or to allow healing by secondary intent is controversial and depends on the type of bite. Old literature regarding management of animal bites speaks of delayed closure or healing by secondary intent due to concerns about infection. However, some recent guidelines now advocate primary definitive repair of injuries, because rates of infection can be higher with delayed closure.[2] Antibiotic prophylaxis should be given for large wounds and hematomas; puncture wounds; cat and human bites (which are at higher risk of infection than dog bites); bites older than 6 hours; and bites in babies, infants, and immunocompromised patients. Prophylaxis in such cases is a combination of extended-spectrum penicillin with β-lactamase inhibitors for 5–7 days.[2] Furthermore, evaluation for tetanus and rabies immunization should be performed as appropriate.

Patients with simple scrapes and abrasions are unlikely to benefit from antibiotic treatment.

Thermal and chemical burns

The management of genital and perineal burns includes cooling the burn for 20 minutes with cold tap water as soon as possible to reduce pain and wound edema. Chemical burns should be treated immediately by irrigation to neutralize the chemicals and prevent further damage. Chemical burns in the vagina can cause stricture, and placing a mold may prevent scarring across the vaginal wall. Additionally, a mixture of a topical antibiotic ointment and estrogen cream has been helpful for minimizing scarring from mucosal burns of the female genital tract.

Psychological factors associated with genital injuries

Young victims of genital injuries and their families should be reassured about the future ability to have sexual relation and bear children. When appropriate, offer unsolicited reassurance of reproductive capacity, as a patient or her family members will not always verbalize these concerns. Children and teens recovering from an isolated genital injury seldom have long-standing psychological trauma from the event. The exception would be an injury that leaves lasting scarring or vaginal stenosis.

Conversely, victims of sexual assault often suffer from post-traumatic stress, anxiety, depression, and anger. Offer specific referrals for professional counseling to all victims of sexual assault. Every hospital should have a defined protocol for collecting forensic evidence in cases of alleged or possible sexual assault. It is useful and important to provide a clear description of the injuries with accompanying image documentation, if available.

CONCLUSION

To better prepare the health-care provider to deal with acute evaluation, diagnosis, and management of pediatric and adolescent gynecologic emergencies, this chapter provided a summary of genital trauma. Genital trauma can range from minor lacerations and bruises of external structures, to massive injuries with pelvic fractures and internal bleeding. Familiarity with common causes allows one to determine if injuries correlate to the story provided. The provider must be equipped with tools to assess the young female during a potentially very emotional time in her life being detailed. The important point to remember is that a majority of times, with proper evaluation and treatment, injuries should heal without long-lasting effects.

REFERENCES

1. Lopez, HN, Focseneanu, MA, Merritt, DF. Genital injuries acute evaluation and management. *Best Pract Res Clin Obstet Gynaecol*. 2018;48:28–39.

2. Agrawal A, Kumar P, Singhal R et al. Animal bite injuries in children: Review of literature and case series. *Int J Clin Pediatr Dent.* 2017;10(1):67–72.

3. Tresh A, Baradaran N, Gaither TW et al. Genital burns in the United States: Disproportionate prevalence in the pediatric population. *Burns,* 2018;44(5): 1366–1371.

4. Nakib G, Calcaterra V, Pelizzo G. Longstanding presence of a vaginal foreign body (battery): Severe stenosis in a 13-year-old girl. *J Pediatr Adolesc Gynecol.* 2017; 30(1):e15–e18.

5. WHO guidelines on the management of health complications from female genital mutilation. World Health Organization. 2016. http://www.who.int/ reproductivehealth/topics/fgm/managementhealth-complications-fgm/en. Accessed January 16, 2018.

6. Abraham M, Kondis J, Merritt DF. Case series: Vaginal rupture injuries after sexual assault in children and adolescents. *J Pediatr Adolesc Gynecol.* 2016;29(3):e49–e52.

Basic dermatology in children and adolescents

10

KALYANI MARATHE and KATHLEEN ELLISON

INTRODUCTION

Dermatology is the study of the skin and adjacent mucosa, hair, and nails. Dermatologic conditions are commonly encountered in all areas of medicine. We discuss the more frequent skin diseases in children and adolescents that may affect the genital area. Accurate descriptions of the clinical features of skin disease are important. A brief overview of common descriptive terms used in dermatology is given in Table 10.1.

DIAPER DERMATITIS AND INFLAMMATORY DERMATOSES

Diaper (nappy) dermatitis can be a persistent and difficult problem in the pediatric outpatient setting; it is estimated that around 50% of infants will develop this condition. While diaper dermatitis is common, it is important to look for clinical findings to help elucidate the etiology of the eruption. Rashes in the diaper area are most commonly due to contact dermatitis, but they can also indicate infection or a cutaneous manifestation of systemic disease.

Contact dermatitis

Contact dermatitis can essentially be divided into two categories: allergic contact dermatitis and irritant contact dermatitis.

Allergic contact dermatitis

Allergic contact dermatitis (ACD) is an acute inflammatory skin reaction that can result from a number of different allergens. The exact incidence of allergic contact diaper dermatitis is unknown, but it is estimated that at any given time, between 7% and 35% of the infant population may be affected.[1] Numerous antigens may be implicated as causing ACD of the diaper area, including dyes, fragrance, elastic, rubber compounds, and materials used to make disposable diapers.[2–5] Methylisothiazolinone, a component of diaper wipes, is also a commonly implicated cause of ACD.[6]

It presents as acute onset of well-demarcated erythematous papules and plaques, often with the presence of small, clear, fluid-filled vesicles. The vesicles may erode and ooze, eventually evolving into more eczematous plaques with lichenification. It is important to note that during the initial sensitization phase, the rash may not become apparent until 5–7 days after initial contact with the allergen. Upon reexposure to the allergen, the rash will typically appear 12–24 hours after contact.

It can occur in areas besides the groin, and the distribution of the rash is a useful clue in diagnosing ACD. Rashes localized to specific parts of the body (i.e., hands, feet, or earlobes) or rashes that have discrete shapes and sharply demarcated borders prompt consideration of ACD (Figure 10.1).

Identification and removal of the inciting allergen is of paramount importance in treating ACD. For ACD in the diaper area, this can be done by changing diaper brands, wipes, and barrier creams to see if relief is obtained. Patch testing can be done in a dermatologist's office, but this type of allergy testing may not be practical or high yield in the infant patient.

For symptomatic relief, topical low-potency corticosteroids such as desonide 0.05% or hydrocortisone 2.5% ointment may be applied twice daily for 2 weeks. Of note, some patients may experience an allergic reaction to certain components of topical steroids; this is an important consideration if the expected relief is not obtained. Additionally, barrier/repair creams, such as zinc oxide paste or white petrolatum, may be effective in expediting healing of affected areas.

Irritant contact dermatitis

Irritant contact dermatitis (ICD) of the diaper area is the most common cause of diaper dermatitis. It is a non-immunologic reaction to various irritants in the diaper environment, including urine, feces, and chemicals. As opposed to the immunologic basis of ACD, ICD results from the direct toxic effect of these agents on the skin when the irritant is in contact with the skin for a prolonged period of time. It can be exacerbated by friction, occlusion, moisture, cracks or fissures in the skin, and cleansing wipes.[7]

ICD can be difficult to clinically distinguish from ACD. Typically, there are discrete areas of erythema that have a glazed appearance and may be surrounded by erythematous papules. It is most evident in the convex areas of skin that are exposed to the offending agent; the inguinal folds and gluteal cleft are usually spared.[3]

The absence of clear, fluid-filled vesicles as seen in ACD steers the clinician toward a diagnosis of ICD; however, blistering and erosions may be seen in severe cases. The presence of punched-out erosions is characteristic of Jacquet erosive diaper dermatitis (Figure 10.2). Granuloma gluteale infantum is another form of severe ICD that usually is triggered by topical steroid use and/or *Candida* infection. It typically presents in the first year of life as oval reddish-brown or reddish-purple nodules or plaques varying from 0.5 to 3 cm.[8]

Table 10.1 Descriptive terms used in dermatology.

Configuration—how skin lesions are arranged

Annular or circinate	Ring shaped, often with an area of central clearing
Confluent	Lesions that merge
Discrete	Lesions that remain distinct and separated
Clustered	Groupings of lesions that are similar in morphology
Guttate	Drop-like
Linear	Occurring in a line
Umbilicated	Lesions that have an area of depression or a "dell" in the central portion

Primary lesions—how to describe various types of skin lesions

Macule	A flat, nonpalpable area of less than 1 cm in diameter that appears different from the surrounding skin
Patch	A flat, nonpalpable area of greater than 1 cm in diameter that appears different from the surrounding skin
Papule	An elevated, palpable, circumscribed lesion that is less than 1 cm in diameter
Plaque	An elevated, palpable, broad lesion that is greater than 1 cm in diameter
Nodule	An elevated, palpable, solid lesion less than 2 cm wide with a deeper component that may extend into the dermis or subcutaneous tissues
Tumor	An elevated, palpable, solid lesion greater than 2 cm wide with a deeper component that may extend into the dermis or subcutaneous tissues
Wheal	A pink to red edematous, inflamed, elevated lesion, often with central clearing
Vesicle	An elevated lesion less than 1 cm in diameter that is filled with fluid
Pustule	An elevated lesion less than 1 cm in diameter that is filled with pus
Bulla	An elevated lesion greater than 1 cm in diameter that is filled with fluid
Abscess	An elevated lesion greater than 1 cm in diameter that is filled with pus

Secondary lesions—how to describe various types of skin lesions

Crust	Dried serum, blood, or exudative remains on the surface of a lesion
Scale	Dry desquamated corneocytes that have been shed onto the surface of a lesion
Fissure	A linear cleavage in the skin
Erosion	Superficial loss of the epidermis that leaves denuded skin
Ulcer	A deeper loss of the epidermis and dermis, and sometimes portions of the subcutaneous tissue
Excoriation	Superficial loss of skin, often due to scratching or trauma
Atrophy	Loss of skin tissue; can be due to epidermal or dermal loss
Lichenification	Thickening of the epidermis with enhanced skin markings from chronic rubbing of the lesion
Induration	Palpable thickening of the dermis

Color

Erythematous	Red; blanchable
Violaceous	Purple
Sclerotic	Scar-like, often having a shiny white to pink appearance; can appear wrinkled

As with ACD, the best treatment is prevention. Frequent diaper changes will minimize irritation from moisture and feces in the diaper area. Eruptions of ICD that persist longer than 3 days can often develop superimposed infection with *Candida*; for this reason, treatment with topical antifungal creams is recommended.[9] The use of barrier pastes with 40% zinc oxide will help prevent recurrences. If the eruption fails to resolve with these treatments, evaluation by a dermatologist is warranted.

Inflammatory dermatoses with infectious etiologies

Candidiasis

Candida albicans, a common yeast, may be found on skin with diaper dermatitis and may cause acute or chronic infection of the skin or the mucous membranes. *C. albicans* is not a normal cutaneous saprophyte but exists in the microflora of the vagina of infant and postpubertal females. Certain systemic medications (antibiotics, corticosteroids, and immunosuppressant medications) as well as the moist and warm environment of the diaper area can alter the normal flora, making infants more susceptible to *Candida* overgrowth.

The presence of beefy, bright red papules and plaques, satellite pustules, and scale are characteristic of infection with *C. albicans*. As opposed to ACD and ICD, *Candida* infection will often involve the intertriginous folds. Other presentations of candidiasis include oral candidiasis, vulvovaginitis, angular cheilitis (perleche), and chronic

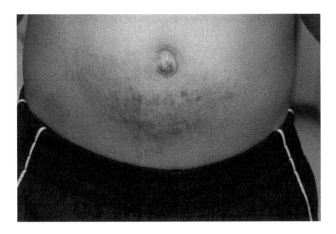

Figure 10.1 Allergic contact dermatitis (ACD) to nickel in a belt buckle. The distribution of involved skin suggests the etiology of the rash. Acute ACD can be seen in the central eczematous plaque; the periphery of this lesion demonstrates lichenification of chronic ACD. (Courtesy of Kalyani Marathe, MD, MPH.)

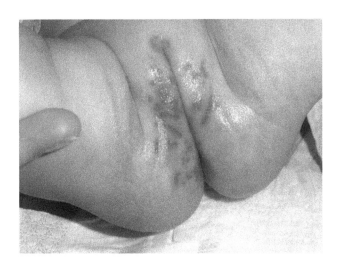

Figure 10.2 Jacquet erosive diaper dermatitis presents as punched-out erosions on a background of irritant contact dermatitis. (Courtesy of Scott A. Norton, MD, MPH.)

paronychia (nail infection). A potassium hydroxide (KOH) wet mount can confirm the presence of *Candida*.

Intertrigo refers to an inflammatory disorder of the skin that is often secondarily infected with *Candida*; this occurs in areas of skin-to-skin contact, known as the intertriginous areas, such as the neck in infants, axillae, and groin. The combination of friction in a moist and warm environment causes inflammation to occur, resulting in macerated erythematous plaques in these areas.

Candidal diaper dermatitis and intertrigo are most effectively treated with a topical antifungal cream applied after diaper changes. Azole antifungal creams, such as miconazole and clotrimazole, are fungicidal rather than fungistatic, so they are more effective than nystatin at treating *Candida* diaper dermatitis. Frequent changing of

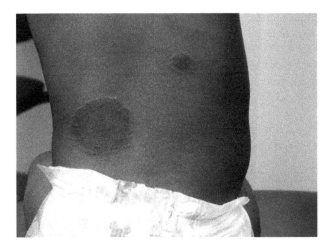

Figure 10.3 Round, scaly plaques with raised edges, characteristic of tinea corporis. (Courtesy of Kalyani Marathe, MD, MPH.)

diapers and dusting powders such as miconazole nitrate 2% powder will also aid in preventing excess moisture in the diaper area. For immunocompromised children or widespread infections, oral antifungals such as fluconazole may be needed. For cases with severe inflammation, adding a topical corticosteroid is indicated (clotrimazole/betamethasone cream). For candidal vulvovaginitis, antifungal vaginal tablets or creams such as clotrimazole or miconazole may be used daily for 3–7 days. A single oral dose of fluconazole 150 mg is also effective for adolescents.[10]

Tinea

Superficial fungal infections can occur anywhere on the skin, including the groin (tinea cruris), body (tinea corporis) (Figure 10.3), face (tinea faciei) (Figure 10.4), and scalp (tinea capitis). Tinea can be caused by a number of different pathogens and presents with scaly erythematous

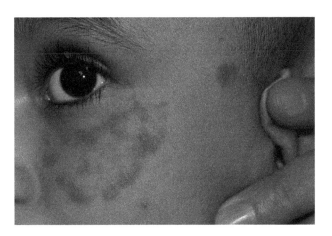

Figure 10.4 Tinea faciei can manifest as a discontinuous erythematous plaque with central clearing and a raised border. (Courtesy of Scott A. Norton, MD, MPH.)

plaques, often with central clearing and a raised border. The plaques can vary in size from less than 1 cm to greater than 10 cm. They are often asymptomatic but can be pruritic. Tinea versicolor can present as hyperpigmented or hypopigmented scaling macules that commonly arise on the scalp, face, or trunk.

Most uncomplicated superficial fungal infections can be treated with a topical antifungal agent. For complicated or widespread infections, a systemic antifungal, such as terbinafine, fluconazole, or itraconazole, may be indicated. However, these agents have not been extensively studied in the neonatal and pediatric populations.[11] Topical or systemic corticosteroids should never be used either alone or in preparations with topical antifungal agents to treat superficial fungal infections, as these preparations can mask, exacerbate, or result in propagation of the fungal infection into the hair follicles.

Perianal streptococcal dermatitis

Perianal streptococcal dermatitis (PSD) is an infection seen in the diaper area caused most commonly by group A ß-hemolytic streptococci (GABHS), gram-positive bacteria. The mean age of onset is 4 years, though it has been reported in children as young as 6 months and as old as 10 years of age.[12] Transmission among family members and in daycare settings has been reported.[12,13]

It presents as a well-defined plaque, which can vary in appearance from a dry pink plaque to bright red moist erythema with overlying maceration. Affected infants and children may have tenderness, discomfort, and sensitivity of the area, rectal pruritus, blood-streaked stools, and constipation. Guttate psoriasis, classically associated with streptococcal pharyngitis, can be related to PSD. Therefore, a thorough anogenital exam should be performed in infants and children presenting with skin findings of guttate psoriasis (discussed later in this chapter). Diagnosis is made clinically, and a culture or rapid strep test can be used to confirm the diagnosis. The differential diagnosis of PSD includes contact dermatitis, candidiasis, seborrheic dermatitis, pinworm infection, and sexual abuse, so a thorough history and examination are warranted.[12] Of note, girls can also become infected with group A vaginal streptococcal vaginitis; this often presents with vulvar erythema and copious watery vaginal discharge.

Oral amoxicillin is the treatment of choice for PSD; penicillin, clindamycin, and erythromycin may also be used, but close attention to regional resistance patterns is recommended, since certain areas have large percentages of streptococcal isolates that have become resistant to macrolide antibiotics.[12,14] Treatment duration should be at least 14 days.[12]

Patients with PSD should be monitored for signs and symptoms of poststreptococcoal glomerulonephritis, including edema, hypertension, and tea-colored urine. A thorough history and physical exam should include examination of the pharynx to identify possible coexisting pharyngitis.

Other inflammatory dermatoses of the groin

Lichen sclerosus

Lichen sclerosus (LS) is an autoimmune chronic inflammatory dermatitis that has bimodal peak incidence in female patients: prepubertal and postmenopausal. Of the prepubertal cases, most have onset around ages 4–6 years.[15] Prevalence rates are estimated at 1:300 to 1:1000 based on referrals to dermatology, though true incidence is unknown.[16] The exact cause of LS is unclear; there is a noted association with autoimmune diseases such as alopecia areata, vitiligo, thyroid disease, and pernicious anemia. However, it is not recommended to screen for these disorders unless other clinical findings raise suspicion. Koebnerization, the formation of a lesion at a site of trauma, occurs with friction or rubbing of the affected area.

It is characterized by vulvar irritation, bleeding, pruritus, dysuria, and dyspareunia. Prepubertal patients often experience constipation, which is more common in pediatric patients with LS than in postmenopausal females. The course waxes and wanes with episodic flares. It classically involves the genital area, although any area of the skin may be affected. On physical exam, white to pink, slightly elevated, flat-topped papules coalesce into well-defined plaques; scarring, atrophy, and follicular plugging can develop within the plaques. Telangiectasias, purpura, linear erosions, and excoriations may also be noted. When the perineal and perianal areas are involved, the classic "figure-of-eight" (hourglass) shape can be seen (Figure 10.5). When the skin becomes atrophic, it can develop a "cigarette paper" texture.[16] On average, patients typically have symptoms of LS 1–2 years prior to diagnosis.[15] Diagnosis in children and adolescents is made clinically; however, a biopsy may be needed to confirm the diagnosis in rare cases. While LS is often thought to be similar in appearance to vitiligo, it can be differentiated using a Wood's lamp. Diseases that present with similar symptoms include allergic or irritant contact dermatitis, lichen planus, discoid lupus, morphea, sexual abuse, and Bowen disease.

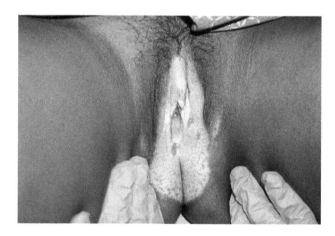

Figure 10.5 Lichen sclerosus, showing classic atrophy and hypopigmentation. Erosions can also be seen. (Courtesy of Kalyani Marathe, MD, MPH.)

The goals of therapy are alleviation of symptoms and prevention of complications such as scarring and labial and clitoral hood adhesions.[16] In premenarchal and adolescent girls, ultrapotent steroids such as clobetasol propionate 0.05% ointment can be used twice a day for 6 weeks; a close follow-up appointment is recommended for reevaluation and discussion about tapering use of the topical steroid. Experts recommend that patients use clobetasol propionate 0.05% ointment twice per week for maintenance therapy rather than abruptly discontinue the topical steroid. Pimecrolimus and tacrolimus, both steroid-sparing agents, have been effective in treating LS but are second-line agents that tend to be more effective maintenance agents once a higher-potency topical steroid has been used to abate the acute flare.[16–18] Scarring may need to be corrected surgically if medical therapy fails. In adolescents (and adults) with chronic, long-standing LS, there is an association with squamous cell and verrucous carcinoma, and proper screening is of great importance. It is unclear if prepubertal or childhood LS predisposes children to neoplasia.

Psoriasis

Psoriasis is a chronic papulosquamous autoimmune disorder that can present in the diaper area as well as other areas of the skin. While immune mediated, it is also multifactorial and driven by both genetic and environmental factors. Koebnerization is a well-known feature of psoriasis and may cause involvement in the diaper area of infants. Other triggering factors can include friction, yeast overgrowth, surgical procedures, and sunburn, among others. The prevalence of pediatric psoriasis is estimated to be around 0.5%–2%.[19]

Lesions start as small red papules, which enlarge to form pink to erythematous plaques with overlying silvery scale (Figure 10.6). The classic distribution is on the extensor surfaces (as opposed to the flexural surfaces in atopic dermatitis); however, lesions can occur anywhere on the body including the genital region. Psoriatic lesions in the

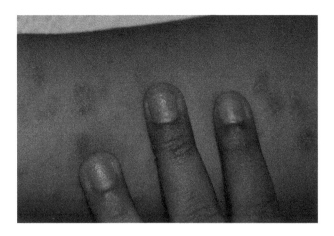

Figure 10.7 Nail pitting and psoriasis. Approximately 50% of patients with psoriasis have nail changes. (Courtesy of Scott A. Norton, MD, MPH.)

diaper area of infants may lack the classic surface scale due to the moist nature of this area. Scalp psoriasis can also be seen in children and adolescents.[19] Patients may also have symptoms of geographic tongue, nail pitting or dystrophy, or arthritis (Figure 10.7). Psoriasis can be pruritic in children.[19]

Guttate psoriasis is a particular subtype that manifests as drop-like 1–2 cm scaly red plaques and often occurs after streptococcal infection of the oropharynx or perianal area. It is important to screen for asymptomatic streptococcal pharyngeal infection with culture and antistreptolysin O (ASO) titer, as many patients report no preceding sore throat. While guttate psoriasis can resolve within a few months, approximately one-third of patients with guttate psoriasis evolve to have chronic plaque psoriasis.

Topical treatments are effective for limited disease and include corticosteroids (low to mid-potency in infants and children), calcineurin inhibitors, and calcipotriene. While tar has been used historically, its odor and phototoxicity make its use less appealing for children.[19] Keratolytic agents such as salicylic acid break down the scale and increase penetration of these topicals. Ultraviolet light, including narrowband ultraviolet-B light, is also very effective in treating psoriasis. Exposure to natural sunlight may help with flares, although sunburn must be avoided, as this can trigger the disease and increase the risk of skin cancer. For widespread involvement or psoriasis that is refractory to topical therapies and/or light, systemic treatment with methotrexate, cyclosporine, or biologic agents may be necessary. These medications require careful follow-up due to their side effect profiles and should be given only by a clinician well versed in their possible side effects and comfortable with monitoring guidelines. Systemic steroids should be avoided because of the risk of a rebound flare and pustular psoriasis on discontinuation.

Atopic dermatitis

Atopic dermatitis is a very common chronic inflammatory skin disorder, with prevalence estimated to be 10%–20% of

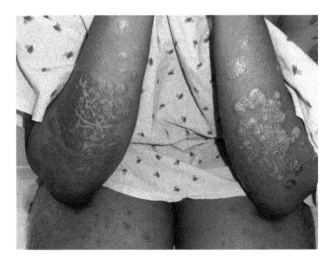

Figure 10.6 Psoriatic plaques with overlying silvery scale in a symmetric distribution. (Courtesy of Scott A. Norton, MD, MPH.)

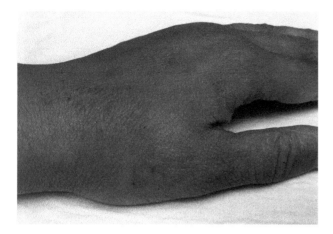

Figure 10.8 Lichenification, eczematous plaques, and excoriations in atopic dermatitis. (Courtesy of Kathleen Ellison, MD.)

children younger than age 10 years.[20] The exact pathogenesis is poorly understood but is likely related to a complex relationship between interrupted epidermal barrier and immune dysregulation of the T cells and Langerhans cells of the skin.[21] Children with atopic dermatitis often have family members with eczema, allergies, and asthma.

Diagnostic features of atopic dermatitis include eczematous dermatitis, pruritus, and a history of a chronic or relapsing-remitting course.[20] The clinical appearance of atopic dermatitis can vary significantly from patient to patient, and the morphology of eczematous dermatitis can depend on the age of the patient. Classic features include the presence of erythematous scaly or lichenified plaques with or without excoriation (Figures 10.8 through 10.10). Atopic dermatitis may also present as hyperkeratotic, follicularly based papules, especially in infants. The cheeks are often involved as well as the flexural surfaces. Diffuse xerosis may be present. Sparing of the diaper area is common; the barrier of the diaper helps to keep the skin in that area moist. This helps differentiate atopic dermatitis from other inflammatory dermatoses of the groin.

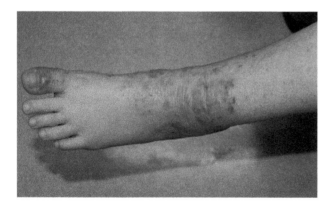

Figure 10.9 Atopic dermatitis: Eczematous plaques with overlying excoriations on the ankle and dorsal foot. (Courtesy of Kalyani Marathe, MD, MPH.)

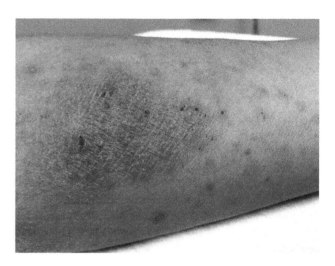

Figure 10.10 Lichenification and papules with overlying excoriations in atopic dermatitis. This patient also has some postinflammatory hyperpigmentation from previous flares of eczema. (Courtesy of Kathleen Ellison, MD.)

Due to the interrupted epidermal barrier as well as impaired local immunity, secondary infection of affected areas with *Staphylococcus aureus* or *Streptococcus pyogenes* is fairly common. Over 90% of eczema patients are colonized with *S. aureus* at the time of an acute flare. Impetigo, characterized by honey-colored crusting, can complicate a flare of eczema. Therefore, topical or oral antibiotics are an essential component of treatment in these patients. Viral diseases such as herpes simplex, hand-foot-and-mouth disease, or molluscum contagiosum may also infect areas of atopic dermatitis.[14]

Atopic dermatitis can have significant psychosocial effects, including stress, decreased participation in sports and recreational activities, low self-esteem, and difficulties in sleeping and focusing in school.[20] Thus, treatment of atopic dermatitis is essential. Affected individuals must be treated with regular moisturization using a thick emollient immediately after bathing and multiple times daily. Mild, nonabrasive soaps and cleansers without fragrances should be used to wash the skin, and bubble baths are discouraged.[20] Patients should avoid wool clothing that could irritate the skin. Topical steroids are an essential tool in managing moderate and severe atopic dermatitis; steroid selection is determined depending on location and severity of the disease. In general, low-potency topical steroids should be used for the face and intertriginous areas or for milder disease. Mid- to high-potency topical steroids may be used on other areas of the body and for more severe symptoms. Steroid-sparing agents, such as topical pimecrolimus and tacrolimus (calcineurin inhibitors) and crisaborole (a phosphodiesterase-4 inhibitor), help control mild to moderate disease; they are useful for maintenance therapy, especially on the face and intertriginous areas. Skin that is routinely treated with topical steroids and areas of thin skin, including the eyelids and intertriginous areas, are at increased risk of side effects. Side effects of topical steroids include allergic contact dermatitis, acne, telangiectasias, erythema, tachyphylaxis, dyspigmentation, and atrophy. Ointments are typically better tolerated than creams, which can cause burning at the site of application. For severe cases of recalcitrant atopic dermatitis, treatment with systemic immunosuppression or ultraviolet light may be necessary.

A common condition associated with atopic dermatitis is keratosis pilaris. Patients may present with many rough, monomorphic, perifollicular papules on the posterior upper arms, the anterior thighs, or the lateral cheeks. This benign condition can be treated with ammonium lactate lotions (AmLactin or LacHydrin), creams containing urea, or creams containing salicylic acid (CeraVe SA).

Hidradenitis suppurativa

Hidradenitis suppurativa is an inflammatory disorder that commonly presents as recurrent tender papules, pustules, and nodules in the anogenital region, inframammary areas, and axillae. This chronic condition occurs secondary to dysregulation of the inflammatory process and subsequent damage of surrounding tissue. The etiology is poorly understood, but genetics, hormones, and obesity leading to occlusion of the follicular orifice may all play a role. While there is significant inflammation in HS, infection is not thought to play a causative role in the etiology of the underlying inflammatory process. However, lesions of HS can become secondarily infected.[22]

Patients complain of painful, inflamed, foul-smelling, draining pustules and abscesses that swell and enlarge. With further progression and inflammation, sinus tracts can form, eventually resulting in extensive scarring. Patients can become embarrassed or socially isolated by their disease, causing significant morbidity. Patients often suffer for several years prior to diagnosis, with the average delay from onset of symptoms to diagnosis being 7.2 years.[23]

Treatment of hidradenitis should be based on individual symptoms. Lifestyle modifications including weight loss and smoking cessation are recommended for HS patients who are overweight or current smokers. Topical antibacterial washes such as benzoyl peroxide and chlorhexidine are often recommended. Topical antibiotics such as clindamycin 1% lotion or solution are also used. Oral antibiotics, especially tetracyclines, are used to reduce inflammation. It has also been suggested that oral zinc gluconate can induce clinical improvement or remission in patients with mild to moderate HS.[24] Biologic medications are now being used for the treatment of HS. Adalimumab is approved for use for moderate to severe HS in adults. Anakinra and ustekinumab are also being studied for the treatment of HS. Carbon dioxide laser treatment has also been effective. For acute, limited flares of hidradenitis or for persistent nodules, intralesional triamcinolone (5–10 mg/mL) is often used for short-term relief of symptoms. However, if infection is suspected, intralesional steroids are contraindicated.[25] While incision and drainage of nodules can provide pain relief, this treatment is associated with recurrence of the lesions.[26]

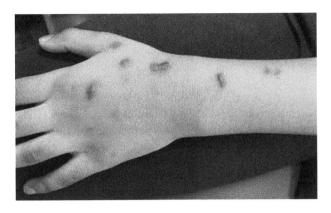

Figure 10.11 Lichen planus often presents as purple papules on the extremities. (Courtesy of Kalyani Marathe, MD, MPH.)

For persistent cases, deroofing of sinus tracts or surgical excision may be necessary.[22]

Lichen planus

Lichen planus is an inflammatory dermatosis of unknown etiology that classically presents as flat-topped, polymorphic, pink to violaceous papules that can vary in size from 0.2 to 1 cm or more (Figure 10.11). The lesions are usually pruritic and commonly occur symmetrically on the flexural surfaces of the extremities as well as the trunk and genitalia; lichen planus can also present on the mucous membranes as a network of delicate white lines referred to as Wickham striae. Koebnerization may be observed. Atypical presentations include bullous, annular, hypertrophic, and vesicular, among others. While the majority of lichen planus cases occur in adults, children comprise 5%–11% of reported cases.[27]

Lichen planus often responds to potent topical corticosteroids. Treatment with narrow-band UVB light can improve symptoms of pruritus.[27] Patients should be screened for hepatitis C, as this has been linked with lichen planus, especially in the adult population.

Urticaria

Urticaria, commonly known as hives, is an IgE-mediated type I hypersensitivity reaction that causes activation of mast cells and release of histamine. This fairly common condition can present anywhere on the skin and can be triggered by infections, drugs, or foods, or may be idiopathic.

Urticaria presents with white or pink, edematous plaques, which are usually round, but sometimes polycyclic in appearance. They can sometimes have central clearing, but they do not have the overlying scale that is characteristic of tinea corporis. A rim of pallor often surrounds pink hives. The size of an individual lesion can vary from less than 1 cm to greater than 10 cm. Lesions may be focal or widespread. Individual lesions rarely last longer than 24 hours, a quality that distinguishes them from lesions of erythema multiforme, which remain fixed in a given location for longer periods of time. While individual lesions of urticaria resolve in less than a day, new lesions can form in the meantime, giving the appearance that individual lesions last for several days. For this reason, it is helpful to trace urticaria with a pen to see if lesions resolve or persist for greater than 24 hours; this can help confirm the diagnosis. Urticaria is usually very pruritic, and patients often complain that the discomfort caused by the intractable itching interferes with their daily activities. If angioedema occurs, emergent evaluation is warranted.

The most effective treatment is identification and elimination of the inciting agent. Antihistamines are usually very helpful in controlling symptoms, and nonsedating H1 blockers such as cetirizine, loratadine, and fexofenadine are often used. Hydroxyzine or diphenhydramine may also be utilized, but these agents often cause sedation and should be administered before bedtime. Antihistamines should be continued through clearance of the urticaria and then gradually tapered. For severe cases, epinephrine or systemic steroids may be indicated.

Others

Other, less common conditions that should be considered in the differential diagnosis of inflammatory disorders of the groin include Langerhans cell histiocytosis, acrodermatitis enteropathica, mastocytosis, erythema multiforme, and pityriasis rosea, among others. A full discussion of these entities is beyond the scope of this chapter. When these conditions are suspected, a skin biopsy is useful in making the proper diagnosis, and evaluation by a dermatologist is warranted.

Infectious diseases

Dermatologic infectious diseases are common in the pediatric and adolescent population because they are easily spread among individuals. Some of the more frequent infections are discussed in the following section. Herpes simplex virus, human papillomavirus, and syphilis are covered in Chapter 17.

Molluscum contagiosum

Molluscum contagiosum is a common cutaneous poxvirus infection in children and a sexually transmitted infection of the genital region in adolescents and adults. In children, infection usually occurs between the ages of 2 and 5 years.[28,29]

The lesions of molluscum are discrete, dome-shaped, umbilicated papules with creamy cores that vary in color from pink to flesh-colored or white. They have a tendency to look translucent or shiny (Figure 10.12). Mollusca vary in size from 1 to 15 mm and can become inflamed and irritated with surrounding dermatitis. Any area of the body may be involved; however, in children, characteristic locations include the axilla, flanks, lower abdominal wall, inner thighs, and face. In adolescents and young adults, molluscum contagiosum often presents in the external genital area. Viral infection can be spread by scratching or shaving over the mollusca. Immunocompetent patients usually have fewer than 20 mollusca, but immunocompromised

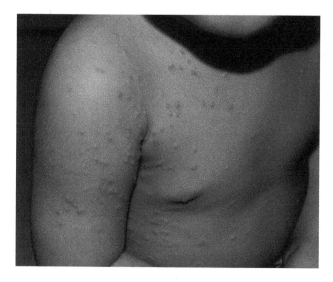

Figure 10.12 Patients with molluscum contagiosum can have multiple discrete shiny papules with creamy cores. (Courtesy of Kalyani Marathe, MD, MPH.)

patients can have extensive, diffuse involvement and can present with giant molluscum.[30]

Molluscum contagiosum cannot be cultured, and the diagnosis is usually made on the basis of clinical appearance. Diagnosis can be confirmed with biopsy, electron microscopy, or ELISA (enzyme-linked immunosorbent assay). Lesions that mimic mollusca include verrucae, varicella, folliculitis, juvenile xanthogranuloma, spitz nevi, and skin tags. In immunocompromised patients, deep fungal infection is included in the differential.[30]

The infection is self-limited and will resolve spontaneously without treatment in most patients. However, patients may scratch or autoinnoculate themselves and cause new lesions. Genital lesions should be treated to prevent spread of infection to sexual partners. Medical or surgical management can be implemented if lesions last longer than expected or become irritated or bothersome. There are several modalities of destructive therapy including curettage, cryotherapy, or laser. Topical therapies include cantharidin, tretinoin cream, imiquimod, and podophyllotoxin cream. Oral cimetidine has also been reported to be helpful in treating molluscum contagiosum.[31] Care should be taken in treating children, as ablative treatments can cause dyspigmentation, scarring, and pain.[30]

Parents of children with active molluscum should be counselled about the contagious nature of the virus. Viral spread has been associated with skin contact, swimming pools, and the sharing of towels.[30] Adolescents with molluscum in the genital area should be screened for other sexually transmitted infections (STIs) and counseled regarding the risk of spread to their sexual partners.

Impetigo

Impetigo is a common, highly contagious superficial skin infection that can easily be spread among family members, in schools, or in day-care settings.[32] While impetigo can

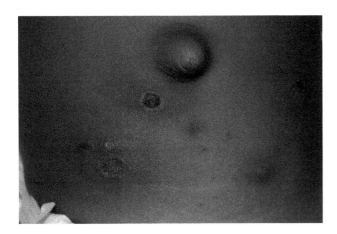

Figure 10.13 Bullous impetigo can present as grouped flaccid bullae with surrounding erythema. (Courtesy of Scott A. Norton, MD, MPH.)

be caused by staphylococcus, streptococcus, or a combination, *S. aureus* is responsible for most cases of impetigo.

Impetigo can present as either bullous or nonbullous. Nonbullous impetigo represents about 70% of all cases and often occurs after skin trauma, such as insect bites, burns, abrasions, or exacerbations of atopic dermatitis. Lesions begin as pustules or vesicles that collapse to reveal a red base. Lesions may develop characteristic overlying honey-colored adherent crust with surrounding erythema. Bullous impetigo is almost always caused by coagulase-positive *S. aureus* and presents as solitary or grouped flaccid bullae. The bullae collapse, leaving a rim of scale surrounding a shallow, erythematous erosion (Figure 10.13).[33]

Diagnosis is made clinically, but nonbullous impetigo can mimic many other cutaneous infections, such as enteroviruses, varicella-zoster virus, and HSV. Bullous impetigo can look similar to nonaccidental trauma (specifically cigarette burns), pemphigus foliaceus, erythema multiforme, thermal injury, or hypersensitivity response to insect bites. Cultures are diagnostic, but it can be difficult to differentiate the pathogenic bacteria from commensal skin organisms.

Most cases of impetigo will resolve spontaneously within 2 weeks. Topical medications can be used if a patient has limited cutaneous involvement and otherwise appears well. However, if patients have systemic symptoms or more generalized skin involvement, oral antibiotics should be used. First-line treatment for uncomplicated, limited infection is topical mupirocin 2% ointment applied three times daily for 7–10 days.[34] For more extensive impetigo, oral cephalexin or clindamycin can be used.[33] In older patients, doxycycline may be used.

If a patient has multiple recurrent episodes of impetigo, the patient may be a carrier of *S. aureus*.[33] Colonizing strains of *S. aureus* can be present in the nares, perianal region, umbilicus, and under the nails. Carriers of *S. aureus* may be treated with topical mupirocin ointment applied directly to these areas three times daily for 2–4 days. Patients can also take bleach baths for 15 minutes twice per week. To make a bleach bath, add 1 teaspoon of regular-strength household bleach for every gallon of bath water; this is approximately 1/4 cup of bleach for half a bathtub of water. Retreatment every few weeks to months may be required because of the risk of recolonization and recurrent impetigo.

Scabies

Scabies is a highly contagious and intensely pruritic infection caused by the mite *Sarcoptes scabiei*. Infection can be seen in all ethnic groups and at all socioeconomic levels, and scabies can be transmitted by skin-to-skin contact as well as contaminated fabrics. The female mite burrows into the skin, lays eggs, and causes the human host to become sensitized to its secretions.

Patients present with 1–2 mm erythematous papules and complain of intense itching. In adults, itching is prominent around the nipples, wrists, finger webs, intergluteal cleft, groin, and axillae. Young children commonly develop lesions on the hands, feet, buttocks, and skinfolds around the neck, but infants can present with a diffuse papular eruption (Figure 10.14).[35,36] Pruritus may persist for up to 6 weeks following treatment.

Evidence of the mite, larvae, or eggs is diagnostic for scabies and can be obtained from skin scrapings or biopsy. Other diseases that can present with similar symptoms and clinical findings include follicular eczema, papular urticaria, and contact dermatitis.

Permethrin 5% cream is the first-line treatment for most patients and is safe to use in infants over 2 months of age and pregnant women. The cream is applied to the entire body from the neck down and washed off in 8–14

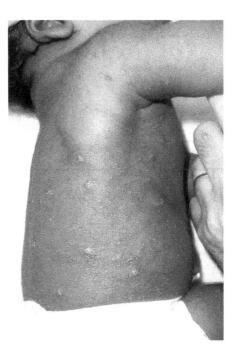

Figure 10.14 Scabies can present as diffuse papules, some with overlying scale, in infants. (Courtesy of Scott A. Norton, MD, MPH.)

hours. Patients should be instructed to ensure that the cream is applied to the webbed spaces, underneath the nails, and in the body folds. A second treatment 7 days later is crucial to kill the eggs that hatched into mites since the first treatment. Lindane cream is an alternative treatment for people unable to tolerate permethrin. However, use of lindane is limited due to resistance and side effects, including neurotoxicity, especially in small children who are prone to increased systemic absorption. For this reason, the use of lindane has been prohibited in some areas of the world. Oral ivermectin is an alternative to permethrin, though the potential side effect of neurotoxicity should be taken into consideration. To symptomatically treat the pruritus, topical midpotency corticosteroids may be used and are often required for several weeks following treatment.

For patients with severe infestations, all bed linens and clothing should be washed in hot water, as mites can live for 24–36 hours away from their host.[37,38] Family members and all close contacts should be treated. (If pregnant, medication safety during pregnancy must be considered.) The risk of reinfestation from fomites in other members of the household is negligible in most scabies infections.

Bedbugs

While bedbugs (species *Cimex lectularius*) are not known to transmit disease, their bites can produce very itchy and urticarial reactions in humans. Bedbugs are brown insects that live in furniture, floors, walls, and the cracks and joints of beds. They feed on human blood at night while their host is sleeping. When a bedbug bites its host, it injects saliva that acts as an anticoagulant, which allows the bug to feed. Proteins in the bug's saliva can induce an allergic response, leading to itching and formation of an urticarial red papule. While it can be difficult to capture a bedbug to confirm diagnosis, bedbug bites classically present in a linear grouped configuration, known as the "breakfast, lunch, and dinner" sign (Figure 10.15). While no treatment is necessary for bedbug bites, a topical steroid such as hydrocortisone 2.5% or desonide 0.05% can improve the symptoms of pruritus. Eradication of bedbugs with

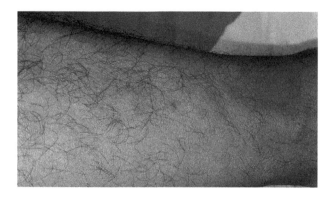

Figure 10.15 Urticarial papules in a linear configuration, characteristic of bedbug bites. (Courtesy of Karl M. Saardi, MD.)

a professional pest control service is recommended. For outbreaks at hotels or public spaces, contact with the local government or Department of Health is recommended.[33]

Cutaneous tumors

Hemangioma

Hemangiomas of infancy are diagnosed by clinical appearance and natural history of the lesion. Infantile hemangiomas, sometimes called strawberry hemangiomas, have a characteristic life cycle—they appear a few weeks after birth. Infantile hemangiomas are benign and regress on their own (as detailed in the following text). Hemangiomas that are fully formed at birth are called congenital hemangiomas: noninvoluting congenital hemangiomas, which do not enlarge or regress, partially involuting congenital hemangiomas, which partially regress, and rapidly involuting congenital hemangiomas, which tend to regress quickly. These congenital hemangiomas do not follow the life cycle of the infantile hemangiomas but are benign. Careful history, as well as possible imaging, can help one differentiate infantile and congenital hemangiomas. Deep hemangiomas can be hard to differentiate from soft tissue tumors such as fibrosarcomas or rhabdomyosarcomas, which are malignant. Magnetic resonance imaging (MRI), computed tomography scan, ultrasound, or surgical pathology may be required for definite diagnosis. Other vascular tumors include pyogenic granuloma, tufted angioma, spindle cell hemangioendothelioma, Kaposi sarcoma, and port-wine stain.

Infantile hemangiomas are the most common vascular tumors of infancy, occurring in about 4%–5% of neonates. Hemangiomas are benign proliferations composed of capillaries, which usually present within the first few weeks of life. There is a slightly higher incidence in girls, Caucasians, premature infants, and infants of multiple gestation.[39,40]

Infantile hemangiomas often appear at birth or in the first few weeks of life as precursor lesions, such as telangiectasias, macular erythematous stains, or bruises. Deeper hemangiomas can present in the first few months of life. Around 1–3 weeks after they appear, hemangiomas enter the proliferative phase and rapidly grow over the first few months of life, though this stage can continue until approximately 1 year of age.[40] After the proliferative phase, there is a stage of stabilization, and then the involution phase begins. Hemangiomas spontaneously involute, at a rate of complete resolution of approximately 10% per year (e.g., 10% at age 1, 20% at age 2, 30% at age 3, etc.).

Superficial hemangiomas have a predilection for the head and neck but can appear at any location, including the oral and genital mucosa. Hemangiomas can vary dramatically in size and depth of involvement. Superficial hemangiomas are located in the papillary dermis and will appear bright red clinically and grow into a firm, rubbery, lobular nodule or plaque (Figure 10.16). Deeper (formerly called cavernous) hemangiomas are located in the reticular dermis or subcutaneous fat and present as ill-defined, compressible,

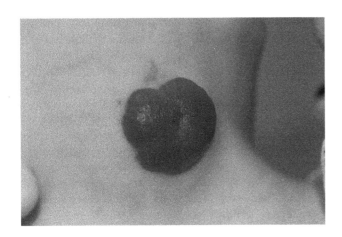

Figure 10.16 Infantile hemangioma. (Courtesy of Kalyani Marathe, MD, MPH.)

skin-colored or reddish-blue lesions. Hemangiomas are typically not painful unless they ulcerate; this occurs in approximately 10% of all hemangiomas.[41]

Hemangiomas follow a benign course; for uncomplicated lesions, observation is recommended. For hemangiomas that ulcerate, disfigure the patient, or start to compress vital structures, the patient should be referred to a dermatologist, and treatment with topical timolol or oral propranolol should be considered. For residual telangiectasias, pulsed-dye laser therapy can be used. Hemangiomas that occur in the lumbosacral region can potentially be associated with spinal, bony, and genitourinary abnormalities and should be investigated accordingly. Hemangiomas that occur in a segmental distribution on the face or neck can be associated with arterial, cardiac, neurologic, and eye abnormalities (PHACE syndrome). When PHACE syndrome is considered in the differential diagnosis, urgent referral to a dermatologist is recommended.

Lymphatic malformations

Microcystic lymphatic malformation is a type of lymphatic malformation that presents at birth as asymptomatic discrete groups of 1–5 mm clear or blood-tinged papules that resemble vesicles. Clinically, these are said to resemble "frog spawn." Another type of lymphatic malformation is a macrocystic lymphatic malformation; this is a larger, deeper malformation made of large cyst-like spaces containing lymphatic fluid.

A diagnosis of lymphatic malformation is usually made on clinical history and physical exam findings. MRI studies are helpful to identify the size of the lesion as well as any compression or involvement of underlying structures.

The preferred treatment of lymphangioma is complete surgical excision, though recurrence rates are high. Carbon dioxide lasers have been used to treat superficial lymphatic malformations, and sclerotherapy has been used to successfully treat deeper lymphatic malformations. If lymphatic malformation is suspected, referral to dermatology is warranted.[42]

Cyst

Cutaneous cysts are common growths that can present anywhere on the body, including the genital area. There are many different types of cysts; however, this section focuses on one of the most common subtypes—epidermal inclusion cysts. Epidermal inclusion cysts are subcutaneous, firm nodules filled with keratin that arise from the infundibulum of the hair follicle.

Epidermal cysts present as firm dome-shaped intradermal or subcutaneous painless nodules that range from 0.5 to 5.0 cm. They are attached to the overlying skin and have a small punctum that looks like an open comedone. Cysts are usually asymptomatic but can become tender and red when infected and inflamed; they may be clinically confused with an abscess.

Epidermal cysts must be differentiated from other cutaneous tumors. Complete excision of the cyst may be performed under local anesthesia; care must be taken to remove the entire cyst wall to avoid recurrence.

Pigmented lesions

Nevi and melanoma

Nevi, or moles, are very common skin neoplasms seen in the pediatric and adolescent population. The primary concern with nevi is their potential for malignant transformation. The likelihood of an individual mole transforming into melanoma is extremely low, and nevi can evolve as the child grows; however, all nevi should be monitored on a regular basis, and biopsy should be considered in nevi that are rapidly changing. Malignant melanoma is rare in the pediatric and adolescent population but still does exist.

Nevi can be congenital or acquired, and the tendency to develop nevi is likely multifactorial, with genetics, sun exposure, and pigmentary skin type all playing a role. Congenital nevi are nevi that are present at birth, and they present as pink or light to dark brown macules and patches (Figure 10.17). They may have some pigment variation, and there may be increased hair on the surface; they can also become more elevated over time. Congenital nevi are

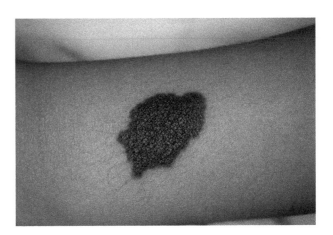

Figure 10.17 Congenital nevus with prominent overlying hair. (Courtesy of Kalyani Marathe, MD, MPH.)

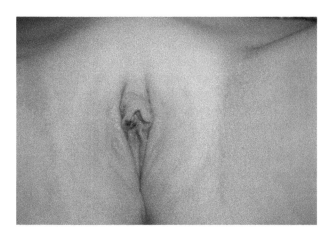

Figure 10.18 Genital nevi are common entities that can present as pink, tan, or brown macules and papules. (Courtesy of Kalyani Marathe, MD, MPH.)

subdivided based on their size: small (<1.5 cm), medium (1.5–19.9 cm), and large/giant (>20 cm). Giant congenital nevi have an increased risk of malignant transformation (around 5%) and should be monitored closely by a dermatologist.[43] Giant congenital nevi can occupy large segments of the body, sometimes involving most of the trunk in a "bathing suit" distribution.

Melanocytic nevi on the clitoris, clitoral hood, labia majora and minora, and perineum are classified as genital nevi. Genital nevi can vary in appearance, from macular to papular, and color can range from pink to tan to brown (Figure 10.18). Approximately 3.5% of children and adolescents have genital melanocytic nevi. Over half of genital melanocytic nevi present before age 2 years, and genital nevi can undergo changes in diameter, size, color, and texture. While genital nevi can be concerning to parents and providers, they are a common finding. Referral to dermatology should be made when the genital nevus changes rapidly or becomes symptomatic. Biopsies should be obtained with caution and only as needed, as they can lead to psychological distress, scarring, and disfigurement.[48]

Dysplastic nevi have a distinct appearance. Clinically, these lesions will have one or more of the features described in monitoring for melanoma (discussed later in this chapter). The presence of one or more of these features does not ensure that the nevus is dysplastic; rather, they must be considered in the context of the individual patient and the particular lesion. A helpful rule of thumb for patients and parents is the "ugly duckling" principle: atypical nevi often stand out from the patient's other moles as being unusual in morphology.

Malignant melanoma usually has one or more of the following features: asymmetry, border irregularity, dark color or variable pigment, large size, and evolution. However, pediatric melanoma can have other findings, often leading to a delayed diagnosis. In one recent study, authors suggested modifying the criteria for suspicion of pediatric melanoma to include lesions that are amelanotic, bleeding, a papule, uniform in color, or new.[44] Melanomas often have a history of rapidly changing shape, size, or features. Amelanotic melanomas are one of the more common presentations in pediatric melanomas, and they can present as pink to red papules; they are difficult to distinguish from a number of other benign lesions, including vascular tumors, Spitz nevi, and adnexal tumors. While incidence of melanoma in the pediatric and adolescent population is low, risk factors include maternal transmission of metastatic melanoma *in utero*, xeroderma pigmentosa, immunosuppression, family history, nevus phenotype, and environmental factors such as ultraviolet radiation.[49] However, most pediatric patients with melanoma have no known risk factors.

Careful history and physical examination are important in diagnosing nevi and melanomas. Consultation with dermatology is warranted in patients with congenital nevi or a history of dysplastic nevi or melanoma. Digital photography may be useful for following individual moles and evaluating for any changes. An excisional biopsy should be performed whenever a nevus is changing, or when the diagnosis or behavior of a particular lesion is in question. This allows histologic evaluation of the entire lesion. The authors recommend sending specimens for histologic evaluation by a dermatopathologist experienced in pigmented lesions. The management of biopsy-proven Spitz nevi remains controversial, as their behavior is uncertain. Many advocate complete removal, while others recommend close surveillance for any changes.[50] Malignant melanoma must be excised with appropriate margins as indicated by the depth of the melanoma on initial biopsy. Sentinel lymph node biopsy may be warranted in certain cases.

Patients and parents should be counseled on the importance of periodic surveillance, sun protection, and characteristics of melanoma. They should also be instructed to have immediate evaluation of any rapidly changing nevi, as this can be a warning sign of dysplasia or malignancy.

Acne

Acne is a very common condition of the pilosebaceous unit of the skin, affecting around 95% of the population in Western cultures, and usually peaking in adolescence.[33] Numerous factors, including genetics, hormones, and the presence of *Propionibacterium acnes*, contribute to the development of acne. An increase in dehydroepiandrosterone sulfate (DHEA-S) correlates with the onset of acne in prepubertal or pubescent females. Increased androgen production leads to sebaceous gland enlargement and greater amounts of sebum production.[51] Benign cephalic pustulosis (often called by its misnomer, neonatal acne) can occur during the first 3 months of life and is due to the influence of maternal androgens and Malassezia yeast. It will resolve without treatment as the maternal hormones become less active with time. Infantile acne, which develops around 6–16 months of age, is uncommon. Unlike neonatal acne, infantile acne has true comedones and can result in scarring. Thus, treatment with topical acne products is indicated, and patients refractory to treatment should be referred to dermatology.[33]

Stress and mechanical occlusion can exacerbate acne. The role of diet in acne pathogenesis remains controversial, but current research suggests diets with high glycemic index are positively associated with the development of acne.[52] Certain medications including systemic steroids, anabolic steroids, lithium, phenytoin, isoniazid, and iodides, among others, can cause the sudden appearance of an acneiform eruption. Endocrinologic abnormalities are well-established causes of acne. A history of hirsutism, irregular menstrual periods, insulin resistance, or deepening of the voice should prompt a further investigation into possible endocrine disturbances that include polycystic ovary syndrome (PCOS). These patients should be screened with lab tests, including serum free and total testosterone, DHEA-S, and 17-hydroxyprogesterone. Glucose intolerance and diabetes screening should also be considered.

The severity of acne can vary, and patients can present with one or both types of acne: comedonal and inflammatory. Noninflammatory acne, also referred to as comedonal acne, is characterized by open and closed follicularly based comedones. Closed comedones may present as 1–2 mm white papules, commonly called whiteheads (Figure 10.19); open comedones appear clinically as blackheads (Figure 10.20). Inflammatory acne consists of papules, pustules, nodules, and cysts. These lesions have the potential for more serious scarring. Patients with acne can have postinflammatory hyperpigmentation, which presents as pink to brown 1–3 mm macules in the areas of former acne after inflammatory papules have resolved. Postinflammatory hyperpigmentation can appear more pronounced in darker skin tones.

When instituting new acne therapy, it is of utmost importance to counsel patients that 2–3 months of consistent use is necessary to determine the efficacy of any therapeutic regimen. Topical treatments are usually effective in patients with primarily comedonal acne. All patients with acne should be started on a topical retinoid such as adapalene, tretinoin, or tazarotene. Topical retinoids normalize the abnormal follicular keratinization that contributes to acne and have anti-inflammatory properties. Patients

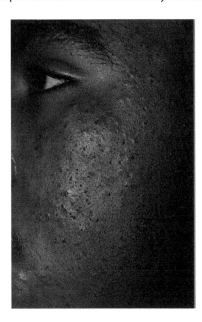

Figure 10.20 Open comedones. (Courtesy of Scott A. Norton, MD, MPH.)

should be warned of potential irritation as well as the possibility of a pustular flare during the first month of use. Adapalene 0.1% has become available over the counter in the United States, but the other topical retinoids require a prescription. It is important to note that tazarotene is a topical medication that is contraindicated with pregnancy, and it requires simultaneous contraception. Azelaic acid, a comedolytic dicarboxylic acid that has modest activity against *P. acnes*, can be prescribed during pregnancy, as it has minimal systemic absorption, and is, therefore, the safest comedolytic to use during pregnancy. Azelaic acid is also helpful as an adjunct to acne therapy in darker-skinned individuals who exhibit postinflammatory hyperpigmentation, as hypopigmentation can be a side effect of this medication.[33]

Topical antibiotics should be used in conjunction with topical retinoids because of their synergistic effects. The antibiotics target *P. acnes*, limiting the inflammatory component of acne. Effective topical antibiotics include clindamycin, erythromycin, and dapsone. Benzoyl peroxide is a product with antibiotic properties that is used as a topical cream, gel, or wash. Common side effects of benzoyl peroxide include irritation as well as bleaching of hair and fabrics. Resistance to antibiotics can occur with prolonged use of any single agent; therefore, a combination of benzoyl peroxide with clindamycin, erythromycin, or dapsone is often most effective in treating acne and limiting resistance. Sodium sulfacetamide is another topical antibacterial with activity against *P. acnes*; it is available as a lotion or wash. This is a particularly helpful adjunct to treat acne in the athlete or patient with oily skin in whom the clinician suspects yeast overgrowth.

For patients with more severe acne or inflammatory cysts and nodules, an oral antibiotic may be indicated, as these have both anti-inflammatory and antibacterial

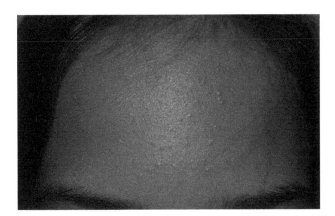

Figure 10.19 Closed comedones can present as multiple monomorphic 1–2 mm papules. (Courtesy of Scott A. Norton, MD, MPH.)

properties. Oral antibiotics should be used in conjunction with topical retinoids (adapalene, tretinoin, and tazarotene) but should not be used with systemic retinoids (isotretinoin). Tetracyclines, doxycycline or minocycline, are the most commonly prescribed antibiotics for acne. Side effects of doxycycline include photosensitivity, gastrointestinal upset, and esophageal erosions. Taking doxycycline with food can diminish the gastrointestinal upset. Side effects of minocycline include vertigo, drug-induced lupus, and, less commonly, hypersensitivity reactions, hepatotoxicity, and interstitial nephritis.[45] Minocycline can also be associated with vestibular toxicity and a blue-black hyperpigmentation, especially within acne scars. Any of the tetracyclines can be associated with pseudotumor cerebri, especially in the setting of concomitant isotretinoin administration, and patients should be counseled appropriately. Tetracyclines should not be used in children younger than 10 years of age because of the potential for tooth discoloration. Erythromycin has also been used to treat acne. However, this is not first-line treatment, as resistance to this medication is more common. Amoxicillin and trimethoprim-sulfamethoxazole are other antibiotics that are sometimes used in resistant cases. The role of any of these antibiotics in decreasing the efficacy of oral contraceptives has not been proven. The only antibiotic to reproducibly reduce oral contraceptive efficacy in well-performed studies is rifampin. For further treatments, see Table 10.2.

Patients with acne thought to be secondary to hormonal disturbances should be managed appropriately. Oral contraceptives may be useful in this setting, and several of these have been approved by the U.S. Food and Drug Administration in treating acne (norgestimate/ethinyl estradiol, norethindrone acetate/ethinyl estradiol with ferrous fumarate, and drospirenone/ethinyl estradiol).[33] Spironolactone can also be effective, as this drug acts as both an androgen receptor blocker and an inhibitor of 5α-reductase. It is important to note that spironolactone is not recommended in pregnancy and can feminize a male fetus. Sexually active patients should be on contraception and counseled accordingly.

Table 10.2 Common acne treatments.

Type and severity of acne	Initial treatments	Common medication side effects	Alternative treatments
Comedonal acne	Topical retinoid (tretinoin 0.025%, 0.05%, or 0.1% depending on the dryness, irritation of skin) nightly	Dryness and irritation of the skin, photosensitivity	Adapalene 0.1% (over-the-counter strength) or 0.3% if unable to tolerate topical retinoid Tazarotene gel if comedones are persistent despite use of tretinoin
	Benzoyl peroxide (face wash, spot treatment) once daily	Irritation of the skin (especially during first 1–2 weeks of use), bleaching of fabrics	Salicylic acid face wash
Inflammatory acne	Treatments for comedonal acne previously mentioned, plus add: Topical clindamycin 1% (gel, lotion, or solution)		
	Treatments for comedonal acne previously mentioned, plus add: oral tetracyclines (doxycycline or minocycline 100 mg twice a day)	Nausea, photosensitivity, pseudotumor cerebri, tooth discoloration when used in patients younger than 10 years, hyperpigmentation (minocycline)	If inflammatory acne is persistent and patient fails traditional treatments, consider use of isotretinoin
Nodulocystic, scarring acne	If patient fails maximum therapies previously mentioned, can consider use of isotretinoin	Many side effects, including xerosis, cheilitis, elevation of cholesterol and liver function tests, teratogenicity	
Hormonal acne—consider when the patient is female, acne is hormonally distributed on the jawline, and acne flares with menses	Spironolactone	Contraindicated in patients with renal dysfunction, hyperkalemia, Addison disease, and those using eplerenone as well as with pregnancy	
	Oral contraceptive pills	Do not use in those with contraindications to oral contraceptive pills	
	Topical retinoids	See previous text	

For patients with severe, nodulocystic acne that does not respond to any of the previously mentioned treatments, isotretinoin, an oral retinoid, may be indicated. Patients who are taking isotretinoin should discontinue all other acne medications, both systemic and topical, and if sexually active, they should be on contraception due to potential teratogenicity. Isotretinoin acts on the sebaceous glands, causing atrophy and reducing sebum production by up to 90%. *Propionibacterium acnes* is unable to thrive, and follicular keratinization becomes normalized. Patients must be monitored carefully with monthly lab tests including a complete blood count, liver function test, fasting lipids, renal function, and pregnancy tests. The most common side effects of isotretinoin are dryness of the skin and mucous membranes. Less common side effects include visual disturbances, nausea, hepatitis, depression, myalgias, headache, pseudotumor cerebri, skeletal hyperostosis, osteoporosis, and premature closure of the epiphyseal plates. The teratogenicity of isotretinoin is well established. Female patients of childbearing potential must receive appropriate counseling and demonstrate appropriate contraceptive measures. The iPledge system is a national registry in the United States for patients taking isotretinoin. This federally managed system aims to enforce appropriate follow-up, patient education, and pregnancy prevention for patients receiving treatment with isotretinoin. Pregnancy should not be attempted until 1 month after discontinuation of therapy.

Health-care providers should not dismiss acne as simply a skin condition that accompanies teenage years, as acne can cause profound psychosocial distress during one's formative years, as well as physical scarring. By intervening early and referring to a dermatologist for refractory disease, providers can improve both the patient's skin and quality of life.

Hair removal

Pubic hair grooming practices, including hair removal, are widespread in the United States. Pubic hair exists as a barrier for vulvar and vaginal irritants and infections. Historically, shaving pubic hair reduced rates of pubic lice. However, women today are increasingly removing their body hair for a variety of reasons. It is thought that popular culture and media portrayal of genitalia normalize hair removal behaviors. A recent study of over three thousand women inquired about the motivation behind grooming of pubic hair. Women noted that they removed pubic hair for hygienic purposes, an improved perception regarding the appearance of genitalia, to promote certain sexual practices, or for a sexual partner's preference. Women also reported grooming or removing pubic hair in anticipation of seeing their health-care provider for a skin or genital exam.[53] Shaving is the most utilized technique for hair removal, as it is inexpensive and can be done in the privacy of one's home, but hair removal creams, depilatories, waxing, electrolysis, and laser hair removal can also be used.

There are risks involved in removal of pubic hair. As pubic hair is a natural barrier to infection, it is thought that its removal can predispose one to imbalances in the microbiome of the vulva. Any trauma to the skin that occurs during hair removal can cause microabrasions of the skin, leading to bacterial or viral infection. However, adverse effects and injuries can occur during and after hair removal. Patients can suffer adverse effects from hair removal ranging from abrasions, contact dermatitis, folliculitis, irritation due to razor (razor burn), or ingrown hairs to potentially more serious effects, including infection of the vulva, folliculitis, postinflammatory pigmentary alteration, and even genital burns from waxing. Vulvar folliculitis can be divided into two categories: mechanical and infectious. Mechanical folliculitis is a sterile inflammation of the hair follicle that occurs when hair is cut below the surface of the epidermis. Infectious folliculitis is most commonly due to the bacteria *S. aureus* or *S. pyogenes*. Viral infections such as warts or molluscum contagiosum can also be locally spread while shaving.[46,47]

For local irritation due to a dull or dry razor (razor burn), one can apply a low-potency topical steroid such as hydrocortisone 1%. Treatment of infectious folliculitis includes a combination of a topical steroid such as hydrocortisone 1% and application of a topical antibiotic, such as clindamycin 1% or mupirocin. Patients can treat superficial abrasions at home, but some patients who sustain lacerations or burns or develop abscesses require medical attention.[47] For treatment failure, bacterial culture and referral to a dermatologist are recommended. It is important to educate patients about safe techniques, risks, and potential adverse effects related to hair removal.

REFERENCES

1. Jordan WE, Lawson KD, Berg RW, Franxman JJ, Marrer AM. Diaper dermatitis: Frequency and severity among a general infant population. *Pediatr Dermatol.* 1986;3:198–207.
2. Klunk C, Domingues E, Wiss K. An update on diaper dermatitis. *Clin Dermatol.* 2014;32(4):477–87.
3. Coughlin CC, Eichenfield LF, Frieden IJ. Diaper dermatitis: Clinical characteristics and differential diagnosis. *Pediatr Dermatol.* 2014;31:19–24.
4. Alberta L, Sweeney SM, Wiss K. Diaper dye dermatitis. *Pediatrics.* 2005;116:450–2.
5. Draelos ZD. Hydrogel barrier/repair creams and contact dermatitis. *Am J Contact Dermat.* 2000;11: 222–5.
6. Admani S, Matiz C, Jacob SE. Methylisothiazolinone: A case of perianal dermatitis caused by wet wipes and review of an emerging pediatric allergen. *Pediatr Dermatol.* 2014;31:350–2.
7. Friedlander SF. Consultation with the specialist: Contact dermatitis. *Pediatr Rev.* 1998;19:165–71.
8. deZeeuw R, van Praag MC, Oranje AP. Granuloma gluteal infantum: A case report. *Pediatr Dermatol.* 2000;17:141–3.
9. Krol A, Krafchik B. Diaper area eruptions. In: Eichenfield L, Frieden I, Esterly N, eds. *Neonatal Dermatology.* 2nd ed. Philadelphia, PA: Saunders Elsevier; 2008:245–66.

10. Paller AS, Mancini AJ. Skin disorders due to fungi. In: Paller AS, Mancini AJ, eds. *Hurwitz Clinical Pediatric Dermatology: A Textbook of Skin Disorders of Childhood and Adolescence*. Philadelphia, PA: Elsevier; 2006:464–8.

11. Smolinski KN, Shah SS, Honig PJ, Yan AC. Neonatal cutaneous fungal infections. *Curr Opin Pediatr.* 2005;17:486–93.

12. Herbst R. Perineal streptococcal dermatitis/disease: Recognition and management. *Am J Clin Dermatol.* 2003;4:555–60.

13. Brilliant LC. Perianal streptococcal dermatitis. *Am Fam Physician.* 2000;61:391–3, 397.

14. Pichichero ME. Group A ß-hemolytic streptococcal infections. *Pediatr Rev.* 1998;19:291–302.

15. Lagerstedt M, Karvinen K, Joki-Erkklia M, Huotari-Orava R, Snellman E, Laasanen SL. Childhood lichen sclerosus – A challenge for clinicians. *Pediatr Dermatol.* 2013;30:444–50.

16. Bercaw-Pratt JL, Boardman LA, Simms-Cendan JS. Clinical recommendation: Pediatric Lichen Sclerosus. *J Pediatr Adolesc Gynecol.* 2014;27(2):111–6.

17. Goldstein AT, Marinoff SC, Christopher K. Pimecrolimus for the treatment of vulvar lichen sclerosus in a premenarchal girl. *J Pediatr Adolesc Gynecol.* 2004;17:35–7.

18. Mashayekhi S, Flohr C, Lewis FM. The treatment of vulvar lichen sclerosus in prepubertal girls: A critically appraised topic. *Br J Dermatol.* 2017;176(2):307–16.

19. Tangtatco JAA, Lara-Corrales I. Update in the management of pediatric psoriasis. *Curr Opin Pediatr.* 2017;29(4):434–42.

20. Krakowski A, Eichenfeld L, Dohil M. Management of atopic dermatitis in the pediatric population. *J Pediatr.* 2008;122(4):812–24.

21. Paller AS, Mancini AJ. Eczematous eruptions in childhood. In: Paller AS, Mancini AJ, eds. *Hurwitz Clinical Pediatric Dermatology: A Textbook of Skin Disorders of Childhood and Adolescence*. Philadelphia, PA: Elsevier; 2006:49–64.

22. Saunte DML, Jemec GBE. Hidradenitis suppurativa advances in diagnosis and treatment. *JAMA.* 2017;318(20):2019–32.

23. Saunte DM, Boer J, Stratigos A et al. Diagnostic delay in hidradenitis suppurativa is a global problem. *Br J Dermatol.* 2015;173(6):1546–9.

24. Brocard A, Knol AC, Khammari A, Dreno B. Hidradenitis suppurativa and zinc: A new therapeutic approach. A pilot study. *Deramatology.* 2007;214(4):325–7.

25. Van der Zee HH, Gulliver W. Medical treatments of hidradenitis suppurativa. *Dermatologic Clin.* 2016;34(1):91–6.

26. Ritz JP, Runkel N, Haier J, Buhr HJ. Extent of surgery and recurrence rate of hidradenitis suppurativa. *Int J Colorectal Dis.* 1998;13:164–8.

27. Payette MJ, Weston G, Humphrey S et al. Lichen planus and other lichenoid dermatoses: Kids are not just little people. *Clin Dermatol.* 2015;33:631–43.

28. Rogers M, Barnetson RSC. Diseases of the skin. In: Campbell AGM, McIntosh N, eds. *Forfar and Arneil's Textbook of Pediatrics*. 5th ed. New York, NY: Churchill Livingstone; 1998:1633–5.

29. van der Wouden JC, Koning S, van Suijlekom-Smit LWA, Berger M, Butler C, Menke J, Gajadin S, Tasche MJA. Interventions for cutaneous molluscum contagiosum. *Cochrane Database Syst Rev.* 2006, Issue 2. Art. No.: CD004767.

30. Chen X, Anstey A, Bugert J. Molluscum contagiosum virus infection. *Lancet Infect Dis.* 2013;13(10): 877–88.

31. Dohil M, Prendiville JS. Treatment of molluscum contagiosum with oral cimetidine: Clinical experience in 13 patients. *Pediatr Dermatol.* 1996;13:310.

32. Hlady WG, Middaugh JP. An epidemic of bullous impetigo in a newborn nursery due to *Staphylococcus aureus*: Epidemiology and control measures. *Alaska Med.* 1986;28:99–103.

33. Habif T. *Clinical Dermatology.* 6th ed. St. Louis, MO: Elsevier; 2016.

34. George A, Rubin G. A systematic review and meta-analysis of treatments for impetigo. *Br J Gen Pract.* 2003;53:480–7.

35. Johnston G, Sladden M. Scabies: Diagnosis and treatment. *BMJ.* 2005;331:619–22.

36. James W, Berger T, Elston D. *Andrews' Diseases of the Skin.* 12th ed. Philadelphia, PA: Elsevier; 2016.

37. Arlian LG, Runyan RA, Achar S, Estes SA. Survival and infectivity of *Sarcoptes scabiei* var. *canis* and var. *hominis. J Am Acad Dermatol.* 1984;11:210–15.

38. Arlian LG, Vyszenski-Moher DL, Pole MJ. Survival of adults and development stages of *Sarcoptes scabiei* var. *canis* when off the host. *Exp Appl Acarol.* 1989;6:181–7.

39. Haggstrom AN, Drolet BA, Baselga E et al. Prospective study of infantile hemangiomas: Demographic, prenatal, and perinatal characteristics. *J Pediatr.* 2007;150:291–4.

40. Leaute-Labreze C, Harper JI, Hoeger PH et al. Infantile hemangioma. *Lancet.* 2017;390(10089):85–94.

41. Chamlin SL, Haggstrom AN, Drolet BA et al. Multicenter prospective study of ulcerated hemangiomas. *J Pediatr.* 2007;151:684–9.

42. Puttgen K, Cohen B. *Neonatal Dermatology, Pediatric Dermatology.* 4th ed. Philadelphia, PA: Saunders Elsevier; 2013, 14–67.

43. Schafer J. Update on melanocytic nevi in children. *Clin Dermatol.* 2015;33(3):368–86.

44. Cordoro KM, Gupta D, Frieden IJ, McCalmont T, Kashani-Sabet M. Pediatric melanoma: Results of a large cohort study and proposal for modified ABCD detection criteria for children. *J Am Acad Dermatol.* 2013;68(6):913–25.

45. Smith K, Leyden JJ. Safety of doxycycline and minocycline: A systematic review. *Clin Ther.* 2005;27:1329–42.

46. DeMaria AL, Flores M, Hirth JM, Berenson AB. Complications related to pubic hair removal. *Am J Obstet Gynecol.* 2014;210(6):528.e1–5.

47. Hodges AL, Holland AC. Prevention and treatment of injuries and infections related to pubic hair removal. *Nurs Womens Health.* 2017;21(4):313–7.

48. Hunt RD, Orlow SJ, Schaffer JV et al. Genital melanocytic nevi in children: Experience in a pediatric dermatology practice. *J Am Acad Dermatol.* 2013;70(3):429–34.

49. Pappo AS. Melanoma in children and adolescents. *Eur J Cancer.* 2003;39:2651–61.

50. Gelbard SN, Tripp JM, Marghoob AA et al. Management of Spitz nevi: A survey of dermatologists in the United States. *J Am Acad Dermatol.* 2002;47:224–30.

51. White GM. Recent findings in the epidemiologic evidence, classification, and subtypes of acne vulgaris. *J Am Acad Dermatol.* 1998;39:S34–7.

52. Cerman AA, Aktas E, Altunay IK et al. Dietary glycemic factors, insulin resistance, and adiponectin levels in acne vulgaris. *J Am Acad Dermatol.* 2016;75(1):155–62.

53. Rowen TS, Gaither TW, Awad MA. Pubic hair grooming prevalence and motivation among women in the United States. *JAMA Dermatol.* 2016;152(10):1106–13.

Pediatric urology

LAUREL SOFER and EMILIE K. JOHNSON

11

INTRODUCTION

Urologic abnormalities often overlap with gynecologic issues in the pediatric population. In this chapter, we focus on topics in pediatric urology that are relevant to the pediatric and adolescent gynecologist. Topics include urinary tract infections and vesicoureteral reflux, interstitial cystitis and bladder pain syndrome, ureteral bud anomalies, bladder exstrophy, and spina bifida.

URINARY TRACT INFECTIONS

Introduction and epidemiology

Urinary tract infections (UTIs) are common in children/adolescents. They account for 0.7% of pediatrician visits annually, 5%–14% of emergency department visits annually, and are the second most common bacterial infections in children.[1,2] The incidence spikes during infancy, toilet training, and at the onset of sexual activity in girls,[3] and 5% of girls will experience a UTI by age 6 years.[2] Febrile UTIs (fUTIs) may be associated with vesicoureteral reflux (VUR) or other anatomic anomalies, which may lead to chronic kidney disease (CKD) and renal scarring. Accurate diagnosis of UTI (Box 11.1) is important to prevent these undesirable sequelae. Additionally, misdiagnosis can lead to overtreatment with antibiotics and unnecessary testing. The remainder of this section focuses on fUTI/pyelonephritis.

Box 11.1 Definitions

- *Uncomplicated UTI*: Occurs in a normal host without structural or functional genitourinary abnormalities, without pregnancy, and without instrumentation (e.g., catheterization)[4]
- *Complicated UTI*: Occurs in hosts with either anatomical urologic abnormality, in pregnancy, or in patients who have undergone instrumentation
- *Bacteriuria*: Bacteria in the urine found on any urine specimen; may be a result of true infection, colonization, or contaminant; may be symptomatic or asymptomatic
- *Pyuria*: White blood cells in the urine; indicates inflammation of the bladder lining
- *Cystitis/afebrile UTI*: Bladder infection, indicated by lower urinary tract symptoms (i.e., dysuria, frequency, urgency, suprapubic pain) with bacteriuria and pyuria
- *Pyelonephritis/fUTI*: Upper UTI (ureter and kidney), indicated by systemic signs/symptoms (i.e., flank pain, fever, chills) with bacteriuria and pyuria; can occur in the presence or absence of cystitis symptoms
- *Urethritis*: Inflammation of the urethra causing pain with voiding or dysuria; usually caused by a sexually transmitted infection; may mimic the symptoms of a UTI

Pathophysiology and risk factors

The pathophysiology of UTI is multifactorial. Young girls and adolescents have peri-urethral bacterial colonization. These bacteria may ascend via the urethra into the bladder due to dysfunctional elimination, instrumentation, and/or voiding abnormalities. Ascent of bacteria to the upper urinary tract may lead to kidney infection/pyelonephritis. Additionally, the virulence properties of different bacteria may contribute to their ability to cause UTI. Other risk factors include young age, female gender, white race, anatomic abnormality (e.g., VUR, ureteropelvic junction obstruction), neurogenic bladder, bowel and bladder dysfunction (BBD), and immunocompromised state.[5]

The evaluation for UTI must include a thorough history and physical. Important components in the history include cystitis/pyelonephritis symptoms, presence of irritability, vomiting and poor feeding, number/type of previous infections, bowel and bladder habits (e.g., constipation or holding of urine or stool), impaired development and coordination indicating occult neurologic disease, prenatal history including abnormal prenatal ultrasounds, history of urologic anatomic abnormalities (i.e., VUR or hydronephrosis), and family history (UTIs, VUR, CKD, and urologic anatomic abnormalities).

Physical exam should be focused on ruling out other causes of fever/symptoms. Vital signs and general appearance will help indicate whether inpatient or outpatient management is most appropriate. A female genitourinary examination is often normal but can demonstrate labial adhesions and/or erythema, or a prolapsed ureterocele. The presence of stool or urine in the child's underwear may indicate a history of BBD. A full neurologic exam should be performed.

Urine specimen collection

Many misdiagnoses of UTIs are due to inadequate or incorrect urine collection. In children who are not toilet trained, a urine sample should be obtained by bladder catheterization or suprapubic aspiration. Bagged specimens have a high false-positive rate and are only valid if the result is negative.[6] If a bagged specimen is obtained and the urinalysis is positive with leukocyte esterase, pyuria, and/or nitrites, then a subsequent urine specimen should be obtained through catheterization or suprapubic aspiration for confirmatory urinalysis and culture. Empiric treatment should generally not be initiated before a catheterized sample is collected. Reliably toilet-trained children may provide a clean midstream voided sample.

Requirements for diagnosis of a UTI

1. A correctly collected urine specimen demonstrating pyuria *and*
2. A positive urine culture with >50,000 colony forming units (CFU)/mL of a single uropathogen[6]

Leukocyte esterase and nitrite positive specimens should raise the suspicion of UTI but are not diagnostic. Proteinuria suggests underlying renal pathology, and hematuria suggests urothelial bleeding or kidney disease.

While an abnormal urinalysis is suggestive of a UTI, the final diagnosis requires a positive urine culture. After confirming reliable collection of the specimen, a bacterial count of >50,000 CFU/mL of a single uropathogen is required to make the diagnosis of UTI.[7] Common organisms include *Escherichia coli*, *Klebsiella*, *Proteus*, *Pseudomonas*, and *Enterococcus*.

Blood tests

Screening for renal dysfunction should be performed (renal function panel) in cases of fUTI/pyelonephritis.[7] If any concern for sepsis, a complete septic workup should be performed according with the guidelines of the patient's institution.

Imaging

Afebrile UTIs do not routinely require further imaging workup unless the child has recurrent UTIs. All children who present with fUTI should have basic urinary tract imaging. The most recent fUTI guidelines from the American Academy of Pediatrics (AAP) were published in 2011 and are targeted for children aged 2–24 months, although they are often applied to other age groups. These guidelines recommend a *renal and bladder ultrasound* (RBUS) to rule out anatomic abnormalities such as hydronephrosis, bladder wall thickening, or bladder abnormalities (e.g., ureterocele). Timing of RBUS depends on the clinical scenario—in a septic, febrile infant, RBUS should be obtained within the first 2 days of treatment. Otherwise, the timing is determined by physician discretion and can often wait until after the acute infection is resolved. For patients who do not respond to antibiotics, imaging should be obtained earlier to rule out a renal abscess.[6]

Voiding cystourethrogram (VCUG) is used to evaluate for anatomic abnormalities, including VUR, in children with fUTI. Figure 11.1 shows an example VCUG demonstrating bilateral VUR. A small catheter is used to fill the bladder with contrast. Fluoroscopic images of the urinary tract are taken during filling and voiding to evaluate for VUR, bladder abnormalities, and urethral pathologies. If a Foley catheter is used, the contrast should be instilled with the balloon deflated.

When and if to perform a VCUG after a first-time fUTI is controversial. The 2011 AAP guidelines recommend obtaining a VCUG if the RBUS reveals hydronephrosis, scarring, or other findings to suggest high-grade reflux or obstructive uropathy, and in atypical circumstances.[6] Other indications include suspicion of VUR or bladder

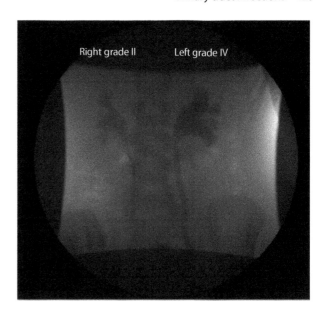

Figure 11.1 Bilateral vesicoureteral reflux (VUR). After radiopaque contrast is instilled through a Foley catheter, VUR is indicated by the presence of contrast in the collecting system, as seen on fluoroscopic images.

pathology, recurrent fUTIs, and a fUTI in a child with a solitary kidney. Urologists have expressed concern about the recommendation to only obtain a VCUG after a second fUTI, citing limitations of the data used to inform the 2011 AAP UTI guidelines, as well as concerns that renal scarring could be prevented in some children if VCUG was performed after a first fUTI.[8]

Radionucleotide cystograms (RNCs) are an alternative to VCUG. Although sensitivity for detection of VUR is higher, RNCs lack the anatomic detail of VCUG. Thus, RNCs are not recommended as the initial screening study for children with fUTI. Indications include follow-up of patients with known VUR, and evaluation of children in whom suspicion of VUR is high who have had a negative VCUG.

Dimercaptosuccinic acid (DMSA) renal scans are used to evaluate for renal scarring and differential renal function. An intravenous catheter is placed, and DMSA radiotracer is injected. DMSA tracer is bound to renal tubules and is not excreted. Renal scarring is suspected when there is a paucity of radiotracer uptake in one region of the kidney, particularly at the poles. Figure 11.2 shows an example of asymmetric differential function. If used to assess for renal scarring, a DMSA renal scan should be obtained no sooner than 3 months after an episode of pyelonephritis, as pyelonephritis can appear similar to scarring within this time period.

Indications for obtaining DMSA renal scans include the following: (1) a diagnosis of pyelonephritis when the clinical picture is unclear; (2) documentation of renal scarring or asymmetric differential function, to guide surgical management for patients with VUR; and (3) initial testing in the "top-down" approach to imaging after fUTI.[9] With this strategy, a VCUG is obtained only if the DMSA renal scan is concerning for renal scarring.

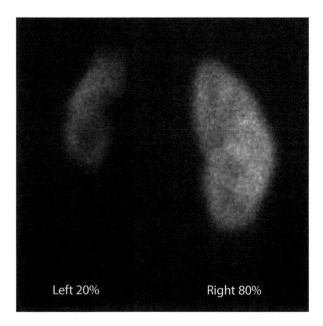

Left 20%   Right 80%

Figure 11.2 Asymmetric differential function in a patient with vesicoureteral reflux during a Dimercaptosuccinic acid renal scan.

Treatment

The initial management of fUTI is hydration, vital sign stabilization, and empiric antibiotics. Antibiotics are administered orally or parenterally, depending on whether patients can tolerate oral intake. The choice of antibiotic therapy should be based on local antimicrobial sensitivity patterns and adjusted according to sensitivities of the culture once results are available. A course of 7–14 days is the recommended treatment duration for a fUTI.[6] Inpatient treatment is indicated in cases of vital sign instability, very young age (<2 months old), immunocompromised condition, inability to tolerate oral medications or fluids, and failure of outpatient treatment.

After completion of antibiotics, priorities include management of BBD, determination of need for prophylactic antibiotics, and assessment/management for VUR and other anatomical abnormalities.

VESICOURETERAL REFLUX

Introduction and epidemiology

VUR is a condition where urine flows retrograde from the bladder to the upper urinary tract (Box 11.2). It is found in about 30%–45% of children presenting with fUTI.[9] It may also be clinically silent and is detected in ~1% of screened neonates.[10] Although VUR is not a cause of UTI, it is thought to be an accelerant of bacteriuria by delivering infected urine to the renal pelvis. Thus, children with VUR are at higher risk of pyelonephritis.

Pathophysiology (primary vesicoureteral reflux)

The ureter develops from the ureteric bud, which branches off the mesonephric duct. This ureteric bud interacts with the urogenital sinus (future bladder). This interaction

---

Box 11.2 Definitions and grading

Primary VUR: Deficiency in the function of the ureterovesicular junction (UVJ)—bladder and ureter are minimally contributory to the overall mechanism.

Secondary VUR: Due to bladder dysfunction overwhelming the UVJ. Common causes of secondary reflux include posterior urethral valves (males), neurogenic bladder and spina bifida, and BBD.[11]

Grading: VUR is graded according to the International Reflux Grading System (Table 11.1), which describes the contour of the ureter, renal pelvis, and calyces according to their appearance on VCUG.[12] The grade at diagnosis contributes to prognosis and rate of resolution. Grades I and II are considered mild, grade III moderate, and grades IV and V severe.

Table 11.1 International reflux grading system.

Grade	Description
I	Into a nondilated ureter
II	Into the pelvis and calyces without dilation
III	Mild to moderate dilation of the ureter, renal pelvis, and calyces with minimal blunting of the fornices
IV	Moderate ureteral tortuosity and dilation of the pelvis and calyces
V	Gross dilation of the ureter, pelvis, and calyces; loss of papillary impressions; and ureteral tortuosity

---

allows for adequate submucosal tunnel length of the intramural ureter, creating a mechanical antireflux mechanism. During bladder filling, the ureter remains compressed to prevent reflux. This requires a tunnel-length-to-ureteral-diameter ratio of 5:1.[13] If this embryologic interaction of the ureter and bladder occurs too soon, the ureter implants superiorly and laterally in the bladder wall, leading to inadequate tunnel length and VUR. If the interaction occurs too late, it leads to an ectopic, obstructed ureter.[14]

Management

VUR management is controversial. General strategies include observation with or without prophylactic antibiotics and surgery. Management goals are to prevent UTIs, minimize renal damage, and avoid unnecessary interventions/procedures.[15]

VUR will often resolve spontaneously over time. The probability of resolution is dependent on clinical presentation (i.e., fUTI versus prenatal hydronephrosis), patient age, sex, laterality, and associated BBD.[16] Probability of resolution can help guide whether expectant management with or without prophylactic antibiotics or surgical treatment is most appropriate for each child.

There are two key studies in pediatric urology related to VUR management. One is the *Swedish Reflux Study*, which compared antibiotic prophylaxis, endoscopic injection therapy, and surveillance in children 1–2 years old with grade III or IV reflux.[17] The rate of new-onset fUTIs was significantly lower in the group of females receiving prophylactic antibiotics, and antibiotics prevented renal scarring in females as well. The second is the *RIVUR Trial* (Renal Scarring in the Randomized Intervention for Children with Vesicoureteral Reflux). This trial randomized children with grades I–IV VUR to antibiotic prophylaxis or placebo for 2 years. Antibiotic prophylaxis significantly lowered the risk of UTI, particularly in children with BBD. Antibiotics did not protect against renal scarring. Children randomized to antibiotic prophylaxis were more likely to present with resistant organisms if they developed a breakthrough UTI.[18]

The American Urological Association (AUA) VUR Guidelines divide management for patients by age.[19] For patients less than 1 year of age, patients are nonverbal, and thus, signs/symptoms of UTI may not be clear. Infants with fUTI and VUR should be prescribed antibiotic prophylaxis. Any infant with VUR grades III–V should also be prescribed antibiotics, even if the infant has not had fUTI.

Patients greater than 1 year of age have a greater likelihood of having BBD, lower likelihood of spontaneous VUR resolution, and can express symptoms. If BBD is present, this should be treated prior to surgical management of VUR. If the patient has had a fUTI, prophylactic antibiotics should be prescribed. Patients older than 1 year may be observed without prophylactic antibiotics if they have no anatomic abnormalities, or history of a fUTI, in the absence of BBD.

Antibiotic prophylaxis is generally indicated for children with moderate or high-grade VUR (grades III–V). Prophylaxis may be considered for any child in whom a VCUG is planned. Antibiotics are generally discontinued if the VCUG is normal. Table 11.2 outlines common prophylactic agents with contraindications and doses.

Surgical management

Decision-making about antireflux surgery is based on the degree of VUR, age and gender of the patient, BBD, and renal scarring.[15] Surgical management options include endoscopic injection and ureteral reimplantation.

Endoscopic injection: Cystoscopic injection of a bulking agent (dextronomer/hyaluronic acid, or Deflux as the only bulking agent approved by the U.S. Food and Drug Administration [FDA]) to elevate and coapt the ureteral

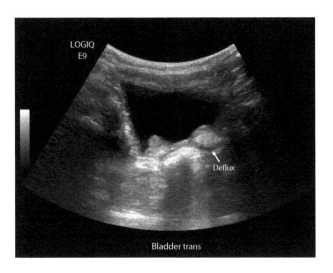

Figure 11.3 Ultrasound appearance of Deflux. Typical appearance of bladder after Deflux injection with hyperintensity on ultrasound of the left ureteral orifice. Often, the shadowing can be stronger and can mimic the appearance of a ureteral stone.

orifice and detrusor tunnel.[20] Resolution rates of endoscopic injection are highest for VUR grades I–III and lower for higher VUR grades (71% grade III, 59% grade IV, and 62% grade V).[21] Potential adverse effects are VUR recurrence and delayed-onset ureteral obstruction. The bulking material can appear as a calcification on ultrasound or CT scan, mimicking the appearance of a UVJ stone. Figure 11.3 shows the typical appearance of Deflux on ultrasound, and Figure 11.4 shows a computed tomography scan where the Deflux mound mimics a distal ureteral stone.

Ureteral reimplantation: Ureters are repositioned in the bladder via open, laparoscopic, or robotic procedures. These procedures elongate the ureteral segment that passes through a submucosal tunnel in the bladder to achieve a 5:1 tunnel-to-ureteral-diameter ratio. The surgery may be performed intravesically (tunnels made after opening the bladder) or extravesically (tunnels made by raising external detrusor flaps). All open techniques are reported to have a greater than 95% success rate.[15] Reported success rates for robotic ureteral reimplantation range from 72% to 99%; this procedure appears to still be in its dissemination phase.[22]

Table 11.2 Prophylactic antibiotics for children with urinary tract infection.

Agent	Contraindications	Prophylactic dose
Trimethoprim/sulfamethoxazole	Age <2 months G6PD deficiency Severe renal or hepatic disease Porphyria	2 mg/kg orally once daily (based on trimethoprim component)
Amoxicillin	No absolute contraindications, except previous severe hypersensitivity reaction	10–15 mg/kg orally once daily
Nitrofurantoin	Age <2 months G6PD deficiency Severe renal disease	1–2 mg/kg orally once daily

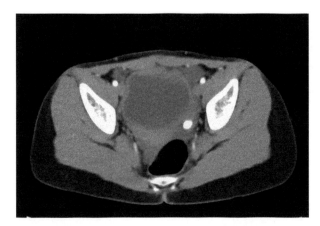

Figure 11.4 Computed tomography scan of patient after Deflux demonstrating calcification of the left ureteral orifice, mimicking a left distal ureteral stone.

BOWEL AND BLADDER DYSFUNCTION

BBD refers to a combination of bladder and bowel complaints that can be subcategorized into lower urinary tract symptoms and bowel dysfunction.[23] Lower urinary tract symptoms include urinary frequency and urgency, dysuria, and incontinence (day and/or night). Other signs of BBD include holding behaviors, sensation of incomplete emptying, urinary retention, postvoid dribbling, spraying of the urinary stream, genital/vaginal pain or itching, constipation, and encopresis (the soiling of stool on underpants in young children due to prolonged holding).[23]

Also known as dysfunctional elimination syndrome, BBD has a strong association with UTIs and VUR. In patients with VUR, about 20%–50% have been found to have concomitant BBD. It is essential to treat BBD prior to addressing VUR, as treatment of BBD reduces the incidence of UTI and improves VUR resolution rates.[24] Treatment of constipation can also reduce UTI incidence in patients without genitourinary anomalies.

Management options in BBD include behavioral therapy, biofeedback (patients >5 years old), neuromodulation, anticholinergics, α-blockers, and constipation management.[25]

INTERSTITIAL CYSTITIS/BLADDER PAIN SYNDROME
Introduction

Interstitial cystitis/bladder pain syndrome (IC/BPS) is most often seen in adults but can also be seen in children/adolescents. Pediatric and adolescent urologists and gynecologists should expect to diagnose one case of IC/BPS annually.[26] A great mimicker of other diseases of the bladder, a high index of suspicion is needed for diagnosis, and the lack of definitive diagnostic criteria can make diagnosis difficult.

The triad of IC/PBS consists of urinary frequency, bladder pain while the bladder is full, and relief of pain with voiding.[27] Patients may present with all three or may only present with one symptom. The median time from initial symptomatology to development of all three symptoms is

2 years.[28] Children with IC/BPS most often present with frequency and/or pain. Common misdiagnoses include UTI, urgency-frequency syndrome, vulvodynia, yeast vaginitis, chronic pelvic pain, and endometriosis.[29]

Evaluation

A recent consensus statement, from a meeting led by the Society for Urodynamics and Female Urology, defines IC/BPS as an unpleasant sensation, perceived to be related to the bladder, associated with lower urinary tract symptoms for more than 6 weeks' duration in the absence of infection or other identifiable causes.[30] There are, however, no definitive diagnostic tests for interstitial cystitis. The AUA recommends the following components: history and physical examination, frequency/volume chart, postvoid residual (to exclude other causes), urinalysis, urine culture (should be negative in IC/PBS), cytology (if smoking history is present), symptom questionnaire, and pain evaluation.

History

Patients with IC have urgency/frequency syndrome and/or pain in the bladder/pelvic area without any other obvious cause for their symptoms. The O'Leary-Sant[31,32] and pelvic pain and urgency/frequency questionnaires[33] are validated IC/PBS questionnaires, but they have not been validated in children. Patients may report symptoms are worse after drinking caffeine, fruit drinks, tomatoes, tomato products, and diet soft drinks, as well as around time of menses, during sexual activity, and while under stress.[27]

Disorders associated with IC/BPS include fibromyalgia, vulvodynia, migraines, allergic reactions, chronic pelvic pain, and gastrointestinal problems.[34] It can present with similar symptoms to chronic pelvic pain, and the bladder should be considered in young women with chronic pelvic pain.[35] It may also present with sexual dysfunction and is strongly correlated with sexual abuse.[36]

Physical exam

A systematic pelvic exam should be performed, including palpation of the anterior vaginal wall, bladder neck, urethra, vestibule, cervix, adnexa, posterior vaginal wall, and rectum. Evaluation of myofascial trigger points should also be performed. Performing a pelvic exam may be difficult in a child or adolescent. In young patients, this may need to be deferred until the patient is under anesthesia in the operating room if cystoscopy is planned.[37]

Diagnostic tests

Cystoscopy should be considered if a diagnosis of IC is suspected, as it may be diagnostic and therapeutic. The bladder should be distended to approximately 70–100 cm of water by raising the irrigation fluid to the appropriate height above the patient. Cystoscopy findings include hypervascular bladder mucosa, linear scarring, glomerulations and ulcers upon bladder emptying, hematuria post cystoscopy, and Hunner ulcers (Figure 11.5).[27]

Hunner ulcers are grossly inflammatory, red, bleeding lesions of the bladder that can be visualized on cystoscopy (see image) and are seen in 10% of all patients with IC/BPS,[38] although in a study of a cohort of young women with IC/BPS, no Hunner ulcers were identified on cystoscopy.[35]

While urine cultures in IC/BPS are typically negative, the patient's symptoms may respond to antibiotic therapy, possibly due to anti-inflammatory properties of antibiotics.[27]

The potassium sensitivity test involves catheterization and intravesical instillation of either saline or potassium chloride, where patients rate their degree of urgency upon instillation of either solution. This test is considered impractical in children/adolescents and has not been validated in these age groups.[27]

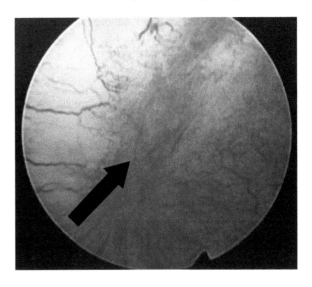

Figure 11.5 Cystoscopic view of Hunner ulcers. (Reproduced with permission from Chennamsetty A et al. *Urology*. 2015;85[1]:74–8.)

Management

The AUA guidelines outline an algorithm for treatment of IC/BPS (Table 11.3). All treatment options are available to patients at any stage of the disease. The AUA suggests following these clinical principles: [39]

- Treatments are ordered from most to least conservative. Surgical treatment is only indicated once other treatments are proved to be ineffective.
- Initial treatment level depends on patient symptom severity, clinical judgment, and patient preference.
- Multiple, simultaneous treatments may be used if it is in the best interest of the patient.
- Ineffective treatments should be stopped.
- Pain management should be considered throughout the course of the treatment plan.

Table 11.3 American Urological Association guidelines for management of interstitial cystitis/bladder pain syndrome.

First line	Fourth line
• Diet modification	• Intradetrusor botulinum toxin A
• General relaxation/stress management	• Neuromodulation
• Pain management	• Pain management
• Patient education	• Treatment of Hunner lesions if found via
• Self-care/behavioral modification	fulguration, resection, or submucosal injection
Second line	**Fifth line**
• Physical therapy techniques	• Cyclosporine
• Oral: amitriptyline, cimetidine, hydroxyzine, pentosan polysulfate	• Pain management
• Intravesical: DMSO (dimethylsulfoxide), heparin, lidocaine	
• Pain management	
Third line	**Sixth line**
• Cystoscopy under anesthesia with hydrodistention	• Urinary diversion with or without cystectomy
• Pain management	• Pain management
	• Substitution cystoplasty

Source: From Hanno PM et al. *J Urol.* 2011;185(6):2162–70. With permission.

- Diagnosis should be reconsidered if there is no improvement in symptoms within a clinically meaningful time frame.

Diet modification and behavioral therapy are often the first steps in management of IC/PBS. The key to diet modification is to determine and avoid trigger foods and beverages, which often include caffeinated beverages, alcohol, dairy products, certain fruits, and foods high in carbohydrates.

Pentosan polysulfate (PPS) is the only FDA-approved medical therapy for IC/PBS, but it has not been studied in children. Hydroxyzine is an antihistamine that is safe for use in children. The combination of PPS plus evening hydroxyzine may be a safe starting point for moderate symptoms of IC/PBS in adolescent females.

Bladder instillations and hydrodistention should be reserved for more severe symptoms. Bladder instillations include heparin, lidocaine, and sodium bicarbonate. Some studies have shown efficacy of hydrodistention in children with relief of symptoms in the majority, but with high recurrence rates and need for multiple procedures.[26,40] Neuromodulation, cystectomy and urinary diversion, and other surgical procedures are rarely indicated, especially in adolescents.

Patients should be informed that the management is challenging, and realistic expectations must be set. Lifelong care and changes in management may be necessary.[37]

Key points in interstitial cystitis/bladder pain syndrome

- IC/BPS is a triad of urinary frequency, bladder pain while the bladder is full, and relief of pain with voiding.
- Diagnosis includes history, physical exam, and exclusion of other causes of symptoms.
- Management options range from conservative medical management to hydrodistention to invasive surgical management.

When to refer to urology:

- Suspicion of diagnosis of IC/BPS.
- Pelvic pain refractory to conservative management.
- Consultation for cystoscopy.

ECTOPIC URETER AND URETEROCELE
Introduction

Ectopic ureter and ureterocele are two urologic conditions that are intimately connected embryologically and can cause UTIs, urinary tract obstruction, and urinary incontinence in children/adolescents. The embryology and anatomical abnormalities associated with these conditions are presented, including the clinical presentation, diagnosis, and management strategies.

Hydronephrosis

Hydronephrosis, often the presenting finding for these ureteral anomalies, is defined as dilation of the renal pelvis and calyces.[41] When hydronephrosis is diagnosed

Box 11.3 The Society for Fetal Urology (SFU) hydronephrosis grading system

- *Grade 1*: Dilation of pelvis only (mild)
- *Grade 2*: Dilation of pelvis and major calyces only (generally mild)
- *Grade 3*: Dilation of pelvis, major and minor calyces (moderate to severe dilation)
- *Grade 4*: Severe dilation with renal parenchymal thinning[42]

Source: Chow JS. et al. *Pediatr Radiol.* 2015;45(6):787–9.

postnatally, different grading systems are used to characterize the dilation (see Box 11.3).

The urinary tract dilation (UTD) system is graded on a three-point scale, based on six ultrasound findings, including renal pelvis diameter, calyceal dilation, parenchymal thickness of the kidney, renal parenchymal appearance, bladder abnormalities, and ureteral abnormalities.

The differential diagnosis of hydronephrosis includes ureteropelvic junction obstruction, VUR, prune belly syndrome, megaureter, duplicated collecting system, ureterocele, ectopic ureter, and multicystic dysplastic kidney.[41]

URETERAL BUD ANOMALIES
Pathophysiology and definitions

An ectopic ureter is one that opens into the bladder in an aberrant location. It may be associated with the upper pole of a duplicated collecting system or a single ectopic ureter. The most common orifice locations are the bladder neck, the proximal or distal urethra, and the vaginal vestibule, but may enter anywhere from the bladder neck to the perineum, including the vagina, cervix, or uterus. If the orifice is beyond the external urinary sphincter, it may cause continuous urinary incontinence in females.[43]

Ureterocele is a version of an ectopic ureter with a cystic dilation of the distal ureter. They may be associated with a duplex or single system. A simple (intravesical) ureterocele is entirely within the bladder and above the bladder neck. In an ectopic (extravesical) ureterocele, a portion is located at or below the bladder neck or urethra; these are typically obstructive.[44]

Presentation

Ureterocele and ectopic ureter may present prenatally, in childhood or in adolescence, and have variable presentations. Presenting symptoms may include fUTI or incontinence. If the patient presents with a fUTI, urgent incision of the ureterocele may be required. If incontinence is the present symptom, this suggests the presence of an ectopic ureter and often presents during toilet training as continuous dribbling from the vaginal vestibule. On imaging, they may present with hydronephrosis and/or as a cystic structure on ultrasound.

Ureterocele prolapse is an atypical physical exam finding, presenting as a mucosal-covered intralabial mass with

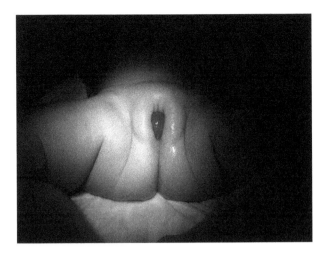

Figure 11.6 Prolapsed ureterocele presenting as an inter-labial mass in a 3-week-old. (Reproduced with permission from Arrabal-Polo MA et al. *J Pediatr.* 2012;161[5]:964.)

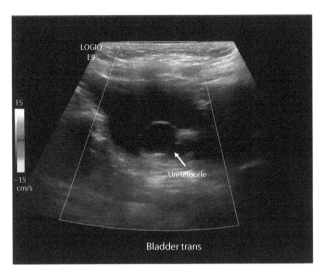

Figure 11.7 Ultrasound appearance of intravesical ureterocele.

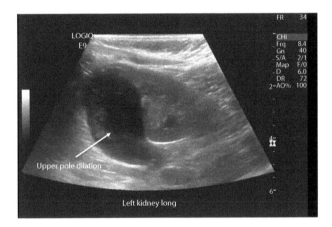

Figure 11.8 Ultrasound appearance of left kidney with duplicated collecting system, hydronephrosis of the upper pole due to obstructing ureterocele.

the patient having difficulty urinating and with reten-tion, requiring immediate intervention (Figure 11.6). Differential diagnosis includes urethral prolapse, imper-forate hymen, and introital tumor. Descriptions of these are provided in more detail elsewhere in the book. These pathologies can usually be differentiated on physical exam and pelvic ultrasound.

Diagnosis and evaluation

Physical examination

Physical exam is often normal. A prolapsing ureterocele is rare but will be prominent at the introitus. A young girl with persistent incontinence may have dribbling from the vagina or perineum, although it is difficult to see an ecto-pic opening in an infant. Examination under anesthesia or endoscopy may be required. One may be able to palpate a hydronephrotic kidney from an ectopic ureter on abdomi-nal examination in an infant.

Imaging

Ultrasound, VCUG, DMSA scan, and diuretic renal scan (MAG-3) are all important in the workup and manage-ment of ureterocele and ectopic ureter.

Ultrasound often demonstrates hydronephrosis of a single or duplicated system in cases of obstruction. A ureterocele appears as a thin-walled, cystic dilation that does not extend beyond the bladder wall. (Figures 11.7 and 11.8 show an intravesical ureterocele with upper tract hydroureteronephrosis.)

DMSA scan provides differential renal function. In duplicated systems, a DMSA can delineate the relative function of the lower and upper pole moieties. VCUG may be used to evaluate for VUR before and/or after interven-tion. A MAG-3 scan may provide both functional and drainage information about the kidney in concern for obstruction. Functional estimation on a MAG-3 scan is slightly less accurate. Finally, while often unnecessary for

the diagnosis, magnetic resonance urography can provide detailed anatomic images for challenging cases. It may be useful in identifying an occult ectopic ureter in an older child with incontinence.

Treatment

Treatment options for ectopic ureter/ureterocele include observation, endoscopic procedures, and surgery. The management strategies are controversial, and all options should be discussed with the patient prior to proceeding. The trend in management has veered away from aggres-sive initial management and toward a more conservative, minimally invasive approach.[45]

Observation is indicated if the patient is asymptomatic, in the absence of high-grade reflux, high-grade ureteral obstruction, or bladder outlet obstruction, and if there is good or absent function in the affected ureterocele moi-ety.[45] In all other scenarios, endoscopic or surgical man-agement is indicated.

Key points on ectopic ureter/ureterocele

- Ectopic ureter and ureterocele are causes of urinary tract obstruction, urinary tract infections, and urinary incontinence.
- Diagnosis is often made prenatally with a fetal ultrasound demonstrating hydronephrosis.
- Ureterocele prolapse is an emergency requiring urgent decompressive management.
- Ectopic ureter is a cause of persistent urinary incontinence in a female.
- Management varies from observation; endoscopic puncture of ureterocele; and open, laparoscopic, or robotic surgery.

When to refer to urology:

- Prenatal diagnosis of ectopic ureter or ureterocele.
- Ectopic ureter/ureterocele with fUTI.
- Ureterocele prolapse.
- Persistent urinary incontinence.

Endoscopic management

Endoscopic puncture or incision of a ureterocele under general anesthesia is the fastest way to achieve decompression, relieve obstruction, and decrease the risk of UTI.[46,47] Endoscopic management may be definitive in the case of a simple (intravesical) ureterocele, but patients with ectopic ureteroceles may require additional surgical interventions. Endoscopic puncture is indicated in the following scenarios: (1) obstructing ureterocele with UTI; (2) obstructing ureterocele with severe hydroureteronephrosis; and (3) intravesical ureterocele with a single, nonrefluxing system.[45]

Surgical management

Surgical management includes both upper and lower tract approaches performed via open, laparoscopic, or robotic techniques.

Upper tract surgery includes removal of the nonfunctional portion of a duplex kidney associated with an ectopic ureter/ureterocele. Lower tract management includes upper-to-lower ureteroureterostomy to bypass distal obstruction and/or ureteral reimplantation.

In the case of ectopic ureter causing persistent incontinence, a nephroureterectomy resolves symptoms in greater than 90% of cases.[48]

BLADDER EXSTROPHY AND EPISPADIAS
Introduction

Exstrophy-epispadias complex (EEC) is a rare condition with anomalies of the genitourinary tract, abdominal wall, and pelvis. It occurs in every 2.2/100,000 births. It is twice as common in males versus females. While the exact cause is unknown, there is a genetic component with siblings of patients with EEC at an increased risk. The EEC has three possible presentations: epispadias, classic bladder exstrophy (CBE), and cloacal exstrophy.[49]

Epispadias

Epispadias is the least severe form of EEC, consisting of a dorsally located urethra, with a closed abdominal wall and bladder. It is caused by failure of the dorsal urethral plate to tubularize. Epispadias is even less common than CBE, occurring in 1/150,000 to 1/300,000 girls. Often, epispadias is associated with bilateral VUR. A large percentage of patients born with epispadias suffer from incontinence. Patients with an epispadias defect closer to the bladder neck tend to have smaller bladder capacity and more severe incontinence.

Female epispadias may be difficult to identify at birth and may not be diagnosed until toilet training becomes delayed.[50] Diagnosis is made by physical exam, which demonstrates incomplete development of the labia minora, an incompletely tubularized urethra, bifid clitoris, and a flat mons pubis (Figure 11.9).

Surgical management

The goal of epispadias surgery is continence, which typically requires bladder neck reconstruction. Correction of the external genital appearance is often performed in the same setting. Surgery most often occurs between 6 and 12 months of age.

Classic bladder exstrophy

CBE is the most common presentation of the EEC. It occurs in 1/10,000 to 1/50,000 live births and is more common in males (2:1). Risk factors include white race, young maternal age, and multiparity. It includes defects of the genitourinary, reproductive, and musculoskeletal systems. Figure 11.10 shows the external appearance of an infant with CBE.

Genitourinary system

Patients with CBE have an abdominal wall defect in the midline with extrusion of the bladder. Many CBE patients

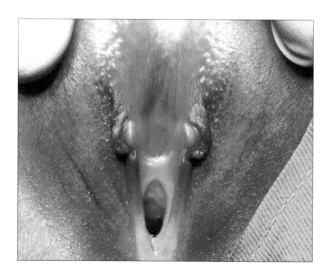

Figure 11.9 Female epispadias with bifid clitoris, flat mons pubis, incomplete development of the labia minora, and an incompletely tubularized urethra.

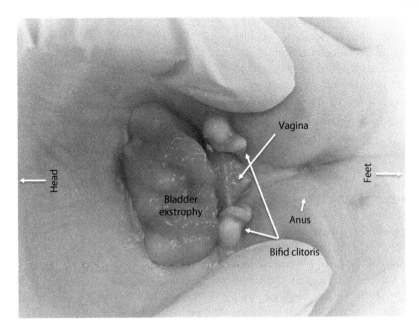

Figure 11.10 Infant girl with CBE: (a) polypoid, exstrophied bladder; (b) bifid clitoris; (c) anteriorly displaced vagina; and (d) anus.

have VUR after bladder closure. Additional renal anomalies associated with bladder exstrophy include horseshoe kidney, UPJ obstruction, and ectopic/pelvic kidney.[51] The dorsal urethra remains open in females with classic bladder exstrophy, creating a wide open bladder neck.

Reproductive system defects

The vagina and introitus are displaced anteriorly, and the vaginal canal is short and narrow. The cervix is lower than in patients without bladder exstrophy. The clitoris is bifid and surrounded by divergent labia. Müllerian anomalies are more common in EEC, including bicornuate and unicornuate uteri. Following surgical repair, 15%–30% of females with classic bladder exstrophy will experience pelvic organ prolapse.[52]

Musculoskeletal and other defects

Patients with CBE and cloacal exstrophy experience diastasis of the pubic rami and divergence of the rectus abdominis muscles. Patients may also have wider sacroiliac joint angles, an inferiorly rotated pelvis, and a large sacrum.[53] These abnormalities, if not corrected, may cause a wobbly gait.

Gastrointestinal/neurologic

More severe forms of EEC are associated with anal sphincter abnormalities, imperforate anus, omphalocele, and other gastrointestinal defects. In addition, 7% of patients with classic bladder exstrophy have an associated spinal abnormality such as spina bifida, scoliosis, or other vertebral anomalies.[49]

Diagnosis

The majority of CBE diagnoses are made on physical exam at birth. An increasing number are being detected prenatally with improved prenatal ultrasonography. Ultrasound may reveal absent bladder filling, widened pubic rami, or small genitalia. Suspicion or diagnosis should prompt referral to a specialized medical center with significant experience managing this EEC. Several consortiums have been developed in the United States to provide surgical education for pediatric urologists around the country and to collaborate on surgical technique.

Surgical repair

Baseline preoperative evaluation should include a renal and bladder ultrasound, VCUG, cystourethroscopy, and urodynamics. The overall goals of surgical repair for CBE are to recreate a normal anatomic and physiologic bladder, bladder neck, and urethra; protect kidney function; minimize incontinence; preserve sexual function; and optimize cosmesis.

There has been a trend in surgical technique from staged repair toward complete primary repair of bladder exstrophy (CPRE) where bladder neck reconstruction is performed at the same time as bladder closure. Closure can be performed right after birth or several months after birth to allow time for families to adjust to the diagnosis, and for a specialized team to be assembled. Ureteral reimplantation, if needed, can be done at the time of bladder neck reconstruction or bladder augmentation.[54]

Complications of CBE repair include dehiscence, inclusion cysts, bladder prolapse, bladder outlet obstruction, urinary leak, and vesicocutaneous fistula formation. Long-term complications include pelvic organ prolapse, incontinence, pelvic pain, and sexual dysfunction. Patients with vesicoureteral reflux are at risk for recurrent urinary tract infections, renal scarring, and ultimately renal failure, if not managed properly. Continence is directly related to the success of the initial bladder closure, as it depends on the final bladder capacity.[49]

Patients with CBE may require additional procedures, including bladder augmentation, to increase bladder capacity. Further bladder neck reconstruction, Botox injection, and sling placement may also be required to achieve continence. A continent urinary diversion, such as a Mitrofanoff procedure, can facilitate catheterization, when needed.

Body image/sexual function

A survey of patients with CBE indicated concerns about social and emotional functioning related to body image.[55] Another survey of adult women with CBE revealed that 84% were sexually active, 42% complained of dyspareunia, and one patient had genital prolapse. All patients suffered from severe sexual dysfunction.[56] Pelvic organ prolapse occurs in about 18%–30% of exstrophy patients, potentially due to the presence of a wider, flatter levator hiatus, shortened horizontal vagina, a narrow introitus, and weak cardinal ligaments.[53] Sexual function, continence, and quality of life all appear improved by repair of pelvic organ prolapse.[57]

Fertility

Due to the high incidence of Müllerian anomalies, adhesions from prior surgeries, and musculoskeletal abnormalities, the rate of spontaneous abortions and preterm delivery is high among patients with CBE. It has been recommended that women with CBE who become pregnant undergo a cesarean delivery, although vaginal deliveries have been reported.[52] The largest series of reported pregnancies in EEC patients includes 52 patients with CBE, 19 of whom became pregnant, leading to 57 total pregnancies. The miscarriage rate was 35%, which is higher than in the general population.[58] Many EEC patients require fertility treatments and *in vitro* fertilization.

SPINA BIFIDA AND NEUROGENIC BLADDER

Introduction

Spina bifida (SB) is the most common nonchromosomal birth defect, affecting multiple organs including the central nervous, musculoskeletal, and genitourinary systems. It occurs in 30/100,000 live births.[59] While the severity of symptoms is variable, many patients with SB have lifelong challenges with incontinence or urinary retention, UTIs, CKD, bowel function, and sexual function.

Pathophysiology

Spina bifida is a neural tube defect caused by failure of the caudal neural tube to fuse normally in early development. The location of the lesion, and therefore the severity of the disease, is dependent on the fusion location and abnormality. The most severe form is open myelomeningocele, manifested by an open, exposed spinal cord and, typically, an Arnold-Chiari malformation of the brain, which leads to a variable clinical presentation.

Risk factors for neural tube defects include family history, young and advanced maternal age, maternal

---

Key points on exstrophy-epispadias complex (EEC)/classic bladder exstrophy (CBE)

- Epispadias is defined by a dorsally located urethral meatus with a closed abdominal wall and bladder.
- CBE is characterized by an open protruding bladder and open abdominal wall with other genitourinary and musculoskeletal abnormalities.
- Management of CBE is shifting toward complete primary closure rather than delayed closure.
- CBE patients require multiple surgical interventions in their lifetime.
- Sexual dysfunction is a complex issue for CBE patients.

When to refer to urology:

- Prenatal or postnatal diagnosis of bladder exstrophy or epispadias.
- Bladder exstrophy or epispadias patient with incontinence.
- Recurrent urinary tract infections in a patient with a history of bladder exstrophy.

---

obesity, maternal diabetes, occupational exposures, and low maternal weight gain. Folic acid deficiency is an additional risk factor that can be prevented by taking a folic acid supplement prior to conception. Antiepileptics, such as valproic acid or carbamazepine, can directly cause neural tube defects unless taken with folic acid supplementation.[60]

Presentation/evaluation

Most cases of SB are detected on prenatal ultrasound. Ultrasound can detect the presence of the defect, location of the lesion, and severity of the lesion, allowing for prenatal consultation and possible management. Termination rates due to prenatal diagnosis of up to 65% have been reported.[61]

Early surgical myelomeningocele closure is critical to optimizing motor, genitourinary, and bowel function. Intrauterine repair has been studied in a randomized, multicenter clinical trial, which demonstrated a decreased need for ventriculoperitoneal shunting and improved motor function outcomes at the expense of increased preterm delivery.[62] The trial has yet to determine the urologic effects of intrauterine repair, but other retrospective studies of prenatal intervention have demonstrated minimal long-term improvement in urinary outcomes.[63]

Postnatal evaluation

Patients with SB should be managed in the neonatal intensive care unit with a dedicated multidisciplinary team. Renal and bladder ultrasound should be performed shortly after birth (before closure) to evaluate kidney anatomy and for urinary retention. Clean intermittent catheterization (CIC)[64] is initiated immediately after birth, with careful measurement of residual urine volumes, gradually decreasing the frequency of catheterization based on volumes. The following are other tests that should be performed in the neonatal period:

- Urinalysis and culture (prior to initiation of CIC)
- Serum creatinine
- Postclosure renal ultrasound
- VCUG
- Urodynamics study

Complications

Genitourinary

The goals of urinary tract management patients with SB are avoidance of UTIs, protection of kidney function and urinary continence, and independence. In general, the higher the level of the lesion, the higher is the severity of the lower urinary tract symptoms. Detrusor sphincter dyssynergia is a dangerous condition that can lead to high bladder pressures and damage to the upper tracts. Early and frequent urodynamic studies are crucial for monitoring patients with SB, as is determining optimal timing for medical and surgical intervention (Box 11.4).

Gastrointestinal

Almost all patients with SB require constipation management. Options for management include enemas, digital stimulation, laxatives, and dietary modification. Refractory constipation may need surgical intervention, such as an antegrade continence enema (ACE) through an abdominal stoma created from the appendix or small bowel. Often, this procedure is performed in conjunction with a urinary continence procedure.

Sexual function and fertility

With improvements in surgical interventions and more patients living into adulthood, many want to engage in intimate relationships.[65] However, more than 50% of patients with SB report they are dissatisfied with their current sex life.[66] Eighty percent of women with SB experience genital sensation, and about 37% have experienced orgasm.[67] However, lack of independence can make engaging in sexual activity difficult. Appropriate sex education is essential for promoting safe sex practices.

Patients with SB are more prone to precocious puberty and early onset of menarche. This can lead to potential

---

Key points on spina bifida

- Spina bifida (SB) is the most common nonchromosomal birth defect, affecting multiple organs including the central nervous, musculoskeletal, and genitourinary systems.
- Interventions that may be performed to optimize urinary function include the following:
  - Clean intermittent catheterization.
  - Medical management (antimuscarinics, antibiotic prophylaxis).
  - Intravesical botulinum toxin injection.
  - Sacral neuromodulation.
  - Deflux subureteric injection.
  - Ureteral reimplantation.
  - Bladder augmentation.
  - Continence catheterizable channels (Mitrofanoff [appendix] or Monti [small bowel]).
- Sexual function and fertility are important issues to address in patients with spina bifida.

When to refer to urology:

- Prenatal or postnatal diagnosis of spina bifida.
- Spina bifida patient with worsening incontinence or recurrent urinary tract infections.
- Spina bifida patient with changes in urinary function.

---

hygienic issues due to lack of mobility and independence. Fertility is possible with SB, and prenatal counseling is paramount, as patients have an increased risk of having a child with SB. This risk is increased if both parents carry the trait. Women with SB who are planning on becoming pregnant should take folic acid for 3 months prior to becoming pregnant and up until at least the 12th week of gestation.[68]

Pregnant women with SB are at an increased risk for UTIs, and use of prophylactic antibiotics during pregnancy has been suggested. Vaginal delivery is possible, and many of these women are at increased risk for pelvic floor dysfunction postpartum. Cesarean delivery may be necessary due to anatomical abnormalities.[69]

SUMMARY

In summary, urologic problems affect female children and adolescents. UTIs are common among this population. In addition to proper diagnosis and management, it is important to consider ureterocele, ectopic ureter, and even IC/BPS in the differential diagnosis of UTI. Pediatric and adolescent gynecologists need to be aware of the rare congenital anomalies that may affect sexual function and reproduction, such as SB and EEC. All of these disorders should be managed in conjunction with a pediatric urology team.

REFERENCES

1. Freedman AL, Urologic Diseases in America Project. Urologic diseases in North America Project: Trends in resource utilization for urinary tract infections in children. *J Urol.* 2005;173(3):949–54.

Box 11.4 Interventions that may be performed to optimize urinary function

- Clean intermittent catheterization
- Medical management (antimuscarinics, antibiotic prophylaxis)
- Intravesical botulinum toxin injection
- Sacral neuromodulation
- Deflux subureteric injection
- Ureteral reimplantation
- Bladder augmentation
- Continence catheterizable channels (Mitrofanoff [appendix] or Monti [small bowel])

2. Becknell B, Schober M, Korbel L, Spencer JD. The diagnosis, evaluation and treatment of acute and recurrent pediatric urinary tract infections. *Expert Rev Anti Infect Ther.* 2015;13(1):81–90.

3. Jackson EC. Urinary tract infections in children: Knowledge updates and a salute to the future. *Pediatr Rev.* 2015;36(4):153–64; quiz 65–6.

4. Foxman B. The epidemiology of urinary tract infection. *Nat Rev Urol.* 2010;7(12):653–60.

5. Traisman ES. Clinical management of urinary tract infections. *Pediatr Ann.* 2016;45(4):e108–11.

6. Subcommittee on Urinary Tract Infection SCoQI, Management, Roberts KB. Urinary tract infection: Clinical practice guideline for the diagnosis and management of the initial UTI in febrile infants and children 2 to 24 months. *Pediatrics.* 2011;128(3): 595–610.

7. Roberts KB. Revised AAP guideline on UTI in febrile infants and young children. *Am Fam Physician.* 2012;86(10):940–6.

8. Wan J, Skoog SJ, Hulbert WC et al. Section on Urology response to new guidelines for the diagnosis and management of UTI. *Pediatrics.* 2012;129(4):e1051–3.

9. Hoberman A, Charron M, Hickey RW, Baskin M, Kearney DH, Wald ER. Imaging studies after a first febrile urinary tract infection in young children. *N Engl J Med.* 2003;348(3):195–202.

10. Hiraoka M, Hori C, Tsukahara H et al. Vesicoureteral reflux in male and female neonates as detected by voiding ultrasonography. *Kidney Int.* 1999;55(4):1486–90.

11. Khoury AE, Bagli DJ. *Vesicoureteral Reflux. Campbell-Walsh Urology.* 4. 11th ed. Philadelphia, PA: Elsevier; 2016:4143–4.

12. Duckett JW, Bellinger MF. A plea for standardized grading of vesicoureteral reflux. *Eur Urol.* 1982;8(2):74–7.

13. Paquin AJ, Jr. Ureterovesical anastomosis: The description and evaluation of a technique. *J Urol.* 1959;82:573–83.

14. Mackie GG, Awang H, Stephens FD. The ureteric orifice: The embryologic key to radiologic status of duplex kidneys. *J Pediatr Surg.* 1975;10(4):473–81.

15. Hajiyev P, Burgu B. Contemporary management of vesicoureteral reflux. *Eur Urol Focus.* 2017;3(2–3):181–8.

16. Estrada CR, Jr., Passerotti CC, Graham DA et al. Nomograms for predicting annual resolution rate of primary vesicoureteral reflux: Results from 2,462 children. *J Urol.* 2009;182(4):1535–41.

17. Brandstrom P, Esbjorner E, Herthelius M, Swerkersson S, Jodal U, Hansson S. The Swedish reflux trial in children: III. Urinary tract infection pattern. *J Urol.* 2010;184(1):286–91.

18. Mattoo TK, Chesney RW, Greenfield SP et al. Renal scarring in the Randomized Intervention for Children with Vesicoureteral Reflux (RIVUR) Trial. *Clin J Am Soc Nephrol.* 2016;11(1):54–61.

19. Peters CA, Skoog SJ, Arant BS, Jr. et al. Summary of the AUA Guideline on Management of Primary Vesicoureteral Reflux in Children. *J Urol.* 2010;184(3): 1134–44.

20. Kim SW, Lee YS, Han SW. Endoscopic injection therapy. *Investig Clin Urol.* 2017;58(Suppl 1):S38–S45.

21. Routh JC, Inman BA, Reinberg Y. Dextranomer/hyaluronic acid for pediatric vesicoureteral reflux: Systematic review. *Pediatrics.* 2010;125(5):1010–9.

22. Timberlake MD, Peters CA. Current status of robotic-assisted surgery for the treatment of vesicoureteral reflux in children. *Curr Opin Urol.* 2017;27(1):20–6.

23. Austin PF, Bauer SB, Bower W et al. The standardization of terminology of lower urinary tract function in children and adolescents: Update report from the standardization committee of the International Children's Continence Society. *Neurourol Urodyn.* 2016;35(4):471–81.

24. Kibar Y, Ors O, Demir E, Kalman S, Sakallioglu O, Dayanc M. Results of biofeedback treatment on reflux resolution rates in children with dysfunctional voiding and vesicoureteral reflux. *Urology.* 2007;70(3):563–6; discussion 6-7.

25. Franco I. Functional bladder problems in children: Pathophysiology, diagnosis, and treatment. *Pediatr Clin North Am.* 2012;59(4):783–817.

26. Close CE, Carr MC, Burns MW et al. Interstitial cystitis in children. *J Urol.* 1996;156(2 Pt 2):860–2.

27. Mattox TF. Interstitial cystitis in adolescents and children: A review. *J Pediatr Adolesc Gynecol.* 2004;17(1):7–11.

28. Driscoll A, Teichman JM. How do patients with interstitial cystitis present? *J Urol.* 2001;166(6):2118–20.

29. Teichman JM, Parsons CL. Contemporary clinical presentation of interstitial cystitis. *Urology.* 2007;69(4 Suppl):41–7.

30. Hanno P, Dmochowski R. Status of international consensus on interstitial cystitis/bladder pain syndrome/painful bladder syndrome: 2008 snapshot. *Neurourol Urodyn.* 2009;28(4):274–86.

31. O'Leary MP, Sant GR, Fowler FJ, Jr., Whitmore KE, Spolarich-Kroll J. The interstitial cystitis symptom index and problem index. *Urology.* 1997;49(5A Suppl):58–63.

32. Lubeck DP, Whitmore K, Sant GR, Alvarez-Horine S, Lai C. Psychometric validation of the O'Leary Sant interstitial cystitis symptom index in a clinical trial of pentosan polysulfate sodium. *Urology.* 2001;57(6 Suppl 1):62–6.

33. Parsons CL, Dell J, Stanford EJ et al. Increased prevalence of interstitial cystitis: Previously unrecognized urologic and gynecologic cases identified using a new symptom questionnaire and intravesical potassium sensitivity. *Urology.* 2002;60(4):573–8.

34. Kennedy CM, Bradley CS, Galask RP, Nygaard IE. Risk factors for painful bladder syndrome in women seeking gynecologic care. *Int Urogynecol J Pelvic Floor Dysfunct.* 2006;17(1):73–8.

35. Rackow BW, Novi JM, Arya LA, Pfeifer SM. Interstitial cystitis is an etiology of chronic pelvic pain in young women. *J Pediatr Adolesc Gynecol.* 2009;22(3):181–5.

36. Peters KM, Killinger KA, Carrico DJ, Ibrahim IA, Diokno AC, Graziottin A. Sexual function and sexual distress in women with interstitial cystitis: A case-control study. *Urology.* 2007;70(3):543–7.

37. Yoost JL, Hertweck SP, Loveless M. Diagnosis and treatment of interstitial cystitis in adolescents. *J Pediatr Adolesc Gynecol.* 2012;25(3):162–71.

38. Simon LJ, Landis JR, Erickson DR, Nyberg LM. The Interstitial Cystitis Data Base Study: Concepts and preliminary baseline descriptive statistics. *Urology.* 1997;49(5A Suppl):64–75.

39. Hanno PM, Burks DA, Clemens JQ et al. AUA guideline for the diagnosis and treatment of interstitial cystitis/bladder pain syndrome. *J Urol.* 2011;185(6):2162–70.

40. Shear S, Mayer R. Development of glomerulations in younger women with interstitial cystitis. *Urology.* 2006;68(2):253–6.

41. Liu DB, Armstrong WR, 3rd, Maizels M. Hydronephrosis: Prenatal and postnatal evaluation and management. *Clin Perinatol.* 2014;41(3):661–78.

42. Sidhu G, Beyene J, Rosenblum ND. Outcome of isolated antenatal hydronephrosis: A systematic review and meta-analysis. *Pediatr Nephrol.* 2006;21(2):218–24.

43. Bisset GS, 3rd, Strife JL. The duplex collecting system in girls with urinary tract infection: Prevalence and significance. *Am J Roentgenol.* 1987;148(3):497–500.

44. Peters CA, Mendehlson, C. *Ectopic Ureter, Ureterocele, and Ureteral Anomalies. Campbell-Walsh Urology,* 4. 11th ed. Philadelphia, PA: Elsevier; 2016:4072–81.

45. Timberlake MD, Corbett ST. Minimally invasive techniques for management of the ureterocele and ectopic ureter: Upper tract versus lower tract approach. *Urol Clin North Am.* 2015;42(1):61–76.

46. Hagg MJ, Mourachov PV, Snyder HM et al. The modern endoscopic approach to ureterocele. *J Urol.* 2000;163(3):940–3.

47. Singh SJ, Smith G. Effectiveness of primary endoscopic incision of ureteroceles. *Pediatr Surg Int.* 2001;17(7):528–31.

48. Plaire JC, Pope JC 4th, Kropp BP et al. Management of ectopic ureters: Experience with the upper tract approach. *J Urol.* 1997;158(3 Pt 2):1245–7.

49. Inouye BM, Tourchi A, Di Carlo HN, Young EE, Gearhart JP. Modern management of the exstrophy-epispadias complex. *Surg Res Pract.* 2014;2014: 587064.

50. Frimberger D. Diagnosis and management of epispadias. *Semin Pediatr Surg.* 2011;20(2):85–90.

51. Ebert AK, Reutter H, Ludwig M, Rosch WH. The exstrophy-epispadias complex. *Orphanet J Rare Dis.* 2009;4:23.

52. Mathews RI, Gan M, Gearhart JP. Urogynaecological and obstetric issues in women with the exstrophy-epispadias complex. *BJU Int.* 2003;91(9):845–9.

53. Stec AA, Pannu HK, Tadros YE, Sponseller PD, Fishman EK, Gearhart JP. Pelvic floor anatomy in classic bladder exstrophy using 3-dimensional computerized tomography: Initial insights. *J Urol.* 2001;166(4):1444–9.

54. Borer JG, Vasquez E, Canning DA et al. Short-term outcomes of the multi-institutional bladder exstrophy consortium: Successes and complications in the first two years of collaboration. *J Pediatr Urol.* 2017;13(3):275 e1–e6.

55. Pennison MC, Mednick L, Rosoklija I et al. Health related quality of life in patients with bladder exstrophy: A call for targeted interventions. *J Urol.* 2014;191(5 Suppl):1553–7.

56. Bujons A, Lopategui DM, Rodriguez N, Centeno C, Caffaratti J, Villavicencio H. Quality of life in female patients with bladder exstrophy-epispadias complex: Long-term follow-up. *J Pediatr Urol.* 2016;12(4):210 e1–6.

57. Everett RG, Lue KM, Reddy SS et al. Patient-reported impact of pelvic organ prolapse on continence and sexual function in women with exstrophy-epispadias complex. *Female Pelvic Med Reconstr Surg.* 2017;23(6):377–81.

58. Deans R, Banks F, Liao LM, Wood D, Woodhouse C, Creighton SM. Reproductive outcomes in women with classic bladder exstrophy: An observational cross-sectional study. *Am J Obstet Gynecol.* 2012;206(6):496 e1–6.

59. Snow-Lisy DC, Yerkes EB, Cheng EY. Update on urological management of spina bifida from prenatal diagnosis to adulthood. *J Urol.* 2015;194(2):288–96.

60. Agopian AJ, Tinker SC, Lupo PJ, Canfield MA, Mitchell LE, National Birth Defects Prevention S. Proportion of neural tube defects attributable to known risk factors. *Birth Defects Res A Clin Mol Teratol.* 2013;97(1):42–6.

61. Cromie WJ. Implications of antenatal ultrasound screening in the incidence of major genitourinary malformations. *Semin Pediatr Surg.* 2001;10(4):204–11.

62. Adzick NS, Thom EA, Spong CY et al. A randomized trial of prenatal versus postnatal repair of myelomeningocele. *N Engl J Med.* 2011;364(11):993–1004.

63. Clayton DB, Tanaka ST, Trusler L et al. Long-term urological impact of fetal myelomeningocele closure. *J Urol.* 2011;186(4 Suppl):1581–5.

64. Winkler TW, Justice AE, Graff M et al. The influence of age and sex on genetic associations with adult body size and shape: A large-scale genome-wide interaction study. *PLOS Genet.* 2015;11(10):e1005378.

65. Cromer BA, Enrile B, McCoy K, Gerhardstein MJ, Fitzpatrick M, Judis J. Knowledge, attitudes and behavior related to sexuality in adolescents with chronic disability. *Dev Med Child Neurol.* 1990;32(7):602–10.

66. Verhoef M, Barf HA, Vroege JA et al. Sex education, relationships, and sexuality in young adults with spina bifida. *Arch Phys Med Rehabil.* 2005;86(5):979–87.

67. Sawyer SM, Roberts KV. Sexual and reproductive health in young people with spina bifida. *Dev Med Child Neurol.* 1999;41(10):671–5.

68. Wilson RD, Davies G, Desilets V et al. The use of folic acid for the prevention of neural tube defects and other congenital anomalies. *J Obstet Gynaecol Can.* 2003;25(11):959–73.

69. Visconti D, Noia G, Triarico S et al. Sexuality, pre-conception counseling and urological management of pregnancy for young women with spina bifida. *Eur J Obstet Gynecol Reprod Biol.* 2012;163(2):129–33.

70. Chennamsetty A, Khourdaji I, Goike J, Killinger KA, Girdler B, Peters KM. Electrosurgical management of Hunner ulcers in a referral center's interstitial cystitis population. *Urology.* 2015;85(1):74–8.

71. Chow JS, Darge K. Multidisciplinary consensus on the classification of antenatal and postnatal urinary tract dilation (UTD classification system). *Pediatr Radiol.* 2015;45(6):787–9.

72. Arrabal-Polo MA, Nogueras-Ocana M, Tinaut-Ranera J, Zuluaga-Gomez A, Arrabal-Martin M. Vulval tumor in an infant: Prolapse of ureterocele. *J Pediatr.* 2012;161(5):964.

Adnexal masses in the neonate, child, and adolescent

12

LISA ALLEN, NATHALIE FLEMING, JULIE STRICKLAND, and HEATHER C. MILLAR

INTRODUCTION

Ovarian cysts and masses are not frequent in children and adolescents but can be present at any age. They most commonly come to attention as a result of pain but may also be diagnosed incidentally or with other symptoms, such as increasing abdominal distension, nausea and vomiting, or signs and symptoms of hormonal production. Management requires knowledge of the pathology that may present at different ages. Fertility-sparing decisions are important for benign lesions, either expectant or surgical ovarian-sparing procedures. The infrequent malignancy requires surgical staging and oncologic consultation for chemotherapy when indicated. This chapter reviews ovarian pathology as it presents in the neonate, child, and adolescent.

FETAL AND NEONATAL OVARIAN CYSTS

The etiology of a fetal or neonatal ovarian cyst is almost universally a functional cyst.[1–3] Only rarely will pathology such as a mature teratoma[1,2,4] or cystadenoma[5] be present. Management of the antenatal or neonatal ovarian cyst requires consideration of ovarian preservation and avoidance of complications, in particular, ovarian torsion, a challenging diagnosis in infancy.

Incidence, etiology, and diagnosis

Primordial follicles are present in the fetal ovary as early as the 20th week of gestational age, peaking at 33 weeks.[2] Ovaries are not quiescent during the antenatal or neonatal period, with small physiologic ovarian cysts of diameter less than 1.4 cm visible in 84% of sonographic images.[6] The detection of clinically relevant ovarian cysts greater than 2 cm is less frequent, being diagnosed in 1:2,625 pregnancies.[7] The pathogenesis of the fetal ovarian cyst is believed to be related to follicular stimulation from placental chorionic gonadotropin (HCG), maternal estrogen, and fetal gonadotropins. Conditions of excess placental HCG secretion or enhanced placental permeability to HCG, such as maternal diabetes mellitus, gestational hypertension, and Rh isoimmunization, are associated with fetal ovarian cysts.[8] However, the majority of fetal and neonatal ovarian cysts occur in the absence of one of the aforementioned conditions.[9,10] Fetal conditions of hypothyroidism and congenital adrenal hyperplasia with 21-hydroxylase or 11β-hydroxylase deficiency in association with neonatal ovarian cysts have also been reported.[10–12] The bilateral rate of ovarian cysts in this age group ranges from 1.4% to 27%.[3,5,9,13–15] At birth, levels of follicle-stimulating

hormone (FSH) rise rapidly due to the withdrawal of maternal estrogen and progesterone sources. This level peaks at 3–4 months of age and then gradually falls thereafter to the low prepubertal levels that will be maintained throughout childhood. The regression of neonatal ovarian cysts over the same time period can be expected. With the increasing use of ultrasound during pregnancy, the majority of recent reports contain series of primarily antenatally diagnosed ovarian cysts.[5,14–22] Antenatal ovarian cysts are reported to be diagnosed at an average of 33 weeks of gestational age[2,9,14] but have been identified as early as 19 weeks.[23] The diagnosis *in utero*, which is based on the findings of a nonperistaltic cystic abdominal structure in a female fetus with otherwise intact urinary and gastrointestinal tracts, must be considered presumptive as confirmation is not feasible until postdelivery; rarely will a neoplasm of the ovary be the etiology of an ovarian lesion at this age. Histopathology assessment of 385 surgically managed fetal cysts comprised only 2.1% cystadenomas and 1.5% teratomas; the remainder were either follicular or theca lutein cysts.[24] The differential diagnosis of an ovarian cystic mass includes mesenteric cysts, intestinal duplication, intestinal obstruction, megacystitis, hydronephrosis, omental cysts, anterior meningomyelocele, lymphangioma, urachal cysts, hydrometrocolpos, and choledochal cysts.[11,14,25] The false-positive rate of *in utero* diagnosis is 7.5%, with the most common misdiagnosis related to gastrointestinal anomalies.[24] Simple cysts are anechoic, unilocular with thin walls. Fetal and neonatal cysts that have become complicated, related to hemorrhage or torsion, are heterogenous on ultrasound, with fluid-debris levels, retracting clots, septations, and solid areas, and may develop dystrophic calcification in their walls[21,26] (Figure 12.1).

In the neonatal period, an ovarian cyst may be diagnosed due to a palpable abdominal mass, symptoms such as respiratory distress, vomiting, irritability, or failure to thrive, or incidentally during imaging for other medical conditions.[18,27]

Natural history, risk, and complications

Given the functional nature of the majority of cysts in infants, resolution of many would be expected with expectant management. While resolution is documented, cyst complications such as torsion and hemorrhage do occur in both the antenatal and neonatal periods, with torsion the most concerning complication due to potential loss of the adnexa.

(a)

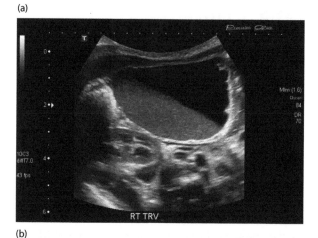

(b)

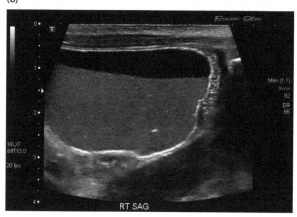

Figure 12.1 Postnatal appearance of antenatal diagnosis of a simple ovarian cyst, but complex by delivery.

There is a significant risk of *in utero* complication when cysts are diagnosed prenatally. A recent systematic review and meta-analysis of 92 articles on fetal ovarian cysts documented an overall torsion rate of 31% with expectant management, with a 20% prenatal torsion rate.[28] *In utero* torsion appears to cause few sequelae for the newborn. Most are asymptomatic, although bowel adhesions,[10] autoamputation,[29–31] and eventual loss of ovarian function are possible sequelae.[16,18] Bilateral ovarian cysts can place the neonate at risk for complete loss of ovarian function.[29] Polyhydramnios[4,11,17,32] has been associated with fetal ovarian cysts. The etiology is speculated to be related to a partial small bowel obstruction or compression of the umbilical cord.[17,32,33] Soft tissue dystocia at delivery from abdominal distention, while possible, is rare; hence, most authors advocate cesarean section for obstetrical indications only.[11] Presumptive diagnosis of antenatal torsion has been shown to be unreliable and does not justify any obstetric intervention to expedite delivery.[34]

Ovarian torsion in the neonate can be difficult to diagnose but is occasionally associated with serious sequelae, including death.[16,35–39] Symptoms from ovarian cysts in neonates include vomiting and failure to thrive due to small bowel obstruction or volvulus from bowel adhesions,[9,13] respiratory distress due to mass effect,[4,32] and anemia or hypovolemic shock due to hemoperitoneum associated with cyst hemorrhage and rupture.[32]

The size of ovarian cysts does affect the likelihood of ovarian torsion, being significantly higher in fetal ovarian cysts larger than 40 mm compared to those smaller than 40 mm, with an odds ratio of 30.8 (95% confidence interval 8.6–110).[24]

Management

Antenatal cysts

The management of both antenatal and postnatal ovarian cysts is not standardized. In only rare cases will interventional therapy be indicated; 54% of all fetal cysts resolve during pregnancy or after birth, with higher rates of resolution of 70% and 85% for simple cysts and cysts <4 cm in size, respectively.[24] Arguments for both expectant and active management have been put forth in the medical literature. The criteria for interventional management are usually based on size and complexity of the cyst during sonographic evaluation.

Given the high rate of *in utero* torsion, consideration has been given to antenatal intervention by aspiration to help avoid this complication.[9] Most centers that perform prenatal aspiration use a criteria of greater than 4–5 cm, and apply antenatal aspiration to simple ovarian cysts only. In a systematic review and meta-analysis of the published literature, the frequency of total torsion (12% versus 39%, $p < 0.001$), prenatal torsion (4% versus 25%, $p < 0.001$), and postnatal surgery (63% versus 8%) were all significantly lower in the aspirated cysts meeting those standard criteria, compared to expectant management. However, the quality of studies included was low, resulting in an inability to make any strong recommendations.[28] One small, open randomized controlled trial has been published on intrauterine ovarian cyst aspiration. Aspiration, performed in 31 pregnancies, was associated with higher rates of *in utero* involution of the cyst and lower rates of oophorectomy compared to the expectant management group.[40] Hemorrhage, preterm labor, premature rupture of membranes, needle injuries to fetal intraabdominal organs, and infection are potential risks of *in utero* aspiration.[41] These risks may be minimal due to the later gestational age at which cysts are diagnosed and, hence, managed.[9] The greatest risk of antenatal aspiration is the risk of misdiagnosis. A policy of routine aspiration of presumed ovarian cysts antenatally may result in aspiration of other intraabdominal cystic masses.[1,9] While careful sonographic imaging will be able to differentiate many of these lesions, antenatal aspiration could result in inadvertent aspiration of a nonovarian etiology. Cyst recurrence may occur after aspiration and is reported at 37.9%.[24]

Neonatal cysts

Expectant management

The risk of malignancy in fetal and neonatal ovarian cysts is extremely low as outlined previously, allowing a nonsurgical approach to be contemplated in their management (Figure 12.2). The following criteria have been suggested

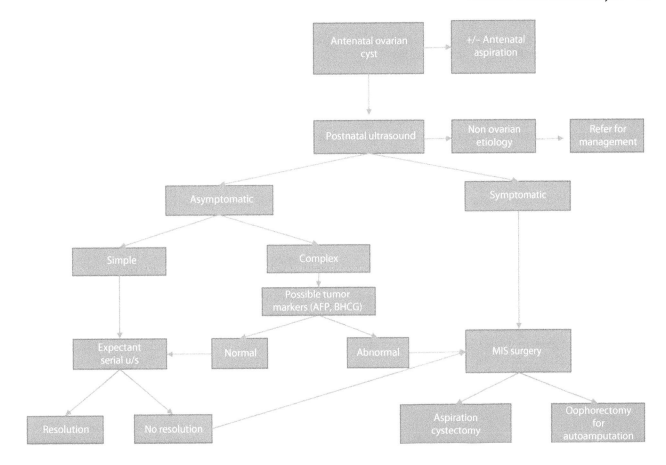

Figure 12.2 Algorithm for management of neonatal ovarian cysts.

as justifying expectant management in the asymptomatic neonate:

1. The cyst is clearly of ovarian origin.
2. There is no solid component on ultrasound beyond septations and debris from hemorrhage.
3. Tumor markers are negative, i.e., α-fetoprotein (AFP), chorionic gonadotropin (βHCG), and lactate dehydrogenase (LDH).
4. The family is willing and able to comply with follow-up.[8]

Cautious interpretation of tumor markers in the newborn is required, with application of age-referenced norms, and, given the low rate of malignancy, could be potentially eliminated as a necessity in the evaluation of cystic lesions at this age.

When expectant management with serial ultrasound follow-up is chosen in the newborn period, several factors affect resolution rates. Complexity and cyst size are most predictive. The odds ratio for resolution is 0.15 for complex cysts versus simple cysts.[24] The time to resolution for complex cysts is also longer than for simple cysts.[14] Many simple cysts will resolve by 6 months of age.[14,17] Final resolution of complex lesions may require up to 16 months.[5,14,18] If surgery is only undertaken for symptoms, inability to continue follow-up, for increasing size or persistence, then up to 81%–100% of cysts diagnosed in the antenatal period resolve without intervention.[14,16,18] Resolution of cysts as large as 8 cm in diameter has been recorded; however,

resolution rates decrease with increasing cyst size dropping to 17%–21% for cysts greater than 6 cm in size.[10,28]

As complexity often represents antenatal torsion, not surprisingly, after complex cyst resolution on imaging, the majority of ipsilateral ovaries will not be visualized, reflecting absence of function.[14,16,18,20] Of the 10 complex cysts followed expectantly by Luzzato et al., only 20% of the children had both ovaries visible after resolution of the complex mass.[14] Enriquez et al. reported on two groups of infants managed in their institution, a retrospective surgical cohort of 9 infants and a prospective expectant cohort of 11 infants, all with prenatal or postnatal diagnosis of ovarian cysts. Of the nonsurgical group, while all cysts involuted between 3 and 15 months of age, 100% of the infants had a single ovary remaining on pelvic ultrasound.[18]

The persistence of a neonatal cyst, especially in the presence of complex elements, should raise the consideration of the rare diagnosis of an ovarian neoplasm, ovarian teratoma, or cystadenoma. In these circumstances, surgical management is indicated.[1,2,4]

Postnatal aspiration

Postnatal aspiration is less commonly employed in comparison with either expectant serial imaging follow-up or surgical therapy, but may have a role in the management of the larger simple ovarian cyst.[14] Aspiration of complex cysts is controversial, because in the rare circumstance of a mature teratoma, aspiration and spillage of cyst contents could theoretically lead to chemical peritonitis and pelvic adhesions. Nonovarian pathology must be excluded before aspiration.

Surgery

Most authors direct surgical management based on the presence of symptoms, and for asymptomatic cysts, a size criterion of >4–5 cm and complexity of the cyst on ultrasound imaging, coupled with lack of resolution with initial expectant management.[3]

When surgery is indicated, the approach to surgery in infants is evolving toward minimally invasive techniques. Laparoscopy,[3,19,31] laparoscopic-assisted minilaparotomy, and minilaparotomy[30] are all reported. Laparoscopy allows an enhanced visualization of the pelvis and abdomen compared with the view obtained through a minilaparotomy incision. Regardless of the approach to surgery, the guiding principle in surgical management of neonatal cysts should be the least aggressive surgery to preserve the maximum normal ovarian tissue.[1] Surgically guided cyst

(a)

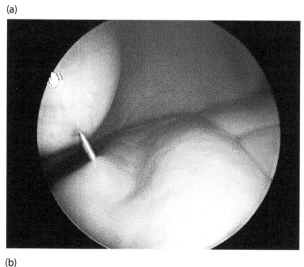

(b)

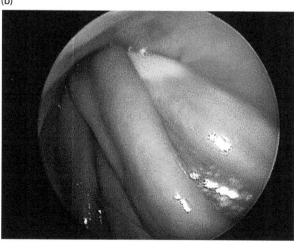

Figure 12.3 Laparoscopic aspiration for decompression of twisted large ovarian cyst. Oophorectomy undertaken after decompression through small abdominal incision.

aspiration, fenestration or unroofing of the cyst, or cystectomy is preferable to oophorectomy in simple ovarian cysts. The autoamputated or necrotic torsed ovary is nonsalvageable and should be managed with oophorectomy (Figure 12.3).

CHILDHOOD OVARIAN CYSTS

Adnexal masses are reported less frequently in childhood than in the adolescent owing to the low levels of gonadotropins. As a result, fewer functional cysts will develop in prepubertal ovaries.[42] Consequently, if an ovarian mass is noted in this age group, a reasonable index of suspicion of neoplasia must be maintained when deciding on the approach to both investigation and management.

Incidence

The incidence of all ovarian masses in childhood is quoted as approximately 2.6 cases/100,000 girls per year.

With the widespread use of ultrasound, ovarian cysts may currently be diagnosed more frequently. Microcysts (<9 mm) and macrocysts (>9 mm) exist within the ovaries of 2- to 9-year-old girls.[43] These simple, small, and transient cysts are not clinically significant, and caution should be applied in attributing symptoms to their presence.

Ovarian neoplasms are said to constitute not more than 1% of all childhood tumors; 8% of all malignant abdominal tumors in children are of ovarian origin.[44] The incidence of neoplasms overall is higher in adolescence compared with childhood, up to 10-fold, but the proportion of malignancies in neoplasms is higher in the first decade of life compared with the second, with a peak at age 6 years of more than 30% and then decreasing to less than 10% by age 14 and down to 2%–4% by age 20[45] (Figure 12.4).

Presentations

Ovarian masses in children may present with abdominal pain, mass effect, or rarely, with endocrine disturbance.[46] Girls have a proportionally long infundibulopelvic ligament and a small unyielding bony pelvis, which may result in symptoms from ovarian pathology being abdominal rather than pelvic in children.

Pain is the most common presenting symptom and is present in over 70% of cases.[47] Acute pain results from a cyst complication of hemorrhage, rupture, or torsion. An ovarian etiology for abdominal pain syndromes in girls must be contemplated and appropriate imaging undertaken.[48] The most common misdiagnosis of a childhood ovarian mass is appendicitis.[48,49] Identification by palpation is less frequent, ranging from 21.7% to 35.7%.[46,50] Associated symptoms may be nonspecific, such as vomiting, fever, anorexia, constipation, weight loss, abdominal distention, urinary frequency, urinary retention, and dysuria. Less commonly, masses present with endocrine manifestations such as isosexual precocious puberty, virilization, and/or vaginal bleeding. Sex cord-stromal tumors traditionally are associated with endocrine manifestations, but other nonneoplastic and neoplastic lesions may

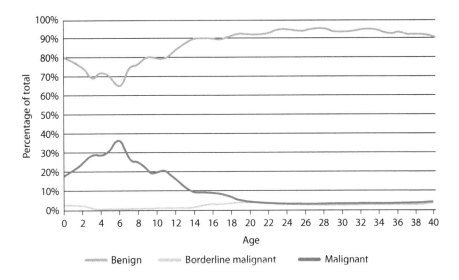

Figure 12.4 Proportion of benign, borderline, and malignant neoplasms over the reproductive ages. (From Hermans AJ et al. *Gynecol Oncol.* 2016;143[1]:93–7. With permission.)

also lead to endocrine disturbance. Follicular cysts, ovarian edema, and germ cell tumors have all been reported in association with hormonal production and symptoms.[42]

Etiology

The differential diagnosis of the adnexal mass in childhood includes functional ovarian cysts, benign and malignant ovarian neoplasms, paratubal or paraovarian cysts, and Müllerian anomalies, as well as nongynecologic pathology (Table 12.1). Functional cysts, however, are very uncommon in children.

All histologic cell lines are described at all ages; however, the proportions change between childhood and adolescence (Figures 12.5 and 12.6). In the child age range, the most common origin for ovarian neoplasms is the germ cell line, accounting for approximately 70% of tumors.[45] Both epithelial and stromal tumors are uncommon in the first decade of life. However, stromal tumors account for a larger proportion of surgical masses between the ages of 2 and 6 years, approximately 20%, before dropping to their low rates in the remainder of the reproductive years (1.5%).[45,51] The most common ovarian neoplasm in children is the mature cystic teratoma.[42,45,46,50,51] The malignant germ cell tumors consist of dysgerminomas, endodermal sinus tumors, immature teratomas, and embryonal carcinomas.[52]

Investigations

The diagnostic approach to a pelvic mass in childhood combines careful physical examination as the initial step, with imaging and possibly the inclusion of tumor markers when malignancy is suspected. Height, weight, and general appearance should be documented. On abdominal examination, the size of the mass is ascertained, and the presence or absence of abdominal tenderness or ascites is noted. As ovarian cysts may be secondary to other medical conditions, a physical examination must address potential related pathology. Café au lait spots on the skin

Table 12.1 Differential diagnosis of pelvic mass in children.

Ovarian
1. Functional
   - Corpus luteum
   - Theca lutein cyst
2. Benign
   - Germ cell (mature cystic teratoma, functional teratoma, gonadoblastoma)
   - Epithelial cystadenoma (serous, mucinous)
   - Stromal (thecoma, fibroma)
3. Low malignant potential
   - Serous
   - Mucinous
4. Malignant
   - Germ cell (dysgerminoma, endodermal sinus tumor, immature teratoma, embryonal, polyembryoma, choriocarcinoma, mixed)
   - Epithelial cystadenocarcinoma (serous, mucinous)
   - Stromal (juvenile granulosa cell tumor, Sertoli-Leydig tumor)
5. Metastatic
   - Lymphoma

Embryologic remnants
   - Paratubal
   - Para-ovarian cysts
   - Adnexal torsion

Müllerian anomaly

Gastrointestinal
   - Mesenteric cyst
   - Appendiceal abscess
   - Intussusception

Urologic
   - Wilms tumor

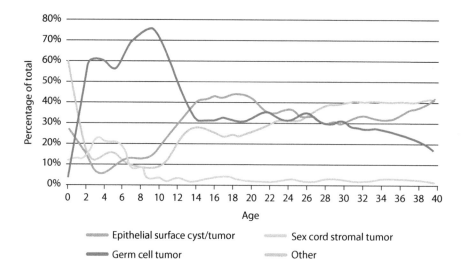

Figure 12.5 Histologic subtypes in surgical specimens over the reproductive ages. (From Hermans AJ et al. *Gynecol Oncol.* 2016;143[1]:93–7. With permission.)

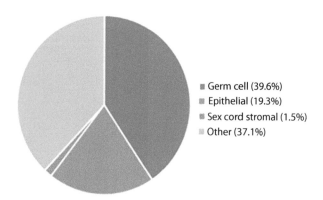

Figure 12.6 Histologic proportion of neoplasms in children. (From Rogers E et al. *JPAG* 2014;27[3]:125–8. With permission.)

may indicate McCune-Albright syndrome, and a thyroid nodule may be related to hypothyroidism. Evaluation for signs of hormonal production with Sexual Maturity Scale staging of the breast and pubic hair is necessary. As tumors may produce either estrogen or androgens, the examiner should look for isosexual precocious puberty and virilization or hirsutism. The external genitalia should be inspected for signs of estrogenization of the hymen and for signs of virilization, such as clitoromegaly.

Imaging is essential in characterization of the ovarian mass. Ultrasound is the initial imaging modality of choice to assess for size, characteristics of the lesion (wall thickness, mural nodules, excrescences, septations, and shadowing), bilaterality, pelvic fluid (hemoperitoneum or ascites), and prepubertal or pubertal appearance of the uterus; it may also identify extra-ovarian disease. Ultrasound Doppler can document the presence or absence of flow to an ovarian lesion. Ultrasound imaging may be complemented by computed tomography (CT) scanning or magnetic resonance imaging (MRI), with MRI preferable due

to the absence of radiation. These modalities are usually only needed if the origin of the mass is not clear on ultrasound or there are features concerning for malignancy, including size, complexity, solid components, ascites, or bilaterality, and are useful at that point to assess for the presence of pelvic or para-aortic lymphadenopathy and extra-ovarian disease.[53]

Tumor markers in childhood should include, as a minimum, AFP, LDH, and βHCG, if malignancy is suspected. These tumor markers are positive in multipotential germ cell tumors (embryonal carcinoma) and extra-embryonal tumors (endodermal sinus tumor and choriocarcinoma) (Table 12.2). A mature or immature teratoma that contains malignant elements may secrete AFP. LDH is positive but nonspecific in dysgerminomas. CA 125, while positive in serous epithelial tumors, is a nonspecific indicator of peritoneal inflammation and has limited value in premenopausal patients. If examination suggests hormonal production by the tumor, determination of serum estrogen and androgen levels can confirm the clinical suspicion. Granulosa cell tumors are indicated by an elevated inhibin level, although this test is not routinely available (Table 12.2).

Management

The management of ovarian cysts in children is dictated by the symptoms, the likelihood of neoplasm, and, in particular, the concern for malignancy. Expectant management with conservative follow-up of nonconcerning ovarian lesions is feasible in children and should be the method of choice in selected cases of simple and/or small ovarian cysts. Expectant management is possible in 41%–80% of masses referred for gynecologic assessment in children and adolescents, although the proportion of children who require surgery is higher than in adolescents.[47,54] While most neoplasms will be 5 cm or larger, the largest cyst

Table 12.2 Tumor markers in childhood ovarian tumors.

Tumor	AFP (α-fetoprotein)	BHCG (β-Human Chorionic Gonadotropin)	Inhibin	LDH (lactate dehydrogenase)	CA125	Androgens
Dysgerminoma	−	−/+	−	−/+	−/+	−
EST (endodermal sinus tumor)	+	−	−	−/+	−/+	−
Immature teratoma	−	−	−	−	−	−
Embryonal carcinoma	−/+	−/+	−	−	−	−
Choriocarcinoma	−	+	−	−	−	−
Mixed GCT (germ cell tumor)	−/+	−/+	−	−	−/+	−
Granulosa cell	−	−	+	−	−	−/+
Sertoli-Leydig	−	−	−/+	−	−	+
Epithelial tumor	−	−	−	−	−/+	−

diameter that resolved in conservative follow-up of ovarian cysts in children was 9.8 cm.[47]

Criteria modified from Warner et al.[55] may be useful in deciding on surgical management:

1. Persistent nonresolving symptoms
2. Suspicion of torsion
3. Signs and symptoms of a large mass associated with complications (hydronephrosis)
4. Concern for neoplasm (see preoperative risk stratification)
5. Unclear origin of mass

As with ovarian masses at other ages, a surgical approach by laparoscopy or laparotomy must be planned. Guiding principles in surgical management of ovarian lesions should be toward ovarian preservation and minimization of adhesion formation to preserve fertility. Surgical management of ovarian lesions by experienced health-care providers is important and has been shown to enhance the likelihood of the patient receiving an ovarian-conserving surgery.[48,56,57]

If there is a low index of suspicion for malignancy, a laparoscopic approach with ovarian cystectomy is the surgical procedure of choice. Occasionally, benign masses may be too large to approach laparoscopically. In these situations, a minilaparotomy incision with surgical decompression of the ovarian cyst is appropriate. Once decompressed, the mass can be exteriorized, and an ovarian cystectomy may be completed. Cystectomy is appropriate for surgical management of epithelial cystadenomas, para-ovarian or para-tubal cysts, and mature cystic teratomas. As mature cystic teratomas may be bilateral in 10% of cases, conservative management is even more important.

Mature cystic teratomas have pathognomonic imaging features that assist with diagnosis: Rokitansky nodules (dense tubercle in the cyst lumen which will have shadowing from its echogenicity), dot-dash sign (sign arising from presence of hairs in different orientations with an appearance of lines and dots), intratumoral fat, fat-fluid levels, as well as calcifications.[58] These findings reflect the presence of various tissue types present from the three germ cell layers—ectoderm, mesoderm, and endoderm—most commonly hair, fat, bone, and teeth. The surgical approach for mature cystic teratomas remains controversial, particularly due to the theoretical risks associated with intraoperative spill. Ovarian cystectomy of dermoid cysts by laparoscopy is associated with higher rates of spill than by laparotomy, ranging from 46% to 100% in pediatric and adolescent surgical series.[59-63] In these same series, with a total of 240 children managed laparoscopically, there were no incidences of chemical peritonitis.[59,61-63] While increased recurrence rates have been reported with laparoscopy over an open approach, this was not replicated in two more recent small studies where recurrent rates were 10% in each.[60,62,64] When obtaining parental consent for laparoscopic treatment of dermoid cysts, the risk of spill and recurrence rate should be discussed. Postoperatively, pelvic ultrasounds should be considered to assess for teratoma recurrence, which is most likely to be identified in the first year after surgery.[64] Recurrence is more common when dermoids are large (>8 cm), bilateral, and multiple.[65]

Surgical staging is paramount for malignant ovarian neoplasms, as stage of disease guides decisions for postoperative adjuvant chemotherapy. Pediatric germ cell tumors are staged using the system developed by the Pediatric Oncology Group. Epithelial tumors are staged according to the International Federation of Gynecology and Obstetrics (FIGO) system for primary carcinoma of the ovary. Rupture of a malignant neoplasm at surgery can result in upstaging of the patient; hence, most suspicious tumors are optimally approached by laparotomy. If a germ cell tumor is suspected, the primary tumor is resected with a unilateral salpingo-oophorectomy without interruption of the ovarian capsule on the surgical field. Intraoperative staging includes collection of ascites or peritoneal washings for cytology, inspection, and palpation of peritoneal surfaces, the contralateral ovary, pelvic and/or para-aortic nodes bilaterally, and omentum with biopsy only for abnormalities. Extensive germ cell tumors should be biopsied for diagnosis, but aggressive surgical procedures are not undertaken at the risk of harm to vital structures due to the effective response observed to multiagent chemotherapy in these tumors. Postoperative chemotherapy with bleomycin, etoposide, and cisplatin has resulted in marked advances in survival compared with previous regimens. Six-year survival rates of 93%–98% are reported for malignant ovarian germ cell tumors after four cycles of BEP.[66] With meticulous staging and careful postoperative monitoring to determine need for salvage chemotherapy, 50%–60% of stage I malignant germ cell tumors can now be managed without the need for postoperative chemotherapy.[67] This emphasizes the importance of preoperative risk stratification, to select patients appropriately for complete surgical staging.

Epithelial cystadenocarcinomas are extremely rare in childhood.[68] Management of these lesions would be as per adult guidelines. Low malignant potential epithelial tumors are managed in young patients with unilateral salpingo-oophorectomy, omental biopsy, and resection of all visible disease. If the lesion is of mucinous histology, an appendectomy is recommended to rule out a synchronous gastrointestinal lesion. Low malignant potential lesions begin to appear in early adolescence, where they comprise 2%–4% of surgical lesions (Figure 12.4) and hence are rarely encountered in children.[45,51]

Stromal cell tumors are often present in an early tumor stage and can be treated effectively with surgery alone, rarely requiring postoperative chemotherapy.

Ovarian function as evidenced not only by ongoing menstruation but also by pregnancy has been documented following fertility-sparing approaches to surgery and platinum-based adjuvant chemotherapy regimens in the treatment of pediatric malignant ovarian tumors.[69]

Risk stratification

In order to choose an appropriate management strategy for both benign and malignant masses in children and adolescents, several algorithms have been developed to guide decisions regarding ovarian-sparing surgery and oophorectomy and, in some situations, whether or not to proceed to surgery at all.[51,54,70]

The components of preoperative risk stratification include imaging features (complexity or solid components, size, ovarian crescent sign, and morphology index) with or without age and germ cell tumor markers.[51,54,70–72] As mentioned previously, the proportion of masses representing malignancy is highest in childhood, with an odds ratio of 3.02 for the ages of 1–8 years.[72] However, published algorithms focus more on imaging features as the main component in decision-making. Completely cystic lesions of any size are rarely malignant; hence, it is appropriate to offer ovarian cystectomy when surgery is required and tumor markers are not required in assessment.[51,70] For complex and/or solid ovarian masses, a size threshold of 8–9 cm is often applied to separate the benign lesions (hemorrhagic cysts, endometriomas, or mature cystic teratomas) from malignant lesions, with consideration of non-ovarian-sparing surgery for the larger complex/solid

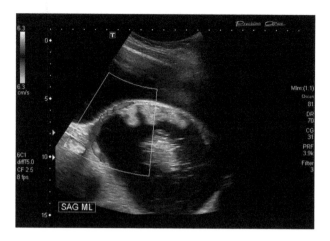

Figure 12.7   Ovarian crescent sign.

lesions where the positive predictive value for malignancy increases to 37%–67%.[51,70] Abnormal tumor markers suggest a germ cell malignancy and usually indicate the need for surgical staging. While size and complexity have an excellent sensitivity for detecting malignancies, strict application of oophorectomy to any larger complex lesion will result in oophorectomies for benign lesions such as larger teratomas or mucinous cystadenomas. The positive predictive value of algorithms may be improved with the introduction of further refined imaging criteria of a morphology index (structural score and volume score) with the presence or absence of an ovarian crescent sign. An ovarian crescent sign is the identification of healthy ovarian tissue adjacent to the mass in the ipsilateral ovary and is more commonly present in benign lesions (Figure 12.7). The structural score assesses wall thickening, echogenicity, septa, presence of papillary projections, complexity, presence of solid components, and extratumoral fluid. The volume score assigns an increasing score to larger volumes >10, >50, >100, >200, and >500 cm^3. When these components are included in three decision tree rules, the positive predictive value of surgically treated masses for malignancy rose to 86% in one study.[54]

A structured and algorithmic approach to the assessment of pediatric and adolescent masses that incorporates imaging features and mass size provides risk stratification to guide decision-making. The age of the patient and the presence of abnormal tumor markers contribute to risk assessment.

ADOLESCENT OVARIAN MASSES

Ovarian cysts overall are more frequently encountered in adolescents when compared with children. However, the proportion of cysts or masses within the ovary that represent either benign neoplasms or malignancy is even lower; hence, management styles in this age group must reflect the propensity toward formation of functional ovarian cysts postmenarche.

Etiology and diagnosis

Functional ovarian cysts often result from the failure of the maturing follicle to ovulate and involute and represent up to 50% of adolescent ovarian cysts.[73] Often these cysts are simple on ultrasound, with thin walls. They are benign and self-limiting and over time will involute. Functional cysts may also reflect the persistence of the corpus luteum.[74,75] Approximately two-thirds to three-quarters of functional cysts will regress within two to three menstrual cycles (10–12 weeks).[76]

Functional cysts may become complicated by hemorrhage. Following ovulation, both the luteinized theca cells and the granulosa cell layer of the follicle become vascularized. These vessels are fragile and may rupture easily, leading to a hemorrhagic cyst.[77] The average diameter of a hemorrhagic ovarian cyst is 3.0–3.5 cm, but they may range up to 8.5 cm on ultrasound.[77] A hemorrhagic ovarian cyst often presents with an abrupt onset of lower abdominal or pelvic pain midcycle or in the luteal phase without fever or leukocytosis. If the cyst wall ruptures, a hemoperitoneum may develop, and peritoneal signs or postural hypotension may be evident on examination. A hemorrhagic cyst has been termed a great imitator, as its appearance on ultrasonography may be confused with an ectopic pregnancy, ovarian neoplasm, or inflammatory process such as a tubo-ovarian abscess.[78] The hallmark of a hemorrhagic ovarian cyst is its evolution over time from acute hemorrhage, through clot retraction, to resolution.[77] While acute pain is often the presentation, the symptoms gradually resolve without intervention, with analgesia often required.

The differential diagnosis of the adolescent functional ovarian cyst includes endometriomas, benign and malignant ovarian neoplasms, disorders of the fallopian tube (hydrosalpinx, paratubal cyst), ectopic pregnancies, or nongynecologic etiologies (peritoneal cysts, periappendiceal abscesses). This is similar to the differential diagnosis in the childhood age range but also includes complications of sexual activity.[75]

Similar to the childhood age group, of the tumors that may present in the adolescent ovary, germ cell tumors predominate, with a benign cystic teratoma the most common neoplasm noted.[50] The incidence of malignancy in adolescents ranges from 2% to 10%, with the incidence decreasing with increasing age.[45,50,73] As mentioned, low malignant potential tumors begin to appear in early adolescence.[45]

Endometriomas have previously been considered quite rare in the adolescent age group; however, more recent series of adolescent patients with surgically confirmed endometriosis document the presence of endometriomas in 19%–34%; hence, an endometrioma should remain in the differential diagnosis of adolescent adnexal masses.[79,80] Symptoms suggestive of endometriosis include dysmenorrhea, chronic acyclic abdominal pain, as well as dyspareunia, dysuria, and pain with defecation.[79,80] Adolescents with endometriosis often have a family history of an affected relative.[80,81]
Paratubal cysts, which are remnants of paramesonephric or mesonephric ducts, have an incidence of 7%–11% in children and adolescents undergoing surgery for adnexal

pathology.[51,82,83] The majority of patients with paratubal cysts will be postmenarcheal, although they are present in childhood. These cystic lesions are located in the mesosalpinx and are asymptomatic unless complicated. They may serve as a lead point for adnexal or fallopian tube torsion. Unilocular, anechoic, or hypoechoic, they are often not accurately diagnosed on imaging with only 26% identified correctly on ultrasound or CT preoperatively.[83] The differential diagnosis includes a cystadenoma, follicular cyst, or nonadnexal pathology, such as a mesenteric cyst. An association with obesity and hyperandrogenism has been suggested.[84]

Management

In the adolescent with an adnexal mass, it is important to illicit a full menstrual and sexual history in addition to the history of the presenting symptoms. The differential diagnosis in this age group includes complications of pregnancy; hence, investigations should include a βHCG in sexually active adolescents. A speculum examination in the sexually active adolescent should be considered, and testing for chlamydia and gonorrhea should be performed; a bimanual examination should be performed to assess for adnexal and/or cervical motion tenderness associated with pelvic inflammatory disease. In an adolescent, an abdominal and pelvic ultrasound is the initial imaging modality of choice; however, in the sexually active adolescent, a transvaginal ultrasound may assist in the diagnosis.[73]

The adolescent ovarian cyst should be managed conservatively. Functional ovarian cysts may be either simple or complex on ultrasound imaging. Given their propensity for resolution in the absence of symptomatology requiring immediate surgical diagnosis (i.e., suspicion of torsion or malignancy), follow-up sonography at 6-week intervals will document resolution in the majority of adolescent ovarian cysts. The use of an oral contraceptive pill does not aid in regression of the functional ovarian cyst[76] but is an option to prevent future cyst formation in an adolescent who experiences recurrent painful hemorrhagic cysts.[85] Instructions should be given to both the adolescent and, if possible, her family during the observation period concerning symptoms of adnexal torsion that should lead them to seek assistance. A hemorrhagic cyst with a frank hemoperitoneum rarely may require surgical management. Patients on anticoagulants or with a bleeding diathesis are at greatest risk.[86]

Surgical management of an adolescent adnexal mass should be considered if there is an absence of regression after two or three menstrual cycles, if there is a suspicion of malignancy or if acute symptomatology is present. Similar to with children, the guiding principle in surgical management should be to maintain future fertility options. The approach to surgery is dependent on the presumptive diagnosis. However, laparoscopy is a reasonable approach to the management of the majority of cysts in this age group. Ovarian cystectomy should be performed unless there is a high index of suspicion of malignancy.

ADNEXAL TORSION

Adnexal torsion involves partial or complete twisting of the ovary and/or fallopian tube around its vascular pedicle, leading to edema, ischemia, and necrosis. Adnexal torsion is reported in approximately 3% of all emergent gynecologic surgeries.[56] Torsion of normal ovaries occurs more commonly in young girls than in women, with 30%–40% of ovarian torsions occurring without a lead point of an adnexal mass in this age group.[87,88] This is thought to be due to an excessively mobile mesovarium or fallopian tube resulting from congenitally long ovarian ligaments or laxity of pelvic ligaments, that resolves in adulthood with growth of the gynecologic structures.[89] When an adnexal mass is present, it is most commonly a benign functional ovarian cyst or teratoma. The right adnexa is more likely to twist than the left, suggesting that the sigmoid colon may help prevent torsion.[90] Torsion of the adnexa results in rapid onset of acute pelvic pain that may be described as colicky or intermittent. It is often associated with nausea and/or vomiting.[91] Clinically, the young woman may appear ill with mild fever, and may have an acute abdomen and palpable pelvic mass.[91] However, some patients have more mild symptoms and an atypical physical exam.

There is no blood test that can definitively diagnose adnexal torsion. An elevated white blood cell count may be found but is not sensitive or specific.[92] B-mode ultrasound is the imaging modality of choice, but it is important to know that ultrasound findings on their own are not diagnostic. A recent meta-analysis of 18 studies in children and adolescents found that morphological criteria on B-mode ultrasound yielded a sensitivity of 92% and a specificity of 96% for torsion.[93] Morphological criteria used varied across the included studies but included absolute or relative ovarian size, heterogeneous echotexture, peripheral cortical follicles dilated with transudative fluid, whirlpool sign (spiraling of the adnexal vessels), fluid debris level in follicular cysts, and the presence of an adnexal mass with ipsilateral non-identification of the ovary. Doppler ultrasound in this meta-analysis was moderately specific (87%) but only 55% sensitive for torsion, meaning that the presence of normal blood flow on Doppler does not exclude the diagnosis of torsion.[93] Naiditch et al. recently reported a positive predictive value (PPV) of 19% and a negative predictive value of 99.5% for transabdominal color Doppler ultrasound in a pediatric sample, using a combination of unilateral enlarged ovary, free pelvic fluid, lack of arterial or venous flow, or a twisted vascular pedicle as diagnostic criteria.[94] Ultrasound is operator dependent, and it is important to know the ultrasound capabilities of one's own institution, in particular, with regard to assessment of gynecologic structures in the pediatric population (Figures 12.8a and b).

Preoperative diagnosis of adnexal torsion in a girl is often challenging and requires a high level of suspicion. There is often a delay in diagnosis as signs and symptoms are similar to other conditions such as appendicitis, constipation, gastroenteritis, inflammatory bowel disease, volvulus, and bowel obstruction.[95] Furthermore, symptoms may mimic urinary causes including pyelonephritis, renal calculi, cystitis, urethritis, or urinary retention.[95] Psychologic causes of abdominal pain should remain a diagnosis of exclusion. Definitive diagnosis of adnexal torsion is based on surgical findings. The difficulty in diagnosis was illustrated in a series of 115 cases of adnexal torsion that revealed correct preoperative diagnosis in only 38% of these patients.[96] Expedient diagnosis is important, however, as a delay or a missed diagnosis may compromise fertility. Unfortunately, there is often a delay in diagnosis of adnexal torsion in a child. The clinical presentation, combined with a high level of suspicion, and possibly imaging, will lead to the probable diagnosis.

(a)

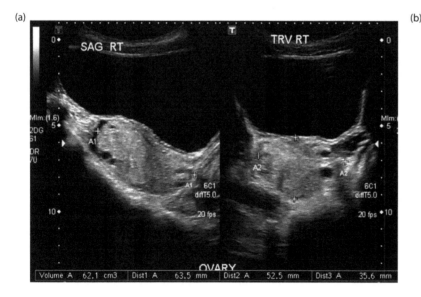

(b)

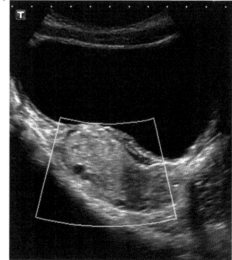

Figure 12.8 (a) and (b) Ultrasound features of ovarian torsion, with an enlarged ovary with peripheralization of follicles, central edema, localized medially (a). Panel (b) demonstrates lack of flow on doppler imaging.

The paradigm has shifted from ovarian removal to adnexal untwisting and ovarian preservation. Conservative management of primary adnexal torsion by untwisting the involved adnexa to preserve ovarian function and prevent adverse sequelae of torsion is the standard of care.[97] Laparoscopic adnexal untwisting will be successful in preserving presumed ovarian function (as demonstrated by follicular development seen on ultrasound) in approximately 74%–93% of cases.[94,98,99] Historically, removal of the affected ovary had been advocated as it was believed that restoring normal anatomy via untwisting could dislodge a clot in the ovarian vein or leave a necrotic vestige.[100] However, pulmonary embolism is reported in only 0.2% of cases with adnexal torsion treated by adnexectomy, yet not more frequently when the adnexa was untwisted.[101] Malignancy is rarely present in the setting of ovarian torsion; in series of ovarian torsion only 1%–1.5% are malignant masses.[87,88]

The decision to proceed with cystectomy at the time of untwisting is dependent on whether the edema of the ovary may lead to a more difficult excision. Interval cystectomy can be considered.[102,103]

Recurrence of ovarian torsion is higher when torsion occurs with a normal adnexa compared to in the presence of a mass (15%–55% versus 3%–6%).[104,105] Oophoropexy, defined as stabilization of ovarian tissue, may prevent recurrence and is performed by pexing the ovary to the ipsilateral uterosacral ligament, the back of the uterus, or the pelvic sidewall (fixation technique) or by shortening the utero-ovarian ligament (plication technique). It is reasonable to consider oophoropexy of the untwisted ovary, contralateral ovary, or both in cases of recurrent torsion, when the ovarian ligament is obviously elongated or when there is no obvious cause for torsion.[89,104,106,107] The most commonly encountered complication of oophoropexy is postoperative fever, and this can be managed conservatively.[108] The effects of oophoropexy on long-term tubal function remain to be demonstrated with the collection of prospective data.

CONCLUSION

Ovarian cysts and masses may present across the ages, from the antenatal period, through childhood, and into adolescence. Functional cysts, neoplasms, and malignancies occur within the ovaries of children and adolescents at varying frequencies. Careful and often conservative management in most circumstances can lead to appropriate ovarian-preserving treatments. The symptomatic ovarian cyst is often due to complications such as hemorrhage and ovarian torsion. Ovarian torsion represents a true surgical emergency, and a high index of clinical suspicion must be maintained to avoid inadvertent delay in therapy.

REFERENCES

1. Heling KS, Chaoui R, Kirchmair F, Stadie S, Bollmann R. Fetal ovarian cysts: Prenatal diagnosis, management and postnatal outcome. *Ultrasound Obstet Gynecol*. 2002;20(1):47–50.

2. Brandt ML, Luks FI, Filiatrault D, Garel L, Desjardins JG, Youssef S. Surgical indications in antenatally diagnosed ovarian cysts. *J Pediatr Surg*. 1991;26(3):276–81; discussion 81–2.

3. Esposito C, Garipoli V, Di Matteo G, De Pasquale M. Laparoscopic management of ovarian cysts in newborns. *Surg Endosc*. 1998;12(9):1152–4.

4. Tsakiri SP, Turk CA, Lally KP, Garg K, Morris B. Atypical Meigs' syndrome in a neonate with ovarian torsion associated with an ovarian dermoid cyst. *Pediatr Surg Int*. 2005;21(5):407–9.

5. Kwak DW, Sohn YS, Kim SK, Kim IK, Park YW, Kim YH. Clinical experiences of fetal ovarian cyst: Diagnosis and consequence. *J Korean Med Sci*. 2006;21(4):690–4.

6. Cohen HL, Shapiro MA, Mandel FS, Shapiro ML. Normal ovaries in neonates and infants: A sonographic study of 77 patients 1 day to 24 months old. *Am J Roentgenol*. 1993;160(3):583–6.

7. Kirkinen P, Jouppila P. Perinatal aspects of pregnancy complicated by fetal ovarian cyst. *J Perinat Med*. 1985;13(5):245–51.

8. Brandt ML, Helmrath MA. Ovarian cysts in infants and children. *Semin Pediatr Surg*. 2005;14(2):78–85.

9. Bagolan P, Giorlandino C, Nahom A et al. The management of fetal ovarian cysts. *J Pediatr Surg*. 2002;37(1):25–30.

10. Chiaramonte C, Piscopo A, Cataliotti F. Ovarian cysts in newborns. *Pediatr Surg Int*. 2001;17(2–3):171–4.

11. Vogtlander MF, Rijntjes-Jacobs EG, van den Hoonaard TL, Versteegh FG. Neonatal ovarian cysts. *Acta Paediatr*. 2003;92(4):498–501.

12. Sahin NM, Bayramoglu E, Cetinkaya S et al. Vaginal bleeding and a giant ovarian cyst in an infant with 21-hydroxylase deficiency. *J Pediatr Endocrinol Metab*. 2018;31(2):229–33.

13. Bagolan P, Rivosecchi M, Giorlandino C et al. Prenatal diagnosis and clinical outcome of ovarian cysts. *J Pediatr Surg*. 1992;27(7):879–81.

14. Luzzatto C, Midrio P, Toffolutti T, Suma V. Neonatal ovarian cysts: Management and follow-up. *Pediatr Surg Int*. 2000;16(1–2):56–9.

15. Cho MJ, Kim DY, Kim SC. Ovarian cyst aspiration in the neonate: Minimally invasive surgery. *J Pediatr Adolesc Gynecol*. 2015;28(5):348–53.

16. Foley PT, Ford WD, McEwing R, Furness M. Is conservative management of prenatal and neonatal ovarian cysts justifiable? *Fetal Diagn Ther*. 2005;20(5):454–8.

17. Comparetto C, Giudici S, Coccia ME, Scarselli G, Borruto F. Fetal and neonatal ovarian cysts: What's their real meaning? *Clin Exp Obstet Gynecol*. 2005;32(2):123–5.

18. Enriquez G, Duran C, Toran N et al. Conservative versus surgical treatment for complex neonatal ovarian cysts: Outcomes study. *Am J Roentgenol*. 2005;185(2):501–8.

19. Dobremez E, Moro A, Bondonny JM, Vergnes P. Laparoscopic treatment of ovarian cyst in the newborn. *Surg Endosc.* 2003;17(2):328–32.

20. Galinier P, Carfagna L, Juricic M et al. Fetal ovarian cysts management and ovarian prognosis: A report of 82 cases. *J Pediatr Surg.* 2008;43(11):2004–9.

21. Kim HS, Yoo SY, Cha MJ, Kim JH, Jeon TY, Kim WK. Diagnosis of neonatal ovarian torsion: Emphasis on prenatal and postnatal sonographic findings. *J Clin Ultrasound.* 2016;44(5):290–7.

22. Manjiri S, Padmalatha SK, Shetty J. Management of complex ovarian cysts in newborns – Our experience. *J Neonatal Surg.* 2017;6(1):3.

23. Meizner I, Levy A, Katz M, Maresh AJ, Glezerman M. Fetal ovarian cysts: Prenatal ultrasonographic detection and postnatal evaluation and treatment. *Am J Obstet Gynecol.* 1991;164(3):874–8.

24. Bascietto F, Liberati M, Marrone L et al. Outcome of fetal ovarian cysts diagnosed on prenatal ultrasound examination: Systematic review and meta-analysis. *Ultrasound Obstet Gynecol.* 2017;50(1):20–31.

25. Meyberg-Solomayer GC, Buchenau W, Solomayer EF et al. Cystic colon duplication as differential diagnosis to ovarian cyst. *Fetal Diagn Ther.* 2006;21(2):224–7.

26. Ozcan HN, Balci S, Ekinci S et al. Imaging findings of fetal-neonatal ovarian cysts complicated with ovarian torsion and autoamputation. *Am J Roentgenol.* 2015;205(1):185–9.

27. Spence JEH, Domingo M, Pike C, Wenning J. The resolution of fetal and neonatal ovarian cysts. *Adolesc Pediatr Gynecol.* 1992;5:27–31.

28. Tyraskis A, Bakalis S, David AL, Eaton S, De Coppi P. A systematic review and meta-analysis on fetal ovarian cysts: Impact of size, appearance and prenatal aspiration. *Prenat Diagn.* 2017;37(10):951–8.

29. Corbett HJ, Lamont GA. Bilateral ovarian autoamputation in an infant. *J Pediatr Surg.* 2002;37(9):1359–60.

30. Ferro F, Iacobelli BD, Zaccara A, Spagnoli A, Trucchi A, Bagolan P. Exteriorization-aspiration minilaparotomy for treatment of neonatal ovarian cysts. *J Pediatr Adolesc Gynecol.* 2002;15(4):205–7.

31. Tseng D, Curran TJ, Silen ML. Minimally invasive management of the prenatally torsed ovarian cyst. *J Pediatr Surg.* 2002;37(10):1467–9.

32. Nussbaum AR, Sanders RC, Hartman DS, Dudgeon DL, Parmley TH. Neonatal ovarian cysts: Sonographic-pathologic correlation. *Radiology.* 1988;168(3):817–21.

33. Valenti C, Kassner EG, Yermakov V, Cromb E. Antenatal diagnosis of a fetal ovarian cyst. *Am J Obstet Gynecol.* 1975;123:216–19.

34. Gohar J, Segal D, Hershkovitz R, Mazor M. Changing sonographic features of fetal ovarian cysts during pregnancy and the neonatal period. *Arch Gynecol Obstet.* 1999;263(1–2):82–3.

35. Cox HD, Campbell RM, Vishniavsky S, Arayata FR. Huge ovarian cyst with torsion in a newborn infant. *VA Med Mon.* 1969;96(2):96–100.

36. Kasian GF, Taylor BW, Sugarman RG, Nyssen JN. Ovarian torsion related to sudden infant death. *CMAJ.* 1986;135(12):1373.

37. Ahmed S. Neonatal and childhood ovarian cysts. *J Pediatr Surg.* 1971;6(6):702–8.

38. Havlik DM, Nolte KB. Sudden death in an infant resulting from torsion of the uterine adnexa. *Am J Forensic Med Pathol.* 2002;23(3):289–91.

39. Karl S, Sen S, Zachariah N, Chacko J, Thomas G. Torted ovarian cyst with lethal bleeding diathesis in an infant. *Pediatr Surg Int.* 1999;15(2):145–6.

40. Diguisto C, Winer N, Benoist G et al. In-utero aspiration vs expectant management of anechoic fetal ovarian cysts: Open randomized controlled trial. *Ultrasound Obstet Gynecol.* 2018;52(2):159–64.

41. Perrotin F, Potin J, Haddad G, Sembely-Taveau C, Lansac J, Body G. Fetal ovarian cysts: A report of three cases managed by intrauterine aspiration. *Ultrasound Obstet Gynecol.* 2000;16(7):655–9.

42. de Silva KS, Kanumakala S, Grover SR, Chow CW, Warne GL. Ovarian lesions in children and adolescents—An 11-year review. *J Pediatr Endocrinol Metab.* 2004;17(7):951–7.

43. Qublan HS, Abdel-hadi J. Simple ovarian cysts: Frequency and outcome in girls aged 2–9 years. *Clin Exp Obstet Gynecol.* 2000;27(1):51–3.

44. Acosta A, Kaplan AL, Kaufman RH. Gynecologic cancer in children. *Am J Obstet Gynecol.* 1972;112(7):944–52.

45. Hermans AJ, Kluivers KB, Janssen LM et al. Adnexal masses in children, adolescents and women of reproductive age in the Netherlands: A nationwide population-based cohort study. *Gynecol Oncol.* 2016;143(1):93–7.

46. Cass DL, Hawkins E, Brandt ML et al. Surgery for ovarian masses in infants, children, and adolescents: 102 consecutive patients treated in a 15-year period. *J Pediatr Surg.* 2001;36(5):693–9.

47. Kirkham YA, Lacy JA, Kives S, Allen L. Characteristics and management of adnexal masses in a Canadian pediatric and adolescent population. *J Obstet Gynaecol Can.* 2011;33(9):935–43.

48. Bristow RE, Nugent AC, Zahurak ML, Khouzhami V, Fox HE. Impact of surgeon specialty on ovarian-conserving surgery in young females with an adnexal mass. *J Adolesc Health.* 2006;39(3):411–6.

49. van Winter JT, Simmons PS, Podratz KC. Surgically treated adnexal masses in infancy, childhood, and adolescence. *Am J Obstet Gynecol.* 1994;170(6):1780–6; discussion 6–9.

50. Templeman C, Fallat ME, Blinchevsky A, Hertweck SP. Noninflammatory ovarian masses in girls and young women. *Obstet Gynecol.* 2000;96(2):229–33.

51. Rogers EM, Casadiego Cubides G, Lacy J, Gerstle JT, Kives S, Allen L. Preoperative risk stratification of adnexal masses: Can we predict the optimal surgical management? *J Pediatr Adolesc Gynecol.* 2014;27(3):125–8.

52. Gribbon M, Ein SH, Mancer K. Pediatric malignant ovarian tumors: A 43–year review. *J Pediatr Surg.* 1992;27(4):480–4.

53. Marro A, Allen LM, Kives SL, Moineddin R, Chavhan GB. Simulated impact of pelvic MRI in treatment planning for pediatric adnexal masses. *Pediatr Radiol.* 2016;46(9):1249–57.

54. Stankovic ZB, Sedlecky K, Savic D, Lukac BJ, Mazibrada I, Perovic S. Ovarian preservation from tumors and torsions in girls: Prospective diagnostic study. *J Pediatr Adolesc Gynecol.* 2017;30(3):405–12.

55. Warner BW, Kuhn JC, Barr LL. Conservative management of large ovarian cysts in children: The value of serial pelvic ultrasonography. *Surgery.* 1992;112(4): 749–55.

56. Hermans AJ, Kluivers KB, Wijnen MH, Bulten J, Massuger LF, Coppus SF. Diagnosis and treatment of adnexal masses in children and adolescents. *Obstet Gynecol.* 2015;125(3):611–5.

57. Trotman GE, Cheung H, Tefera EA, Darolia R, Gomez-Lobo V. Rate of oophorectomy for benign indications in a children's hospital: Influence of a gynecologist. *J Pediatr Adolesc Gynecol.* 2017;30(2):234–8.

58. Sahin H, Abdullazade S, Sanci M. Mature cystic teratoma of the ovary: A cutting edge overview on imaging features. *Insights Into Imaging.* 2017;8(2):227–41.

59. Templeman CL, Hertweck SP, Scheetz JP, Perlman SE, Fallat ME. The management of mature cystic teratomas in children and adolescents: A retrospective analysis. *Human Reproduction.* 2000;15(12):2669–72.

60. Laberge PY, Levesque S. Short-term morbidity and long-term recurrence rate of ovarian dermoid cysts treated by laparoscopy versus laparotomy. *J Obstet Gynaecol Can.* 2006;28(9):789–93.

61. Childress KJ, Santos XM, Perez-Milicua G et al. Intraoperative rupture of ovarian dermoid cysts in the pediatric and adolescent population: Should this change your surgical management? *J Pediatr Adolesc Gynecol.* 2017;30(6):636–40.

62. Yousef Y, Pucci V, Emil S. The relationship between intraoperative rupture and recurrence of pediatric ovarian neoplasms: Preliminary observations. *J Pediatr Adolesc Gynecol.* 2016;29(2):111–6.

63. Savasi I, Lacy JA, Gerstle JT, Stephens D, Kives S, Allen L. Management of ovarian dermoid cysts in the pediatric and adolescent population. *J Pediatr Adolesc Gynecol.* 2009;22(6):360–4.

64. Rogers EM, Allen L, Kives S. The recurrence rate of ovarian dermoid cysts in pediatric and adolescent girls. *J Pediatr Adolesc Gynecol.* 2014;27(4):222–6.

65. Harada M, Osuga Y, Fujimoto A et al. Predictive factors for recurrence of ovarian mature cystic teratomas after surgical excision. *Eur J Obstet Gynecol Reprod Biol.* 2013;171(2):325–8.

66. Billmire D, Vinocur C, Rescorla F et al. Outcome and staging evaluation in malignant germ cell tumors of the ovary in children and adolescents: An intergroup study. *J Pediatr Surg.* 2004;39(3):424–9; discussion-9.

67. Billmire DF, Cullen JW, Rescorla FJ et al. Surveillance after initial surgery for pediatric and adolescent girls with stage I ovarian germ cell tumors: Report from the Children's Oncology Group. *J Clin Oncol.* 2014;32(5):465–70.

68. Hazard FK, Longacre TA. Ovarian surface epithelial neoplasms in the pediatric population: Incidence, histologic subtype, and natural history. *Am J Surg Pathol.* 2013;37(4):548–53.

69. Nishio S, Ushijima K, Fukui A et al. Fertility-preserving treatment for patients with malignant germ cell tumors of the ovary. *J Obstet Gynaecol Res.* 2006;32(4):416–21.

70. Madenci AL, Levine BS, Laufer MR et al. Preoperative risk stratification of children with ovarian tumors. *J Pediatr Surg.* 2016;51(9):1507–12.

71. Papic JC, Finnell SM, Slaven JE, Billmire DF, Rescorla FJ, Leys CM. Predictors of ovarian malignancy in children: Overcoming clinical barriers of ovarian preservation. *J Pediatr Surg.* 2014;49(1):144–7; discussion 7–8.

72. Oltmann SC, Garcia N, Barber R, Huang R, Hicks B, Fischer A. Can we preoperatively risk stratify ovarian masses for malignancy? *J Pediatr Surg.* 2010;45(1):130–4.

73. Deligeoroglou E, Eleftheriades M, Shiadoes V et al. Ovarian masses during adolescence: Clinical, ultra-sonographic and pathologic findings, serum tumor markers and endocrinological profile. *Gynecol Endocrinol* 2004;19(1):1–8.

74. Murray S, London S. Management of ovarian cysts in neonates, children and adolescents. *Adolesc Pediatr Gynecol.* 1995;8:64–70.

75. Strickland JL. Ovarian cysts in neonates, children and adolescents. *Curr Opin Obstet Gynecol.* 2002;14(5):459–65.

76. Grimes DA, Jones LB, Lopez LM, Schulz KF. Oral contraceptives for functional ovarian cysts. *Cochrane Database Syst Rev.* 2014;29(4):CD006134.

77. Jain KA. Sonographic spectrum of hemorrhagic ovarian cysts. *J Ultrasound Med.* 2002;21(8):879–86.

78. Yoffe N, Bronshtein M, Brandes J, Blumenfeld Z. Hemorrhagic ovarian cyst detection by transvaginal sonography: The great imitator. *Gynecol Endocrinol.* 1991;5(2):123–9.

79. Smorgick N, As-Sanie S, Marsh CA, Smith YR, Quint EH. Advanced stage endometriosis in adolescents and young women. *J Pediatr Adolesc Gynecol.* 2014;27(6):320–3.

80. Audebert A, Lecointre L, Afors K, Koch A, Wattiez A, Akladios C. Adolescent endometriosis: Report of a series of 55 cases with a focus on clinical presentation and long-term issues. *J Minim Invasive Gynecol.* 2015;22(5):834–40.

81. Roman JD. Adolescent endometriosis in the Waikato region of New Zealand—A comparative cohort study with a mean follow-up time of 2.6 years. *Aust N Z J Obstet Gynaecol.* 2010;50(2):179–83.

82. Bosnali O, Moralioglu S, Cerrah-Celayir A. Occurrence of paratubal cysts in childhood: An analysis of 26 cases. *Turk J Pediatr.* 2016;58(3):266–70.

83. Muolokwu E, Sanchez J, Bercaw JL et al. The incidence and surgical management of paratubal cysts in a pediatric and adolescent population. *J Pediatr Surg.* 2011;46(11):2161–3.

84. Muolokwu E, Sanchez J, Bercaw JL et al. Paratubal cysts, obesity, and hyperandrogenism. *J Pediatr Surg.* 2011;46(11):2164–7.

85. Steinkampf MP, Hammond KR, Blackwell RE. Hormonal treatment of functional ovarian cysts: A randomized, prospective study. *Fertil Steril.* 1990; 54(5):775–7.

86. Kayaba H, Tamura H, Shirayama K, Murata J, Fujiwara Y. Hemorrhagic ovarian cyst in childhood: A case report. *J Pediatr Surg.* 1996;31(7):978–9.

87. Spinelli C, Buti I, Pucci V et al. Adnexal torsion in children and adolescents: New trends to conservative surgical approach—Our experience and review of literature. *Gynecol Endocrinol.* 2013;29(1):54–8.

88. Hubner N, Langer JC, Kives S, Allen LM. Evolution in the management of pediatric and adolescent ovarian torsion as a result of quality improvement measures. *J Pediatr Adolesc Gynecol.* 2017;30(1):132–7.

89. Crouch NS, Gyampoh B, Cutner AS, Creighton SM. Ovarian torsion: To pex or not to pex? Case report and review of the literature. *J Pediatr Adolesc Gynecol.* 2003;16(6):381–4.

90. Beaunoyer M, Chapdelaine J, Bouchard S, Ouimet A. Asynchronous bilateral ovarian torsion. *J Pediatr Surg.* 2004;39(5):746–9.

91. Breech LL, Hillard PJ. Adnexal torsion in pediatric and adolescent girls. *Curr Opin Obstet Gynecol.* 2005;17(5):483–9.

92. Anders JF, Powell EC. Urgency of evaluation and outcome of acute ovarian torsion in pediatric patients. *Arch Pediatr Adolesc Med.* 2005;159(6):532–5.

93. Bronstein ME, Pandya S, Snyder CW, Shi Q, Muensterer OJ. A meta-analysis of B-mode ultrasound, Doppler ultrasound, and computed tomography to diagnose pediatric ovarian torsion. *European J Pediatr Surg.* 2015;25(1):82–6.

94. Naiditch JA, Barsness KA. The positive and negative predictive value of transabdominal color Doppler ultrasound for diagnosing ovarian torsion in pediatric patients. *J Pediatr Surg.* 2013;48(6):1283–7.

95. Canning DA. Evaluation of the pediatric urologic patient. In: Walsh PC, Retik AB, Vaughan ED, Wein AJ, eds. *Campbell's Urology.* 8th ed. Philadelphia, PA: Elsevier Science; 2002:1812–32.

96. Argenta PA, Yeagley TJ, Ott G, Sondheimer SJ. Torsion of the uterine adnexa. Pathologic correlations and current management trends. *J Reprod Med.* 2000;45(10):831–6.

97. Rody A, Jackisch C, Klockenbusch W, Heinig J, Coenen-Worch V, Schneider HP. The conservative management of adnexal torsion—A case-report and review of the literature. *Eur J Obstet Gynecol Reprod Biol.* 2002;101(1):83–6.

98. Aziz D, Davis V, Allen L, Langer JC. Ovarian torsion in children: Is oophorectomy necessary? *J Pediatr Surg.* 2004;39(5):750–3.

99. Walker SK, Lal DR, Boyd KP, Sato TT. Management of pediatric ovarian torsion: Evidence of follicular development after ovarian preservation. *Surgery.* 2018;163(3):547–52.

100. Jones H, Jones G, eds. *Novak's Textbook of Gynecology.* 10th ed. Baltimore, MD: Williams & Wilkins; 1981.

101. McGovern PG, Noah R, Koenigsberg R, Little AB. Adnexal torsion and pulmonary embolism: Case report and review of the literature. *Obstet Gynecol Surv.* 1999;54(9):601–8.

102. Cohen SB, Wattiez A, Seidman DS et al. Laparoscopy versus laparotomy for detorsion and sparing of twisted ischemic adnexa. *JSLS.* 2003;7(4):295–9.

103. Oelsner G, Cohen SB, Soriano D, Admon D, Mashiach S, Carp H. Minimal surgery for the twisted ischaemic adnexa can preserve ovarian function. *Human Reproduction.* 2003;18(12):2599–602.

104. Comeau IM, Hubner N, Kives SL, Allen LM. Rates and technique for oophoropexy in pediatric ovarian torsion: A single-institution case series. *J Pediatr Adolesc Gynecol.* 2017;30(3):418–21.

105. Smorgick N, Melcer Y, Sarig-Meth T, Maymon R, Vaknin Z, Pansky M. High risk of recurrent torsion in premenarchal girls with torsion of normal adnexa. *Fertil Steril.* 2016;105(6):1561–5 e3.

106. Righi RV, McComb PF, Fluker MR. Laparoscopic oophoropexy for recurrent adnexal torsion. *Hum Reprod.* 1995;10(12):3136–8.

107. Kives S, Gascon S, Dubuc E, Van Eyk N. No. 341—Diagnosis and management of adnexal torsion in children, adolescents, and adults. *J Obstet Gynaecol Can.* 2017;39(2):82–90.

108. Templeman C, Hertweck SP, Fallat ME. The clinical course of unresected ovarian torsion. *J Pediatr Surg.* 2000;35(9):1385–7.

Breast disorders in children and adolescents

13

NIRUPAMA K. DE SILVA and MONICA HENNING

INTRODUCTION

Many congenital and neoplastic breast disorders present in childhood and adolescence. Though the vast majorities are benign, any breast anomaly is significant for young girls and their families. As breast development in adolescents is an important marker of transition to adulthood, alterations in normal development can have significant psychological effects.[1] Patients with breast disorders should be promptly diagnosed and counseled on the significance of the anomaly so that potential treatments can ensue in a timely manner. Such efforts permit minimal physical and/ or emotional sequelae to the patient.[2]

NORMAL BREAST MATURATION

Development of the breast begins at approximately 35 days of gestation, when the ectoderm on the anterior body wall thickens into a ridge known as the "milk line," "milk ridge," or "Hughes lines."[3] This ridge of tissue extends from the area of the developing axilla to the area of the developing inguinal canal. The ridge above and below the area of the pectoralis muscle recedes while *in utero* between weeks 7 and 10,[4] leaving the mammary primordium, which is the origin of the lactiferous ducts.[5,6] The initial lactiferous ducts form between week 10 and 20 and become interspersed through the developing mesenchyme, which becomes the fibrous and fatty portions of the breast.[6] Finally, the areola develops at a pectoral position along the milk line at 20 weeks' gestation, while the nipple appears later in development.[4]

Thelarche, the onset of pubertal breast development, is hormonally mediated. Thelarche normally occurs between the ages of 8 and 13, with an average age of 10.3 years,[7] but the timing is influenced by race and can be affected by other outside influences. Research suggests that at all ages, normal thelarche is more advanced in African American girls than white girls. In a landmark study by Herman-Giddens, they report that approximately 15% of white girls have thelarche between the ages of 8 and 9, whereas 48% of African American children experience thelarche at this age. In the study, the mean age of onset of breast development for African American girls was 8.9 years, while the average age of thelarche in white females was approximately 10 years of age.[8] Other risk factors associated with earlier puberty include adiposity and Mexican American ethnicity.[9] The Breast Cancer and the Environment Research Program, a prospective cohort of more than 1200 girls, observed the onset of thelarche at younger ages (ages 8.8 for African American girls and 9.3 for Caucasian females) than noted previously, and confirmed differences associated with race/ethnicity and increased adiposity.[10]

Once thelarche is initiated, adipose tissue and the lactiferous ducts grow in response to estrogen. Progesterone stimulation results in lobular growth and alveolar budding.[11] The normal development of the breast, which occurs over a period of approximately 4 years, is classified by the five sexual maturity stages. (Table 13.1) Maturation can sometimes occur asymmetrically due to fluctuation of the hormonal environments and variation in end-organ sensitivity.[12] Lack of development by age 13 years is considered delayed and warrants an evaluation.[9] Menarche usually occurs approximately 2 years after initiation of breast development.[7]

Breast self-awareness

There is lack of consensus among health-care providers regarding breast self-examination (BSE) for adults, and currently BSE is not recommended for patients younger than 20 years of age with an average risk of breast cancer. This is based on the fact that the impact of performing

Table 13.1 Sexual Maturity Rating (Tanner staging) for breast development.

Stage	
1 (preadolescent)	Elevation of the breast papilla only
2	Elevation of the breast bud and papillae as a small mound
	Enlargement of the areola diameter
	Areola becomes more pink
3	Further enlargement of the breast and areola with no separation of their contours
	Montgomery tubercules appear
4	Further enlargement with projection of the areola and papilla to form a secondary mound above the level of the breast
5 (mature stage)	Projection of the papilla only, resulting from recession of the areola to the general contour of the breast
	Erectile areolar tissue

Source: From Duflos C et al. In: Sultan C, ed. *Pediatric and Adolescent Gynecology: Evidence-Based Clinical Practice.* Vol. 7. Basel, Switzerland: Karger; 2004:183–96; and Templeman C, Hertweck SP. *Obstet Gynecol Clin North Am.* 2000;27:19–34. See also Figure 1.5.

regular BSE on rates of breast cancer diagnosis has not been proven.[13] In addition, BSE may increase the rate of breast biopsy for benign breast lumps.[14] However, adolescents should be aware of how their breasts normally look and feel and should be advised to report changes to their health-care provider.[13] This enables the adolescent to contribute to her health care, helps the adolescent to accept her body, and provides an opportunity for discussion of issues related specifically to women's health. Teenagers with a history of malignancy, radiation to the chest, or family history of *BRCA1* or *BRCA2* gene defects deserve early SBE teaching in addition to the routine breast exams from their health-care provider.[2]

For those that choose to or need to begin to perform BSE, patients may have difficulty recognizing normal, and possibly abnormal, breast tissue. It is helpful for the adolescent to perform her first BSE on the same day that she had a normal examination in the office so that she has a baseline examination for comparison.[1] A web-based guide to breast health for teenagers that includes information on self-examination of the breasts is available at https://youngwomenshealth.org/2014/02/27/breast-self-exam-and-cancer-risks/.[15]

THE CLINICAL BREAST EXAMINATION

Examination of the newborn includes assessment of breast size, nipple position, presence of accessory nipples, and nipple discharge.[1] Examination of the prepubertal female also includes inspection and palpation of the chest wall for masses, deformities, pain, nipple discharge, and/or signs of premature thelarche. The Sexual Maturity Rating should also be assessed through palpation in order to distinguish from prepubertal fat deposition.

When evaluating an adolescent, a discussion of breast self-awareness should be part of the examination. The performance of a routine clinical breast exam is not currently recommended by all societies for asymptomatic adult women with an average risk of cancer,[16] and there is no consensus to date on this topic for adolescent females. Thus, discussions of breast awareness have replaced routine clinical breast examination secondary to a concern that examination may be of low yield. When clinical examinations occur for the adolescent without complaints or concerns, such as in situations of patient or family preference, they should be done after a discussion with the patient of the limitations of the exam and should focus on development and appearance. The Sexual Maturity Rating should be noted (Table 13.1), and the examiner should evaluate for signs of breast asymmetry, deficits within the breast, skin changes, and/or nipple discharge. If the patient has complaints or concerns, or signs of a breast abnormality are noted when development is assessed, then a full clinical breast exam is warranted.

When a full clinical breast exam is warranted, it should be performed with the patient in the supine position; the arm ipsilateral to the breast that is being examined should be placed over the patient's head.[1] The breast tissue is examined with the flat finger pads using the vertical strip method, concentric circular method, or in a clockwise fashion like the spokes on a wheel.[1] A complete breast examination also includes evaluation for symmetry and/or skin abnormalities, as well as palpation for axillary, supraclavicular, and infraclavicular lymphadenopathy. In addition, the areola should be compressed to assess for nipple discharge. Complete breast exam recommendations for documentation in the adolescent have been made available elsewhere.[17]

DISORDERS OF BREAST DEVELOPMENT
Premature thelarche

Although normal thelarche occurs between 8 and 13 years of age, premature thelarche can occur as early as 1 year of age and, rarely, may even persist from birth,[18] and can be symmetric or asymmetric. Although the vast majority of patients with premature thelarche have no associated medical problems, evaluation for pathology is warranted.

Hypothyroidism can be associated with premature thelarche and should be considered if other symptoms are present.[19] Premature thelarche may be the first symptom of precocious puberty, particularly in girls older than 2 years of age.[18] A complete evaluation is recommended in all cases of suspected premature thelarche to rule out precocious puberty.[12] Precocious puberty occurs in up to 18% of girls with premature thelarche who are followed over time.[20] Serial examinations, with particular emphasis on growth velocity, secondary sexual characteristics such as pubic hair, pigmentation of the labia or areola, or vaginal bleeding, are imperative to identify precocious puberty in girls with premature thelarche.[6,18] Radiographs to estimate bone age are appropriate if precocious puberty is suspected.[20]

Unless there are associated signs of precocious puberty, the parents should be reassured and the child followed expectantly.[11] Ninety percent of patients with isolated premature thelarche will have resolution of breast enlargement 6 months to 6 years after diagnosis.[21] Long-term follow-up has shown that patients with isolated premature thelarche develop normal breasts at puberty and are at no increased risk for disorders or tumors of the breast.[21]

Amastia and hypomastia

Lack of initiation of breast development by age 13 is considered delayed.[7] Complete absence of the breast and nipple-areolar complex, or amastia, is rare and is thought to occur from lack of formation or obliteration of the milk line.[5] Hypomastia is a deficiency in mammary tissue.

Amastia can be associated with syndromes of more diffuse ectodermal anomalies such as congenital ectodermal dysplasia.[5,22] It can also be associated with anomalies of the underlying mesoderm, such as abnormal pectoralis muscle seen in Poland syndrome.[5,23] Bilateral amastia is associated with other congenital anomalies in 40% of patients.[22] Systemic diseases and endocrine disorders can be associated with lack of estrogen and thus lack of or delayed breast development.

Amastia or hypomastia can also result from injuries sustained during thoracotomy, chest tube placement,

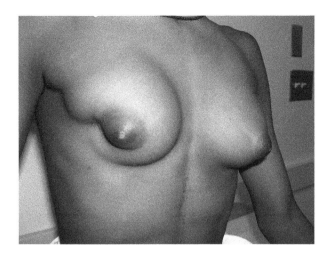

Figure 13.1 Breast deformity from placement of a neonatal chest tube.

inappropriate biopsy of the breast bud, radiotherapy, or severe burns.[6] Because the nipple complex does not normally develop until later in gestation, it can be quite hard to identify in the premature infant. As a result, placement of chest tubes or central lines can inadvertently injure the developing breast (Figure 13.1).

Polymastia and polythelia

Supernumerary breast tissue, most commonly accessory nipples, occurs in approximately 1%–2% of the population.[3,5] A complete accessory breast is termed *polymastia* (Figure 13.2). Supranumerary nipples are referred to as *polythelia*. The abnormally placed tissue is almost universally located in the axilla or just inferior to the normally positioned breast along the embryonic milk line.[5] The normal axillary extension of breast tissue (the tail of Spence) should not be confused with supernumerary breast tissue. True ectopic breast tissue, or breast tissue found outside the normal milk line, is exceedingly rare but has been reported on the face, back, and perineum, and in the midline of the anterior torso.[5,24,25]

Up to 65% of children with supernumerary breast tissue have a single accessory nipple or breast, and 30%–35% have two.[5] The largest number of reported supernumerary structures is 10.[5] Some studies have suggested the association of polythelia with abnormalities of the urinary tract and congenital heart disease, although this is debated by other authors.[3,6,22] Polymastia may warrant surgical excision in girls to prevent painful swelling during pregnancy. Resection of accessory nipples is occasionally warranted for cosmetic reasons.

Congenital anomalies of the nipple

Athelia is defined as the presence of breast tissue with the absence of the nipple (Figure 13.3). This is not infrequent in accessory breasts but is very rare in the normal location.[5] Anomalies of the nipple that have been described include bifid nipples, intra-areolar polythelia (also called dysplastic divided nipples)[22] (Figure 13.4), and inverted nipples.

Inverted nipples can occur in up to 10% of females.[26] They may predispose patients to infections, which can usually be prevented by careful attention to hygiene of the recessed area. Inverted nipples can cause difficulty with breastfeeding, problems with sexuality, and/or aesthetic dissatisfaction. Due to such reasons, some patients may undergo surgical correction of the inversion. Surgical correction is possible, and Hernandez Yenty et al.[27] recommend duct preservation surgical techniques. In their review, studies reported that 96% of patients who tried to breastfeed after treatment were successful.[27]

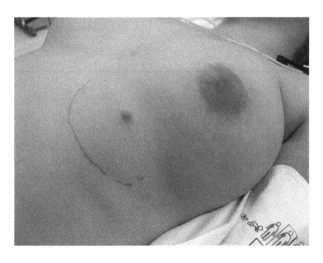

Figure 13.2 Polymastia. This complete breast, with nipple complex, is located in the most common position, just below the normal breast.

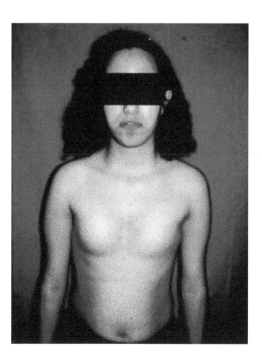

Figure 13.3 Athelia. (From Ishida LH et al., *Br J Plast Surg.* 2005;58[6]:833–7. With permission.)

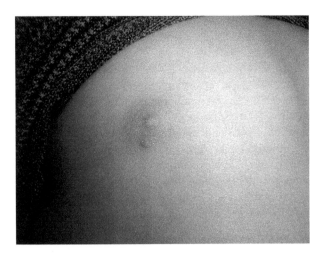

Figure 13.4 Intra-areolar polythelia, which is also called a dysplastic divided nipple.

Breast asymmetry and hypomastia

Asymmetry is often used to describe a difference in breast size. Some degree of asymmetry is normal in women. Asymmetry may be more pronounced during puberty, while the breasts are developing, due to fluctuation of the hormone environment and end-organ sensitivity.[28] When one breast is distinctly different in appearance, patients may desire evaluation. In individuals with breast asymmetry, a thorough clinical breast examination is warranted to evaluate for pathology, and counseling is imperative.

Significant hypomastia may be associated with connective tissue disorders or mitral valve prolapse.[6] Breast hypoplasia may also occur after chest wall irradiation, after trauma to the breast bud, in the presence of hypogonadotropic hypogonadism, with an intersex disorder, or with congenital adrenal hyperplasia, or with 17-hydroxylase deficiency.[1]

Unilateral hypoplasia has been reported in association with a Becker nevus of the breast, which on examination will appear as a clear, brown stain.[6] This hamartoma has been reported to have increased androgenic receptors, which likely explains the hypomastia.[6]

While the adolescent should be evaluated for unilateral hypoplasia or amastia/hypomastia, a breast mass, or significant asymmetry, if no underlying cause is found and psychological impairment is not a concern, then expectant management for the asymmetry is warranted until breast growth is complete. Counseling is imperative in cases of such asymmetry, as it is important for young teens to know that anxiety about breast growth is common, that malignancy is rare, that asymmetry of unknown etiology may resolve or become less prominent with continued breast development, and that most of these clinical situations will not require future surgical intervention.[1] Until the asymmetry becomes less prominent, adolescents should be made aware that they can wear padded bras or prosthetic inserts to obtain symmetry, especially if the asymmetry is the cause of low self-esteem[29] Should

the asymmetry persist, and still be concerning once breast growth is complete, then referral for surgical intervention with a qualified breast provider is appropriate.

Tuberous breasts

Tuberous breasts are a congenital abnormality that is often recognized at puberty. In this condition, the base of the breast is limited, and the hypoplastic breast tissue "herniates" into the areolar complex.[20] This gives the breast the "appearance of a tuberous plant root"[1] (Figure 13.5). The condition may be unilateral or bilateral, and the etiology is unknown but has been described in cases of induction of secondary sexual characteristics via endogenous hormones. Other research has described an anatomic defect to this condition based on the abnormal development of a particular fascial plane.[1] Once emotional and physical maturity has occurred, referral for plastic surgery to correct the areolar complex and augment the hypoplastic breast is an option.

Macromastia

Excessively large breasts are referred to as macromastia. The differential of macromastia in the adolescent includes juvenile hypertrophy, pregnancy, tumors of the breast, and excessive endogenous or exogenous levels of estrogen and/or progesterone.[28] D-Penicillamine and marijuana have also been reported as exogenous etiologies of macromastia[28] (Table 13.2).

(a)

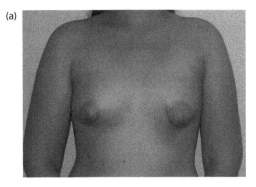

(b)

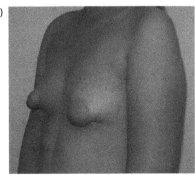

Figure 13.5 Tuberous breasts (a, front view; b, three-quarters view). (From Divasta AD, Weldon C, Labow Bl. The breast: Examination and lesions. In: Emans SJ, Laufer MR, eds. *Emans, Laufer, Goldstein's Pediatric and Adolescent Gynecology*. Chapter 22. Philadelphia, PA: Wolters Kluwer Health; 2011. With permission.)

Table 13.2 Differential diagnosis of macromastia.

Juvenile hypertrophy
Tumors of the breast
  Giant fibroadenoma
  Hamartoma[62]
  Cystosarcoma phyllodes
  Carcinoma
Hormonally active tumors
  Ovarian granulosa cell tumor
  Ovarian follicular cysts
  Adrenal cortical tumors
Exogenous hormones
  Estrogen
  Testosterone
  Gonadotropins
  Corticosterone
Medications
  D-Penicillamine
  Marijuana
Pregnancy

Juvenile or virginal hypertrophy: Spontaneous massive growth of the breast in the adolescent, which may be unilateral or bilateral, is thought to be the result of excessive end-organ sensitivity to gonadal hormones.[28] The number of hormonal receptors in the hypertrophic breast tissue is normal, as are serum estradiol levels.[6,28] An autoimmune etiology has been suggested by some authors because of an occasional association with Hashimoto thyroiditis, rheumatoid arthritis, and myasthenia gravis.[6]

Breast growth in patients with juvenile hypertrophy is rapid, begins shortly after thelarche, and can be dramatic, resulting in breasts that weigh up to 50 pounds each.[20] Spontaneous resolution is very rare.[28] Skin changes, such as peau d'orange and even necrosis, may occur during phases of rapid growth.[28]

Treatment depends on whether breast growth has been completed. If the patient is still growing, progestins or antiestrogen medications can be used to control breast growth.[20] If this is unsuccessful, or if breast growth has been completed, breast reduction surgery is necessary.[28] Patients should be counseled that lactation may be affected by juvenile hypertrophy, particularly after breast reduction surgery, but that there is no increased risk of breast cancer.[28]

INFECTIONS OF THE BREAST

Mastitis is the most common infection of the breast. It is most common in lactating females. It can also occur in nonlactating females, including young infants and adolescents, though it is rare. The prevalence of mastitis in these groups is not known, and the etiology is unclear,[30] though some hypothesize that both populations have slightly enlarged breast tissue.[31]

Neonatal mastitis is an infection that usually occurs in term or near-term infants[32] within the first week of life.[31] It affects female infants twice as often as males, and approximately 50% of infants with neonatal mastitis will develop a breast abscess.[32] Adolescents may develop nonpuerperal mastitis or a breast abscess as a result of irritation of the skin (through shaving or nipple stimulation), a foreign body (e.g., piercing), or infection of an epidermal cyst.[20]

The initial therapy of all breast infections is antibiotics and analgesics.[32] One study suggests that infants need to be treated with parenteral antibiotics, while adolescents can be sufficiently treated with oral antibiotics.[30] Adolescent girls with mastitis may also achieve symptomatic relief with breast support.[20] Ultrasound is recommended to differentiate cellulitis from abscess because drainage is appropriate when an abscess is identified.[33] Aspiration of the mass may assist with clinical and bacteriologic diagnosis,[1] and may be indicated every 48 hours until resolution.[33]

Although *Staphylococcus aureus* is the offending organism in almost all cases, in infants, infections with group A streptococcus, enterococcus, and anaerobic streptococci have been reported.[1] While dicloxacillin or amoxicillin-clavulanic acid are common antibiotics prescribed,[1] the incidence of methicillin-resistant *Staphylococcus aureus* (MRSA) has also become significant enough to warrant using antibiotics that have activity against MRSA, such as clindamycin, trimethoprim/sulfamethoxazole, or vancomycin.[34] Gram-negative coverage, particularly in newborns, may be indicated until culture results are obtained.

Whether in an infant or an older child, small abscesses should initially be aspirated with a needle, using ultrasound guidance if necessary, and reevaluated as antibiotic therapy is continued.[20] Larger or persistent abscesses may need incision and drainage.[20] If incision and drainage are performed, a small, periareolar incision is indicated. Such procedures should be performed in a center with experience in the management of prepubertal breast masses, given that in the prepubertal child, probing and disrupting the tissue should be kept to a minimum to avoid any injury to the underlying breast bud, hypoplasia, or scarring.[35,36]

NIPPLE DISCHARGE
Bloody discharge

The differential diagnosis of bloody discharge in children and adolescents includes mammary duct ectasia, chronic cystic mastitis, intraductal cysts, and intraductal papillomas. In adolescent athletes, bloody discharge may also be due to chronic nipple irritation (jogger's nipple) or cold trauma (cyclist's nipple).[37] Another important cause of bloody or brownish discharge in adolescents is discharge from the ducts of Montgomery (on the edge of the areola, not through the nipple). As inflammation and infection may play a role in cases of bloody nipple discharge in the nonadult population, a culture of the discharge is recommended as the first step in the treatment algorithm for this problem. If the culture is positive, appropriate antibiotics should be initiated.[33]

Mammary duct ectasia is a condition of benign dilatations of the subareolar ducts resulting in inflammation and fibrosis. This is thought to be an anomaly of duct development that results in "pleats" of obstructing epithelium in the lumen of the duct.[6] This obstruction can lead to bacterial overgrowth and abscess, most commonly with *S. aureus*.[11] Other proposed etiologies include chronic inflammation of the periductal stroma with duct obliteration, trauma, and autoimmune reaction.[33] Patients with mammary duct ectasia typically present with a bloody discharge and may also have a retroareolar mass or breast enlargement. Ductal ectasia often resolves spontaneously.[6,11] There may be recurrences that usually respond to conservative therapy. Surgical excision may be indicated for persistent or recurrent symptoms or for an associated persistent cyst.[11] In girls, the excision should be limited to any identified cyst, with great care taken to not injure the underlying breast bud.

Intraductal papillomas are rare, subareolar lesions that are often difficult to palpate. Clinically they present with bloody discharge and breast enlargement.[19] They arise from proliferation of the mammary duct epithelium and are bilateral in 25% of patients. Cytology of the bloody discharge shows ductal cells. Local excision is curative.

In adolescents, cysts of Montgomery, which result from obstruction of the ducts of Montgomery, resolve spontaneously. They are discussed further later in this chapter.

Nipple piercing

Body art, including piercings, is becoming increasingly popular among adolescents. Carroll found that 27% of surveyed participants in one adolescent clinic reported piercings.[38] Another study of 12- to 22-year-old females in an adolescent clinic found that 36.7% of female adolescents had a piercing other than the earlobe.[39]

The most common reasons adolescents claim to get piercings include making a personal statement, reasons of fashion or self-acceptance, an improved perception of appearance and thus self-esteem, or as a rite of passage.[39–41] In some studies, adolescents with multiple piercings have been associated with high-risk behaviors.[39,42] Carroll documented an increase in drug use, distorted eating behaviors, and/or suicidal ideation among adolescents with tattoos or body piercings compared to nonparticipants.[38] Suris et al. noted that adolescent females with multiple piercings were more likely to have multiple sex partners, undergo higher-risk sex practices, be regular smokers, and have more regular use of drugs.[43] Thus, piercing may be a sign to the health-care provider of adolescents who may be more likely to participate in high-risk behaviors.

Along with the increase in nipple piercing is an increase in the risk of complications. Before nipple and areolae piercings, adolescents should be counseled about the lengthy time required for complete healing and the risk of delayed infection.[44] The most common risks include infection, bleeding, pain, hematoma, cyst formation, allergic reactions, and/or development of a keloid.[44] Infection is the most common health problem with *Staphylococcus*

aureus being the most reported causative organism.[39–41] Unusual organisms, such as *Actinomyces*, have also been reported with piercings and should be considered in this population.[33]

Local infection is reported at rates of 10%–30%[41] and can be treated with soap and warm compresses, while the piercing is in place. Topical ointment is not recommended as it is not considered effective and can delay healing. Oral antibiotics may be required depending on severity, and intravenous antibiotics may be required to treat systemic complications including endocarditis, toxic shock, or septic arthritis.[39] Rarely, abscess formation may occur and require antibiotics and/or incision and drainage. In such cases, the piercing may have to be removed and a sterile replacement placed.

There is a potential transmission of viral hepatitis and human immunodeficiency virus through body piercing.[40,41] Transmission can occur via use of contaminated needles or via sharing piercings with other persons with exposure to such infections.[45] Accordingly, patients with postpiercing infections should also get screening for hepatitis B and C, and HIV. They should also have a glucose screen, as diabetes mellitus can increase the risk of infection.[44]

Adolescents who plan to get a piercing should be given information regarding safe piercing strategies. Also, practitioners should ensure they are up to date with immunizations (tetanus, hepatitis B) and are aware of the potential complications. Last, patients should be aware that piercing should not affect subsequent breastfeeding.[41]

Galactorrhea

Milky discharge from the neonatal breast is a normal response to fetal prolactin levels, which peak at birth (Figure 13.6). In an adolescent, nonpuerperal lactation can be classified as neurogenic, hypothalamic, pituitary, endocrine, drug-induced, or idiopathic in origin.[46] Discharge from the areolar glands of Montgomery in the

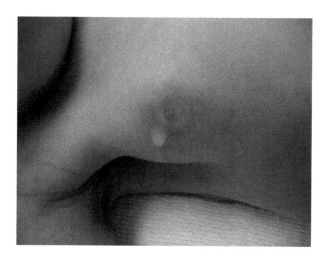

Figure 13.6 Normal breast bud and milky discharge in a neonate.

adolescent can be normal and should not be confused with galactorrhea.

Neurogenic lactation occurs as a result of disorders of the chest wall, thorax, or breast. Neurogenic lactation has been reported after thoracotomy, burns or injuries to the chest wall, herpes zoster, or chronic stimulation of the nipple.[46] Pituitary tumors, especially prolactinomas, are the most common hypothalamic or pituitary cause of galactorrhea, while the most common endocrine cause of galactorrhea in adolescents is hypothyroidism.[46] A wide variety of drugs have also been implicated in causing galactorrhea. The most common drugs are dopamine receptor blockers and catecholamine-depleting agents,[20,46] though oral contraceptive pills can cause this symptom as well.[19] Other common causes of galactorrhea in the adolescent include suckling or self-manipulation. Idiopathic or benign galactorrhea is a diagnosis of exclusion.

Patients with galactorrhea require a careful history and physical exam directed at the possible etiologies of galactorrhea. If there is a question as to whether the discharge is true galactorrhea, it should be sent for fat staining. Patients often present with menstrual abnormalities, specifically oligomenorrhea or amenorrhea. Laboratory studies should include serum prolactin, follicular-stimulating hormone (in those with menstrual abnormalities), and thyroid function studies.[46]

Treatment includes instruction to avoid nipple stimulation or other behaviors that can promote the discharge. Treatment is directed by results of history, physical exam, and lab studies. If the discharge is felt to be due to drugs, the offending medication should be discontinued, hypothyroidism treated, and/or prolactin tumors managed with appropriate medical or surgical care.

BREAST MASSES
Overview of clinical management of breast masses

Although breast malignancy is rare in children or adolescents, breast abnormalities in this population are quite common. Evaluation starts with a thorough history and physical exam. Ultrasound can be used as an adjunct when needed and is the technique of choice in adolescents. Mammography is not indicated in the adolescent patient as it is very hard to interpret due to the large amount of fibroglandular tissue present,[11] and the developing breast tissue is more sensitive to radiation.[12]

Asymptomatic breast masses that are small or consistent with a benign lesion (such as a fibroadenoma) on imaging can be observed. If the mass is cystic on examination and/or on ultrasonography, aspiration may be indicated. If the fluid obtained is clear, it may be discarded as the cytologic results have not been found to be clinically useful. If the fluid is bloody, it may be sent for cytologic examination.[47] If after aspiration the mass collapses, it may be assumed to be a cyst and can be reevaluated in 3 months.[1]

When aspiration is not possible or unproductive, or masses are hard, nonmobile, enlarging, or a source of anxiety, the patient should have the mass evaluated by biopsy or excision.[1] Fine needle aspiration (FNA) is a relatively safe diagnostic procedure. Because malignancy is minimal in this population, excision of breast masses is performed through a periareolar incision for cosmetic reasons. Excision or FNA is best done by a practitioner appropriately trained in surgical management of the breast.

Prepubertal breast masses

Neonatal breast hypertrophy is a normal response to maternal estrogen and occurs in both boys and girls in the first weeks of life. Stimulation, such as attempting to squeeze the breast to promote the discharge, may result in persistence of the hypertrophied tissue. Neonatal breast hypertrophy resolves spontaneously, and no treatment is necessary.

Initial breast development at the onset of thelarche starts with a firm, disc-like area of tissue under the areolar complex that can be mistaken for a "mass." This is often initially unilateral.[11] This is almost universally a normal, physiologic process, and the treatment is expectant management. Unilateral thelarche has also been reported as a side effect of cimetidine and is reversible with stopping this medication.[48] Excisional biopsy is contraindicated, as this can result in injury to the developing breast and subsequent deformity of asymmetry of the breast. If warranted, a FNA with cytology is preferred over biopsy.[49]

Hemangiomas and lymphangiomas can involve the developing breast (Figure 13.7). Although hemangiomas may involute after an initial growth spurt, compression of the breast bud during rapid growth can lead to injury and subsequent breast deformity. The diagnosis is usually made on physical examination but can be confirmed with ultrasound or MRI. If there is doubt about the diagnosis, an FNA may be indicated. Rapid growth of hemangiomas may require resection (if technically possible) or treatment with steroids in order to protect the developing breast bud

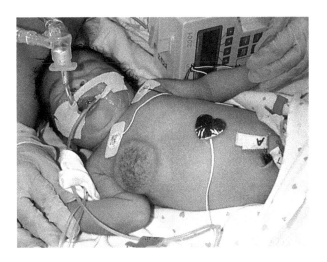

Figure 13.7 Hemangioma of the breast in a newborn infant.

from compression and injury.[11,50] In girls, the risk of injuring the breast bud by resection must be weighed against injury to the breast bud from the enlarging hemangioma or lymphangioma. An MRI may aid in determining the ability to resect the lesion and, hence, the risk-to-benefit ratio of surgical management. Surgical resection of the lesion, with protection of the normal breast tissue, is indicated for complications of the lesion, such as ulceration or hemorrhage.[11]

Other soft tissue or metastatic tumors of the breast are rare but can present in the prepubertal child (Table 13.3). The majority of lesions will be benign; however, if the diagnosis is uncertain, FNA or open biopsy may be indicated.[11]

Benign masses in the adolescent girl

Benign masses seen in postpubertal girls include fibrocystic changes, fibroadenomas, phyllodes tumors, retroareolar cysts (or cyst of Montgomery), hamartomas, adenomas, papillomas, and/or trauma (Table 13.4).

Table 13.3 Differential diagnosis of the prepubertal breast mass.

Unilateral breast bud development (premature thelarche)
Due to medications (Cimetidine)
Hemorrhagic cyst[12]
Abscess[12]
Lymphangioma[12]
Hemangioma[12]
Lipoma[12]
Metastatic tumor
Galactocele

Table 13.4 Differential diagnosis of the postpubertal breast mass in girls.

Fibrocystic changes
Fibroadenoma
Phyllodes tumor
Retroareolar cysts/cyst of Montgomery
Duct ectasia
Fat necrosis
Vascular lipoma[12]
Subareolar neuroma[12]
Hamartoma[62]
Abscess[12]
Lymphangioma[12]
Hemangioma[12]
Lipoma[12]
Adenoma of the nipple
Juvenile papillomatosis
Trauma
Juvenile secretory carcinoma
Ductal carcinoma
Metastatic disease

Fibrocystic changes

Fibrocystic changes in the breast can result in both localized masses and pain in the breast (also termed *mastalgia*). Patients should be reassured that this is a normal variant of female physiology with these changes reported in 50% of women of reproductive age and 90% of women on autopsy.[20] These patients tend to present with pain before menses and have relief after menses.[1] Physical examination alone usually suffices to make this diagnosis, since in most patients there is significant change with serial examinations done at different points in the menstrual cycle. Ultrasound may be helpful if the diagnosis is equivocal, but mammography is not indicated. The treatment of mastalgia includes a properly fitted and firm brassiere and nonsteroidal anti-inflammatory drugs (NSAIDS). Oral contraceptives have been reported to improve symptoms in 70%–90% of women.[20] Treatments with vitamin E and evening primrose oil and avoidance of caffeine are unproven but popular.[20]

Fibroadenoma

The most common mass seen in adolescent girls is the fibroadenoma. These masses usually occur in late adolescence but can occur as early as 1–2 years before menarche.[51] Fibroadenomas are most often located in the upper outer quadrant of the breast and are more common in African American patients.[11] The average size is 2–3 cm, but they can become very large.[20] Fibroadenomas greater than 5 cm are referred to as giant fibroadenomas (Figure 13.8).

Fibroadenomas are felt to develop because of a local exaggerated response to estrogen stimulation.[11] The natural history of these lesions includes an initial period of growth, when the mass will double in size over 6–12 months, and then stabilization of the mass may occur. Only 5% of fibroadenomas develop more rapid growth,[52] and it is reported that regardless of histologic type, 10%–40% of breast masses in adolescents will resolve completely.[53]

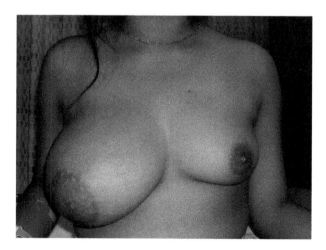

Figure 13.8 Giant fibroadenoma, mimicking juvenile hypertrophy, in an adolescent girl.

Ten percent of patients have bilateral lesions.[20] Up to 25% of girls will have multiple fibroadenomas, a condition that can be called fibroadenomatosis.[6] The lesions may enlarge slightly during the menstrual cycle.[11] The physical examination is usually diagnostic, as these lesions are well circumscribed, have a "rubbery" consistency, and are mobile and nontender. In equivocal cases, an ultrasound is the imaging modality of choice.[54] Mammography is not indicated in the adolescent patient.[53]

Because of the minimal risk of malignancy in adolescents (less than 0.1% risk in adolescents[53]), the low percentage of lesions with rapid growth, and the reports of spontaneous resolution, fibroadenomas <5 cm can be observed for at least one or two menstrual cycles.[55] If the lesion remains stable, then the practitioner and patient can decide between the options of serial observation versus excisional biopsy.

Both observation and resection of persistent lesions can be justified in adolescence. The decision to proceed with excision is based on family anxiety, family history of breast cancer, and the patient's age. While conservative management without surgery is acceptable for nonrapidly changing firm masses suspected to be a fibroadenoma,[1] as girls approach adulthood, and the risk of breast cancer therefore increases, most clinicians may recommend excision of persistent masses.[11] Also, if there is growth of the lesion or the lesion is larger than 5 cm, excisional biopsy is warranted.[55] Families should be counseled that the biopsy or excision may result in cosmetic changes to the breast. Persistent local pain following removal of a fibroadenoma has also been reported.[56] FNA, which is important in women old enough to be at risk for carcinoma of the breast, is not necessary or indicated in adolescent girls with smaller masses.

Giant fibroadenomas

Fibroadenomas >5 cm are termed *giant fibroadenomas*. On examination, these may be softer than the typical fibroadenoma and may even resemble normal surrounding breast tissue.[20] There may be dilated veins over the surface of the breast, and the skin overlying the mass may be warm to the touch[20] (Figure 13.8). Giant fibroadenomas should be excised as they cannot be distinguished from cystosarcoma phyllodes by physical examination, mammography, or sonography.[57] In addition, these tumors have been reported to double in size rapidly on occasion. FNA and core needle biopsy can be helpful for planning the operative approach if the histology leads to a definitive diagnosis of cystosarcoma phyllodes. However, it is very difficult to distinguish between a fibroadenoma and cystosarcoma phyllodes on aspiration or needle biopsy, so a negative result should not affect the decision to operate.[57]

Incisions for excision of a giant fibroadenoma can be problematic. As previously noted, whenever possible, a periareolar incision should be used. Large lesions can be removed through a periareolar incision by placing them in a bag and then morcellating prior to removal.[58] The excision of a large fibroadenoma can result in significant deformity of the breast, and patients should be counseled prior to removal of the tumor.

Phyllodes tumors

Phyllodes tumors were first described by Johannes Muller in 1838 who coined the term "cystosarcoma phylloides." This term is misleading, as these tumors are rarely cystic and do not have the malignant potential of most sarcomas.[55] For that reason, they are better termed *phyllodes tumors*. Phyllodes tumors are stromal neoplasms that are histologically classified as benign, intermediate, or malignant.[11] The distinction is largely semantic, as benign lesions can metastasize and may recur locally. The median age of presentation is 45 years of age; however, they have been reported to occur in girls as young as 10 years old.[55,59]

The diagnosis is difficult to make prior to biopsy, as the exam may resemble a giant fibroadenoma. Large tumors may cause skin stretching, venous distention, and skin ulceration. If the nipple complex is involved, there may be a bloody discharge. Ultrasound findings, which are suggestive, but not diagnostic, include lobulations, a heterogeneous echo pattern, and absence of microcalcifications.[57]

Some authors have reported that adolescents with malignant phyllodes tumors have a more "benign" course than adults regardless of histologic type.[55] The treatment of these benign and malignant tumors is breast-sparing, total surgical excision with adequate margins of normal tissue. Await and see approach can be safely considered in cases with positive surgical margins.[60]

There is a 15% risk of local or distant recurrence, which is more common with incomplete excision and with malignant or borderline groups. Reexcision is indicated if adequate margins were not obtained at the first surgery.[55] Systemic recurrence has been reported in 10% of patients and is more common in malignant tumors. Metastases can occur in lung, bone, and the abdominal viscera and usually occur without lymph node involvement.[55] Isolated reports of palliation from single or multiple chemotherapeutic agents in the treatment of distant recurrences have been reported, but, in general, adjuvant therapy plays a limited role in successful treatment.[55]

Overall, the 5-year survival rate for malignant phyllodes tumors in adults is approximately 80%. Because adolescents may have a biologically less aggressive tumor than adults, their prognosis may be better, although confirmatory data are not available.[55]

Retroareolar cysts/cysts of Montgomery

Montgomery tubercles are the small papular projections on the edge of the areola and are related to the glands of Montgomery that may serve a role during lactation.[20] In adolescents, these glands can become obstructed and present as either acute inflammation (62%) or an asymptomatic mass (38%).[61] The diagnosis of these retroareolar cysts, also referred to as cysts of Montgomery, is primarily clinical but can be confirmed with ultrasound. Ultrasound will most commonly demonstrate a single cystic lesion, usually unilocular, located in the expected retroareolar location.

The most common presentation of patients with retroareolar cysts is acute inflammation with localized tenderness, erythema, and swelling under the areola, extending into the breast tissue.[61] Conservative treatment with oral antibiotics, directed at *Staphyloccocus*, and NSAIDs usually results in resolution of the acute inflammation within 7 days.[61] Following this nonoperative treatment, an asymptomatic mass is usually present. Patients with retroareolar cysts may describe a brownish, bloody discharge from one of the Montgomery tubercles, particularly with compression of the mass. In the absence of persistent infection or other complications, the long-term treatment of the retroareolar cysts is observation with serial physical examination and, if needed, repeat ultrasound examination. Over 80% of these cysts resolve spontaneously, although this may take up to 2 years.[61] Patients should be instructed to not compress the area, as this may prevent resolution of the mass. Only rarely is drainage of a persistent abscess necessary. Resection may be indicated if the mass persists more than 2 years or if the diagnosis is in question.[20]

Other benign breast masses

A variety of rare benign tumors of the breast have been described in adolescents and young adults and include hamartomas, adenomas of the nipple, juvenile papillomatosis, and trauma.

Hamartomas of the breast are a rare tumor composed of the normal components of the breast that can present as unilateral macromastia. They have also been called lipofibromas, adenolipomas, and fibroadenolipomas.[62] Approximately 11 cases have been reported in women under 18 years of age.[63] The treatment of hamartomas is total excision.

Adenomas of the nipple are very rare but have been reported to occur in children and adolescents. Common presentations can include complaints of nodules, enlargement of the nipple, discharge, or erosions, but most people are asymptomatic. Nipple adenomas should be distinguished from Paget disease and intraductal papillomas, as well as breast cancer. They are treated by local excision.[64]

Juvenile papillomatosis is a benign, localized, proliferative lesion usually seen in girls over 10 years of age.[65] Juvenile papillomatosis usually presents with a mass, similar to a fibroadenoma, in one breast. When resected, this is a well-demarcated mass with multiple cysts separated by fibrous stroma, giving it a "Swiss cheese" appearance.[66] Juvenile papillomatosis is considered a marker for increased breast cancer risk in family members, but not necessarily in the patient, unless recurrent.[65] However, in situ and invasive carcinoma, which is usually juvenile secretory carcinoma, has been reported in up to 15% of cases of juvenile papillomatosis.[67] The treatment of juvenile papillomatosis is total resection, with preservation of the normal breast.[65]

Trauma can result in lesions that resemble either an infection or a mass in adolescents. Trauma can cause a breast mass or even a hematoma, and after resolution, scarring may remain. Further, fat necrosis that occurs after trauma can resemble a solid mass in the breast. This has been reported following sports injuries, seat belt injury, abuse, as well as with other direct blows to the breast.[1,68]

Plastic surgery in the adolescent population

There has been an increased interest in cosmetic surgery of the breast during the adolescent years.[69] This can be attributed to our society's emphasis on beauty and self-improvement, as well as easy access to plastic surgery. The media and plastic surgery reality television shows have also exposed the adolescent population to aesthetic surgery and altered patient's perceptions of such operations.[70,71]

The ultimate role of plastic surgery is to alter body image and thus improve a patient's quality of life. The teenage years are a time of sudden changes, and in some patients, there are concerns that a new, unappealing feature has developed, at an age where there is the greatest concern about being attractive. It has been shown that one's body image affects the amount of success that can be achieved. Thus, it is not surprising that such invasive procedures to improve appearance, when condoned by parents, can be free of emotional turmoil and sequelae.[70]

The key to successful plastic surgery in the adolescent is based on appropriate patient selection. Proper patient management involves selecting mature candidates with clear and realistic expectations who are free of psychopathology. Appropriate candidates should be able to freely articulate what they are seeking via surgery, have realistic expectations, and clearly describe why they are motivated to have surgery. They must also be mature enough to tolerate the discomfort of surgery postoperatively. Finally, parents' expectations must be congruent.[70] Patients suspected of having body dysmorphic disorder, eating disorders, or personality disorders should be evaluated to ensure that they are not requesting surgery for psychological, pathologic reasons.

Proper informed consent is also imperative. Informed consent for reduction mammoplasty includes a possible inability for future breastfeeding, scarring, and/or nipple numbness.[72] Informed consent should include the risks and complications of implants as well as promoting an awareness that breast implants may affect future breastfeeding, or require additional surgeries, and that mammography may require additional imaging.[73]

One can argue that adolescents overestimate their deformities and thus are requesting surgery inappropriately. A study in the United Kingdom of adolescents and their motivations for plastic surgery revealed that when adolescents request plastic surgery intervention, they do have realistic appearance perceptions, and they are truly suffering appearance-related burden.[74] For instance, reduction mammoplasty can improve an adolescent's appearance and functional status for female adolescents with extremely large breasts. Plastic surgery surveys always show a very high degree of patient satisfaction with the breast reduction procedure, with over 94% with evidence that patients increase physical activity, fit into clothes better, and have improved self-esteem.[70] Similarly, a patient with asymmetric breasts may require either unilateral breast reduction or augmentation or both, and these procedures can have similar patient success with appropriate candidate selection. The best time for surgery is after breast development has stabilized.

One of the most commonly requested procedures in the adolescent population is breast augmentation. Teenage patients account for approximately 4% of breast augmentations.[75] When breast augmentation is done for purely aesthetic reasons, it is discouraged prior to the age of 18 unless there is careful and thoughtful discussion with the patient and family. The U.S. Food and Drug Administration (FDA) considers aesthetic breast augmentation for patients less than 18 years of age to be an off-label use. The FDA comments that reasons that they take this position include that (a) teens and their parents may not realize the risks associated with breast implants, (b) the teen's body may not have finished developing, and (c) the teen needs to be psychologically ready to handle surgery.[76]

The American Society of Plastic Surgeons has also adopted guidelines for appropriate selection of adolescents for aesthetic breast surgery. Such guidelines are based on the hope that breast development will be finished and maturity of patients will be ensured, as not all teenagers who seek aesthetic surgery are well suited for such surgery. They state that the adolescent candidate for purely aesthetic breast augmentation should be at least 18 years of age, have the physical and emotional maturity, and should have a realistic understanding of the potential results, and the possible risks (such as additional surgical procedures).[69] Currently, the FDA has approved only the use of saline-filled implants in patients younger than 22 years of age.

MALIGNANT TUMORS OF THE BREAST
Primary breast cancer

The risk of primary breast cancer is small in the adolescent population. This risk is increased if there is a significant family history or mutations in the *BRCA1* and *BRCA2* genes, although most of these malignant tumors will not present until the patient is at least in her 20s. Girls who have mutations in one of these genes have a 3.2% risk of breast cancer at age 30 years[20] and a 45%–85% risk by age 70.[77] Screening in adolescence is currently *not* recommended.

Primary carcinoma of the breast has been reported in 39 children between the ages of 3 and 19 years.[11,78] Over 80% of these patients were diagnosed with juvenile secretory carcinoma, with the remainder having intraductal carcinoma. Juvenile secretory carcinoma has been reported in association with juvenile papillomatosis.[11] Juvenile secretory carcinoma often has a thick-walled capsule, which may cause the lesion to appear cystic on ultrasound.[78]

Primary sarcoma of the breast is rare in all age groups and exceedingly rare in children. Rhabdomyosarcoma can occur as a primary tumor of the breast, usually in adolescent girls. They are usually rapidly growing, mobile masses with no skin involvement. Histologically, these are usually

alveolar.[79] Liposarcoma has been reported within a phyllodes tumor of the breast in an adolescent patient.[80] These tumors may appear encapsulated but should be treated by wide local excision.[59] Fibrosarcoma and malignant fibrous histiocytoma may be the most common soft tissue sarcoma of the breast.[59] Other, rare primary sarcomas of the breast include fibrosarcoma, fibrous histiocytoma, leiomyosarcoma, and osteogenic sarcoma.[59] Primary non-Hodgkin lymphoma of the breast has also been reported in children.[81]

The triple assessment (palpation, ultrasound examination, and core needle biopsy) is currently considered the gold standard for evaluation of breast masses in women younger than 30 years of age.[82] There is no accepted guideline for management of breast carcinoma in children. Treatment ranges from excisional biopsy to radical mastectomy. Whenever possible, prepubertal girls should be treated initially with wide local excision.[49] Estrogen and progesterone receptors should be determined. Local recurrence is treated by reexcision, or complete mastectomy. For advanced cases, modified radical mastectomy followed by radiation and chemotherapy for axillary metastasis is a widely accepted approach. Postoperative radiation reduces local recurrences.[49] Prior to treatment with radiation or chemotherapy for breast cancer or other malignancies in an adolescent, the practitioner should discuss options for fertility preservation. In single females, oocyte cryopreservation should be considered and can be carried out with the help of a reproductive medicine specialist.[83] Ovarian tissue cryopreservation is currently considered experimental but may be the only option for very young adolescents and prepubertal children to enable them to have their own genetic offspring. See Chapter 26 regarding fertility preservation options.

Secondary breast cancer

Chest wall radiation, usually given to treat Hodgkin lymphoma, increases the lifetime risk for breast cancer.[84] This is particularly true for girls who are 10–16 years of age at the time they receive radiation, as this is a period of rapid breast growth.[85] Girls with Hodgkin disease who require radiotherapy of the chest have an increased risk of breast cancer (82 times), with almost 40% of patients ultimately developing breast cancer. The median time from radiation therapy to diagnosis of the breast cancer is 20 years.[85] Angiosarcoma of the breast has also been reported in adult women following external beam radiation for breast conservation.[59] Due to this risk, for women treated for pediatric cancer with chest radiation of 20 Gy or more, the Children's Oncology Group recommends annual surveillance mammography and MRI starting at age 25 years or 8 years after completion of radiation therapy, whichever occurs last.[86]

It is now also known that women not exposed to chest radiotherapy who survive childhood sarcoma or leukemia have an increased risk of breast cancer at a young age. The data suggest high-dose alkylating agents and anthracycline chemotherapy increase the risk of breast cancer.[87]

Metastasis to the breast

Cancer metastatic to the breast has been reported in children with primary hepatocellular carcinoma, Hodgkin lymphoma, non-Hodgkin lymphoma, neuroblastoma, and rhabdomyosarcoma, particularly the alveolar variant.[12,81] Other, less common tumors that have been reported to metastasize to the breast in children include histiocytosis, medulloblastoma, renal carcinoma, and neuroblastoma.[88] Bilateral breast disease occurs in 30% of children with rhabdomyosarcoma metastatic to the breast.[88] Ultrasound is the diagnostic tool of choice, as it can often differentiate these lesions from the more common benign lesions.[88]

REFERENCES

1. Davista AD, Weldon C, Labow BI. The breast: Examination and lesions. In: Sydor A, ed. *Pediatric and Adolescent Gynecology.* 6th ed. Philadelphia, PA: Lippincott Williams & Wilkins; 2012:405–20.
2. De Silva NK, Brandt ML. Disorders of the breast in children and adolescents, Part 1: Disorders of growth and infections of the breast. *J Pediatr Adolesc Gynecol.* 2006;19:345–9.
3. Grossl, NA. Supernumerary breast tissue: Historical perspectives and clinical features. *South Med J.* 2000;93:29–32.
4. Dreifuss SE, Macisaac ZM, Grunwaldt LJ. Bilateral congenital amazia: A case report and systemic review of the literature. *J Plast Reconstr Aesthet Surg.* 2014; 67(1):27–33.
5. Skandalakis JE, Gray SW, Ricketts R et al. The anterior body wall. In: Skandalakis JE, Gray S, eds. *Embryology for surgeons: The Embryological Basis for the Treatment of Congenital Anomalies.* Baltimore, MD: Williams and Wilkins; 1994:539–93.
6. Duflos C, Plu-Bureau G, Thibaud E et al. Breast diseases in adolescents. In: Sultan C, ed. *Pediatric and Adolescent Gynecology: Evidence-Based Clinical Practice.* Vol. 7. Basel, Switzerland: Karger; 2004:183–96.
7. Pitts SA, Gordon CM. The physiology of puberty. In: Emans SJ, Laufer MR, ed. *Pediatric and Adolescent Gynecology.* 6th ed. Philadelphian, PA: Lippincott Williams and Wilkins; 2012:100–13.
8. Herman-Giddens ME, Slora EJ, Wasserman RC et al. Secondary sexual characteristics and menses in young girls seen in office practice: A study from the pediatric research in office settings network. *Pediatrics.* 1997;99:505–12.
9. Rosenfield RL, Lipton RB, Drum ML. Thelarche, pubarche and menarche attainment in children with normal and elevated body mass index. *Pediatrics.* 2009;123(1):84–8.
10. Biro FM, Greenspan LC, Galvez MP et al. Onset of breast development in a longitudinal cohort. *Pediatrics.* 2013;132(6):1019.
11. West KW, Rescorla FJ, Scherer LR 3rd et al. Diagnosis and treatment of symptomatic breast masses in the pediatric population. *J Pediatr Surg.* 1995;30:182–7.
12. Bock K, Duda VF, Hadji P et al. Pathologic breast conditions in childhood and adolescence: Evaluation by sonographic diagnosis. *J Ultrasound Med.* 2005;24:1347–54.
13. American Cancer Society. American Cancer Society Recommendations for the Early Detection of Breast Cancer. https://www.cancer.org/cancer/breast-cancer/screening-tests-and-early-detection/american-cancer-society-recommendations-for-the-early-detection-of-breast-cancer.html. Accessed January 15, 2018.
14. Thomas DB, Gao DL, Ray RM et al. Randomized trial of breast self-examination in Shanghai: Final results. *J Natl Cancer Inst.* 2002;94:1445–57.
15. Center for Young Women's Health. https://youngwomenshealth.org/2014/02/27/breast-self-exam-and-cancer-risks//. Accessed April 22, 2019.
16. Practice Bulletin Number 179: Breast Cancer Risk Assessment and Screening in Average-Risk Women. *Obstet Gynecol.* 2017;130(1):e1–e16.
17. LeBlond R. *Examination of the Breast and Nipples.* New York, NY: McGraw-Hill; MedSchool 101, 2012. https://www.youtube.com/watch?v=dfhvF9HJTwQ. Accessed April 22, 2019.
18. Verrotti A, Ferrari M, Morgese G et al. Premature thelarche: A long-term follow-up. *Gynecol Endocrinol.* 1996;10:241–7.
19. Greydanus DE, Matytsina L, Gains M. Breast disorders in children and adolescents. *Prim Care Clin Office Prac.* 2006;33:455–502.
20. Templeman C, Hertweck SP. Breast disorders in the pediatric and adolescent patient. *Obstet Gynecol Clin North Am.* 2000;27:19–34.
21. Van Winter JT, Noller KL, Zimmerman D et al. Natural history of premature thelarche in Olmsted County, Minnesota, 1940 to 1984. *J Pediatr.* 1990;116:278–80.
22. Merlob P. Congenital malformations and developmental changes of the breast: A neonatological view. *J Pediatr Endocrinol Metab.* 2003;16:471–85.
23. Fokin AA, Robicsek, F. Poland's syndrome revisited. *Ann Thorac Surg.* 2002;74:2218–25.
24. Koltuksuz U, Aydin E. Supernumerary breast tissue: A case of pseudomamma on the face. *J Pediatr Surg.* 1997;32:1377–8.
25. Leung W, Heaton JP, Morales A. An uncommon urologic presentation of a supernumerary breast. *Urology.* 1997;50:122–4.
26. Gould DJ, Nadeau MH, Macias LH et al. Inverted nipple repair revisited: A 7 year experience. *Aesthet Surg J.* 2015;35(2):156–64.
27. Hernandez Yenty QM, Jurgens WJ, van Zuijlen PP et al. Treatment of the benign inverted nipple: A systemic review and recommendation for future therapy. *Breast.* 2016;29:82–9.
28. O'Hare PM, Frieden IJ. Virginal breast hypertrophy. *Pediatr Dermatol.* 2000;17:277–81.

29. Desilva NK. Breast development and disorders in the adolescent female. *Best Pract Res Clin Obstet Gynaecol*. 2018;48:40–50.

30. Stricker T, Navratil F, Forster I et al. Nonpuerperal mastitis in adolescents. *J Pediatr*. 2006;148:278–81.

31. Faden H. Mastitis in children from birth to 17 years. *Pediatr Infect Dis J*. 2005;24:1113.

32. Efrat M, Mogilner JG, Iujtman M et al. Neonatal mastitis—Diagnosis and treatment. *Isr J Med Sci*. 1995;31:558–60.

33. Warren R, Degnim AC. Uncommon benign breast abnormalities in adolescents. *Semin Plast Surg*. 2013;27:26–8.

34. Stevens DL, Bisno AL, Chambers HF et al. Practice guidelines by the Infectious Diseases Society of America. *Clin Infect Dis*. 2014;59:147–8.

35. Barren JM. Breast lesions. In: Fleisher GR, Lodus S, Henretig FM, eds. *Textbook of Pediatric Emergency Medicine*. 5th ed. Philadelphia, PA: Lippincott Williams and Wilkins; 2006:193.

36. Schwarz RJ, Shrestha R. Needle aspiration of breast abscess. *Am J Surg*. 2001;182:117.

37. Loud KJ, Micheli LJ. Common athletic injuries in adolescent girls. *Curr Opin Pediatr*. 2001;13:317–22.

38. Carroll ST, Riffenburgh RH, Roberts TA et al. Tattoos and body piercings as indicators of adolescent risk-taking behaviors. *Pediatrics*. 2002;109:1021–7.

39. Braverman PK. Body art: Piercing, tattooing, and scarification. *Adolesc Med*. 2006;17:505–19.

40. Gold MA, Schorzman CM, Murray PJ et al. Body piercing practices and attitudes among urban adolescents. *J Adolesc Health*. 2005;36:352.e17–24.

41. Marcer H, Finlay F, Jordan N. Body piercing in school children: A review of the issues. *Community Pract*. 2006;79:328–30.

42. Deschesnes M, Fines P, Demers S. Are tattooing and body piercing indicators of risk-taking behaviours among high school students? *J Adolesc*. 2006;29:379–93.

43. Suris JC, Jeannin A, Chossis I et al. Piercing among adolescents: Body art as a risk marker. *J Fam Pract*. 2007;56:126–30.

44. Breuner CC, Levine DA, Committee on Adolescence. Adolescent and young adult tattooing, piercing and scarification. *Pediatrics*. 2017;140(4):e20171962.

45. Daniel RA, Sheha T. Transmission of hepatitis C through swapping body jewelry. *Pediatrics*. 2005;116(5):1264–5.

46. Rohn RD. Galactorrhea in the adolescent. *J Adolesc Health Care*. 1984;5:37–49.

47. Hindle WH, Arias RD, Florentine B et al. Lack of utility in clinical practice of cytologic examination of nonbloody cyst fluid from palpable breast cysts. *Am J Obstet Gynecol*. 2000;182:1300–5.

48. Bosman JM, Bax NM, Wit JM. Premature thelarche: A possible adverse effect of cimetidine treatment. *Eur J Pediatr*. 1990;149:534–5.

49. Ahmed ST, Singh SK, Mukherjee S et al. Breast carcinoma in a prepubertal girl. *BMJ Case Rep*. 2014;2014.

50. Akyuz C, Yaris N, Kutluk MT et al. Management of cutaneous hemangiomas: A retrospective analysis of 1109 cases and comparison of conventional dose prednisolone with high-dose methylprednisolone therapy. *Pediatr Hematol Oncol*. 2001;18:47–55.

51. Tiryaki T, Senel E, Hucumenoglu S et al. Breast fibroadenoma in female adolescents. *Saudi Med J*. 2007;28(1):137–8.

52. Hanna RM, Ashebu SD. Giant fibroadenoma of the breast in an Arab population. *Australas Radiol*. 2002;46:252–6.

53. Ezer SS, Oguzkurt P, Ince E et al. Surgical treatment of the solid breast masses in female adolescents. *J Pediatr Adolesc Gynecol*. 2013;2013:31–5.

54. Jayasinghe Y. Preventative care and evolution of the adolescent with the breast mass. *Semin Plast Surg*. 2013;27:13–8.

55. Parker SJ, Harries SA. Phyllodes tumours. *Postgrad Med J*. 2001;77:428–35.

56. Siegal A, Kaufman Z, Siegal G. Breast masses in adolescent females. *J Surg Oncol*. 1992;51:169–73.

57. Chao TC, Lo YF, Chen SC et al. Sonographic features of phyllodes tumors of the breast. *Ultrasound Obstet Gynecol*. 2002;20:64–71.

58. Rojananin S, Ratanawichitrasin A. Limited incision with plastic bag removal for a large fibroadenoma. *Br J Surg*. 2002;89:787–8.

59. Alabassi A, Fentiman IS. Sarcomas of the breast. *Int J Clin Pract*. 2003;57:886–9.

60. Spitaleri G, Toesca A, Botteri E et al. Breast phyllodes tumor: A review of literature and a single center retrospective series analysis. *Crit Rev Oncol Hematol*. 2013;88:427–36.

61. Huneeus A, Schilling A, Horvath E et al. Retroareolar cysts in the adolescent. *J Pediatr Adolesc Gynecol*. 2003;16:45–9.

62. Weinzweig N, Botts J, Marcus E. Giant hamartoma of the breast. *Plast Reconstr Surg*. 2001;107:1216–20.

63. Chang HL, Lerwill MF, Goldstein AM. Breast hamartomas in adolescent females. *Breast J*. 2009;15(5):515–20.

64. Tao W, Kai F, Yue Hua L. Nipple adenoma in an adolescent. *Pediatr Dermatol*. 2010;27(4):399–401.

65. Rice HE, Acosta A, Brown RL et al. Juvenile papillomatosis of the breast in male infants: Two case reports. *Pediatr Surg Int*. 2000;16:104–6.

66. Kafadar MT, Anadolulu Z, Anadolulu AI et al. Juvenile papillomatosis of the breast in a pre-pubertal girl: An uncommon diagnosis. *Eur J Breast Health*. 2018;14(1):51–3.

67. Dehner LP, Hill DA, Deschryver K. Pathology of the breast in children, adolescents, and young adults. *Semin Diagn Pathol*. 1999;16:235–47.

68. Williams HJ, Hejmadi RK, England DW et al. Imaging features of breast trauma: A pictorial review. *Breast*. 2002;11:107–15.

69. Committee Opinion 686. Breast and Labial Surgery in Adolescents. *Obstet Gynecol*. 2017;129(1):235.

70. McGrath MH, Schooler WG. Elective plastic surgical procedures in adolescence. *Adolesc Med*. 2004;15:487–502.

71. Crockett RJ, Pruzinsky T, Persing JA. The influence of plastic surgery "reality TV" on cosmetic surgery patient expectations and decision making. *Plast Reconstr Surg*. 2007;120:316–24.

72. McGrath MH, Mukerji S. Plastic surgery and the teenage patient. *J Pediatr Adolesc Gynecol*. 2000;13:105–18.

73. U.S. Food and Drug Administration. Risks of breast implants. https://www.fda.gov/MedicalDevices/ProductsandMedicalProcedures/ImplantsandProsthetics/BreastImplants/ucm064106.htm#Breastfeeding. Accessed January 22, 2018.

74. Simis KJ, Koot JM, Verhulst FC et al. Assessing adolescents and young adults for plastic surgical intervention: Pre-surgical appearance ratings and appearance-related burdens as reported by adolescents and young adults, parents and surgeons. *Br J Plast Surg*. 2000;53:593–600.

75. Rohrich RJ, Cunningham BL, Jewell ML et al. Teenage breast augmentation: Validating outcome data and statistics in plastic surgery. *Plast Reconstr Surg*. 2005;115:943–4.

76. American Society of Plastic Surgeons. Policy statement: Breast augmentation in teenagers. https://www.plasticsurgery.org/documents/Health-Policy/Positions/policy-statement_breast-augmentation-in-teenagers.pdf. Accessed January 18, 2018.

77. Committee on Practice Bulletins–Gynecology, Committee on Genetics, Society of Gynecologic Oncology. Practice Bulletin 182: Hereditary breast and ovarian cancer syndrome. *Obstet Gynecol*. 2017;130(3):e110–26.

78. Murphy JJ, Morzaria S, Gow KW et al. Breast cancer in a 6-year-old child. *J Pediatr Surg*. 2000;35:765–7.

79. Binokay F, Soyupak SK, Inal M et al. Primary and metastatic rhabdomyosarcoma in the breast: Report of two pediatric cases. *Eur J Radiol*. 2003;48:282–4.

80. Jimenez JF, Gloster ES, Perrott LJ et al. Liposarcoma arising within a cystosarcoma phyllodes. *J Surg Oncol*. 1986;31:294–8.

81. Rogers DA, Lobe TE, Rao BN et al. Breast malignancy in children. *J Pediatr Surg*. 1994;29:48–51.

82. Shannon C, Smith IE. Breast cancer in adolescents and young women. *Eur J Cancer*. 2003;39:2632–4.

83. Sonmezer M, Oktay K. Fertility preservation in young women undergoing breast cancer therapy. *Oncologist*. 2006;11:422–34.

84. Raj KA, Marks LB, Prosnitz RG. Late effects of breast radiotherapy in young women. *Breast Dis*. 2005–2006;23:53–65.

85. Gold DG, Neglia JP, Dusenbery KE. Second neoplasms after megavoltage radiation for pediatric tumors. *Cancer*. 2003;97:2588–96.

86. Henderson TO, Amsteram A, Bhatia S et al. Systemic review: Surveillance for breast cancer in women treated with chest radiation for childhood, adult or young adult cancer. *Ann Intern Med*. 2010;152(7):444–55.

87. Henderson TO, Moskowitz CS, Chou JF et al. Breast cancer risk in childhood cancer survivors without a history of chest radiotherapy: A report from the childhood cancer survivor study. *J Clin Oncol*. 2016;34(9):910–8.

88. Chateil JF, Arboucalot F, Perel Y et al. Breast metastases in adolescent girls: US findings. *Pediatr Radiol*. 1998;28:832–5.

89. Ishida LH, Alves HR, Munhoz AM et al. Athelia: Case report and review of the literature. *Br J Plast Surg*. 2005;58(6):833–7.

90. Divasta AD, Weldon C, Labow BI The breast: Examination and lesions. In: Emans SJ, Laufer MR, eds. *Emans, Laufer, Goldstein's Pediatric and Adolescent Gynecology*. Chapter 22. Philadelphia, PA: Wolters Kluwer Health; 2011.

Menstrual disorders and blood dyscrasias in adolescents

14

LISA MOON, GISSELLE PEREZ-MILICUA, KATHRYN STAMBOUGH,
and JENNIFER E. DIETRICH

INTRODUCTION

Menstrual cycle dysfunction is a common complaint at adolescent clinical visits. Abnormal uterine bleeding (AUB) is defined as a change from the normal menstrual cycle pattern, which can include an alteration in frequency, duration, volume, or other bleeding characteristics, and can be further classified as heavy menstrual bleeding (HMB) or intermenstrual bleeding (IMB). The average age of menarche is 12–13 years.[1] Normal menstrual frequency occurs every 21–45 days with intercycle variation, over a 1-year span, of 2–20 days.[2] Bleeding should be 7 days or less in duration, and the volume of normal bleeding is $\leq$80 cc of blood loss per menstrual cycle (Table 14.1).[3] Although cycle irregularity is common in the first several years after menarche due to the increased incidence of anovulatory cycles with immaturity of the hypothalamic-pituitary-ovarian axis, approximately 90% of adolescent cycles will fall into the previous parameters. The prevalence of heavy menstrual bleeding in adult women is 10%–20%, and the incidence in adolescents is thought to be higher (37%).[4,5] Guidelines recommend an approach to the evaluation and management of abnormal uterine bleeding to include consideration of nine main categories arranged according to the acronym PALM-COEIN, which encompasses structural and nonstructural pathologies (Table 14.2).[2]

In addition to PALM-COEIN, there are a couple of additional considerations in the evaluation and management of AUB in the adolescent patient. All reproductive-aged patients should first be evaluated for pregnancy, with either urine or serum HCG testing. Positive testing should prompt further evaluation for any pregnancy-related causes of bleeding, such as spontaneous abortion or ectopic pregnancy. Sexually transmitted infection testing including *Chlamydia trachomatis* and *Neisseria gonorrhoeae* should also be performed in sexually active patients, as cervicitis can present with intermenstrual and postcoital bleeding. A broader differential diagnosis for bleeding

from the genitourinary tract in the pediatric and adolescent population can also include vaginal foreign body or trauma. The aforementioned causes are reviewed in other chapters, and the remainder of this chapter focuses on the diagnoses included in the PALM-COEIN system.

STRUCTURAL ABNORMALITIES (PALM)

Structural abnormalities that can lead to AUB include polyps (P), adenomyosis (A), leiomyomas (L), and malignancy and hyperplasia (M). The incidence of structural abnormalities in adolescents with AUB is low (<2%).[6,7] Given the overall low incidence of structural abnormalities as the etiology for AUB in adolescents, in the absence of dysmenorrhea, pelvic imaging should be reserved for individuals who fail medical management. Of primary importance in the management of AUB, and in the diagnosis of a structural abnormality in an adolescent, is preservation of fertility. Therefore, medical management should be first line before considering surgical treatments. If pursued, surgical management should ideally be fertility sparing.

Endometrial hyperplasia and malignancy are rare diagnoses in the adolescent population in the absence of hereditary syndromes such as Cowden syndrome and Lynch syndrome. Most reports of endometrial malignancy in adolescents consist of case studies.[8,9] However, obesity and chronic anovulation are known risk factors for hyperplasia and malignancy.[10] One case report that examined 54 adolescent patients age 13–20 years with AUB demonstrated an incidence of 29.6% of endometrial hyperplasia with only one case of atypia.[11] Endometrial sampling should be reserved for adolescents with a history of unopposed estrogen, failed medical management, and

Table 14.1 Signs suggestive of heavy bleeding >80 mL per menstrual cycle.

- Changing a pad or tampon every 1–2 hours
- Use of double hygiene protection
- Frequent soiling of clothes or bed sheets
- Blood clots greater than 1 inch in diameter
- Affects quality of life

Source: Haamid F et al. *J Pediatr Adolesc Gynecol.* 2017;30(3):335–40.

Table 14.2 The PALM-COEIN approach to differential diagnosis of abnormal uterine bleeding.

PALM (structural causes)	• Polyp (AUB-P) • Adenomyosis (AUB-A) • Leiomyoma (AUB-L) • Malignancy or hyperplasia (AUB-M)
COEIN (nonstructural causes)	• Coagulopathy (AUB-C) • Ovulatory dysfunction (AUB-O) • Endometrial (AUB-E) • Iatrogenic (AUB-I) • Not yet classified (AUB-N)

Source: Munro MG et al. *Int J Gynecol Obstet.* 2011;113:3–13.

persistent AUB.[12] Classically, the approach to the management of endometrial malignancy has been surgical, with hysterectomy and bilateral salpingo-oophorectomy ($\pm$ lymphadenectomy reserved for individuals with intermediate to high-risk factors). However, recent literature has supported the use of progestin-only therapy in individuals with stage I disease in whom fertility preservation is desired. Patients should undergo extensive counseling regarding the limited data for both cancer-related and pregnancy-related outcomes in medically managed individuals with endometrial malignancy.[9,13] In adolescents diagnosed with this condition, consultation with a surgeon experienced in the management of endometrial cancer, such as a gynecologic oncologist, is advised.

NONSTRUCTURAL ABNORMALITIES (COEIN)

The predominant causes of AUB in adolescents arise from nonstructural abnormalities, with ovulatory dysfunction and coagulopathies being the most common.

Coagulopathies (C)

The second most common cause of heavy menstrual bleeding in the adolescent population is a bleeding disorder.[14] Although bleeding disorders are rare in the general population, the incidence in adolescents presenting with heavy menstrual bleeding can be up to 30%, with von Willebrand disease being the most common disorder.[15,16] While some patients may have a previously known diagnosis of a bleeding disorder, many patients present for the first time at the age of menarche with significant vaginal bleeding.[17] It is important while taking the patient's history to keep in mind the red flags for bleeding disorders (Table 14.3).[3]

Initial workup of HMB in the adolescent population should include initial history screening for bleeding disorders. Patients with risk factors for bleeding as well as those exhibiting positive red flags on the basis of history

should be evaluated for bleeding disorders, including von Willebrand panel and coagulation studies.[18] Platelet function disorders are the second most common type of bleeding disorder in adolescents; therefore, platelet aggregation studies should be considered in the workup as well.[14,19] Bleeding disorder testing can be affected by several factors, which need to be taken into consideration when initiating workup on a patient. Von Willebrand factor levels can be affected by acute bleeding episodes, stress, specimen handling, and doses of estrogen greater than 50 μg.[18] Testing for von Willebrand disease can be performed while the patient is taking combined hormonal therapy, such as oral contraceptives, as these typically only contain 30–35 μg of estrogen, but ideally, assessment should take place during the placebo interval. Platelet function testing can be altered by recent nonsteroidal anti-inflammatory drug use, specimen handling, or selective serotonin reuptake inhibitor use.[18] Regardless of the results, von Willebrand testing and platelet function analysis are frequently performed at least twice to confirm the results. Additional workup for rarer conditions should be undertaken by a hematologist and can include dysfibrinogenemia panel, fibrinolysis testing, coagulation factor assays, and further platelet function testing.[18] It is also important to keep in mind that some chronic medical diseases, such as renal dysfunction and liver disease, can affect platelet functioning and bleeding profile as well, and may lead to coagulopathy. Thyroid dysfunction, and in particular, hypothyroidism, can also affect the coagulation cascade and lead to bleeding dysfunction.[20]

Management of heavy menstrual bleeding in the setting of a bleeding disorder can include both hormonal (i.e., combined therapies or progestin-only therapies) and nonhormonal treatment (i.e., aminocaproic acid or tranexamic acid weight-based), with many patients requiring dual therapy (Table 14.4).[3,4] Optimal outcomes are achieved when patients are treated in a multidisciplinary setting with both a hematologist and clinician with adolescent gynecology expertise.[21] In patients who have a known bleeding disorder prior to menarche, it is

Table 14.3   Bleeding disorder red flags.

- Prolonged bleeding from trivial wounds lasting more than 15 minutes
- Heavy, prolonged, or recurrent bleeding after surgery
- Heavy, prolonged, or recurrent bleeding after dental procedures or tooth extraction
- Bruising with minimal or no trauma, especially resulting in a lump, one to two times per month
- Nosebleeds lasting more than 10 minutes or requiring medical attention one to two times per month
- Unexplained bleeding from the gastrointestinal tract
- Anemia requiring iron therapy or transfusions
- Heavy menstrual bleeding
- Family history of bleeding disorders such as von Willebrand disease or hemophilia
- Family history of hysterectomy at a young age
- Postpartum hemorrhage

Source: Haamid F et al. *J Pediatr Adolesc Gynecol.* 2017;30(3):335–40.

Table 14.4   Hormonal and nonhormonal treatment options for heavy menstrual bleeding in bleeding disorders.

Estrogen-containing methods	Progesterone-only methods	Nonhormonal methods
• IV estrogen	• Progestin-only pills	• Tranexamic acid
• Combined oral contraceptive pills	• Depot medroxyprogesterone acetate injections	• Aminocaproic acid
• Contraceptive patch	• Levonorgestrel intrauterine system	• DDAVP (desmopressin acetate)
• Contraceptive vaginal ring		

Source: Haamid F et al. *J Pediatr Adolesc Gynecol.* 2017;30(3):335–40; Bradley LD, Gueye N-A. *Am J Obstet Gynecol.* 2016;214:31–44.

important to have an action plan in place for when their first menses occur to prevent significant anemia and potential hospitalization.[22]

Ovulatory dysfunction (O)

Ovulatory dysfunction refers to abnormal ovulation, which can be either absent or irregular, also known as anovulation or oligo-ovulation, respectively. Without ovulation, the corpus luteum fails to form; therefore, progesterone secretion from the ovary is minimized.[23] The endometrium then becomes unstable as it continues to be stimulated by unopposed estrogen. The clinical result is irregular shedding of the endometrium with unpredictable bleeding and variable flow.

In order to have normal ovulation and normal menstrual cycles, the hypothalamic-pituitary-ovarian (HPO) axis needs to be intact. Therefore, abnormalities at any level of the HPO axis can result in ovulatory dysfunction and AUB. Puberty is a physiologic cause of AUB-O, as the HPO axis is initially immature and is unable to maintain a stable endometrium with a functional hormonal feedback mechanism.[23] Immaturity of the HPO axis is a common cause of AUB-O, and it typically resolves after 2–3 years postmenarche, with up to 60%–80% of menstrual cycles becoming ovulatory by the third year.[23] Another common cause of AUB-O in adolescents is polycystic ovary syndrome (PCOS). One study revealed that PCOS was the most common etiology in adolescents who were hospitalized due to abnormal bleeding.[24] There are many other causes of ovulatory dysfunction that should also be considered in the differential diagnosis of AUB (Table 14.5).[24]

To narrow the differential diagnosis, a thorough history and physical examination must be performed. In AUB-O, most patients will report irregular menses or amenorrhea. They may also deny cyclical symptoms such as breast tenderness, increased vaginal discharge, abdominal bloating, and cramping.[23] A general review of systems is also important to identify endocrinopathies. A review of systems should include stressors, changes in weight, hot or cold intolerance, exercise habits, eating disorders, visual changes, headaches, syncopal episodes, acne, hirsutism, acanthosis nigricans, history of radiation or chemotherapy, among others.[25] Physical examination should include

height, weight (body mass index), fat distribution, vital signs, clinical signs of hyperandrogenism, thyroid masses, breast development assessment (Tanner stage), and pelvic examination, when indicated.[25]

Laboratory testing for ovulatory dysfunction, especially in the setting of clinical hyperandrogenism, may include a prolactin level, total or free testosterone levels, dehydroepiandrosterone sulfate (DHEAS), 17-hydroxyprogesterone (17-OHP), androstenedione, thyroid-stimulating hormone (TSH), follicle-stimulating hormone (FSH), and/or luteinizing hormone (LH).[23,26] If PCOS is suspected, an evaluation for glucose metabolism and hypercholesterolemia should be performed.[26]

When AUB-O is a result of an endocrinopathy, the underlying disorder should be addressed and treated first. Hyperthyroidism can lead to oligomenorrhea and amenorrhea, while hypothyroidism can cause heavy or frequent menses, although perhaps to a lesser degree than previously thought, and may also result in irregular or absent cycles[27]; correction of abnormal thyroid hormone levels can facilitate return of normal menstruation. Medical management can usually achieve regulation of menses.[23] Options for medical management include combination hormonal therapies containing estrogen and progesterone, and progesterone-only options for those who have contraindications to estrogen. Combination hormonal therapies are available in combined oral contraceptive (COC) pills, transdermal patches, or vaginal rings, while progestin-only options include pills (i.e., medroxyprogesterone acetate, norethindrone acetate, or megestrol acetate), depot medroxyprogesterone acetate injection, and the levonorgestrel-releasing intrauterine device (IUD).[1] In PCOS, COCs are the treatment of choice due to the reduction in ovarian androgen production and improvements in clinical hyperandrogenism.[26] Lifestyle modifications are also strongly recommended as the initial step in treatment in patients with PCOS, as weight loss can improve menstrual irregularities.[26]

Endometrial (E)

An endometrial etiology for AUB is more likely in the setting of regular menstrual cycles, suggesting ovulation, and the absence of other underlying causes. Given the increased incidence of anovulation as the etiology for AUB in the adolescent population, endometrial causes for AUB in the adolescent are rare. Chronic endomyometritis has been suggested as an etiology of AUB, although data on the association are limited.[2,28] Evaluation for chronic endomyometritis involves testing for *Neisseria gonorrhea* and *Chlamydia trachomatis* and endometrial biopsy, which classically demonstrates plasma cells. Treatment includes doxycycline 100 mg twice daily for a 10–14 day course.[29]

Iatrogenic (I)

Iatrogenic causes of AUB include medications that directly affect the endometrium, interfere with the coagulation cascade, and influence the HPO axis. In the adolescent

Table 14.5 Causes of anovulation.

Physiologic	Pathologic
• Adolescence	• Hyperandrogenic anovulation
• Pregnancy	• Hypothalamic dysfunction
• Lactation	• Hyperprolactinemia
• Perimenopause	• Thyroid disease
	• Primary pituitary disease
	• Premature ovarian failure
	• Iatrogenic
	• Medications

Source: Maslyanskaya S et al. *J Pediatr Adolesc Gynecol.* 2017;30(3): 349–55.

population, more common etiologies of iatrogenic AUB include the administration of combined estrogen-progesterone or progestin-only hormonal therapy. Unscheduled or breakthrough bleeding (BTB) in the adolescent taking combined hormonal methods, such as oral contraceptive pills, transdermal patches, or the vaginal ring, are likely secondary to missed or late dosing or poor compliance with the medications.[30] In addition, unscheduled bleeding may occur in adolescents attempting continuous rather than cyclic administration of combined hormonal methods. Management of AUB in this setting includes improved adherence or transition to an alternative method on which compliance is less reliant on the adolescent, specifically long-acting reversible contraception (LARC) or progestin-only injections.

Unscheduled bleeding is expected in the first 3–6 months after progestin-only IUD and may be longer with an implant insertion. In the absence of another underlying etiology for AUB (IUD displacement, pregnancy, sexually transmitted infection, or structural or other nonstructural condition), first-line management should be reassurance. If the bleeding is bothersome, a short course of nonsteroidal anti-inflammatory drugs (5–7 days) or hormonal therapy (if medically eligible) with low-dose combined hormonal contraceptive method or estrogen (10–20 days) can be helpful. Last, if the bleeding persists and the adolescent finds it unacceptable, transition to an alternate hormonal therapy may be warranted.[31]

The use of medications that affect the coagulation cascade, specifically anticoagulants, is frequently seen in adolescents with medical comorbidities that include cardiac disease or a history of venous thromboembolic disease, which requires either treatment or prophylaxis against the formation of clot. These medications, such as warfarin, heparin, and low molecular weight heparin, affect systemic hemostasis and, therefore, present as AUB in the adolescent.[2] Management should be the same as for other coagulopathies, with careful consideration of their medical comorbidities and done closely with the assistance of other medical services, including hematology.

A number of medications affect the HPO axis and thus affect ovulation. Some of the more common medications include dopamine agonists, tricyclic antidepressants, and phenothiazines.[2] A careful medication history should be part of the evaluation and management of all adolescents with AUB. Management should be done in close consultation with the prescribing physician, carefully balancing the risks and benefits of the offending medication and the adolescent's medical comorbidity with alternative therapies.

Not yet classified (N)

The category of not yet classified should be reserved for uterine pathology that has not definitively been identified to result in AUB (arteriovenous malformations and myometrial hypertrophy) and for other disorders that have not yet been identified and would only be defined by biochemical or molecular biology assays.[2] The incidence of this etiology in the presentation of AUB in the adolescent is extremely unlikely and should be reserved for rare cases in which an extensive evaluation has failed to reveal any other etiology.

CONCLUSION

Abnormal uterine bleeding is a common complaint in the adolescent population, with a broad differential diagnosis. Once pregnancy has been excluded, common causes of AUB can be divided into structural and nonstructural causes as outlined in the PALM-COEIN system, with nonstructural causes predominating. A variety of hormonal and nonhormonal therapies can be effective in treating menstrual dysfunction, with duration of treatment dependent on the underlying cause. Management is focused on conservative medical therapies, as preservation of fertility in this population is of utmost importance.

REFERENCES

1. Menstruation in girls and adolescents: Using the menstrual cycle as a vital sign. Committee Opinion No. 651. American College of Obstetricians and Gynecologists. *Obstet Gynecol*. 2015;126:e143–6.
2. Munro MG, Critchley HOD, Broder MS, Fraser IS, FIGO Working Group on Menstrual Disorders. FIGO classification system (PALM-COEIN) for causes of abnormal uterine bleeding in nongravid women of reproductive age. *Int J Gynecol Obstet*. 2011;113:3–13.
3. Haamid F, Sass AE, Dietrich JE. Heavy menstrual bleeding in adolescents. *J Pediatr Adolesc Gynecol*. 2017;30(3):335–40.
4. Bradley LD, Gueye N-A. The medical management of abnormal uterine bleeding in reproductive-aged women. *Am J Obstet Gynecol*. 2016;214:31–44.
5. Friberg B, Ornö AK, Lindgren A, Lethagen S. Bleeding disorders among young women: A population-based prevalence study. *Acta Obstet Gynecol Scand*. 2006;85:200–6.
6. Pecchioli Y, Oyewumi L, Allen LM, Kives S. The utility of routine ultrasound in the diagnosis and management of adolescents with abnormal uterine bleeding. *J Pediatr Adolesc Gynecol*. 2017;30(2):239–42.
7. Claessens EA, Cowell CA. Acute adolescent menorrhagia. *Am J Obstet Gynecol*. 1981;139:277–80.
8. Gerli S, Spanò F, Di Renzo GC. Endometrial carcinoma in women 40 year old or younger: A case report and literature review. *Eur Rev Med Pharmacol Sci*. 2014;18:1973–8.
9. Gałczyński K, Nowakowski Ł, Rechberger T, Semczuk A. Should we be more aware of endometrial cancer in adolescents? *Dev Period Med*. 2016;20:169–73.
10. Elizondo-Montemayor L, Hernández-Escobar C, Lara-Torre E, Nieblas B, Gómez-Carmona M. Gynecologic and obstetric consequences of obesity in adolescent girls. *J Pediatr Adolesc Gynecol*. 2017;30:156–68.

11. Lee MH, Kim MK, Ahn EH, Moon MJ. Risk factors for endometrial hyperplasia in adolescent girls with irregular menstrual bleeding. *J Pediatr Adolesc Gynecol*. 2009;22:e18.

12. Diagnosis of abnormal uterine bleeding in reproductive-aged women. Practice Bulletin No. 128: American College of Obstetricians and Gynecologists. *Obstet Gynecol*. 2012;120:197–206.

13. Endometrial cancer. Practice Bulletin No. 149. American College of Obstetricians and Gynecologists. *Obstet Gynecol*. 2015;125:1006–26.

14. Karaman K, Ceylan N, Karaman E et al. Evaluation of the hemostatic disorders in adolescent girls with menorrhagia: Experiences from a tertiary referral hospital. *Indian J Hematol Blood Transfus*. 2016;32:356–61.

15. Kulkarni R. Improving care and treatment options for women and girls with bleeding disorders. *Eur J Haematol*. 2015;95(Suppl. 81):2–10.

16. Díaz R, Dietrich JE, Mahoney D, Yee DL, Srivaths LV. Hemostatic abnormalities in young females with heavy menstrual bleeding. *J Pediatr Adolesc Gynecol*. 2014;27:324–9.

17. Sanders YV, Fijnvandraat K, Boender J et al. Bleeding spectrum in children with moderate or severe von Willebrand disease: Relevance of pediatric-specific bleeding. *Am J Hematol*. 2015;90:1142–8.

18. Zia A, Rajpurkar M. Challenges of diagnosing and managing the adolescent with heavy menstrual bleeding. *Thromb Res*. 2016;143:91–100.

19. Mills HL, Abdel-Baki MS, Teruya J et al. Platelet function defects in adolescents with heavy menstrual bleeding. *Haemophilia*. 2014;20:249–54.

20. Squizzato A, Romualdi E, Büller HR, Gerdes VEA. Clinical review: Thyroid dysfunction and effects on coagulation and fibrinolysis: A systematic review. *J Clin Endocrinol Metab*. 2007;92:2415–20.

21. Zia A, Lau M, Journeycake J et al. Developing a multidisciplinary Young Women's Blood Disorders Program: A single-centre approach with guidance for other centres. *Haemophilia*. 2016;22(2):199–207.

22. Dowlut-McElroy T, Williams KB, Carpenter SL, Strickland JL. Menstrual patterns and treatment of heavy menstrual bleeding in adolescents with bleeding disorders. *J Pediatr Adolesc Gynecol*. 2015;28:499–501.

23. Management of abnormal uterine bleeding associated with ovulatory dysfunction. Practice Bulletin No. 136. American College of Obstetricians and Gynecologists. *Obstet Gynecol*. 2013;122:176–85.

24. Maslyanskaya S, Talib HJ, Northridge JL, Jacobs AM, Coble C, Coupey SM. Polycystic ovary syndrome: An under-recognized cause of abnormal uterine bleeding in adolescents admitted to a children's hospital. *J Pediatr Adolesc Gynecol*. 2017;30(3):349–55.

25. Gray S, Emans S. Abnormal vaginal bleeding in the adolescent. In: Emans SJ, Laufer MR, eds. *Emans, Laufer, Goldstein's Pediatric and Adolescent Gynecology*. 6th ed. Philadelphia, PA: Lippincott Williams and Wilkins; 2012:159–67.

26. Kamboj MK, Bonny AE. Polycystic ovary syndrome in adolescence: Diagnostic and therapeutic strategies. *Transl Pediatr*. 2017;6:248–55.

27. Kakuno Y, Amino N, Kanoh M et al. Menstrual disturbances in various thyroid diseases. *Endocr J*. 2010;57:1017–22.

28. Pitsos M, Skurnick J, Heller D. Association of pathologic diagnoses with clinical findings in chronic endometritis. *J Reprod Med*. 2009;54:373–7.

29. Johnston-MacAnanny EB, Hartnett J, Engmann LL, Nulsen JC, Sanders MM, Benadiva CA. Chronic endometritis is a frequent finding in women with recurrent implantation failure after *in vitro* fertilization. *Fertil Steril*. 2010;93:437–41.

30. Endrikat J, Gerlinger C, Plettig K et al. A meta-analysis on the correlation between ovarian activity and the incidence of intermenstrual bleeding during low-dose oral contraceptive use. *Gynecol Endocrinol*. 2003;17:107–14.

31. Curtis KM, Jatlaoui TC, Tepper NK et al. U.S. Selected Practice Recommendations for Contraceptive Use, 2016. *MMWR Recomm Rep Morb Mortal Wkly Rep Recomm Rep*. 2016;65:1–66.

Polycystic ovary syndrome and hyperandrogenism in adolescents

15

ANDREA E. BONNY and ASMA JAVED CHATTHA

INTRODUCTION

Originally described by Stein and Leventhal in seven women with the constellation of hirsutism, obesity, amenorrhea, and enlarged bilateral polycystic ovaries,[1] polycystic ovary syndrome (PCOS) is now known to be the most common endocrine disorder in women. It affects up to 15% of women depending on the diagnostic criteria applied and is associated with impaired reproductive health, infertility, psychosocial dysfunction, metabolic syndrome, cardiovascular disease, and increased cancer risk.[2]

Despite its high prevalence, much remains unknown regarding this disorder. This is particularly true in adolescents, where normal pubertal features overlap with the PCOS phenotype, confounding identification of the syndrome. Controversy remains regarding the etiopathogenesis, diagnostic criteria, and recommendations for PCOS in adolescents. Recent literature has recognized these deficiencies, and evidence-based expert consensus statements and recommendations have become more available.

Although a timely diagnosis of PCOS offers an opportunity for meaningful intervention, overdiagnosis can result in unnecessary treatment and potential anxiety for patient and family.[3] As such, it behooves the practitioner to critically understand the current literature regarding PCOS in adolescents and to closely follow up and reevaluate all adolescents with features of this syndrome.

PATHOPHYSIOLOGY

PCOS is a complex disorder with likely multifactorial etiology. Genetic, metabolic, and environmental factors interact in various degrees leading to the heterogeneity in PCOS symptoms. The earliest pathophysiologic hypothesis proposed functional ovarian hyperandrogenism, and multiple subsequent studies have corroborated this theory.[4] The functional ovarian hyperandrogenism is a primary abnormality, and not secondary to another disorder. Early work also revealed the presence of an elevated luteinizing hormone (LH) to follicle-stimulating hormone (FSH) ratio in PCOS. This led to the understanding that altered neuroendocrine gonadotropin secretion is a hallmark of the disorder.[5] Over the ensuing decades, several studies further elucidated the complex interaction between hyperinsulinemia and elevated testosterone, even independent from exogenous obesity, in the pathogenesis of PCOS.[6,7]

Although the source of hyperandrogenism in PCOS has been debated, both the ovaries and adrenal glands likely play a role, the latter to a lesser extent. The observation that hyperandrogenism persists when ovarian steroidogenesis is blocked with a long-acting gonadotropin-releasing hormone (GnRH) agonist or when adrenal steroidogenesis is inhibited with the use of long-acting corticosteroids, establishes that both organs contribute to the PCOS phenotype.[8–10]

Serum anti-Müllerian hormone (AMH) levels reflect the pool of growing follicles.[11] Across the age span and Tanner stages, females with PCOS have higher AMH concentrations than controls.[12] Although its contribution to pathophysiology is largely unknown, it is likely a consequence of elevated intrafollicular concentrations of androgens, resulting in growth of multiple small follicles. This is likely the basis of the polycystic ovarian morphology (PCOM) seen on ultrasound.

Genetic factors

Heritable factors in the development of PCOS include hyperandrogenemia, insulin resistance, insulin secretory defects, altered neuroendocrine functioning, and PCOM. Ovarian steroidogenic hyperresponsiveness, in the absence of a steroidogenic block, is the fundamental underlying biochemical abnormality. This leads to elevated 17-hydroxyprogesterone and androstenedione in response to GnRH agonist stimulation. Ovarian steroidogenic hyperresponsiveness points to a possible underlying genetic basis in terms of altered cytochrome P450c17 enzyme activity.[13] Cytochrome P450c17 (CYP17A1) is the rate-limiting enzyme for androgen synthesis in the gonads and adrenal cortex.[14] The expression of CYP17A1 is dependent on tropic hormone stimulation by LH in the ovary and by corticotropin (ACTH) in the adrenal cortex.[15,16] Theca cells of the ovary, which express CYP17A1, produce androgens in response to LH, but this action is modulated by factors including estradiol, insulin, and IGF-1 concentrations, resulting in functional ovarian hyperandrogenism.[17] Prevailing high concentrations of insulin, acting via insulin receptors on thecal cells, directly upregulate testosterone production from androstenedione; a concept that has been supported by the absence of these changes in transgenic mice lacking the insulin receptor on theca cells.[18,19]

Genome-wide association studies have revealed overexpression of a protein (DENND) in theca cells, producing an in vitro PCOS phenotype.[20] Other genes identified by genome-wide association studies include FSHR, LHCGR, RAB5B/SUOX, INSR, THADA, YAP1, HMGA2, and SUMO1P1.[21]

In summary, with regard to the genetic basis of development of PCOS phenotype, both desensitization/modulation to trophic stimulation from LH by insulin and other factors, as well as upregulated androgen biosynthesis in a paracrine fashion within the theca cells of the ovary, are seminal events in the pathophysiology of the condition.

Metabolic and environmental factors

The primary environmental factors contributing to the development of PCOS on a predisposing genetic background include prenatal androgen exposure, intrauterine growth restriction, and postnatally acquired obesity, with or without its commonly occurring comorbidity of insulin resistance. Comprehensive animal model studies in monkeys reveal that environmental factors leading to an eventual PCOS phenotype may begin as early as *in utero*.[22,23] Female nonhuman primates exposed to androgen excess early in gestation exhibit increased LH concentrations, ovulatory dysfunction, hyperandrogenism, insulin resistance, and polycystic ovaries.[22,23] Prenatal androgen exposure may alter the hypothalamic-pituitary-ovarian axis, resulting in higher concentrations of LH and changes in LH sensitization at the level of the ovarian theca cells, resulting in functional ovarian hyperandrogenism.[24,25] Intrauterine fetal growth restriction may contribute to an increased prevalence of premature adrenarche, hyperandrogenism, and insulin resistance in girls.[26,27] Rapid weight gain during the peripubertal years in females born small for gestational age and unremitting obesity in females born large for gestational age may accelerate deposition of visceral obesity, insulin resistance, and premature adrenarche through early activation of the hypothalamic-pituitary-ovarian axis and development of PCOS phenotype.[28]

PCOS has been included in the spectrum of diseases speculated to arise from a "two-hit" hypothesis. On the background of genetic predisposition, lifestyle factors such as rapid peripubertal weight gain and visceral adiposity contribute to the full-blown phenotype of PCOS.[29,30]

DIAGNOSTIC CRITERIA AND DEFINITIONS

There are currently three widely used diagnostic criteria for the diagnosis of PCOS in adults, all of which require the exclusion of other etiologies of androgen excess and anovulatory infertility (Table 15.1). The first were introduced by the National Institutes of Health (NIH) in 1990 and required clinical and/or biochemical evidence of hyperandrogenism in the presence of oligo- or chronic anovulation (Table 15.1).[31]

Many experts in the field felt these initial NIH diagnostic criteria did not fully represent the scope of the PCOS phenotype. As such, in 2003, the European Society of Human Reproduction and Embryology and the American Society for Reproductive Medicine (ESHRE/ASRM) criteria were developed, which included PCOM as a diagnostic marker.[32] The ESHRE/ASRM criteria, often called the Rotterdam criteria, require the presence of two of three of the following: oligo- or chronic anovulation, clinical and/or biochemical signs of hyperandrogenism, and polycystic ovaries. The criteria to define polycystic ovaries were the presence of 12 or more follicles in each ovary measuring 2–9 mm in diameter and/or increased ovarian volume (>10 cm^3). The Rotterdam guidelines allowed for the diagnosis of PCOS in women without evidence of androgen excess (Table 15.1).

Table 15.1 Summary of diagnostic criteria for polycystic ovary syndrome in adults.

Guideline	PCOS diagnosis
1990 National Institutes of Health	Presence of both: 1. Clinical and/or biochemical hyperandrogenism 2. Oligo- or anovulation Requires exclusion of other etiologies of androgen excess and anovulation
2003 Rotterdam	Presence of at least two of the three following: 1. Clinical and/or biochemical hyperandrogenism 2. Oligo- or anovulation 3. Polycystic ovarian morphology[a] Requires exclusion of other etiologies of androgen excess and anovulation
2006 Androgen Excess Society	Presence of clinical and/or biochemical hyperandrogenism with at least one of the two following: 1. Oligo- or anovulation 2. Polycystic ovarian morphology[a] Requires exclusion of other etiologies of androgen excess and anovulation
2012 National Institutes of Health	Recommend upholding the Rotterdam criteria with identification of the following distinct PCOS phenotypes: 1. Androgen excess/ovulatory dysfunction 2. Androgen excess/polycystic ovaries 3. Ovulatory dysfunction/polycystic ovaries 4. Androgen excess/ovulatory dysfunction/polycystic ovaries

Abbreviation: PCOS, polycystic ovarian syndrome.

[a] Defined as the presence of 12 or more follicles in each ovary measuring 2–9 mm in diameter and/or increased ovarian volume (>10 mL).

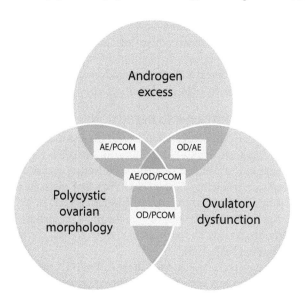

Figure 15.1 Venn diagram depicting polycystic ovary syndrome phenotypes. (AE, androgen excess; OD, ovulatory dysfunction; PCO, polycystic ovary.) (Reproduced with permission from Javed A et al. *Curr Opin Obstet Gynecol.* 2016;28[5]:373–80.)

The inclusion of women without evidence of hyperandrogenism proved controversial. Thus, in 2006, the Androgen Excess Society (AES) established its own diagnostic criteria requiring hyperandrogenism, associated with either oligo-anovulation or polycystic ovaries (Table 15.1).[33]

In 2012, the NIH convened an Evidence-based Methodology Workshop of PCOS and reviewed all previously published diagnostic criteria. Final recommendations were to uphold the broad, inclusionary Rotterdam criteria, while encouraging providers and researchers to begin specifically identifying the distinct PCOS phenotype (Figure 15.1).

Historically, the adult diagnostic criteria have been utilized for adolescents. However, overlap between normal pubertal findings and signs and symptoms of PCOS has made this challenging. Physiologic anovulation, menstrual irregularity, and signs of hyperandrogenism (e.g., acne) can be common in the peripubertal period.[34] Normative testosterone levels are ill defined in this age group.[35] In a prospective cohort study of postmenarcheal adolescent girls, Hickey et al. found significant discrepancies in the prevalence of PCOS when each of the three major adult diagnostic guidelines were applied: 18.5% using Rotterdam criteria, 5% using AES criteria, and 3.1% using NIH criteria.[36] To address these concerns, attempts have been made to develop adolescent-specific diagnostic criteria and recommendations (Table 15.2).

In 2010, Carmina and colleagues recommended that all three features, i.e., hyperandrogenism, chronic anovulation, and polycystic ovaries, should be present for a confirmed diagnosis of PCOS in an adolescent.[37] Furthermore, they suggested that the diagnosis of PCOS be considered

only in girls at least 2 years postmenarche. These recommendations are complicated by normal adolescent ovarian morphology, which overlaps with that of PCOM.[38,39]

Separate recommendations for the diagnosis of PCOS in adolescents were then included in the 2013 Endocrine Society Clinical Practice Guideline.[40] These recommendations concluded that anovulatory symptoms and polycystic ovaries were not sufficient for a diagnosis of PCOS in adolescents, as both of these findings can be evident in normal pubertal development. Hyperandrogenism was felt to be central to the presentation in this age group. As such, the diagnostic criteria put forth for adolescents required clinical and/or biochemical evidence of androgen excess in the presence of persistent oligomenorrhea. The definition of "persistent" was not clear, but menstrual irregularities present 2 years beyond menarche were stated to be noteworthy.

In 2015 and 2017, international pediatric endocrinology societies (PES) were invited to evaluate current criteria for PCOS diagnosis in adolescents.[3,41] Similar to the 2013 Endocrine Society Guidelines, the PES consensuses concluded that ovarian imaging for PCOM (determined by transvaginal imaging, which is not commonly performed in nonsexually active adolescents) can be deferred until high-quality data are available. The 2015 report further concluded that in adolescents, there were no compelling criteria to define PCOM, that an ovarian volume >12 cm³ (by formula for a prolate ellipsoid) could be considered enlarged, and that follicle counts should not be utilized to define PCOM in this population. Based on these recommendations, the diagnosis of PCOS in adolescents currently hinges on evidence of ovulatory dysfunction and androgen excess.[3,41] Given that confirming a firm diagnosis of PCOS can be difficult, particularly in the early adolescent years, deferring a definitive diagnosis of PCOS while providing symptom treatment and regular follow-up is an acceptable alternative.

CLINICAL PRESENTATION
Menstrual irregularity

Unlike adult women who often present with concerns around infertility, menstrual irregularity is a frequent complaint of adolescents with PCOS. Various patterns of menstrual irregularity may be seen, including primary amenorrhea (absence of menarche by 15 years of age or 2–3 years after breast budding), secondary amenorrhea (more than 90 days without a period with history of prior menstrual periods), oligomenorrhea, or excessive uterine bleeding.[3] Accounting for 33% of admissions, PCOS was the most common underlying etiology identified among adolescents hospitalized with abnormal uterine bleeding and heavy menstrual bleeding.[42]

It is important that the clinician be able to differentiate between physiological anovulation, which is normal in the adolescent period, and true ovulatory dysfunction. It is statistically uncommon for adolescents to remain amenorrheic for more than 90 days, even in the first gynecologic

Table 15.2 Recommendations for diagnosis of polycystic ovary syndrome in adolescents.

Guideline	PCOS diagnosis recommendations
2010 Carmina	Presence of all three of the following: 1. Hyperandrogenism • Acne and alopecia are *not* evidence of HA • Hirsutism must be progressive to be evidence of HA 2. Chronic anovulation • Must be present for at least 2 years 3. Polycystic ovaries • If diagnosed by abdominal ultrasound must include increased ovarian size (>10 cm³)
2013 Endocrine Society	Presence of both: 1. Clinical and/or biochemical HA • Acne in isolation is *not* evidence of HA • Alopecia should be used cautiously in PCOS diagnosis 2. Persistent oligomenorrhea • Persistent not clearly defined, but menstrual irregularity present for 2 years is noteworthy Noted that the Rotterdam ultrasound criteria for PCOM are not validated for adolescents
2015 Pediatric Endocrine Societies	Presence of both: 1. Clinical and/or biochemical HA • Moderate to severe hirsutism is evidence of HA • Persistent acne unresponsive to topical therapy suggests HA • Persistent elevation of serum total and/or free testosterone provides the clearest support for HA 2. Ovulatory dysfunction evidenced by: • Consecutive menstrual intervals >90 days even in the first year postmenarche • Menstrual intervals persistently <21 days or >45 days, 2 or more years postmenarche • Lack of menses by 15 years or 2–3 years after thelarche Endorsed deferring diagnostic evaluation for PCOM until better quality-consistent data are available.
2017 Pediatric Endocrine Societies	Required: 1. Irregular menses/oligomenorrhea 2. Evidence of clinical and/or biochemical HA Optional: 1. PCOM Endorsed generally waiting 2 years after menarche for diagnosis

Abbreviations: HA, hyperandrogenism; PCOM, polycystic ovarian morphology; PCOS, polycystic ovarian syndrome.

year,[43,44] and by 3 years after menarche, the 5th and 95th percentiles for menstrual cycle length are 20.2 and 53.5 days, respectively.[43] Furthermore, the persistence of menstrual irregularities is an additional indicator of possible underlying pathology, such as PCOS.

The 2015 PES consensus put forth the following recommendations as evidence of true ovulatory dysfunction in an adolescent (Table 15.2): (1) consecutive menstrual intervals greater than 90 days, even in the first year after menarche; (2) menstrual intervals persistently less than 21 days or more than 45 days, 2 or more years after menarche; and (3) lack of menses by 15 years, or 2–3 years after breast budding.[3]

Signs of androgen excess

Hirsutism and acne may be clinical indicators of androgen excess in an adolescent, and the severity and progression of both of these features should be carefully followed. Hirsutism, defined as excessive, coarse, terminal hairs distributed in a male-like fashion, must be distinguished from hypertrichosis or excessive vellus hair distributed in a nonsexual pattern. PCOS is the most common cause of hirsutism among adolescent females.[45] However, not all patients with PCOS will present with this clinical finding. The severity of hirsutism does not correlate well with circulating androgens,[46] and ethnic/genetic differences can impact the development and severity of this feature.[47,48] The risk of underlying androgen excess is increased when hirsutism is associated with other PCOS findings, such as menstrual irregularities.[49]

The Ferriman-Gallwey scoring system has been used to quantify the degree of hirsutism in adults (Figure 15.2).[50,51] Its usefulness in early adolescence when sexual hair is still developing is not clear. It is generally agreed that isolated mild hirsutism is not clinical evidence of hyperandrogenism in early adolescence. Moderate to severe hirsutism and progressive hirsutism have both been endorsed as signs of androgen excess among adolescents (Table 15.2).[3,37]

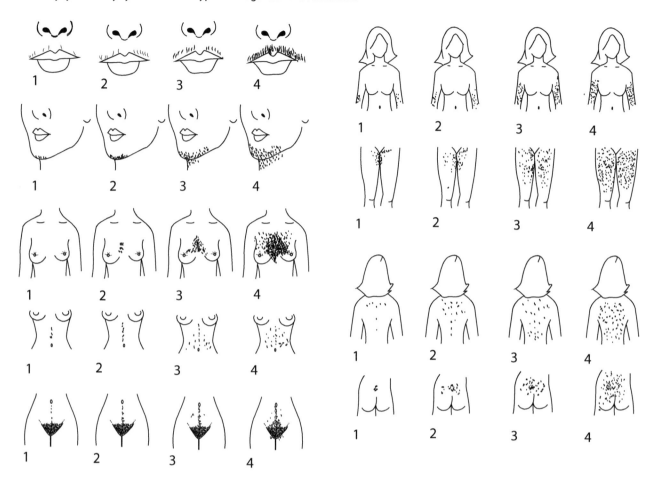

Figure 15.2 Ferriman-Gallwey hirsutism scoring system. Each of nine body areas is assigned a score from 0 (absence of terminal hairs) to 4 (extensive terminal hair growth), and these separate scores are summed to provide a total hirsutism score. (Reproduced with permission from Hatch R et al. *Am J Obstet Gynecol.* 1981;140[7]:815–30.)

Acne, a common finding in adolescence, is also frequently seen in adolescents with PCOS and may be the only pilosebaceous manifestation of androgen excess.[52,53] Although comedonal acne is common in adolescent females, moderate or severe comedonal acne (i.e., 10 or more facial lesions) in early puberty or moderate inflammatory acne through the peri-menarcheal years is uncommon (<5% prevalence).[54,55] While experts have disagreed on whether acne can be utilized as a marker of hyperandrogenism in adolescence,[37,40] recent consensus recommended evaluation for the presence of androgen excess in adolescents with persistent acne that is poorly responsive to topical therapy.[3] An updated document from this consensus group further suggested that severe cystic acne could be used in concert with irregular menses and other evidence of hyperandrogenism for the diagnosis of PCOS.[41] Alopecia can also signal hyperandrogenism but is rare in adolescents and is generally not recommended as diagnostic criteria of PCOS in adolescents (Table 15.2).

Premature adrenarche (PA) in childhood may also signal increased risk of PCOS in adolescence.[56,57] It is defined as the development of pubic hair before the age of 8 years in girls, regardless of race or ethnicity, with no other signs of sexual development. It is the result of an early increase in adrenal androgen production and is associated with hyperinsulinemia and obesity.[58] It is currently not known what proportion of girls with PA will go on to develop PCOS; however, continued prospective monitoring of girls with PA is endorsed with exclusion of congenital adrenal hyperplasia and Cushing syndrome if features are suggestive.[41,59]

Presenting clinical features can vary significantly in patients with PCOS. Efforts to bring attention to clinical and endocrinological differences have resulted in subclassification of PCOS into four distinct phenotypes (Figure 15.1). These phenotypes allow for further specification of patients with PCOS. Clinical correlation allows discernment of "ovulatory" versus "anovulatory" PCOS patients. Notably, not only the presence, but also the source, of androgen excess appears to have metabolic implications. Adrenal hormone excess in PCOS (as reflected by elevated DHEA-S concentrations) as compared to ovarian androgen excess has been shown to be associated with a better metabolic profile.[60]

Signs of metabolic comorbidity

Obesity and acanthosis nigricans are common clinical findings in patients with PCOS,[61] but neither are considered diagnostic criteria. Although highly prevalent,

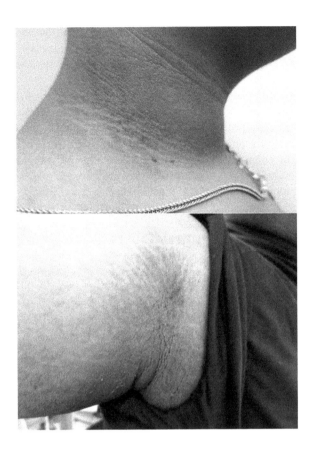

Figure 15.3 Acanthosis nigricans of neck (top) and axilla (bottom). (Reproduced with permission from Ng HY. *Adolesc Health Med Ther* 2017;8:1–10.)

overweight and obesity are not universally found among adolescents with PCOS. However, even nonobese adolescents with PCOS have been found to have twice as much abdominal fat as the reference population.[62,63] The presence of acanthosis nigricans, a velvety hyperpigmented thickening of the skin, particularly in intertriginous areas such as the neck and axilla (Figure 15.3) signals underlying insulin resistance and hyperinsulinemia.

LONG-TERM HEALTH CONSEQUENCES

PCOS is associated with long-term health risks that can impact almost every aspect of the adolescent and young woman's life. Metabolic, oncologic, reproductive, sleep, and psychiatric sequela have been reported.[64] Obesity is present in 35%–60% of women with PCOS, which can further exaggerate the metabolic consequences of the condition.[65,66]

Metabolic consequences

Impaired glucose tolerance and diabetes

Insulin resistance is common in PCOS, affecting up to 60%, and is found even in lean women with this syndrome.[67] Deficiencies in insulin action stimulate higher LH-mediated androgen secretion from ovarian thecal cells. Although insulin resistance is independent of obesity/overweight status, weight gain (particularly accumulation of visceral adiposity) contributes to a more severe

phenotype. The presence of obesity in adolescents with PCOS is associated with a higher risk for impaired glucose metabolism and a threefold to sevenfold increased risk of developing type 2 diabetes.[68–70] A concomitant increased risk of gestational diabetes has also been established in women with PCOS.[71,72]

Dyslipidemia and cardiovascular disease

PCOS is inherently associated with accumulation of several risk factors for early cardiovascular disease.[73] Whether this translates into a higher risk of myocardial infarction and/or death is still under study, but growing evidence points to an increase in stroke, myocardial infarction, and mortality, independent of obesity status. A recent meta-analysis found the body mass index (BMI) adjusted relative risk for coronary heart disease (CHD) or stroke was 1.55 in patients with PCOS compared to women without PCOS.[74] An earlier report found an increase in coronary artery disease severity in women with PCOM versus those with normal ovaries.[75] To varying degrees, both hyperandrogenism and chronic anovulation, features intrinsic to PCOS, may also be independent risk factors for increased risk of cardiovascular disease.[76,77] These findings were corroborated in the Nurse's Health Study as well; wherein, women with oligomenorrhea had a higher incidence of both fatal and nonfatal cardiovascular disease.[78]

Dyslipidemia prevalence approaches 70% in PCOS.[79] Both hyperinsulinemia and obesity exacerbate the propensity to have abnormal lipids.[80] The pattern of dyslipidemia in PCOS demonstrates decreased levels of high-density cholesterol lipoprotein (HDL-C), increased levels of low-density lipoprotein cholesterol (LDL-C), and elevated levels of triglycerides, all of which are well known to be independent risk factors of cardiovascular disease.[81–83] In addition, both insulin resistance and chronic unopposed estrogen concentrations have been thought to be responsible for accelerated cardiovascular disease in PCOS.[64]

Due to the lack of a singular definition of PCOS, rarity of cardiovascular events in premenopausal women, and paucity of long-term prospective studies on metabolic consequences, it is difficult to establish the extent of increased risk conferred by PCOS. However, it is safe to surmise that the PCOS population is at increased risk of several cardiovascular and metabolic health consequences. Although nonalcoholic fatty liver disease (NAFLD) may occur frequently in PCOS, thus far it has been difficult to establish with certainty if there is added risk beyond the obesity inherent to most cases of PCOS.[84]

Cancer risk in PCOS

Endometrial cancer

Due to chronic anovulation and unopposed estrogen, risk of endometrial hyperplasia and eventual carcinoma is higher, both in theory and proven in research endeavors.[85,86] Other risk factors inherently present in the majority of women with PCOS, such as obesity, long-term use of estrogen, infertility, nulliparity, hypertension, and diabetes, are additive risk factors for endometrial cancer.[87] Menstrual cycles longer than 3 months apart have been associated with endometrial hyperplasia and carcinoma.[85] Although estimates vary, the increased risk could be up to three times higher.[88] Interestingly, elevated circulating androstenedione concentrations have also been associated with endometrial cancer risk.[89]

Breast and ovarian cancer

It has not been established whether there is an increased risk of breast cancer in women with PCOS. To date, most studies have not established an increased risk of breast cancer,[86,90] despite there being several risk factors for breast cancer present in this population, including obesity and infertility. Generally reassuring data exist with regard to ovarian cancer with most of the increased risk arising in the setting of fertility treatments and induced ovulations, wherein the risk of ovarian cancer in PCOS may be higher than in controls.[91]

Reproductive implications

From conception to delivery, PCOS presents a challenge to pregnancy. It is the most common cause of anovulatory infertility. Almost 90% of anovulatory women seeking fertility treatment may have underlying PCOS. Even after becoming pregnant, women with PCOS are at higher risk than those without PCOS of developing gestational diabetes, having a large for gestational age infant, developing hypertension and preeclampsia, as well as having spontaneous abortions and preterm delivery.[92,93]

Psychiatric comorbidity

It is increasingly being recognized that adolescents and young women with PCOS are at increased risk of mood disorders, independent of obesity status. Recent meta-analyses have reported this finding, noting that women with PCOS may be three times more likely to suffer from anxiety and depression as compared to those without PCOS.[94] Lower BMI does tend to correlate with improvement in anxiety and depression scores.[95] Past research has demonstrated that hirsutism, low self-esteem, and poor body image are also associated with psychological distress and decreased health-related quality of life in women with PCOS.[96,97]

Sleep-related complications

Sleep-related dysfunction has been well established in adolescents and women with PCOS and exceeds the projected range due to weight abnormalities. Although initially restricted to reports of obstructive sleep apnea,[98] other sleep-related pathology, such as insomnia and excessive daytime sleepiness, is increasingly being reported. These findings are only partially accounted for by body weight and depressive symptoms.[99,100]

EVALUATION

PCOS is a diagnosis of exclusion, and the clinical evaluation commences with a search for disorders mimicking the condition. These include, but are not limited to, other causes of hyperandrogenism and oligo/anovulation such as late-onset congenital adrenal hyperplasia, adrenal or ovarian tumors, hyperprolactinemia, thyroid dysfunction, and premature ovarian failure.[101]

Detailed history and physical examination are the first steps toward establishment of a PCOS diagnosis. History should specifically query about age at menarche; menstrual cycle length; ovulatory symptoms; birth weight; weight changes; dietary history; premature adrenarche/pubarche; presence of hirsutism, recalcitrant acne, or hidradenitis suppurativa; and detailed family history of diabetes, infertility, or recurrent miscarriages. History of low birth weight with excessive catch-up growth is particularly noteworthy. During the physical examination, the clinician should make note of signs of acanthosis nigricans, hirsutism, acne, and/or male pattern baldness. Assessment of weight, height, and visceral adiposity, utilizing the waist-to-hip ratio, is also important.[102]

Laboratory evaluation is done to exclude the presence of thyroid dysfunction and hyperprolactinemia and to evaluate for the presence of hyperandrogenemia. Despite inconsistencies in reliable specialized assays for common androgen measurements, particularly in the pediatric age,[103] it is recommended to obtain free and/or total testosterone, 17-hydroxyprogesterone and dehydroepiandrosterone sulfate (DHEA-S) concentrations to exclude other causes of androgen excess.[104] Although androgen concentrations are somewhat reflective of underlying hyperandrogenism, there is often poor correlation between clinical signs and symptoms of androgen excess and serum androgen levels. This is likely due to the inability to accurately quantify the bioactive percentage of the hormones.[105]

Screening for associated metabolic and mental health comorbidities is also recommended. The presence of insulin resistance is nearly universal in adolescents and women with PCOS, ranging from 50% to 70%.[106,107] Based on the 2013 Endocrine Society Clinical Practice Guideline, it is recommended to obtain an oral glucose tolerance test (OGTT), consisting of a fasting and 2-hour glucose level using a 75 g oral glucose load, to screen for impaired glucose tolerance and type 2 diabetes in adolescents and adult women with PCOS.[40] A fasting lipid panel is also recommended to evaluate for lipid abnormalities.[108,109] Dyslipidemia, regardless of BMI, is often characterized by hypertriglyceridemia, decrease in high-density lipoprotein (HDL)-cholesterol and increase in low-density lipoprotein (LDL)-cholesterol which is the precursor to sex steroid synthesis. Although concern for and awareness of the high prevalence of NAFLD should exist, routine screening with liver function tests is currently not recommended. Reliable testing for insulin resistance is not easily performed, and given the lack of inclusion for the diagnosis of any published criteria, testing for insulin levels is also not recommended. The use of validated screening tools to rule out mood-related disorders and sleep-disordered breathing is essential. Common laboratory tests and their indications are summarized in Table 15.3.

Table 15.3 Common laboratory tests for evaluation of polycystic ovary syndrome.

Laboratory test	Indication
TSH ± Free T4	Exclude thyroid dysfunction
Prolactin	Exclude hyperprolactinemia
Free and/or total testosterone	Evaluate for hyperandrogenism
Dehydroepiandrosterone sulfate (DHEA-S)	Exclude other causes of HA
17-Hydroxyprogesterone	Exclude other causes of HA
Oral glucose tolerance test	Screening for IGT and type 2 diabetes
Fasting lipid profile	Screening for dyslipidemia

Abbreviations: HA, hyperandrogenism; IGT, impaired glucose tolerance.

Pelvic ultrasonography is generally considered optional in the evaluation of adolescents with features consistent with PCOS. Pelvic ultrasonography is not required for diagnosis in this age group; however, it may be indicated based on clinical features to rule out other underlying pathology.[104] Three-dimensional magnetic resonance imaging (MRI) has recently been evaluated as a diagnostic imaging modality for adolescents with suspected PCOS.[110] MRI may prove to be a superior modality for characterizing polycystic ovaries in this population (Figure 15.4).

MANAGEMENT

The cornerstone of management of PCOS remains a healthy lifestyle, which can have broad benefits for adolescents with this syndrome (Table 15.4). Decrease in body weight, particularly abdominal fat, reduces serum testosterone, insulin resistance, and hirsutism in women with PCOS.[111] Increased menstrual regularity is also seen with weight loss.[112] Lifestyle interventions resulting in even a 5% weight loss can decrease risk of dyslipidemia and metabolic and cardiovascular risk.[112]

Use of combined hormonal contraceptives (CHCs) can be particularly helpful for managing menstrual irregularity and decreasing the risk of endometrial hyperplasia or carcinoma. CHCs can also decrease signs of androgen excess, such as hirsutism, acne, and alopecia.[66] At least 6 months of treatment may be needed to see a full response. After at least 6 months of CHC therapy, antiandrogens can be added if further improvement in symptoms is necessary.[66]

CHCs reduce symptoms of PCOS via several mechanisms. They promote negative feedback on LH, causing lowered ovarian androgen production. They also decrease free androgen concentrations by increasing the production of sex-hormone-binding globulin in the liver. They may also inhibit peripheral conversion of testosterone to dihydrotestosterone, as well as reduce adrenal androgen production.[113] Use of CHCs with lower androgenic potential, such as norethindrone, desogestrel, and norgestimate,

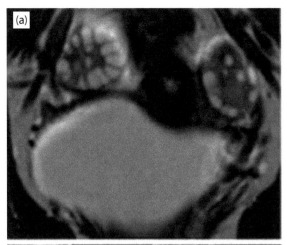
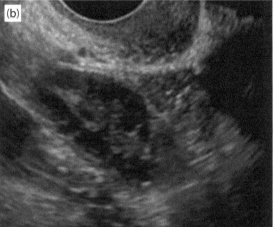
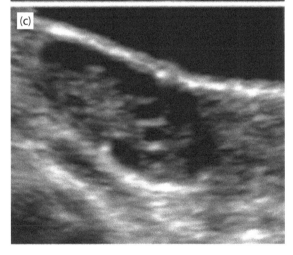

Figure 15.4 Ovarian morphology. (a) Magnetic resonance imaging (MRI), (b) transvaginal ultrasound, (c) transabdominal ultrasound. (a) Coronal view by MRI of an ovary in an adolescent subject with polycystic ovarian syndrome (PCOS). Follicles (hyperintense) are clearly demarcated from stroma (hypointense). (b,c) Ultrasound images from adolescent subjects with PCOS, with (b) representing a transvaginal image and (c) representing a transabdominal image. Follicles are visualized in black (hypoechoic), with stroma appearing more hyperechoic. Distinguishing individual follicles by ultrasound is difficult, precluding a follicle count. (Reproduced with permission from Kenigsberg LE et al. *Fertil Steril*. 2015;104[5]:1302–9.)

Table 15.4 Potential benefits of current polycystic ovary syndrome (PCOS) treatment modalities.

Treatment	Irregular menses	Androgen excess	Hirsutism	Acne	Insulin resistance	Obesity	Dyslipidemia	Endometrial hyperplasia/ carcinoma	Comment
Lifestyle interventions[a]	X	X	X	*	X	X	X	X	First-line therapy for overweight/ obese adolescents
Combined hormonal contraceptives	XX	X	X	X				XX	First-line therapy for menstrual irregularities
Metformin and/or thiazolidinediones	*	X	X	*	XX	X	X		Recommended for PCOS patients with impaired glucose tolerance refractory to lifestyle changes
Antiandrogens	X	X	X	X					Spironolactone best studied
Cosmetic hair removal			X						Photoepilation recommended first line for localized hirsutism

Note: X, potential for benefit; XX, potential for high benefit; *, may be helpful but insufficient evidence exists.
a Weight loss and intense exercise.

is preferred.[66] Drospirenone containing CHC can act as weak androgen receptor antagonists but can precipitate hyperkalemia, particularly in those on concurrent therapy with spironolactone, and may have an increase in incidence of deep vein thrombosis.[114]

Metformin and/or thiazolidinediones have been recommended for women with PCOS with type 2 diabetes or impaired glucose tolerance who do not improve with lifestyle changes.[40] These agents can reduce insulin concentrations and improve androgenic symptoms by causing a concomitant decline in testosterone levels. A recent meta-analysis of randomized controlled trials evaluating the use of metformin versus CHC for the treatment of PCOS in adolescents found metformin to be as effective as CHC for treatment of hirsutism. Metformin was found to be superior for weight reduction and improved dysglycemia, and CHC was preferable for menstrual regulation. The authors stressed, however, that overall quality of current data is poor.[115]

Antiandrogens can be used in combination with CHC or metformin to achieve further improvement in cutaneous symptoms. Spironolactone is most commonly used. It functions as an aldosterone antagonist in addition to directly inhibiting 5α-reductase activity, decreasing active androgen concentrations at hair follicles.[113] Spironolactone doses are started at 25 mg and adjusted over time while monitoring for hyperkalemia. The highest recommended dose is 200 mg daily. Combination metformin and spironolactone has been found to be superior to either drug alone in improving menstrual irregularity, hirsutism, serum androgen levels, and insulin resistance.[116] Finasteride is an antiandrogen that blocks hepatic 5α-reductase, reducing conversion of testosterone to dihydrotestosterone.[117] Intermittent low-dose oral finasteride was found to be effective for treatment of hirsutism in adolescent girls with PCOS or idiopathic hirsutism.[118] Importantly, both spironolactone and finasteride must be used in combination with effective contraception in sexually active adolescents due to teratogenic potential.

A cosmetic hair removal process can offer more immediate results for patients without need for prescription. Electrolysis and laser hair removal therapies are becoming increasingly popular and affordable. Eflornithine is a prescription topical cream effective for removal of unwanted facial hair in females.[66] It inhibits the enzyme ornithine decarboxylase at the hair follicle, reducing the rate of hair growth. Eflornithine combined with laser therapy resulted in more rapid reduction in facial hair as compared to laser treatment alone.[119,120] Drawbacks include need for indefinite use to maintain efficacy and lack of coverage by most insurance plans in the United States.

Although infertility is rarely a complaint of adolescents with PCOS, treatment options for infertility are worth noting. Weight loss is first-line therapy, with some studies reporting that even a 5%–10% reduction in weight can result in increased ovulation rate and subsequent pregnancies.[121] Bariatric surgery has also been shown to improve cycle regularity and increase spontaneous conception.[122–125]

Emotional support and psychological counseling are beneficial for adolescents with PCOS to manage psychiatric comorbidities. Optimal management of the adolescent with PCOS consists of a multidisciplinary team that can include a gynecologist or adolescent medicine specialist, endocrinologist, psychiatrist, psychologist, dermatologist, nutritionist, and primary care provider.

SUMMARY

Despite being the most common endocrine disorder in women, much remains unknown about PCOS. Nevertheless, evidence-based expert recommendations have recently become more available, aiding the clinician with the diagnosis and management of PCOS in adolescents. Although the presence of polycystic ovaries is a key diagnostic criterion in adults, there is currently no convincing standard for defining PCOM in adolescents. As such, the diagnosis of PCOS in adolescents currently hinges on evidence of ovulatory dysfunction and androgen excess. However, a definitive diagnosis of PCOS is not needed to initiate treatment in an adolescent. Treatment may decrease the risk of future comorbidity, even in the absence of a definitive diagnosis. Deferring diagnosis, while providing symptom treatment and regular/frequent follow-up of symptomology, is a recommended option. Treatment goals are to improve quality of life and long-term health outcomes, and treatment options should be individualized to the presentation, needs, and preferences of each patient.

REFERENCES

1. Stein I, Leventhal M. Amenorrhea associated with bilateral polycystic ovaries. *Am J Obstet Gynecol.* 1935;29:181–91.
2. Fauser BC, Tarlatzis BC, Rebar RW et al. Consensus on women's health aspects of polycystic ovary syndrome (PCOS): The Amsterdam ESHRE/ASRM-Sponsored 3rd PCOS Consensus Workshop Group. *Fertil Steril.* 2012;97:28–38, e25.
3. Witchel SF, Oberfield S, Rosenfield RL et al. The diagnosis of polycystic ovary syndrome during adolescence. *Horm Res Paediatr.* 2015.
4. Rosenfield RL, Ehrmann DA. The pathogenesis of polycystic ovary syndrome (PCOS): The hypothesis of PCOS as functional ovarian hyperandrogenism revisited. *Endocr Rev.* 2016;37:467–520.
5. Yen SS, Vela P, Rankin J. Inappropriate secretion of follicle-stimulating hormone and luteinizing hormone in polycystic ovarian disease. *J Clin Endocrinol Metab.* 1970;30:435–42.
6. Dunaif A, Segal KR, Futterweit W, Dobrjansky A. Profound peripheral insulin resistance, independent of obesity, in polycystic ovary syndrome. *Diabetes.* 1989;38:1165–74.
7. Barbieri RL, Makris A, Randall RW, Daniels G, Kistner RW, Ryan KJ. Insulin stimulates androgen accumulation in incubations of ovarian stroma obtained from women with hyperandrogenism. *J Clin Endocrinol Metab.* 1986;62:904–10.

8. Barnes RB, Rosenfield RL, Burstein S, Ehrmann DA. Pituitary-ovarian responses to nafarelin testing in the polycystic ovary syndrome. *N Engl J Med.* 1989;320:559–65.

9. Rittmaster RS, Thompson DL. Effect of leuprolide and dexamethasone on hair growth and hormone levels in hirsute women: The relative importance of the ovary and the adrenal in the pathogenesis of hirsutism. *J Clin Endocrinol Metab.* 1990;70:1096–102.

10. Lachelin GC, Judd HL, Swanson SC, Hauck ME, Parker DC, Yen SS. Long term effects of nightly dexamethasone administration in patients with polycystic ovarian disease. *J Clin Endocrinol Metab.* 1982;55:768–73.

11. Andersen CY, Lossl K. Increased intrafollicular androgen levels affect human granulosa cell secretion of anti-Mullerian hormone and inhibin-B. *Fertil Steril.* 2008;89:1760–5.

12. Song DK, Oh JY, Lee H, Sung YA. Differentiation between polycystic ovary syndrome and polycystic ovarian morphology by means of an anti-Mullerian hormone cutoff value. *Korean J Intern Med.* 2017;32:690–8.

13. Rosenfield RL, Barnes RB, Cara JF, Lucky AW. Dysregulation of cytochrome P450c 17α as the cause of polycystic ovarian syndrome. *Fertil Steril.* 1990;53:785–91.

14. Miller WL, Tee MK. The post-translational regulation of 17,20 lyase activity. *Mol Cell Endocrinol.* 2015;408:99–106.

15. Magoffin DA. Evidence that luteinizing hormone-stimulated differentiation of purified ovarian thecal-interstitial cells is mediated by both type I and type II adenosine 3′,5′-monophosphate-dependent protein kinases. *Endocrinology.* 1989;125:1464–73.

16. Blasio AM D, Voutilainen R, Jaffe RB, Miller WL. Hormonal regulation of messenger ribonucleic acids for P450scc (cholesterol side-chain cleavage enzyme) and P450c17 (17α-hydroxylase/17,20-lyase) in cultured human fetal adrenal cells. *J Clin Endocrinol Metab.* 1987;65:170–5.

17. McAllister JM, Byrd W, Simpson ER. The effects of growth factors and phorbol esters on steroid biosynthesis in isolated human theca interna and granulosa-lutein cells in long term culture. *J Clin Endocrinol Metab.* 1994;79:106–12.

18. Du X, Rosenfield RL, Qin K. KLF15 Is a transcriptional regulator of the human 17ß-hydroxysteroid dehydrogenase type 5 gene. A potential link between regulation of testosterone production and fat stores in women. *J Clin Endocrinol Metab.* 2009;94:2594–601.

19. Wu S, Divall S, Nwaopara A et al. Obesity-induced infertility and hyperandrogenism are corrected by deletion of the insulin receptor in the ovarian theca cell. *Diabetes.* 2014;63:1270–82.

20. McAllister JM, Modi B, Miller BA et al. Overexpression of a DENND1A isoform produces a polycystic ovary syndrome theca phenotype. *Proc Natl Acad Sci U S A.* 2014;111:E1519–27.

21. Casarini L, Brigante G. The polycystic ovary syndrome evolutionary paradox: A genome-wide association studies-based, in silico, evolutionary explanation. *J Clin Endocrinol Metab.* 2014;99:E2412–20.

22. Abbott DH, Nicol LE, Levine JE, Xu N, Goodarzi MO, Dumesic DA. Nonhuman primate models of polycystic ovary syndrome. *Mol Cell Endocrinol.* 2013;373:21–8.

23. Xita N, Tsatsoulis A. Review: Fetal programming of polycystic ovary syndrome by androgen excess: Evidence from experimental, clinical, and genetic association studies. *J Clin Endocrinol Metab.* 2006;91:1660–6.

24. Abbott DH, Barnett DK, Bruns CM, Dumesic DA. Androgen excess fetal programming of female reproduction: A developmental aetiology for polycystic ovary syndrome? *Hum Reprod Update.* 2005;11:357–74.

25. Abbott DH, Tarantal AF, Dumesic DA. Fetal, infant, adolescent and adult phenotypes of polycystic ovary syndrome in prenatally androgenized female rhesus monkeys. *Am J Primatol.* 2009;71:776–84.

26. Ibanez L, Diaz R, Lopez-Bermejo A, Marcos MV. Clinical spectrum of premature pubarche: Links to metabolic syndrome and ovarian hyperandrogenism. *Rev Endocr Metab Disord.* 2009;10:63–76.

27. Ibanez L, Valls C, Potau N, Marcos MV, de Zegher F. Polycystic ovary syndrome after precocious pubarche: Ontogeny of the low-birthweight effect. *Clin Endocrinol (Oxf).* 2001;55:667–72.

28. Ibanez L, Lopez-Bermejo A, Callejo J et al. Polycystic ovaries in nonobese adolescents and young women with ovarian androgen excess: Relation to prenatal growth. *J Clin Endocrinol Metab.* 2008;93:196–9.

29. Diamanti-Kandarakis E, Christakou C, Palioura E, Kandaraki E, Livadas S. Does polycystic ovary syndrome start in childhood? *Pediatr Endocrinol Rev.* 2008;5:904–11.

30. O'Brien RF, Emans SJ. Polycystic ovary syndrome in adolescents. *J Pediatr Adolesc Gynecol.* 2008;21:119–28.

31. Zawadzki JK, Dunaif A. Diagnostic criteria for polycystic ovary syndrome: Towards a rational approach. In: Dunaif A, Givens JR, Haseltine F, Merriam GR, eds. *Polycystic Ovary Syndrome.* Boston, MA: Blackwell Scientific; 1992:377–84.

32. The Rotterdam ESHRE/ASRM-sponsored PCOS consensus workshop group. Revised 2003 consensus on diagnostic criteria and long-term health risks related to polycystic ovary syndrome (PCOS). *Hum Reprod.* 2004;19:41–7.

33. Azziz R, Carmina E, Dewailly D et al. Positions statement: Criteria for defining polycystic ovary syndrome as a predominantly hyperandrogenic syndrome: An Androgen Excess Society guideline. *J Clin Endocrinol Metab.* 2006;91:4237–45.

34. Blank SK, Helm KD, McCartney CR, Marshall JC. Polycystic ovary syndrome in adolescence. *Ann N Y Acad Sci.* 2008;1135:76–84.

35. Fanelli F, Gambineri A, Mezzullo M et al. Revisiting hyper- and hypo-androgenism by tandem mass spectrometry. *Rev Endocr Metab Disord*. 2013;14:185–205.

36. Hickey M, Doherty DA, Atkinson H et al. Clinical, ultrasound and biochemical features of polycystic ovary syndrome in adolescents: Implications for diagnosis. *Hum Reprod*. 2011;26:1469–77.

37. Carmina E, Oberfield SE, Lobo RA. The diagnosis of polycystic ovary syndrome in adolescents. *Am J Obstet Gynecol*. 2010;203:201, e1–5.

38. Villarroel C, Merino PM, Lopez P et al. Polycystic ovarian morphology in adolescents with regular menstrual cycles is associated with elevated anti-Mullerian hormone. *Hum Reprod*. 2011;26:2861–8.

39. Codner E, Villarroel C, Eyzaguirre FC et al. Polycystic ovarian morphology in postmenarchal adolescents. *Fertil Steril*. 2011;95:702–6, e1–2.

40. Legro RS, Arslanian SA, Ehrmann DA et al. Diagnosis and treatment of polycystic ovary syndrome: An Endocrine Society clinical practice guideline. *J Clin Endocrinol Metab*. 2013;98:4565–92.

41. Ibanez L, Oberfield SE, Witchel S et al. An international consortium update: Pathophysiology, diagnosis, and treatment of polycystic ovarian syndrome in adolescence. *Horm Res Paediatr*. 2017;88:371–95.

42. Maslyanskaya S, Talib HJ, Northridge JL, Jacobs AM, Coble C, Coupey SM. Polycystic ovary syndrome: An under-recognized cause of abnormal uterine bleeding in adolescents admitted to a children's hospital. *J Pediatr Adolesc Gynecol*. 2017;30:349–55.

43. Treloar AE, Boynton RE, Behn BG, Brown BW. Variation of the human menstrual cycle through reproductive life. *Int J Fertil*. 1967;12:77–126.

44. Diaz A, Laufer MR, Breech LL. Menstruation in girls and adolescents: Using the menstrual cycle as a vital sign. *Pediatrics*. 2006;118:2245–50.

45. Plouffe L, Jr. Disorders of excessive hair growth in the adolescent. *Obstet Gynecol Clin North Am*. 2000;27:79–99.

46. Yildiz BO, Bolour S, Woods K, Moore A, Azziz R. Visually scoring hirsutism. *Hum Reprod Update*. 2010;16:51–64.

47. Li R, Qiao J, Yang D et al. Epidemiology of hirsutism among women of reproductive age in the community: A simplified scoring system. *Eur J Obstet Gynecol Reprod Biol*. 2012;163:165–9.

48. Engmann L, Jin S, Sun F et al. Racial and ethnic differences in the polycystic ovary syndrome metabolic phenotype. *Am J Obstet Gynecol*. 2017;216:493, e1–e13.

49. Hawryluk EB, English JC, 3rd. Female adolescent hair disorders. *J Pediatr Adolesc Gynecol*. 2009;22:271–81.

50. Hatch R, Rosenfield RL, Kim MH, Tredway D. Hirsutism: Implications, etiology, and management. *Am J Obstet Gynecol*. 1981;140:815–30.

51. Martin KA, Chang RJ, Ehrmann DA et al. Evaluation and treatment of hirsutism in premenopausal women: An Endocrine Society clinical practice guideline. *J Clin Endocrinol Metab*. 2008;93:1105–20.

52. Chen WC, Zouboulis CC. Hormones and the pilosebaceous unit. *Dermatoendocrinol*. 2009;1:81–6.

53. Lowenstein EJ. Diagnosis and management of the dermatologic manifestations of the polycystic ovary syndrome. *Dermatol Ther*. 2006;19:210–23.

54. Lucky AW, Biro FM, Simbartl LA, Morrison JA, Sorg NW. Predictors of severity of acne vulgaris in young adolescent girls: Results of a five-year longitudinal study. *J Pediatr*. 1997;130:30–9.

55. Eichenfield LF, Krakowski AC, Piggott C et al. Evidence-based recommendations for the diagnosis and treatment of pediatric acne. *Pediatrics*. 2013;131(Suppl. 3):S163–86.

56. Ibanez L, Dimartino-Nardi J, Potau N, Saenger P. Premature adrenarche—Normal variant or forerunner of adult disease? *Endocr Rev*. 2000;21:671–96.

57. Ibanez L, Potau N, Virdis R et al. Postpubertal outcome in girls diagnosed of premature pubarche during childhood: Increased frequency of functional ovarian hyperandrogenism. *J Clin Endocrinol Metab*. 1993;76:1599–603.

58. Diaz A, Bhandari S, Sison C, Vogiatzi M. Characteristics of children with premature pubarche in the New York metropolitan area. *Horm Res*. 2008;70:150–4.

59. Oberfield SE, Sopher AB, Gerken AT. Approach to the girl with early onset of pubic hair. *J Clin Endocrinol Metab*. 2011;96:1610–22.

60. Nofal A A, Viers LD, Javed A. Can the source of hyperandrogenism in adolescents with polycystic ovary syndrome predict metabolic phenotype? *Gynecol Endocrinol*. 2017;33:882–7.

61. Buggs C, Rosenfield RL. Polycystic ovary syndrome in adolescence. *Endocrinol Metab Clin North Am*. 2005;34:677–705, x.

62. Coviello AD, Legro RS, Dunaif A. Adolescent girls with polycystic ovary syndrome have an increased risk of the metabolic syndrome associated with increasing androgen levels independent of obesity and insulin resistance. *J Clin Endocrinol Metab*. 2006;91:492–7.

63. Lee S, Gungor N, Bacha F, Arslanian S. Insulin resistance: Link to the components of the metabolic syndrome and biomarkers of endothelial dysfunction in youth. *Diabetes Care*. 2007;30:2091–7.

64. Daniilidis A, Dinas K. Long term health consequences of polycystic ovarian syndrome: A review analysis. *Hippokratia*. 2009;13:90–2.

65. Teede HJ, Joham AE, Paul E et al. Longitudinal weight gain in women identified with polycystic ovary syndrome: Results of an observational study in young women. *Obesity (Silver Spring)*. 2013;21:1526–32.

66. Badawy A, Elnashar A. Treatment options for polycystic ovary syndrome. *Int J Womens Health*. 2011;3:25–35.

67. Legro RS, Kunselman AR, Dodson WC, Dunaif A. Prevalence and predictors of risk for type 2 diabetes mellitus and impaired glucose tolerance in polycystic

ovary syndrome: A prospective, controlled study in 254 affected women. *J Clin Endocrinol Metab.* 1999;84:165–9.

68. Wijeyaratne CN, Balen AH, Barth JH, Belchetz PE. Clinical manifestations and insulin resistance (IR) in polycystic ovary syndrome (PCOS) among South Asians and Caucasians: Is there a difference? *Clin Endocrinol (Oxf).* 2002;57:343–50.

69. Gopal M, Duntley S, Uhles M, Attarian H. The role of obesity in the increased prevalence of obstructive sleep apnea syndrome in patients with polycystic ovarian syndrome. *Sleep Med.* 2002;3:401–4.

70. Palmert MR, Gordon CM, Kartashov AI, Legro RS, Emans SJ, Dunaif A. Screening for abnormal glucose tolerance in adolescents with polycystic ovary syndrome. *J Clin Endocrinol Metab.* 2002;87:1017–23.

71. Rizzo M, Berneis K, Spinas G, Rini GB, Carmina E. Long-term consequences of polycystic ovary syndrome on cardiovascular risk. *Fertil Steril.* 2009;91:1563–7.

72. Sharma A, Yousef M. Recent development in polycystic ovary syndrome. In: Studd J, ed. *Progress in Obstetrics and Gynecology*; 2005:227–39.

73. Wild S, Pierpoint T, McKeigue P, Jacobs H. Cardiovascular disease in women with polycystic ovary syndrome at long-term follow-up: A retrospective cohort study. *Clin Endocrinol (Oxf).* 2000;52:595–600.

74. de Groot PC, Dekkers OM, Romijn JA, Dieben SW, Helmerhorst FM. PCOS, coronary heart disease, stroke and the influence of obesity: A systematic review and meta-analysis. *Hum Reprod Update.* 2011;17:495–500.

75. Birdsall MA, Farquhar CM, White HD. Association between polycystic ovaries and extent of coronary artery disease in women having cardiac catheterization. *Ann Intern Med.* 1997;126:32–5.

76. Solomon CG, Hu FB, Dunaif A et al. Menstrual cycle irregularity and risk for future cardiovascular disease. *J Clin Endocrinol Metab.* 2002;87:2013–7.

77. Gorgels WJ, v d Graaf Y, Blankenstein MA, Collette HJ, Erkelens DW, Banga JD. Urinary sex hormone excretions in premenopausal women and coronary heart disease risk: A nested case-referent study in the DOM-cohort. *J Clin Epidemiol.* 1997;50:275–81.

78. Solomon CG, Hu FB, Dunaif A et al. Long or highly irregular menstrual cycles as a marker for risk of type 2 diabetes mellitus. *JAMA.* 2001;286:2421–6.

79. Legro RS, Kunselman AR, Dunaif A. Prevalence and predictors of dyslipidemia in women with polycystic ovary syndrome. *Am J Med.* 2001;111:607–13.

80. Mather KJ, Kwan F, Corenblum B. Hyperinsulinemia in polycystic ovary syndrome correlates with increased cardiovascular risk independent of obesity. *Fertil Steril.* 2000;73:150–6.

81. Reaven GM. Banting lecture 1988. Role of insulin resistance in human disease. *Diabetes.* 1988;37:1595–607.

82. Dejager S, Pichard C, Giral P et al. Smaller LDL particle size in women with polycystic ovary syndrome compared to controls. *Clin Endocrinol (Oxf).* 2001;54:455–62.

83. Austin MA, Breslow JL, Hennekens CH, Buring JE, Willett WC, Krauss RM. Low-density lipoprotein subclass patterns and risk of myocardial infarction. *JAMA.* 1988;260:1917–21.

84. Gutierrez-Grobe Y, Ponciano-Rodriguez G, Ramos MH, Uribe M, Mendez-Sanchez N. Prevalence of non-alcoholic fatty liver disease in premenopausal, postmenopausal and polycystic ovary syndrome women. The role of estrogens. *Ann Hepatol.* 2010;9:402–9.

85. Cheung AP. Ultrasound and menstrual history in predicting endometrial hyperplasia in polycystic ovary syndrome. *Obstet Gynecol.* 2001;98:325–31.

86. Royal College of Obstetricians and Gynaecologists. Long-term consequence of polycystic ovary syndrome. *Green-top Guideline No. 33,* 2014:1–15.

87. Wild RA. Long-term health consequences of PCOS. *Hum Reprod Update.* 2002;8:231–41.

88. Balen A, Rajkhowa R. Health consequences of polycystic ovary syndrome. In: Balen A, ed. *Reproductive Endocrinology for the MRCOG and Beyond.* London, UK: RCOG Press; 2003:99–107.

89. Potischman N, Hoover RN, Brinton LA et al. Case-control study of endogenous steroid hormones and endometrial cancer. *J Natl Cancer Inst.* 1996;88:1127–35.

90. Pierpoint T, McKeigue PM, Isaacs AJ, Wild SH, Jacobs HS. Mortality of women with polycystic ovary syndrome at long-term follow-up. *J Clin Epidemiol.* 1998;51:581–6.

91. Rossing MA, Daling JR, Weiss NS, Moore DE, Self SG. Ovarian tumors in a cohort of infertile women. *N Engl J Med.* 1994;331:771–6.

92. Sirmans SM, Parish RC, Blake S, Wang X. Epidemiology and comorbidities of polycystic ovary syndrome in an indigent population. *J Investig Med.* 2014;62:868–74.

93. Salley KE, Wickham EP, Cheang KI, Essah PA, Karjane NW, Nestler JE. Glucose intolerance in polycystic ovary syndrome—A position statement of the Androgen Excess Society. *J Clin Endocrinol Metab.* 2007;92:4546–56.

94. Blay SL, Aguiar JV, Passos IC. Polycystic ovary syndrome and mental disorders: A systematic review and exploratory meta-analysis. *Neuropsychiatr Dis Treat.* 2016;12:2895–903.

95. Barry JA, Kuczmierczyk AR, Hardiman PJ. Anxiety and depression in polycystic ovary syndrome: A systematic review and meta-analysis. *Hum Reprod.* 2011;26:2442–51.

96. Borghi L, Leone D, Vegni E et al. Psychological distress, anger and quality of life in polycystic ovary syndrome: Associations with biochemical, phenotypical and socio-demographic factors. *J Psychosom Obstet Gynaecol.* 2017;1–10.

97. Kaczmarek C, Haller DM, Yaron M. Health-related quality of life in adolescents and young adults with polycystic ovary syndrome: A systematic review. *J Pediatr Adolesc Gynecol.* 2016;29:551–7.

98. Vgontzas AN, Legro RS, Bixler EO, Grayev A, Kales A, Chrousos GP. Polycystic ovary syndrome is associated with obstructive sleep apnea and daytime sleepiness: Role of insulin resistance. *J Clin Endocrinol Metab.* 2001;86:517–20.

99. Moran LJ, March WA, Whitrow MJ, Giles LC, Davies MJ, Moore VM. Sleep disturbances in a community-based sample of women with polycystic ovary syndrome. *Hum Reprod.* 2015;30:466–72.

100. Franik G, Krysta K, Madej P et al. Sleep disturbances in women with polycystic ovary syndrome. *Gynecol Endocrinol.* 2016;32:1014–7.

101. Kyritsi EM, Dimitriadis GK, Kyrou I, Kaltsas G, Randeva HS. PCOS remains a diagnosis of exclusion: A concise review of key endocrinopathies to exclude. *Clin Endocrinol (Oxf).* 2017;86:1–6.

102. Goodman NF, Bledsoe MB, Cobin RH et al. American Association of Clinical Endocrinologists medical guidelines for the clinical practice for the diagnosis and treatment of hyperandrogenic disorders. *Endocr Pract.* 2001;7:120–34.

103. Albrecht L, Styne D. Laboratory testing of gonadal steroids in children. *Pediatr Endocrinol Rev.* 2007;5(Suppl 1):599–607.

104. Bremer AA. Polycystic ovary syndrome in the pediatric population. *Metab Syndr Relat Disord.* 2010;8:375–94.

105. Nisenblat V, Norman RJ. Androgens and polycystic ovary syndrome. *Curr Opin Endocrinol Diabetes Obes.* 2009;16:224–31.

106. Dunaif A. Insulin resistance and the polycystic ovary syndrome: Mechanism and implications for pathogenesis. *Endocr Rev.* 1997;18:774–800.

107. Yildiz BO, Haznedaroglu IC, Kirazli S, Bayraktar M. Global fibrinolytic capacity is decreased in polycystic ovary syndrome, suggesting a prothrombotic state. *J Clin Endocrinol Metab.* 2002;87:3871–5.

108. Gambineri A, Pelusi C, Vicennati V, Pagotto U, Pasquali R. Obesity and the polycystic ovary syndrome. *Int J Obes Relat Metab Disord.* 2002;26:883–96.

109. Wild RA, Carmina E, Diamanti-Kandarakis E et al. Assessment of cardiovascular risk and prevention of cardiovascular disease in women with the polycystic ovary syndrome: A consensus statement by the Androgen Excess and Polycystic Ovary Syndrome (AE-PCOS) Society. *J Clin Endocrinol Metab.* 2010;95:2038–49.

110. Kenigsberg LE, Agarwal C, Sin S et al. Clinical utility of magnetic resonance imaging and ultrasonography for diagnosis of polycystic ovary syndrome in adolescent girls. *Fertil Steril.* 2015;104:1302–9, e1–4.

111. Moran LJ, Hutchison SK, Norman RJ, Teede HJ. Lifestyle changes in women with polycystic ovary syndrome. *Cochrane Database Syst Rev.* 2011;CD007506.

112. Lass N, Kleber M, Winkel K, Wunsch R, Reinehr T. Effect of lifestyle intervention on features of polycystic ovarian syndrome, metabolic syndrome, and intima-media thickness in obese adolescent girls. *J Clin Endocrinol Metab.* 2011;96:3533–40.

113. Polycystic ovary syndrome. ACOG Practice Bulletin No. 194. American College of Obstetricians and Gynecologists. *Obstet Gynecol.* 2018;131:e157–71.

114. Risk of venous thromboembolism among users of drospirenone-containing oral contraceptive pills. Committee Opinion No. 540. American College of Obstetricians and Gynecologists. *Obstet Gynecol.* 2012;120:1239–42.

115. Khalifah RA A, Florez ID, Dennis B, Thabane L, Bassilious E. Metformin or oral contraceptives for adolescents with polycystic ovarian syndrome: A meta-analysis. *Pediatrics.* 2016;137.

116. Ganie MA, Khurana ML, Nisar S et al. Improved efficacy of low-dose spironolactone and metformin combination than either drug alone in the management of women with polycystic ovary syndrome (PCOS): A six-month, open-label randomized study. *J Clin Endocrinol Metab.* 2013;98:3599–607.

117. Bates GW J, Propst AM. Polycystic ovarian syndrome management options. *Obstet Gynecol Clin North Am.* 2012;39:495–506.

118. Tartagni MV, Alrasheed H, Damiani GR et al. Intermittent low-dose finasteride administration is effective for treatment of hirsutism in adolescent girls: A pilot study. *J Pediatr Adolesc Gynecol.* 2014;27:161–5.

119. Smith SR, Piacquadio DJ, Beger B, Littler C. Eflornithine cream combined with laser therapy in the management of unwanted facial hair growth in women: A randomized trial. *Dermatol Surg.* 2006;32:1237–43.

120. Hamzavi I, Tan E, Shapiro J, Lui H. A randomized bilateral vehicle-controlled study of eflornithine cream combined with laser treatment versus laser treatment alone for facial hirsutism in women. *J Am Acad Dermatol.* 2007;57:54–9.

121. Homburg R. The management of infertility associated with polycystic ovary syndrome. *Reprod Biol Endocrinol.* 2003;1:109.

122. Eid GM, Cottam DR, Velcu LM et al. Effective treatment of polycystic ovarian syndrome with Roux-en-Y gastric bypass. *Surg Obes Relat Dis.* 2005;1:77–80.

123. Jamal M, Gunay Y, Capper A, Eid A, Heitshusen D, Samuel I. Roux-en-Y gastric bypass ameliorates polycystic ovary syndrome and dramatically improves conception rates: A 9-year analysis. *Surg Obes Relat Dis.* 2012;8:440–4.

124. Pritts EA. Letrozole for ovulation induction and controlled ovarian hyperstimulation. *Curr Opin Obstet Gynecol.* 2010;22:289–94.

125. Holzer H, Casper R, Tulandi T. A new era in ovulation induction. *Fertil Steril.* 2006;85:277–84.

126. Javed A, Chelvakumar G, Bonny AE. Polcystic ovary syndrome in adolescents: A review of past year evidence. *Curr Opin Obstet Gynecol.* 2016;28(5):373–80.

127. Ng HY. Acanthosis nigricans in obese adolescents: Prevalence, impact, and management challenges. *Adolesc Health Med Ther.* 2017;8:1–10.

Adolescent contraception

16

HANNA GOLDBERG, JASMINE MULTANI, and SARI KIVES

INTRODUCTION

Contraception is a crucially important adolescent health issue. Although there has been a slight decrease in adolescent pregnancy rates and decrease in the age of first intercourse across North America, data from 2015 still indicate that 24% of ninth graders (aged 14–15 years) and 57.2% of twelfth graders (aged 17–18 years) have had sexual intercourse.[1,2,3] According to data from 2014, 53% of females and 45% of males discussed contraception or sexually transmitted infections (STIs) with their partner before having sexual intercourse for the first time. Oral contraceptive pills (OCPs) and condoms were the most common choices of contraception used.[4] Nonetheless, 22% of adolescent females and 14% of adolescent males indicated that they did not use contraception with first intercourse.[4] In addition, 17% of adolescent males and 13% of adolescent females in the United States report at least four previous sexual partners, highlighting the role of contraception not only for protection from pregnancy but also in prevention of STIs. Canadian data from 2010 are similar, with 30% of 15- to 17-year-olds and 68% of 18- to 19-year-olds having had sexual intercourse; 39% of adolescent males and 25% of adolescent females reported more than one partner in the preceding year, and 27% of males and 37% of females reported not using condoms.[5]

Approximately 57 per 1000 American women between the ages of 15 and 19 will experience a pregnancy.[6] Overall, 20% of all adolescent pregnancies will occur within the first month of coitus, and 50% within the first 6 months. Many adolescents will delay seeking contraception for as long as 12 months or more following sexual debut. Reasons include anxiety that their parents will find out,

their sense of invincibility or misconceptions about contraception methods, and the extent of evaluation they anticipate before initiating contraception.[7,8] Dialogue and education around contraception should therefore become part of the routine health exchange with the adolescent before the initiation of sexual activity.[7] The discussion should also include screening for medical and psychosocial concerns and ruling out coercive sexual activity. The adolescent's thoughts in regard to contraception should be explored, and any misconceptions should be dispelled.[8] Despite initiating contraception, continuation rates for shorter-term methods such as the OCP over 1 or 2 years have been described to be as low as 12% and 2%, respectively. The reasons most commonly cited for discontinuation are running out of pills or forgetting to take them. Close follow-up with the adolescent after the initiation of contraception is therefore crucial to adherence.[8]

Discussing contraception with adolescents can often be problematic. The medical team and adolescent need to work together to find a method that will be successful. Ideally, the medical professional should be skilled in interactions with the adolescent age group.[8] Education needs to be age-appropriate and tailored to the concrete thought processes of the adolescent. Encounters should be kept interactive and should encourage dialogue. The adolescent must participate in the exchange and demonstrate her cognitive abilities in selecting her contraceptive.[9] Discussions regarding the effectiveness of each individual method should be included (Table 16.1).

Merely handing out contraception to adolescents and not educating them about contraception use and pregnancy prevention has been shown to be insufficient for

Table 16.1 Effectiveness of family planning methods.

Family planning method	Pregnancy per 100 women in first 12 months of use	
	Effectiveness with typical use	Effectiveness with perfect use
Male condom	14	3
Female condom	21	5
Diaphragm	10.4	7.9
Spermicide	28	18
Combined oral contraceptive pill	9	0.3
Depot medroxyprogesterone acetate	0.3	0.3
Etonorgestrel implant	0.05	0.05
Progestin-only pill	9	0.3
Copper intrauterine device	1.26	1.26
Levonorgestrel intrauterine system	0.09	0.09

improving compliance in this age group.[1] Sexual activity may be linked to other risk-taking behaviors.[10,11] Education and discussion about sexual activity is important and has not been shown to increase the rates of sexual activity among adolescents.[1] More comprehensive youth development programs, which also provide information and counseling around life goals, career planning, and self-esteem, may be successful in reducing teen pregnancy rates.[1]

Confidentiality is an extremely important factor in communicating with adolescents; 25% of adolescents have indicated that they would avoid contacting a healthcare provider about a sensitive topic if they felt that their parents would find out. Therefore, health care around contraception should be provided in a confidential and nonjudgmental environment.[9] The parents and/or primary caregivers can also have an active role in educating their adolescents about contraception needs. In fact, adolescents who have open conversations about these topics with their parents and families are less likely to engage in unprotected intercourse or become pregnant.[12] Greater parental supervision is associated with increased use of contraceptives. In addition, greater warmth in parental relationships leads to increased likelihood of young women discussing contraception with their male partners.[12] The relationship between the adolescent and parent should be assessed, and the adolescent should be encouraged to openly involve her parents in her health concerns, if appropriate. In addition, the attitudes of the partner, as well as the greater social and cultural context, should be considered to ensure a successful choice of contraceptive.[12]

Despite similar characteristics of the youth in the United States and the European Union (EU), significant differences in pregnancy rates are seen. In the EU, the average pregnancy rate is 27.8 per 1000.[13] Data suggest that neither the initiation nor frequency of sexual activity differ, but rather the level of utilization of contraception is higher in the EU. Education and awareness as well as availability of contraceptive services in the EU most likely contribute to the differences seen in pregnancy rates. These differences should be considered when developing comprehensive programs for contraception in teens.[14,15]

Abstinence

While options for all forms of contraception should be discussed with an adolescent, abstinence should be encouraged as the healthiest method of preventing both pregnancy and STIs. Abstinence after a previous experience of sexual activity (secondary abstinence) should also be encouraged as an acceptable choice.[7,16] Adolescents should have the opportunity to discuss which behaviors are safe and how to communicate effectively with their partners about which sexual activities they feel comfortable engaging in.[16] Abstinence-only programs have specifically not been shown to reduce age at first intercourse; therefore, any counseling or program on abstinence should also provide education about other methods of contraception.[1,7]

Intrauterine device contraception

In North America, intrauterine contraceptive (IUC) use is increasing and is now estimated to be up to 9.3%.[17-19] There are two types of IUC currently available in the United States and Canada: the copper intrauterine device (IUD) and the levonorgestrel-releasing intrauterine system (LNG-IUS). There are four types of LNG-IUS available in the United States: Mirena, Liletta, Kyleena, and Skyla. Mirena and Kyleena are available in Canada. Each LNG-IUS varies with respect to daily levonorgestrel release and duration of use (Table 16.2). Although long-acting reversible contraceptives (LARCs) are approved by the U.S. Food and Drug Administration (FDA) for 3–10 years of use depending on method chosen, current research is underway on extended duration beyond the FDA limits, and evidence for use beyond the FDA-approved times is available (Table 16.3).

Both types of IUCs (LNG-IUS and copper IUD) are highly effective and reversible methods of contraception. Overall contraceptive failure is reported to be 1.26 per 100 women-years for the copper IUD and 0.09 per 100 woman-years for the LNG-IUS.[20,21] The mechanism of action for both IUCs includes prevention of fertilization and potential inhibition of implantation.[22,23] The copper IUD also affects sperm transport and sperm motility so that fertilization rarely occurs.[24-26] The LNG-IUS causes

Table 16.2 Levonorgestrel intrauterine systems.

Brand name	Total dose	Daily dose	Duration of use
Mirena	52 mg	20 mcg	Up to 5 years
Liletta	52 mg	19.5 mcg initially 17 mcg at 1 year 14.8 mcg at 2 years 12.9 mcg at 3 years 11.3 mcg at 4 years	Up to 4 years
Kyleena	19.5 mg	17.5 mcg 9.8 mcg after 1 year	Up to 5 years
Skyla	13.5 mg	14 mcg 6 mcg after 1 year	Up to 3 years

Table 16.3 Duration of contraceptive efficacy of long-acting reversible contraceptive methods.

	Approved by U.S. Food and Drug Administration (years)	Recent studies (years)	Failure rate (per 100 woman-years)
Copper IUD			
ParaGard	10	12	2.2
LNG-IUD 52 mg			
Mirena	5	7	0.5
LNG-IUD 52 mg			
Liletta	4	5	0.5
Etonorgestrel Implant 68 mg			
Nexplanon	3	5[a]	0.6
Sterilization			1.9

Source: With permission from NASPAG resources for clinicians, Mt. Royal, NJ. https://c.ymcdn.com/sites/www.naspag.org/resource/resmgr/pdf's/Extended_Use_LARCs-_NASPAG_T.pdf.

Abbreviations: IUD, intrauterine device; LNG-IUD, levonorgestrel-releasing intrauterine device.

[a] Body mass index less than 30.

endometrial decidualization and glandular atrophy, and thickening of cervical mucus, which may create a barrier to sperm penetration.[27,28] Ovulation may also be suppressed.[29,30]

Although physicians have traditionally been reluctant to prescribe an IUC to the adolescent population, age alone is not an absolute contraindication to the IUC. In fact, the World Health Organization (WHO) categorizes the IUC as class 2 for individuals less than or equal to age 20. The American College of Obstetricians and Gynecologists (ACOG) also supports the use of these methods as safe and effective first-line options for adolescents.[31] The IUC should be considered particularly in adolescents most at risk for unplanned pregnancy, including those who are already parents or have failed or refused other methods of birth control.

Absolute contraindications to the IUC include pregnancy; current, recurrent, or recent (within the past 3 months) pelvic inflammatory disease (PID) or STI; severely distorted cavity; unexplained vaginal bleeding; cervical or endometrial cancer awaiting treatment; malignant trophoblastic disease; copper allergy (for copper IUCs); pelvic tuberculosis; and breast cancer (for LNG-IUS).[32,33]

The WHO states that IUCs do not protect against STIs, including HIV. For those at risk for STIs, the correct and consistent use of condoms is recommended.[32]

While STI screening should be performed in adolescents at high risk for STIs, IUC insertion should not be delayed for pending STI results unless the adolescent is symptomatic or shows signs of infection.[33] In general, STI screening can be performed at the time of insertion.[33]

The increased risk of upper tract disease is predominantly limited to the 20 days following insertion of the IUC according to the WHO.[28] After insertion, the risk of infection is related to exposure to STIs and not to the device itself.[34] The overall risk of PID in the first 90 days has been found to be 0.54%.[35] Some studies suggest the LNG-IUS may actually protect against PID.[20,36]

This protection is felt to be secondary to the progestin effect on the cervical mucus but still must be further corroborated.

If the adolescent is diagnosed with PID following IUC insertion, the IUC can be left *in situ* unless there is no clinical improvement after 48–72 hours of appropriate antibiotic therapy. Routine antibiotic prophylaxis is not recommended at time of insertion; however, if the adolescent is found to have chlamydia and/or gonorrhea on preinsertion screening, the patient should be appropriately treated, and the IUC can remain in place.[33]

Other risks following IUC insertion include perforation, which is a rare complication occurring at a rate of 0.6 per 1000 insertions.[37,38] Expulsion can also occur and appears to be most common the first year (2%–10%), especially in the first 3 months.[20,39] The risk of expulsion does not appear to be higher with nulliparity, size of endometrial cavity, or concomitant use of tampons or menstrual cups.[39] Insertion may also be more difficult in the nulliparous patient and adolescent. Preinsertion anti-inflammatories can be provided for analgesia. A paracervical block may also be considered, as it has been shown to decrease pain in a placebo-controlled trial in adolescents.[41] However, the routine use of Misoprostol to soften the cervix is not recommended for assisting with insertion.[42] Although the absolute risk of ectopic pregnancy is lower due to reduced fertilization, 15%–50% of pregnancies that occur with an IUC *in situ* are ectopic, and this must thus be ruled out.[43,44] If an intrauterine pregnancy is confirmed, removal of the IUC is recommended.[45] IUCs do not increase the risk of infertility.[46]

The LNG-IUS has a high rate of reduction of bleeding and dysmenorrhea. Up to 16%–35% of recipients of the LNG-IUS will become amennorrheic after 1 year of use.[20,47,48] Women with heavy menstrual bleeding prior to LNG-IUS insertion have noted reductions in menstrual blood loss of 74%–98%, favorable effects in hemoglobin levels, and improved health-related quality of life.[49] Other noncontraceptive benefits of the LNG-IUS and copper IUD include the decreased risk of endometrial cancer.[33]

Adolescents must also be counseled about the nuisance, irregular bleeding that occurs most frequently in the first few months following insertion of an LNG-IUS. The copper IUD, in contrast, can increase menstrual loss by up to 65%,[50,51] as well as both bleeding and spotting. This IUC may therefore be less acceptable to the adolescent. Discontinuation of the IUC due to pain or bleeding is higher in a younger population.[14,20,52]

Implantable contraceptives

The implantable contraceptive is a single 4 mm by 2 mm rod, 68 mg etonorgestrel implant, which is placed discretely under the skin on the inner upper arm during a small procedure in the physician's office and releases 40 μg of etonorgestrel daily. The implant can be used for up to 3 years. The pearl index is 0.05 pregnancies per 100 woman-years provided that insertion is on days 1–5 of the menstrual cycle.[53] The primary mechanism of action is inhibition of ovulation as well as thickening of cervical mucus and thinning of the endometrial lining.[33] The invisible nature of the implant and reduced requirement for adherence make it a particularly good choice for adolescents who are seeking long-term contraception.[33] Contraindications and side effects are very similar to other progestin methods of contraception, with the exception of bone density, as the implant does not impact unfavorably on bone density.[33] Menstrual irregularities are the most common side effect seen with the implant and other progestin methods of contraception. Headache, emotional lability, acne, breast pain, abdominal pain, and weight gain have also been described.[54–56] Studies have also indicated a 1% rate of complications associated with the site of implant insertion, such as erythema, swelling, hematoma, pain, and difficult insertion.[54,57] Removal complications were only 1.7% and included problems of fibrosis, broken implant, and difficulty finding the implant.[58]

Immediate postpartum use of long-acting reversible contraceptives

LARCs consist of IUCs and the contraceptive implant.[31] LARC is the most effective form of contraception, with effectiveness rates of greater than 99%. Up to one-third of postpartum mothers will become pregnant again in the first 2 years postpartum.[59–61]

Placement of LARC in the immediate postpartum period before hospital discharge can play an important role in the prevention of unwanted short-interval pregnancies in adolescents.[62] Immediate postpartum use of LARC should be discussed with the patient prenatally,[62] including benefits and potential risks.

Immediate postpartum IUD insertion should be performed within 10 minutes of placental delivery in both vaginal and cesarean births.[62] The IUD may be placed at the fundus of the uterus manually or with a ring or Kelly forceps. At the time of cesarean section, the strings should be placed into the cervix prior to closing the uterus. The technique of contraceptive implant insertion does not differ in the immediate postpartum period.[62]

Risk of IUD expulsion is higher in the immediate postpartum period. There is also a theoretical negative impact of LARC on milk production,[62] but there is no evidence that immediate postpartum use of levonorgestrel IUD or etonorgestrel affects milk supply or quality of breastfeeding (Medical Eligibility Criteria level 2 for both). Benefits of immediate postpartum use of LARCs include preventing unintended or short-interval pregnancies and circumventing the need to attend a postpartum visit for insertion of the LARC.[62] Contraindications to immediate postpartum use of IUD include chorioamnionitis, endometritis, and postpartum hemorrhage.[62] There are no additional contraindications to immediate postpartum use of contraceptive implants.

Depot medroxyprogesterone acetate

Depot medroxyprogesterone acetate (DMPA) is a progestin-only intramuscular injectable contraceptive administered every 11–15 weeks. A dose of 150 mg is ideally initiated during the first 7 days of the woman's menstrual cycle to achieve almost immediate contraceptive effect (<24 hours), and it is repeated every 3 months.[63–65] It is a highly effective (failure rate less than 0.3% per year), safe, convenient, and reversible method of contraception.[22,32,66–70] The mechanism of action is primarily the prevention of ovulation, but decidualization of the endometrium and thickening of cervical mucus also provide supplemental action.[71] Effective plasma concentrations of DMPA are sustained for at least 14 weeks, and ovulation is suppressed for an average of 18 weeks.[72] Fertility can be delayed for up to 9 months following discontinuation due to DMPA's very effective suppression of the hypothalamic-pituitary axis. More recently, DMPA has also become available in a subcutaneous formulation (104 mg).

Same-day injection or "quick start" of DMPA has been reported as a safe and effective alternative to the standard prescribing practice of restricting initiation of DMPA to menstruation.[73,74] If DMPA is given after the first 7 days of the menstrual cycle, the adolescent should be counseled to use backup contraception for the next 7 days.[33] Pregnancy should be ruled out at the time of DMPA injection as well as 3–4 weeks following quick-start initiation.[33] This method of administration is felt to enhance access to contraception without putting the patient at increased risk for pregnancy while she is waiting for her next menstrual cycle.[74]

If an adolescent presents late for injection, DMPA should still be given; however, pregnancy must first be ruled out, and a backup method of contraception should be used for 7 days. Emergency contraception should also be considered.[33] Additionally, a pregnancy test should be performed 3–4 weeks following a late injection.

DMPA is also useful in treating adolescents with medical conditions, where estrogen would be contraindicated (migraine headaches and anticonvulsant medications). DMPA has very few contraindications, and the majority do not apply to the adolescent population. Absolute contraindications to DMPA are rare but include pregnancy (known or suspected) and current diagnosis of breast cancer. Relative contraindications include unexplained vaginal bleeding, severe liver cirrhosis, acute viral hepatitis, benign hepatic adenoma, and malignant hepatoma.[32] Venous thromboembolism (VTE) is not considered a contraindication to DMPA use according to the 2015 WHO guidelines.[75] Additionally, DMPA can be used immediately after delivery in adolescents who are breastfeeding, with no significant reduction in breast milk or adverse effects on infant growth and development.[33]

Side effects attributed to DMPA include weight gain, breakthrough bleeding, and potential bone mineral density (BMD) loss. More recent literature, however, does not demonstrate an increase in depressive symptoms in DMPA users.[76-78]

Published studies on weight changes have been inconsistent. Some studies report weight gain changes as high as 9 kg in 2 years or less.[66,79-82] The product monograph indicates average weight gains of 2.5 kg after the first year of use, 3.7 kg after the second year of use, and 6.3 kg after the fourth year of use.[83] More recently, a prospective study demonstrated that this substantial increase in weight is composed entirely of increases in fat mass and not lean mass.[84,85] The mechanisms by which DMPA increases weight are unknown but are felt to be secondary to appetite stimulation.[85] Regardless, informed counseling about the potential weight changes must be included when prescribing DMPA to the adolescent population. Excessive weight gain is reported to appear more frequently in adolescents who experience greater than 5% weight gain after the first 6 months of use.[86]

Breakthrough bleeding may be the most common reason for discontinuation of DMPA, particularly in the adolescent. Irregular bleeding may occur in as many as 25%–50% of users in the first 6–12 months of dosing. Counseling is therefore paramount at the time of prescribing DMPA. Increasing the DMPA dose and shortening the interval between doses are no longer recommended.[33] Rather, if breakthrough bleeding persists beyond 3–6 months, other causes should first be investigated.[33] Therapeutic options for irregular bleeding include supplemental estrogen, such as 0.625–1.25 mg of conjugated equine estrogen (CEE) per day for 28 days, 1–2 mg of 17β-estradiol per day for 28 days, or transdermal 17β-estradiol per day for 25 days. Additionally, administration of a nonsteroidal anti-inflammatory drug (NSAID) twice daily for 5 days, adding an oral contraceptive pill for 1–3 months, and administration of tranexamic acid (500 mg twice daily) for 5 days may be considered.[33] Unfortunately, none of these methods is completely satisfactory; fortunately, amenorrhea occurs in 55%–60% of DMPA users at 12 months[66,69,87-89] and up to 68% of DMPA users at greater than 1 year. Many teenagers perceive this as an appealing feature of the medication, which may contribute to their compliance.

Continuation rates of DMPA, despite its ease of administration, are similar to those of the OCP and range from 63% to 70% at 6 months.[87,90] Quick-start administration of DMPA has shown similar continuation rates at both 6 months and 1 year.[74,91]

DMPA received a black box warning from the FDA in 2004 regarding its potential negative effect on BMD. The adult literature does suggest that DMPA is associated with a reduction in BMD. Overall, DMPA users have lower mean BMD than nonusers. Studies specifically in adolescents also confirm these findings.[92-95] This difference in BMD in DMPA users is felt to be a loss in BMD in adolescent users compared with gains in adolescent nonusers and ranges from 2% to 3% for the first year of DMPA use. One study found that new adolescent users in fact lose more BMD than continuing users, and the adjusted mean change in BMD decreases with increasing DMPA use.[95] This decrease is most rapid in the first 2 years of use and appears to be largely reversible once the DMPA is discontinued.[33,96] It is unknown, however, if adolescents ultimately achieved similar peak bone mass to that they would have achieved if they had avoided DMPA. Importantly, the clinical significance of reduction in BMD is unknown. It is unclear if this decrease in BMD is a good surrogate marker for subsequent fracture risk, particularly among the adolescent population. As such, it is no longer recommended to perform routine evaluation of BMD in DMPA users.[33] In addition, the loss of BMD is analogous to changes in BMD that occur during both pregnancy and lactation, which are effectively prevented by use of DMPA in the sexually active adolescent.[97]

The Society for Adolescent Medicine and ACOG continue to endorse the use of DMPA with the following provisions: explain the benefits and potential risks, inform patients of the possible risk for bone loss, understand individual risk profile for osteopenia, recommend 1300 mg calcium carbonate plus 600 IU vitamin D and daily weight-bearing exercise, and finally, do not restrict DMPA use to 2 years.[98,99] Furthermore, the adolescent should be counseled to decrease caffeine and alcohol intake, and smoking cessation should be encouraged.[33] The WHO also suggests that the advantages of using DMPA generally outweigh the theoretical safety concerns regarding fracture risk in the adolescent population (under 18 years of age).[100] Ultimately, there should be no restriction on the duration of use in the adolescent population.[33] The overall risks and benefits of continuing DMPA should be discussed on a regular basis with the patient and her family.[33]

Noncontraceptive clinical benefits of DMPA include management of dysmenorrhea, endometriosis, protection against endometrial hyperplasia and endometrial cancer, protection against ovarian cancer, reduction of premenstrual syndrome and chronic pelvic pain, decreased risk of PID, decreased risk of myomas, and a reduction in sickle cell crisis and seizures.[33,101] DMPA has been shown to raise the seizure threshold and thus to lower seizure frequency in epileptic patients.[102] DMPA also offers a unique advantage to the adolescent with special needs who requires menstrual suppression.

Combined oral contraceptive pill

Over the last 4 decades that the combined oral contraceptive (COC) pills have been in use, the hormonal doses have decreased, and newer, less androgenic progestins have been developed. COCs can be classified as either monophasic, which contain the same dose of hormones daily, or triphasic, in which the amount of progestin varies over the 21 days.[7,16] Current formulations include the following: 21 days followed by 7 days of placebo pills or no pills, 24 days followed by 4 days of placebo pills, 24 days followed by 2 days of ethinyl estradiol only and 2 days of placebo pills, 26 days followed by 2 days of placebo pills, and 84 days followed by 7 days of no pills or 7 days of ethinyl estradiol only.[33] To allow for fewer hormone-free intervals, COCs may also be prescribed in an extended or continuous regimen.[33]

COCs work in a variety of ways to prevent conception. They exert a negative feedback on gonadotropin-releasing hormone (GnRH), thus preventing ovulation via inhibition of luteinizing hormone (LH) and follicle-stimulating hormone (FSH). In addition, cervical mucus is thickened, the endometrium is thinned, and tubal transport is delayed, all of which further decrease the probability of conception.[7,16]

With ideal use, the COC is 99.7% effective at pregnancy prevention within the first year; with typical use the efficacy is 91%.[53] Poor compliance, however, limits efficacy. Adolescent users of the COC have failure rates of up to 15% in the first year of use due to missed pills; 28% of 15- to 17-year-old users of the COC report missing two or more pills in their most recent cycle (compared with 13% of those 18 and older).[1,7] Patients should therefore be advised how to manage missed pills (Table 16.4), how to access and use emergency contraception, and to use condoms.[7] The highest risk of ovulation occurs when the hormone-free interval is extended beyond 7 days.[33]

Table 16.4 How to manage missed combined oral contraceptive pills.

Number of pills missed	Recommendation
1	Take immediately.
≥2 within first 2 weeks of pack	Two pills should be taken daily for the next 2 days.
	Backup contraception should be used for 7 consecutive days.
≥2 within third week of pack	Remainder of pack should be discarded, and a new pack should be started.
	Backup contraception should be used for 7 consecutive days.
≥3 at any time	Remainder of pack should be discarded, and a new pack should be started.
	Backup contraception should be used for 7 consecutive days.

Adolescents with medical conditions need to be assessed as to whether they are at increased risk from the COC. The WHO has developed four categories of safety for use of COCs (Table 16.5)[7,75]:

Category 4 includes absolute contraindications:

- Personal history of thromboembolic disease
- Known hypercoagulability
- Pregnancy
- Severe hypertension
- Active breast cancer
- Migraine with aura (as defined by the International Headache Society)
- Active liver disease
- Cerebrovascular disease
- Diabetes with end-organ damage
- Congenital heart disease complicated by structural lesions with turbulent flow or cardiac stents
- Cerebrovascular disease
- Less than 4 weeks postpartum if breastfeeding
- Less than 21 days postpartum if not breastfeeding
- Major surgery with prolonged immobilization
- Systemic lupus erythematosus (positive antiphospholipid antibodies)
- Solid-organ transplantation with complications[7,33,75]

Category 3 contraindications where the risk may outweigh the benefit include the following:

- 3–6 weeks' postpartum
- VTE on anticoagulation therapy with no other risk factors for VTE
- Adequately controlled hypertension
- Symptomatic gallbladder disease
- Diabetes with microvascular and macrovascular complications
- Certain anticonvulsant use
- Rifampicin or rifabutin use[33,75]

Serious adverse reactions to the COC are rare and occur less frequently in the adolescent population than in older adults.[7] Common adverse reactions include nausea, which typically subsides within the first one or two cycles. *Candida* vaginitis is also more common in users of the

Table 16.5 World Health Organization (WHO) categories of medical eligibility criteria for contraceptive use.

Category	Recommendation
1	A condition for which there is no restriction for the use of the contraceptive method
2	A condition where the advantages of using the method generally outweigh the theoretical or proven risks
3	A condition where the theoretical or proven risks usually outweigh the advantages of using the method
4	A condition that represents an unacceptable health risk if the contraceptive method is used

COC; it can be treated without discontinuing the COC. Despite the concerns of adolescents, the current formulations of the COC are not associated with inherent weight gain, but patients must be advised to monitor their food consumption and exercise regimes.[16,103]

The risk of a VTE event decreases with duration of use and amount of estrogen per dose.[104] As such, VTE risk has decreased with the development of lower-dose COCs. It is still increased in users of the COC compared with the general population, with a relative risk of between 3 and 6, and the highest risk in the first year of use.[105,106] The absolute risk in the healthy adolescent population is still extremely low, in the range of 1.6–5.0 events per 10,000 women. Case control and retrospective cohort studies have suggested an increased risk in VTE in women using COCs containing third- and fourth-degree progestins.[107] Well-designed prospective cohort studies have failed to demonstrate this increased risk; therefore, any risk of venous thromboembolism (VTE) attributable to different progestin and estrogen dosing in low-dose COCs does not currently justify preferential prescribing.[33,108,109] The risk of mortality from arterial or venous events attributable to the COC, for women aged 20–24, is 1 in 370,000 users.[106] There is no significant concern for increase in myocardial infarction (MI) or stroke in nonsmokers under age 35 using the COC.[110]

Medications that interact with combined hormonal contraceptives (CHCs) include phenytoin, phenobarbetol, primidone, and carbamazepine.[111] These medications interact with cytochrome P450 to decrease serum concentration of estrogen, thereby reducing the efficacy of CHCs.[111] Additionally, CHC induces metabolism of lamotrigine, thereby reducing lamotrigine levels and reducing seizure control.[111]

There are many noncontraceptive benefits to use of the COC, including the following:

- Predictable menses
- Lighter menses
- Decreased rates of dysmenorrhea
- Decreased formation of ovarian cysts
- Decreased rates of PID
- Decreased rates of ectopic pregnancy
- A protective effect for endometriosis
- Improved acne[112] and hirsutism
- Reduction in lifetime rates of fibrocystic breast disease[7,16,110]
- Decreased rates of affective symptomatology of premenstrual syndrome (PMS) and premenstrual dysphoric disorder (PMDD)
- Decreased rates of endometrial and ovarian cancers[110]
- Reduced risk of colorectal cancer[110]

While there may be a small increased risk of breast cancer in young female COC users, the absolute risk is very small and may be due to delay of the first full-term pregnancy rather than COC use itself.[113] While studies are equivocal as to whether COCs exert a positive effect on BMD, there are no studies indicating a detrimental effect. Some studies do indicate less increase in BMD in adolescents using 20 μg ethinyl estradiol COCs compared with adolescent nonusers of the COC.[110,114] Previous studies, however, have only examined BMD as a primary endpoint rather than a fracture risk. Therefore, it remains unknown whether the effect of COC on BMD is clinically relevant.[115]

Despite many misconceptions on the part of adolescents, there are no routine laboratory tests required before initiation of the COC. Screening for thrombophilias in a healthy patient, without significant family history, is not cost-effective for preventing DVT.[7] In addition, a pelvic examination is not required before initiation of the COC. In adolescents, the COC can be used for an indefinite period of time without pelvic examination; in a sexually active teen, routine STI screening can be performed without a pelvic exam (see Chapter 17), and the first exam may be delayed until cervical cancer screening is indicated or if the patient has an indication (Chapter 3). This delay allows for the establishment of a successful relationship with the adolescent and has been shown to increase the likelihood of follow-up. All patients who initiate the COC, however, must have a blood pressure measurement. This is the only mandatory examination required prior to starting the COC.

On average, 45%–66% of adolescent users will discontinue the COC during the first year. Younger adolescent age is associated with poorer adherence. Many adolescents will identify the immediate consequence of a minor side effect while ignoring the long-term benefit of contraception. Careful education, dispelling myths about the COC, and close follow-up are therefore important components of counseling and treatment initiation.[16,116] The quick-start method, in which the pill is initiated in the office in the presence of the health-care provider (rather than waiting for a Sunday start or starting with menses) is associated with better adherence over time.[116] Some small studies have found success with daily electronic reminders to adolescents.[117] New formulations of the COC that have been designed to enhance adherence include formulations containing iron, those with drospirenone (a spironolactone-like progestin), those that have just a 4-day placebo regimen, and chewable, flavored pills.[118]

With increasing numbers of overweight adolescents and increasing rates of obesity in the adolescent population, the potential impact of body weight on COC efficacy has become increasingly more concerning. Recently, there have been several studies investigating the impact of body weight on the efficacy of COC; however, the data are conflicting. A meta-analysis of seven clinical trials found that pregnancy rate was higher in obese compared to nonobese women (AHR 1.44 [1.06–1.95]).[119] A randomized controlled trial found a small increased risk; however, this finding was not significant.[120] Two prospective cohort studies and one clinical trial found that body weight had no impact on the efficacy of COC.[121–123] While most well-designed studies fail to demonstrate a decreased COC efficacy with increasing weight, there may be a small increase in contraceptive failure in women with a body mass index greater than 30.[33]

Transdermal combined hormonal contraception

Recognizing the difficulties associated with daily adherence to a pill, development efforts have been aimed at contraceptive methods that are equally safe and effective but require less vigilance. A weekly contraceptive patch has been available in North America since 2001. The patch is 1.5 inches and contains ethinyl estradiol and norelgestromin, with daily absorption equivalent to 20 μg ethinyl estradiol and 150 μg norelgestromin.[124,125] Steady drug concentrations have been shown through the 1-week period of wear.[126]

The patch is typically placed weekly for 3 weeks and then left off for 1 week, during which a withdrawal bleed occurs. It can be placed anywhere on the torso, excluding the breasts, such as the lower abdomen, buttocks, or upper outer arm; sites should be rotated to avoid skin irritation.[124–127] In studies using over 70,000 patches, only 4.7% required replacement due to partial or complete detachment. In an adolescent study, 21% experienced a patch coming off completely, and 32% experienced a patch peeling partially in the corner.[124] Women can maintain all normal activities, including all forms of bathing and water sports, and the patch has also been shown to maintain adhesion in various weather conditions.[125,126,128,129] While the patch is designed to last for 7 days, if forgotten, there is sufficient medication that it can be left in place for up to 9 days. If a patch is detached for less than 24 hours, it can be replaced in the same location or replaced with a new patch if the adhesive no longer works. If the patch is removed for more than 24 hours, contraceptive efficacy may be lost.[7,124–126]

Contraindications, side effects profile, and noncontraceptive benefits are similar to those of the COC; there are noted increased rates of breast discomfort and local skin irritation but less breakthrough bleeding with the patch.[130] There is no clinically significant effect on patient weight gain.[124,131,132] However, women over 90 kg were shown to have increased pregnancy rates compared with thinner women and thus are thought to be poorer candidates for this method of contraception.[7,132] In 2005 and 2006, the FDA issued warnings with regard to the contraceptive patch, indicating 60% increased estrogen exposure and a possible twofold increase in VTE in users of this product as compared with the COC. Subsequently, studies investigating the association between the patch and VTE demonstrated conflicting results. Three studies found no significant increased risk of thromboembolic events among contraceptive patch users.[133–135] A more recent case-control study, which was an extension of an earlier study, continued to demonstrate a twofold increased risk of VTE.[136] The estimated frequency of VTE in women who use the contraceptive patch is 5.3 per 10,000 women, which is similar to COC users.[130]

As the patch is replaced weekly, it has particular appeal in the adolescent population over the COC, which must be remembered daily. Studies in this population indicate good acceptance of the method, excellent cycle control, and adherence rates greater than those observed with the COC.[124,125,128,137] In one cross-sectional study, 97% of adolescents were either very or somewhat satisfied with the patch, and 93% would recommend it to a friend.[124]

Vaginal combined hormonal ring

The contraceptive ring is an ethylene-vinylacetate copolymer that offers sustained, slow release of 15 μg ethinyl estradiol and 120 μg etonorgestrel daily over 3 weeks. The ring has an outer diameter of 54 mm and cross-sectional diameter of 4 mm.[138,139] The advantages of the method include the rapid absorption of steroid through the vaginal mucosa, the constant release rate of the medication, and the privacy of the method.[140] The ring is placed vaginally, starting on days 1–5 of the cycle, for 3 weeks, and then removed for 1 week, during which a withdrawal bleed occurs.[138] There are no contraindications or difficulties in use of the device in conjunction with tampons or with barrier or spermicidal contraceptives.[138,141,142] If the ring is dislodged for less than 3 hours, it can be replaced without any interruption in contraceptive efficacy. If it is removed for more than 3 hours, contraceptive efficacy may be lost, and a backup method of contraception should be used for 7 days.[83] Ovulation is suppressed for at least 28 days after insertion of the vaginal contraceptive ring if left in place continuously.[33]

The mechanism of action is identical to that of the COC, and studies have indicated complete suppression of ovulation in study patients as assessed on ultrasound as well as measurements of serum FSH and LH. A matched pairs analysis demonstrated that the vaginal ring induces greater ovarian suppression compared to COC.[138,143] Efficacy, side effect profile, and contraindications are again similar to those of the COC, and there is no effect on patient weight gain.[7,144,145] Nausea, acne, and emotional lability may be reduced in ring users.[130] Rates of irregular bleeding (<5%) are also lower than those noted with the COCs, and significantly more patients experience regular withdrawal bleeds than with COCs.[128,138,139,146] The duration of menstrual bleeding is also significantly shortened in women using the ring as compared to the patch.[33] Some increased leukorrhea and vaginal irritation have been described.[7,138] With regard to changes in vaginal flora, studies have been conflicting. While some studies noted no changes in vaginal flora, at least two studies found an increased number of lactobacilli in the vaginal flora.[147,148] Increased lactobacilli could be protective against cervicovaginal infection and sexually transmitted infections.[147]

The vaginal ring has been well accepted by all ages in clinical trials, with 53% switching to the vaginal ring from another method, and 90% indicating that they would recommend it to others.[138] The vaginal ring may have poor uptake in the adolescent population, as adolescents are typically uncomfortable with inserting contraceptive methods into the vagina. An empty tampon applicator can be used to insert the vaginal ring for those who are uncomfortable about using their fingers to do so.[128] While the ring can remain *in situ* safely during intercourse and is only felt (but not thought to be bothersome) by 15% of women and 30% of partners, it can also be removed for up to 3 hours around intercourse and then rinsed with water and reinserted.[138–140]

Continuous combined hormonal contraception

More recently, there has been increased interest in the use of combined hormonal contraception (CHC) in an extended or continuous regimen in which hormones are taken for longer than 21 days. The traditional regimen of 21 hormonally active days followed by 7 hormonally free days was developed to mimic the natural "lunar" cycle and to be morally permissible.[149] The 7-day pill-free interval is not necessary for contraceptive efficacy or physiologic purposes. It simply produces scheduled monthly bleeding in most users by withdrawing the hormones. This monthly or periodic withdrawal bleed is not the same as menstruation. The doctrine that women using contraception need a menstrual cycle for health-related reasons is changing, and reversible amenorrhea is becoming more acceptable to most women.[150,151] Previous studies have shown that 59%–70% of women were interested in not menstruating every month.[152–154] Physician views on prescribing extended cycles of CHCs are also shifting to accommodate patients' requests, and to treat gynecologic conditions exacerbated during the hormone-free interval.[155] Gynecologists routinely recommend and prescribe extended regimens as compared with pediatricians, internists, and family physicians.[155]

Common gynecologic conditions including dysmenorrhea, endometriosis, menstrual migraines, and heavy menstrual bleeding can easily be treated with an extended or continuous hormonal regimen. Moreover, a continuous hormonal regimen has been shown to be associated with fewer menstrual symptoms compared to a cyclic regimen by eliminating the hormone-free interval.[156] Continuous combined hormonal regimens are also effective methods of menstrual suppression in the special needs population. In addition to the medical benefits of reversible amenorrhea, many patients are interested in altering the menstrual cycle simply to have fewer menses. In recent studies of adolescents, conducted in both the United States and Europe, there was a clear preference demonstrated to menstruate less frequently rather than monthly or never again.[157,158]

No consensus exists on the optimal length for extending the pill-free interval. Sequences of 63 days on and 7 hormone-free days (63/7) and 84 days on and 7 hormone-free days (84/7) are common regimens described in the literature, along with continuous 365-day regimens. At present, it is up to the prescribing physician and patient to select the optimal regimen. In the United States, there are dedicated products for extended contraception, which include 84/7 regimens and a 365-day regimen. While any cyclic product can be used, monophasic pills are usually prescribed in a continuous fashion with few adverse side effects.[159] Extending or continuous cycling with the transdermal patch and vaginal ring have also been shown to be effective alternatives to cyclical use with similar side effects.[160,161]

Breakthrough bleeding is often the most common reason for discontinuing an extended or continuous regimen. In a Cochrane review comparing continuous or extended regimens to a cyclic regimen, most bleeding outcomes showed either no major difference between groups or less bleeding and/or spotting with continuous dosing.[162–164] More recently, a flexible extended regimen of 20 μg ethinyl estradiole/3 mg drospirenone (24–120 days of hormonal pills with a 4-day no pill interval) has been shown to be associated with significantly fewer bleeding/spotting days compared to a 21/7 formulation and 24/4 formulation.[165,166] Furthermore, studies have demonstrated that 84/7 (7-day interval of ethinyl estradiol) formulation is associated with significantly reduced bleeding/spotting compared to 84/7 (7-day no pill interval) formulations.[167] The institution of a 3-day hormone-free interval only has been found to be an effective treatment for breakthrough bleeding in patients specifically on a continuous regimen.[168]

Participant adherence and contraceptive efficacy appear to be very similar to both cyclic and continuous regimens.[162,169] Nevertheless, the most frequently forgotten pills are the first few days of the new pack and the last few days of the previous pack. An extended or continuous regimen decreases the total number of hormone-free intervals and is associated with less ovulation and greater sustained ovarian suppression.[170] This favorable effect would potentially decrease the number of high-risk days.[155]

One frequent patient and physician concern about a continuous or extended regimen is the possibility of endometrial "build-up" with an extended administration of both estrogen and progestin on the endometrium. However, continuous pill administration maintains a progestin-dominant effect, resulting in a thin and decidualized endometrium. A recent study confirmed this progestin effect, as all subjects on ultrasound had endometrial stripe measurements less than 5 mm.[164]

Short-term adverse events are similar to conventional 21/7 cyclical regimens.[162] Long-term data on the safety of an extended regimen are not available. Safety data on use of a cyclic regimen, however, have been clearly demonstrated, and as such, continuous pill use appears to be a reasonable alternative approach.

Progestin-only pill

The progestin-only pill (POP) consists of a daily pill containing 0.35 mg of norethindrone. The pill is taken daily, and there are no placebo pills. The POP works as a contraceptive primarily by thickening cervical mucus.[171–173] It also prevents fertilization by inhibiting sperm penetration and impairing sperm motility and tubal cilia activity.[174–176] Importantly, it does not reliably prevent ovulation (50% of POP users).[177] It has similar efficacy as the COC, with 0.3% failure rate with perfect use and 9% failure rate with typical use.[53] The half-life of the pill is also short, requiring not only that it be taken on a daily basis, but that it be taken regularly exactly every 24 hours (efficacy can be lost if the pill is missed by more than 3 hours). The narrower therapeutic index and requirement for very strict adherence make this a poor choice of contraceptive for most adolescents; however, it is an option for those with medical contraindications to estrogen.[7] Contraindications are similar to those of DMPA with the addition of malabsorptive bariatric surgery procedures.[33] As with any progesterone-only method, the most common side effect of the POP is menstrual irregularities.[11]

Male barrier method: The male condom

With the advent of newer forms of contraception, barrier contraceptive use as a primary method of birth control has declined.[178] As a group, their use poses a challenge in that they are all coitus dependent; however, they can be used selectively and have minimal or no side effects in comparison with other forms of contraception.[178]

Male condoms are the second most popular form of contraception in the United States (next to the OCP) and the one most commonly used at first intercourse, likely due to the lack of need for a visit to a health-care provider.[1] According to a recent National Survey of Family Growth, 35.6% of 15- to 19-year-old women and 53.5% of 15- to 19-year-old men use a condom every time they engage in sexual intercourse.[179] School condom distribution programs have been associated with equal rates of sexual activity and small but significantly increased rates in condom use.[1] Perfect condom use is associated with an efficacy rate of approximately 97%, although typical use is associated with an 86% efficacy rate.[16,178] Contrary to previous beliefs, spermicide-coated condoms are associated with increased risks of *Escherichia coli* urinary tract infections (UTIs) through alterations in vaginal flora and are no longer recommended.[180]

Condoms require compliance on the part of the male partner and must be used with each act as well as throughout the entire duration of intercourse. Correct use includes leaving a reservoir in the tip of the condom during application, holding the condom during withdrawal of the penis, and removing the condom from the erect penis, as well as avoiding the use of an expired condom.[8,178,181]

Condoms are inexpensive and available over-the-counter and are therefore an easily accessible form of contraception.[8] Patients can further be advised to obtain condoms ahead of time and keep them in a convenient location in the event they are needed, but always out of direct light and extreme heat.[181]

Latex condoms are best for STI protection in comparison with natural materials (such as lamb cecum) and should be recommended for all penetrative sexual activity (i.e., vaginal, anal, and oral) in addition to any other forms of contraception that are used; dental dams should be advised for STI protection in female receptive oral intercourse.[8] For individuals who are allergic to latex, nonlatex condoms are now available: polyisoprene, polyurethane, silicone, and lambskin. Polyurethane condoms and other nonlatex condoms have significantly higher failure rates and pregnancy probabilities when compared to their latex counterparts.[182,183] They are associated with a significantly increased chance of breakage and slippage as compared to latex condoms, but no difference in typical-use failure rates.[184] Polyisoprene condoms are made of synthetic latex and are also safe for those with latex allergies. There are no data of the contraceptive effectiveness; however, they are considered to be comparable to latex condoms due to similar structural makeup.[185] Lambskin condom use is contraindicated in those with lanolin sensitivity, and lambskin condoms do not protect against HIV. Polyurethane condoms may be associated with improved sensation for the male partner.[178]

Female barrier methods

Currently available female barrier methods include the diaphragm, diverse cervical caps and shields, the sponge, and the female condom.[178] In general, adolescents are uncomfortable with the idea of placing barrier methods in the vagina, and these methods are therefore unpopular in this age group. Typically, adolescents are inconsistent users of female barrier methods, and discontinuation rates average 55% over 1 year.[8] The highly motivated adolescent, however, may find significant success with these methods.[16] Individuals choosing a female barrier method are more likely to be in monogamous relationships and motivated to use a method that must be contemplated with each act of intercourse.[127,186] There have been associations of barrier methods with toxic shock syndrome with prolonged placement. Barrier methods are also associated with higher rates of UTIs, possibly related to higher rates of *E coli* colonization and pressure on the urethra preventing complete bladder emptying.[178] Additionally, they are more complicated to use and are less effective than their hormonal counterparts. All of these reasons likely contribute to their decreased rates of use over time.[186]

The diaphragm, which has a failure rate of 7.9% with perfect use and 10.4% with typical use at 6 months, is a rubber cup with a flat or coil spring rim or wide seal, and is designed to fit in the vagina and cover the cervix.[54] It traditionally was fitted by a health-care provider, who measured the distance between the posterior vaginal fornix and the pubic symphysis. A 60–80 mm diaphragm suits most adolescent women well. The diaphragm should be refitted after any pregnancy or pregnancy termination, if the user was virginal at first fitting, after a 10 lb or more weight change, if vaginismus is experienced, and on an annual basis. More recently, a one-size-only diaphragm has become available. It measures 67 mm in width and 75 mm in length and fits most women.

Diaphragms are used in conjunction with spermicide, which should be placed in the cup of the diaphragm before intercourse; additional spermicide should be placed in the vagina with each additional act of intercourse. The diaphragm can be placed up to 2 hours before intercourse and must remain in place for a minimum of 6 hours and a maximum of 24 hours after intercourse.[178,186] Efficacy is decreased with frequent coitus, numerous partners, younger age, use of oil-based lubricants, poor instructions for use, prior failure of contraceptive, and ambivalence about pregnancy.[16] Some studies have indicated that diaphragms are associated with a decreased risk of STIs. However, this may not be due to the method itself, but may be more related to the fact that it is often used in association with spermicide and that many diaphragm users are older, well educated, and in monogamous relationships.[178]

The cervical cap is smaller than the diaphragm and fits over the cervix, staying in place by suction. The only cervical cap available is made of silicone and shaped like a sailor's cap with a strap for removal such that spermicide can be put on the anticervical side. It comes in three sizes, fitted on the basis of the patient's obstetrical history. It can be left in place for up to 48 hours and is associated with fewer UTIs than the diaphragm. The cervical cap has been shown to be less effective than the diaphragm with a failure rate of 13.5% at 6 months.[187]

There are no absolute contraindications to using the diaphragm or cervical cap. The relative contraindications are limited to latex allergy (not applicable to silicone-based barriers), silicone allergy, or history of toxic shock syndrome.[188]

A silicone vaginal barrier contraceptive, also known as a shield, is another form of barrier contraceptive. It comes in one size and therefore does not need to be fitted by a health-care professional. It has a reservoir for spermicide, a central valve that relieves positive pressure and allows for drainage of cervical secretions, and a loop to aid in removal.[186] Being silicone, it is a suitable barrier method for individuals who are allergic to latex. Efficacy rates are similar to those seen with the diaphragm and may also be lower in parous women.[178,186]

The sponge is a disposable, single-use polyurethane sponge 3 inches in diameter and 1.5 inches thick, which contains 1 g of nonoxynol-9 and is inserted vaginally and does not need to be fitted.[16,186] It is moistened before insertion to activate the spermicide (125–150 mg nonoxynol-9 is released over 24 hours) and has a dimple on one side that sits against the cervix and a strap on the other side for removal. The sponge acts as a physical barrier, releases spermicide, and absorbs sperm; all of these methods decrease the exposure of sperm to the cervix. It can be placed up to 24 hours before intercourse, can be used for multiple acts of intercourse, and should stay *in situ* for 6 hours after intercourse, for a total of 30 hours. To decrease rates of toxic shock syndrome, it is also recommended that the sponge not be used during menstruation, postpartum, or after an abortion.[186] It has similar efficacy to the diaphragm, although like the cervical cap, decreased efficacy is noted in parous women. After being taken off the market in 1995, it has now been available again since 2005.[16,178,186] The failure rate is 9% in nulliparous women and 20% in parous women with perfect use and 12% and 24% with typical use, respectively.[53,189] The single absolute contraindication for the sponge is being at high risk for HIV due to the increased risk of vaginal and cervical irritation with nonoxynol-9 use.[188] The relative contraindications are limited to allergy to nonoxyl-9, being HIV positive, use of antiretroviral therapy, and a history of toxic shock syndrome.[188]

The female condom is a female-initiated method of both contraception and STI prevention. The female condom is a single-use polyurethane sheath, 78 mm wide and 170 mm long, with a ring at either end. It is prelubricated on the inside with a spermicidal lubricant, and one ring is placed in the vagina before intercourse and the other open ring sits outside the vagina to allow for intercourse. It can be placed in the vagina up to 8 hours before intercourse.[178] It has been shown to reduce rates of STI transmission in women whose partners refuse to use a male condom.[16] The female condom can be placed autonomously and is safe to use for those with a latex sensitivity.[190] It should not, however, be used in conjunction with a male condom, as the two can adhere to each other and become displaced.[178] While clinical evidence is limited, the polyurethane sheath as well as the small amount of protection provided over the perineum should provide STI protection similar to that observed with the male condom. The 12-month pregnancy rate for perfect use is 5% and typical use is 21%.[53] Slippage is a problem noted specifically with the female condom, and cost can be prohibitive to its use.[178] There are no absolute contraindications to the female condom, but relative contraindications include nitrile polymer allergy or abnormal vaginal anatomy that may pose difficulty with satisfactory placement.[188]

Vaginal spermicides

Vaginal spermicides consist of a spermicidal agent (most commonly nonoxynol-9) with a carrier method such as a cream, foam, tablet, jelly, or film and can be purchased without a prescription. Patients should be advised to allow the film or tablet to dissolve before intercourse and should also be reminded to use a fresh dose of spermicide before each act of intercourse. Vaginal spermicides are not as effective as other forms of contraception, with a failure rate of 28% with typical use and 18% with perfect use.[53] They can be used alone; however, they are more often used in conjunction with other male and female barrier methods. Currently, there is no evidence to support the use of spermicides against STIs.[191] Vaginal spermicides used alone do not decrease rates of HIV transmission. In fact, nonoxynol-9 has also been associated with increased rates of HIV transmission in Kenyan sex trade workers as a result of increased irritation and abrasions to the vagina.[178] Vaginal odor, irritation, yeast infections, UTIs, and allergic reactions are the primary side effects. In addition, the spermicide may leak out of the vagina after intercourse.[8,16,178]

Miscellaneous methods

The rhythm method, Billings method, and calculations of basal body temperature can all be used by the highly motivated adolescent to identify the body's physiologic changes and thus the most fertile period of the cycle. They can then avoid sexual activity during these times. Due to the high degree of motivation required, this method is not applicable to most adolescents, and failure rates of these methods over time are quite high (6%–38%).[16] However, in low-resource areas, the rhythm method can be quite helpful. Lactational amenorrhea is not a reliable method, especially if the infant is over 6 months of age or if breastfeeding is not exclusive and the woman has resumed menses.[16] Coitus interruptus or withdrawal is a technique that is also unreliable and relies on the male partner's ability and willingness to withdraw before ejaculation; these concepts are not realistic for many adolescent males. Furthermore, there is no protection against STI with any of these methods.[16]

Emergency contraception

Emergency contraception is an option that all too few adolescents are aware of and which is advocated by all too few providers of contraception. In one survey of providers specifically trained in the care of adolescents, only 80% provided the emergency contraceptive pill (ECP) when prescribing contraception. Of those who did, many were misguided or misinformed in its use, such as not providing it to teens who would choose to keep a pregnancy or providing it only within 48 hours of unprotected intercourse.[1] In one study, 7% of ECP users went on to have subsequent pregnancies, indicating that those who use ECP should be identified as being at increased risk for pregnancy in the future.[1] Provision of emergency contraception should also involve discussion of a longer-term method of contraception if one is not already in use, or reevaluation of the current method.[192]

Emergency contraceptive methods are designed to be used after an act of unprotected intercourse, or when a chosen method of contraception fails (e.g., a broken condom), to prevent pregnancy from that act of intercourse. Methods of emergency contraception include ECP (Yuzpe), levonorgestrel [LNG] and ulipristal acetate [UPA]) and postcoital insertion of the copper IUD (Table 16.6). The mechanisms of action differ depending on type of emergency contraceptive, but generally involve inhibition or delay of ovulation, or prevention of implantation or fertilization.[7,16,193] Emergency contraceptives do not disrupt an established pregnancy and do not increase the risk of an ectopic pregnancy.[193]

In general, the pregnancy rate following emergency contraception use is between 0.01% and 3.2%.[194–197] However, efficacy differs depending on type of emergency contraceptive and decreases with time from intercourse (with the exception of UPA).[7,127,198] The only contraindication to the use of any method of emergency contraception is a known, previously established pregnancy.[192] The patient should also be advised that her subsequent menstrual cycle can be altered, starting earlier than usual (21 days).[16,33] Despite the large number of users of ECP, there are no reports of major adverse outcomes.[192] Increased provision of ECPs has not been shown to reduce adherence to longer-term contraceptive methods.[199]

There are currently three FDA-approved versions of ECP.[192] The first is the Yuzpe method, which consists of any combination of COCs containing 100 μg ethinyl estradiol and 500 μg levonorgestrel or norgestrel, taken twice, 12 hours apart.[1,128,199,200] The most common side effects are nausea (50%) and emesis (20%). For these reasons, many clinicians will provide an antiemetic along with the ECP; a repeat dose should be taken if there is emesis within 2 hours of taking either dose.[16]

A second available ECP consists of two pills of 0.75 mg LNG taken 12 hours apart or one pill of 1.5 mg of LNG. Studies have shown that both dosing methods are equally as effective in preventing unplanned pregnancy.[7,199,201] It should be taken as soon as possible following unprotected intercourse, as its efficacy decreases with time.[202] The risk of pregnancy has been shown to be five times more likely when it is administered 5 days following unprotected intercourse compared to within 24 hours.[202] Backup contraception should be used 7 days following use of LNG, even if the adolescent has resumed birth control.[203]

Table 16.6 Emergency contraception.

Emergency contraceptive	Dose	Timing of emergency contraceptive administration	Rate of pregnancy at 72 hours	Side effects
Yuzpe	Combined oral contraceptive containing 100 μg ethinyl estradiol and 500 μg levonorgestrel or norgestrel, taken twice, 12 hours apart	Effective up to 3 days (72 hours); ideally taken within 24 hours	3.2%	Frequently causes nausea and vomiting
Levonorgestrel	Two pills of 0.75 mg levonorgestrel 12 hours apart or one pill of 1.5 mg	Effective up to 5 days (120 hours) after intercourse; ideally taken within 72 hours	2.7%	May cause nausea
Ulipristal acetate	One pill of 30 mg	Effective up to 5 days (120 hours) after intercourse)	0.9%	Interferes with hormonal contraception
Copper IUD		Effective up to 7 days after intercourse	0.01%	May cause heavy bleeding and cramping

In randomized trials, it was shown to be slightly more effective than the estrogen-containing methods. It is 95% effective if used within 24 hours and 85% if used between 24 and 48 hours as compared with the Yuzpe method at 77% and 36%, respectively.[7,204,205] The efficacy of LNG has been shown to decrease with increasing body weight (BMI >30).[206] Despite its decreased efficacy in women with a BMI >30, LNG should not be withheld.[33] Because the LNG pills do not involve the use of estrogen, nausea is also less common.[16] For these reasons, LNG is preferred over estrogen-containing methods, where the choice is available.

A third and more recently available ECP is UPA, which was approved by the FDA in 2010 and must be prescribed by a physician for use.[207] UPA is prescribed as a 30 mg dose that can be taken within 120 hours of sexual intercourse.[208] UPA is a selective progesterone receptor modulator that acts as an antagonist and partial agonist at the progesterone receptor site.[208] In contrast to levonorgestrel, UPA has been shown to prevent follicular rupture despite rising LH levels in the late follicular phase.[208] An analysis of pooled data from three randomized trials of contraception regimens demonstrated that UPA was significantly more effective at delaying ovulation for at least 5 days (58.8%) compared to levonorgestrel (14.6%). UPA has also been shown to be more efficacious compared to LNG in women with a BMI >30.[205] Backup contraception should be used for the first 5 days following UPA and an additional 14 days after starting CHC and POP, as it can interfere with the effectiveness of CHC and POP.[40,209]

In addition to the ECP, insertion of a copper IUD up to 7 days after ovulation (generally accepted as up to 5 days after unprotected intercourse to avoid calculation difficulties) is also a highly effective method of emergency contraception. It has been estimated to have an efficacy of up to 100%.[210] Despite its high efficacy, the copper IUD is rarely recommended in clinical practice.[211] One barrier to the prescription of the copper IUD includes the disruption of outpatient clinic flow to accommodate its insertion. Additionally, unlike the other methods, the copper IUD is not cost effective when used only for emergency contraception. However, it can, of course, thereafter be used for long-term contraception for up to 12 years.[192,200] The risk of exposure to STIs should not preclude the use of the copper IUD for emergency contraception, particularly in the adolescent population. In high-risk individuals, the copper IUD can be removed after use as an emergency contraceptive. Side effects are the same as those associated with a copper IUD inserted at any other time and include abdominal cramping and pain, vaginal bleeding, and spotting.[200] The LNG-IUS is not presently licensed for use for emergency contraception.[199]

Future directions

Contraception development persists with an emphasis on manufacturing novel formulations that will provide safe and effective contraceptive options that are increasingly convenient to use, thus enhancing adherence. Products currently under development include a progesterone-only pill with a longer half-life that is capable of suppressing ovulation more reliably, a vaginal ring that can be used for an entire year (replaced after a monthly withdrawal bleed), biodegradable implants that would not require removal, as well as new female barrier methods.[118,128] Vaginal rings that provide protection against HIV and STIs in addition to contraception are also currently being developed.[211] Research is also underway to investigate how to improve injectable contraceptives by lengthening the periods of effectiveness (greater than or equal to 6 months) and making self-administration possible.[212] Although currently, hormonal methods are not available over the counter in the United States, increased efforts are underway to allow access without a prescription to reliable hormonal contraception.

REFERENCES

1. Polaneczky M. Adolescent contraception. *Curr Opin Obstet Gynecol.* 1998;10:213–9.
2. Statistics Canada. Table 102-4503—Live births, by age of mother, Canada, Provinces and territories, annual, CANSIM (database). http://www5.statcan.gc.ca/cansim/a05?lang=eng&id=1024503.
3. Ethier KA, Kann L, McManus T. Sexual intercourse among high school students – 29 states and United States overall, 2005–2015. *MMWR.* 2018;66(51,52):1393–7.
4. Kaiser HJ, Family Foundation. Sexual health of adolescents and young adults in the United States. 2014.
5. Rotermann M. Sexual behaviour and condom use of 15- to 24-year-olds in 2003 and 2009/2010. *Health Rep.* 2012;23(1):1–5.
6. Guttmacher Institute. U.S. Teenage Pregnancies, Births and Abortions, 2010: National Trends by Age, Race and Ethnicity; May 2014.
7. Rimsza ME. Counseling the adolescent about contraception. *Pediatr Rev.* 2003;24:162–70.
8. Brill SR, Rosenfeld WD. Contraception. *Med Clin North Am.* 2000;84:907–25.
9. Davis AJ. Adolescent contraception and the clinician: An emphasis on counseling and communication. *Clin Obstet Gynecol.* 2001;44:114–21.
10. Tripp J, Viner R. Sexual health, contraception, and teenage pregnancy. *BMJ.* 2005;330:590–3.
11. Ornstein RM, Fisher MM. Hormonal contraception in adolescents: Special considerations. *Paediatr Drugs.* 2006;8:25–45.
12. Short MB, Yates JK, Biro F, Rosenthal SL. Parents and partners: Enhancing participation in contraception use. *J Pediatr Adolesc Gynecol.* 2005;18:379–83.
13. Part K, Moreau C, Donati S, Gissler M, Fronteira I, Karro H, The Reprostat Group. Teenage pregancies in the European Union in the context of legislation and youth sexual and reproductive health services. *ACTA Obstetrica et Gynecol.* 2013;92:1395–140.
14. Facts in Brief. *Facts on Sex Education in the United States.* New York, NY: Allan Guttenmacher Institute; 2007.

15. Darroch JE, Singh S, Frost JJ, the Study Team. Differences in teenage pregnancy rates among five developed countries: The role of sexual activity and contraceptive use. *Fam Plann Perspect*. 2001;33:244–50, 281.

16. Greydanus DE, Patel DR, Rimsza ME. Contraception in the adolescent: An update. *Pediatrics*. 2001;107:562–73.

17. United Nations Department of Economic and Social Affairs, Population Division. *World Contraception Use 2015*. New York, NY: UN DoEaSA; 2015. http://www.un.org/en/development/desa/population/publications/dataset/contraception/wcu2015.shtml. Accessed June 29, 2015.

18. Mosher WD, Martinez GM, Chandra A, Abma JC, Willson SJ. Use of contraception and use of family planning services in the United States: 1982–2002. *Adv Data*. 2004;350:1–36.

19. Martin K, Wu Z. Contraceptive use in Canada: 1984–1999. *Fam Plann Perspect*. 2000;32:65.

20. Andersson K, Odlind V, Rybo G. Levonorgestrel-releasing and copper-releasing (Nova T) IUDs during five years of use: A randomized comparative trial. *Contraception*. 1994;49:56–72.

21. Winner B, Peipert JF, Zhao Q et al. Effectiveness of long-acting reversible contraception. *N Engl J Med*. 2012;366:1998e2007.

22. Videla-Rivero L, Etchepareborda JJ, Kesseru E. Early chorionic activity in women bearing inert IUD, copper IUD and levonorgestrel-releasing IUD. *Contraception*. 1987;36:217–26.

23. Stanford JB, Mikolajczyk RT. Mechanisms of action of intrauterine devices: Update and estimation of postfertilization effects. *Am J Obstet Gynecol*. 2002;187:1699–708.

24. Sivin I. IUDs are contraceptives, not abortifacients: A comment on research and belief. *Stud Fam Plann*. 1989;20:355–9.

25. Ortiz ME, Croxatto HB, Bardin CW. Mechanisms of action of intrauterine devices. *Obstet Gynecol Surv*. 1996;51(12 Suppl):S42–51.

26. Wilcox AJ, Weinberg CR, Armstrong EG, Canfield RE. Urinary human chorionic gonadotropin among intrauterine device users: Detection with a highly specific and sensitive assay. *Fertil Steril*. 1987;47:265–9.

27. Critchley HO, Wang H, Jones RL et al. Morphological and functional features of endometrial decidualization following long-term intrauterine levonorgestrel delivery. *Hum Reprod*. 1998;13:1218–24.

28. Jonsson B, Landgren BM, Eneroth P. Effects of various IUDs on the composition of cervical mucus. *Contraception*. 1991;43:447–58.

29. Nilsson CG, Lahteenmaki PL, Luukkainen T. Ovarian function in amenorrheic and menstruatig users of a levonorgestrel-releasing intrauterine device. *Fertil Steril*. 1984;41:52–5.

30. Barbosa I, Bakos O, Olsson SE, Odlind V, Johansson ED. Ovarian function during use of a levonorgestrel-releasing IUD. *Contraception*. 1990;42:51–66.

31. Adolescents and long-acting reversible contraception: implants and intrauterine devices. ACOG Committee Opinion No. 735. American College of Obstetricians and Gynecologists. *Obstet Gynecol* 2018;131:e130–9.

32. World Health Organization. *Improving Access to Quality Care in Family Planning: Medical Eligibility Criteria for Contraceptive Use*. 2nd ed. Geneva, Switzerland: WHO; 2001.

33. Black A, Guilbert E. Canadian contraception consensus part 4 of 4 Chapter 9: Combined hormonal contraception. *J Obstet Gynaecol Can*. 2017;39(4):229–68.

34. Farley TM, Rosenberg MJ, Rowe PJ, Chen JH, Meirik O. Intrauterine devices and pelvic inflammatory disease: An international perspective. *Lancet*. 1992;339:785–8.

35. Sufrin CB, Postlethwaite D, Armstrong MA, Merchant M, Wendt JM, Steinauer JE. *Neisseria gonorrhea* and *Chlamydia trachomatis* screening at intrauterine device insertion and pelvic inflammatory disease. *Obstet Gynecol*. 2012;120:1314e21.

36. Toivonen J, Luukkainen T, Allonen H. Protective effect of intrauterine release of levonorgestrel on pelvic infection: Three years' comparative experience of levonorgestrel- and copper-releasing intrauterine devices. *Obstet Gynecol*. 1991;77:261–4.

37. WHO Scientific Group. Mechanism of action, safety and efficacy of intrauterine devices. *World Health Organ Tech Rep Ser*. 1987;753:1–91.

38. Harrison-Woolrych M, Ashton J, Coulter D. Uterine perforation on intrauterine device insertion: Is the incidence higher than previously reported? *Contraception*. 2003;67:53–6.

39. Madden T, McNicholas C, Zhao Q, Secura GM, Eisenberg DL, Peipert JF. Association of age and parity with intrauterine device expulsion. *Obstet Gynecol*. 2014;124:718e26.

40. Black A, Guilbert E, Costescu D, Dunn S, Fisher W, Kives S et al. Canadian Contraception Consensus (Part 1 of 4): Chapter 3 – Emergency Contraception. *J Obstet Gynaecol Can*. 2015;37(10 Suppl):S20–S28. doi: 10.1016/S1701-2613(16)39372-0.

41. Akers AY, Steinway C, Sonalkar S, Perriera LK, Schreiber C, Harding J, Garcia-Espana JF. Reducing pain during intrauterine device insertion: A randomized controlled trial in adolescents and young women. *Obstet Gynecol*. 2017;130(4):795–802.

42. Waddington A, Reid R. More harm than good: The lack of evidence for administering misoprostol prior to IUD insertion. *J Obstet Gynaecol Can*. 2012;34:1177e9.

43. Heinemann K, Reed S, Moehner S, Do Minh T. Comparative contraceptive effectiveness of levonorgestrel-releasing and copper intrauterine devices: The European Active Surveillance Study for Intrauterine Devices. *Contraception*. 2015;91:280e3.

44. Nelson A, Apter D, Hauck B et al. Two low-dose levonorgestrel intrauterine contraceptive systems: A randomized controlled trial. *Obstet Gynecol.* 2013;122: 1205e13.

45. Brahmi D, Steenland MW, Renner RM, Gaffield ME, Curtis KM. Pregnancy outcomes with an IUD *in situ*: A systematic review. *Contraception.* 2012;85: 131–9.

46. Hubacher D, Lara-Ricalde R, Taylor DJ, Guerra-Infante F, Guzman- Rodriguez R. Use of copper intrauterine devices and the risk of tubal infertility among nulligravid women. *N Engl J Med.* 2001;345:561e7.

47. Ronnerdag M, Odlind V. Health effects of long-term use of the intrauterine levonorgestrel-releasing system. A follow-up study over 12 years of continuous use. *Acta Obstet Gynecol Scand.* 1999;78:716–21.

48. Luukkainen T, Allonen H, Haukkamaa M et al. Effective contraception with the levonorgestrel-releasing intrauterine device: 12-month report of a European multicenter study. *Contraception.* 1987;36: 169–79.

49. Andersson JK, Rybo G. Levonorgestrel-releasing intrauterine device in the treatment of menorrhagia. *Br J Obstet Gynaecol.* 1990;97:690e4.

50. Milsom I, Andersson K, Jonasson K, Lindstedt G, Rybo G. The influence of the Gyne-T 380S IUD on menstrual blood loss and iron status. *Contraception.* 1995;52:175–9.

51. Larsson G, Milsom I, Jonasson K, Lindstedt G, Rybo G. The long-term effects of copper surface area on menstrual blood loss and iron status in women fitted with an IUD. *Contraception.* 1993;48:471–80.

52. Suhonen S, Haukkamaa M, Jakobsson T, Rauramo I. Clinical performance of a levonorgestrel-releasing intrauterine system and oral contraceptives in young nulliparous women: A comparative study. *Contraception.* 2004;69:407–12.

53. Trussell J. Contraceptive failure in the United States. *Contraception.* 2011;83:397–404.

54. Darney P, Patel A, Rosen K, Shapiro LS, Kaunitz AM. Safety and efficacy of a single-rod etonogestrel implant (Implanon): Results from 11 international clinical trials. *Fertil Steril.* 2009;91:1646e53.

55. Blumenthal PD, Gemzell-Danielsson K, Marintcheva-Petrova M. Tolerability and clinical safety of Implanon. *Eur J Contracept Reprod Health Care.* 2008;13(Suppl):29e36.

56. Urbancsek J. An integrated analysis of nonmenstrual adverse events with Implanon. *Contraception.* 1998;58(6 Suppl):109Se15S.

57. Meirik O, Brache V, Orawan K et al. A multi-center randomized clinical trial of one-rod etonogestrel and two-rod levonorgestrel contraceptive implants with nonrandomized copper-IUD controls: Methodology and insertion data. *Contraction.* 2013;87:113e20.

58. Organon USA News and Events. FDA approves Implanon (etonorgestrel implant) 68 mg. The first and only truly implantable contraceptive. July 18, 2006.

59. Templeman CL, Cook V, Goldsmith LJ, Powell J, Hertweck SP. Postpartum contraceptive use among adolescent mothers. *Obstet Gynecol.* 2000;95:770–6.

60. Guttmacher Institute. *Teen Sex and Pregnancy: Facts in Brief.* New York, NY: Alan Guttmacher Institute; 1999.

61. Stevens-Simon C, Kelly L, Kulick R. A village would be nice but … it takes a long-acting contraceptive to prevent repeat adolescent pregnancies. *Am J Prev Med.* 2001;21:60–5.

62. Immediate postpartum long-acting reversible contraception. Committee Opinion No. 670. American College of Obstetricians and Gynecologists. *Obstet Gynecol.* 2016;128:e32–7.

63. Petta CA, Faundes A, Dunson TR et al. Timing of onset of contraceptive effectiveness in Depo-Provera users. Part I. Changes in cervical mucus. *Fertil Steril.* 1998;62:252e7.

64. Petta CA, Faundes A, Dunson TR et al. Timing of onset of contraceptive effectiveness in Depo-Provera users. Part II. Effects on ovarian function. *Fertil Steril.* 1998;70:817e20.

65. Mishell DR Jr. Pharmacokinetics of depot medroxyprogesterone acetate contraception. *J Reprod Med.* 1996;41(5 Suppl):381e90.

66. Schwallie PC, Assenzo JR. Contraceptive use—Efficacy study utilizing medroxyprogesterone acetate administered as an intramuscular injection once every 90 days. *Fertil Steril.* 1973;24:331–9.

67. Cromer BA, Lazebnik R, Rome E et al. Double-blinded randomized controlled trial of estrogen supplementation in adolescent girls who receive depot medroxyprogesterone acetate for contraception. *Am J Obstet Gynecol.* 2005;192:42–7.

68. Hatcher RA Trussell J, Stewart F et al. *Contraceptive Technology.* 17th ed. New York, NY: Ardent Media; 1998.

69. Said S, Omar K, Koetsawang S et al. A multi-centred phase III comparative clinical trial of depot-medroxyprogesterone acetate given three-monthly at doses of 100 or 150 mg: 1. Contraceptive efficacy and side effects. World Health Organization Task Force on Long-Acting Systemic Agents for Fertility Regulation. Special Programme of Research, Development and Research Training in Human Reproduction. *Contraception.* 1986; 34:223–35.

70. Toppozada HK, Koetsawang S, Aimakju VE et al. Multinational comparative clinical trial of long-acting injectable contraceptives: Norethisterone enanthate given in two dosage regimens and depot-medroxyprogesterone acetate. Final report. *Contraception.* 1983;28:1–20.

71. Guillebaud J. *Contraception: Your Question Answered*. 2nd ed. New York, NY: Churchill Livingstone; 1993:261–85.

72. Kaunitz AM. Long-acting injectable contraception with depot medroxyprogesterone acetate. *Am J Obstet Gynecol*. 1994;170:1543–9.

73. Westhoff C, Kerns J, Morroni C et al. Quick start: Novel oral contraceptive initiation method. *Contraception*. 2002;66:141–5.

74. Nelson AL, Katz T. Initiation and continuation rates seen in 2-year experience with same day injections of DMPA. *Contraception*. 2007;75:84–7.

75. World Health Organization. *Medical Eligibility Criteria for Contraceptive Use*. 5th ed. Geneva, Switzerland: World Health Organization; 2015.

76. Gupta N, O'Brien R, Jacobsen LJ et al. Mood changes in adolescents using depot-medroxyprogesterone acetate for contraception: A prospective study. *J Pediatr Adolesc Gynecol*. 2001;14:71e6.

77. Cromer BA, Smith RD, Blair JM, Dwyer J, Brown RT. A prospective study of adolescents who choose among levonorgestrel implant (Norplant), medroxyprogesterone acetate (Depo-Provera), or the combined oral contraceptive pill as contraception. *Pediatrics*. 1994;94:87e94.

78. Westhoff C, Truman C, Kalmuss D et al. Depressive symptoms and Depo-Provera. *Contraception*. 1998;57:237e40.

79. Espey E, Steinhart J, Ogburn T, Qualls C. Depo-Provera associated with weight gain in Navajo women. *Contraception*. 2000;62:55–8.

80. Bahamondes L, Del Castillo S, Tabares G et al. Comparison of weight increase in users of depot medroxyprogesterone acetate and copper IUD up to 5 years. *Contraception*. 2001;64:223–5.

81. Danli S, Qingxiang S, Guowei S. A multicentered clinical trial of the long-acting injectable contraceptive Depo Provera in Chinese women. *Contraception*. 2000;62:15–8.

82. Matson SC, Henderson KA, McGrath GJ. Physical findings and symptoms of depot medroxyprogesterone acetate use in adolescent females. *J Pediatr Adolesc Gynecol*. 1997;10:18–23.

83. Black A, Francoeur D, Rowe T et al. Canadian contraception consensus. *J Obstet Gynaecol Can*. 2004;26:143–56, 158–74.

84. Clark MK, Dillon JS, Sowers M, Nichols S. Weight, fat mass, and central distribution of fat increase when women use depot-medroxyprogesterone acetate for contraception. *Int J Obes (Lond)*. 2005;29:1252–8.

85. Rees HD, Bonsall RW, Michael RP. Pre-optic and hypothalamic neurons accumulate [3H]medroxyprogesterone acetate in male cynomolgus monkeys. *Life Sci*. 1986;39:1353–9.

86. Bonny AE, Lange HL, Rogers LK, Gothard DM, Reed MD. A pilot study of depot medroxyprogesterone acetate pharmacokinetics and weight gain in adolescent females. *Contraception*. 2014;89(5):357–60.

87. Polaneczky M, Guarnaccia M, Alon J, Wiley J. Early experience with the contraceptive use of depot medroxyprogesterone acetate in an inner-city clinic population. *Fam Plann Perspect*. 1996;28:174–8.

88. Belsey EM. Task Force on Long-Acting Systemic Agents for Fertility Regulation. Menstrual bleeding patterns in untreated women and with long-acting methods of contraception. *Adv Contracept*. 1991;7:257–70.

89. Sangi-Haghpeykar H, Poindexter AN 3rd, Bateman L, Ditmore JR. Experiences of injectable contraceptive users in an urban setting. *Obstet Gynecol*. 1996;88:227–33.

90. Lim SW, Rieder J, Coupey SM, Bijur PE. Depot medroxyprogesterone acetate use in inner-city, minority adolescents: Continuation rates and characteristics of long-term users. *Arch Pediatr Adolesc Med*. 1999;153:1068–72.

91. Rickert VI, Tiezzi L, Lipshutz J et al. Depo now: Preventing unintended pregnancies among adolescents and young adults. *J Adolesc Health*. 2007;40:22–8.

92. Cromer BA, Blair JM, Mahan JD, Zibners L, Naumovski Z. A prospective comparison of bone density in adolescent girls receiving depot medroxyprogesterone acetate (Depo-Provera), levonorgestrel (Norplant), or oral contraceptives. *J Pediatr*. 1996;129:671–6.

93. Lara-Torre E, Edwards CP, Perlman S, Hertweck SP. Bone mineral density in adolescent females using depot medroxyprogesterone acetate. *J Pediatr Adolesc Gynecol*. 2004;17:17–21.

94. Cromer BA, Stager M, Bonny A et al. Depot medroxyprogesterone acetate, oral contraceptives and bone mineral density in a cohort of adolescent girls. *J Adolesc Health*. 2004;35:434–41.

95. Scholes D, LaCroix AZ, Ichikawa LE, Barlow WE, Ott SM. Change in bone mineral density among adolescent women using and discontinuing depot medroxyprogesterone acetate contraception. *Arch Pediatr Adolesc Med*. 2005;159:139–44.

96. Harel Z, Johnson CC, Gold MA et al. Recover of bone mineral density in adolescents following the use of depot medroxyprogesterone acetate contraceptive injections. *Contraception*. 2010;81(4):281–91.

97. Curtis KM, Martins SL. Progestogen-only contraception and bone mineral density: A systematic review. *Contraception*. 2006;73:470–87.

98. Committee on Adolescence. Contraception for adolescents. *Pediatrics*. 2014;134(4):e1244–56.

99. Cromer BA, Scholes D, Berenson A et al. Depot medroxyprogesterone acetate and bone mineral density in adolescents – The Black Box Warning: A Position Paper of the Society for Adolescent Medicine. *J Adolesc Health*. 2006;39:296–301.

100. d'Arcanques C. WHO statement on hormonal contraception and bone health. *Wkly Epidemiol Rec*. 2005;80:302–4.

101. Cullins VE. Noncontraceptive benefits and therapeutic uses of depot medroxyprogesterone acetate. *Reprod Med.* 1996;41(5 Suppl):428–33. Review.

102. Mattson RH, Cramer JA, Caldwell BV, Siconolfi BC. Treatment of seizures with medroxyprogesterone acetate: Preliminary report. *Neurology.* 1984;34:1255–8.

103. Gallo MF, Lopez LM, Grimes DA, Schulz KF, Helmerhorst FM. Combination contraceptives: Effects on weight. *Cochrane Database Syst Rev.* 2006;1:CD003987.

104. Lidegaard O, Lokkegaard E, Svendsen AL, Agger C. Hormonal contraception and risk of venous thromboembolism: National follow-up study. *BMJ.* 2009;339:b2890.

105. World Health Organization Collaborative Study of Cardiovascular Disease and Steroid Hormone Contraception. Cardiovascular disease and the use of oral and injectable progestogen-only contraceptives and combined injectable contraceptives: Results of an international, muticenter, case-control study. *Contraception.* 1998;57:315–24.

106. Middeldorp S. Oral contraceptives and the risk of venous thromboembolism. *Gend Med.* 2005;2(Suppl A):S3–9.

107. Risk of venous thromboembolism among users of drospirenone-containing oral contraceptive pills. Committee Opinion No. 540. American College of Obstetricians and Gynecologists. *Obstet Gynecol.* 2012;120:1239–42.

108. Dinger JC, Heinemann LA, Kuhl-Habich D. The safety of a drospirenone- containing oral contraceptive: Final results from the European Active Surveillance Study on oral contraceptives based on 142,475 women-years of observation. *Contraception.* 2007;75:344e54.

109. Dinger J, Bardenheuer K, Heinemann K. Cardiovascular and general safety of a 24-day regimen of drospirenone-containing combined oral contraceptives: Final results from the International Active Surveillance Study of Women Taking Oral Contraceptives. *Contraception.* 2014;89:253e63.

110. Burkman R, Schlesselman JJ, Zieman M. Safety concerns and health benefits associated with oral contraception. *Am J Obstet Gynecol.* 2004;190:S5–S22.

111. Johannessen SI, Landmark CJ. Antiepileptic drug interactions – Principles and clinical implications. *Current Neuropharmacology.* 2010;8:254–67.

112. Arowojolu AO, Gallo MF, Lopez LM, Grimes DA, Garner SE. Combined oral contraceptive pills for treatment of acne. *Cochrane Database Syst Rev.* 2007;24:CD004425.

113. Kahlenborn C, Modugno F, Potter DM, Severs WB. Oral contraceptive use as a risk factor for premenopausal breast cancer: A meta-analysis. *Mayo Clin Proc.* 2006;81:1290–302.

114. Martins SL, Curtis KM, Glasier AF. Combined hormonal contraception and bone health: A systematic review. *Contraception.* 2006;73:445–69.

115. Nappi C, Bifulco G, Tommaselli GA, Gargano V, Di Carlo C. Hormonal contraception and bone metabolism: A systematic review. *Contraception.* 2012;86:606–21.

116. Pons JE. Hormonal contraception compliance in teenagers. *Pediatr Endocrinol Rev.* 2006;3:164–6.

117. Hillard PJ. Contraceptive behaviors in adolescents. *Pediatr Ann.* 2005;34:794–802.

118. Masimasi N, Sivanandy MS, Thacker HL. Update on hormonal contraception. *Cleve Clin J Med.* 2007;74:186, 8–90, 93–4 passim.

119. Yamazaki M, Dwyer K, Sobhan M, Davis D, Kim MJ, Soule L, Willett G, Yu C. Effect of obesity on the effectiveness of hormonal contraceptives: An individual participant data meta-analysis. *Contraception.* 2015;92:445–52.

120. Burkman RT, Fisher AC, Wan GJ, Barnowski CE, LaGuardia KD. Association between efficacy and body weight or body mass index for two low-dose oral contraceptives. *Contraception.* 2009;79:424–7.

121. Dinger JC, Cronin M, Mohner S, Schellschmidt I, Minh TD, Westhoff C. Oral contraceptive effectiveness according to body mass index, weight, age, and other factors. *Am J Obstet Gynecol.* 2009;201:263.e1–9.

122. McNicholas C, Zhao Q, Secura G, Allsworth JE, Madden T, Peipert JF. Contraceptive failures in overweight and obese combined hormonal contraceptive users. *Obstet Gynecol.* 2013;121:585–92.

123. Westhoff CL, Torgal AH, Mayeda ER, Petrie K, Thomas T, Dragoman M, Cremers S. Pharmacokinetics and ovarian suppression during use of a contraceptive vaginal ring in normal-weight and obese women. *Am J Obstet Gynecol.* 2012;207:39.e1–6.

124. Harel Z, Riggs S, Vaz R et al. Adolescents' experience with the combined estrogen and progestin transdermal contraceptive method Ortho Evra. *J Pediatr Adolesc Gynecol.* 2005;18:85–90.

125. Burkman RT. The transdermal contraceptive system. *Am J Obstet Gynecol.* 2004;190(Suppl 4):S49–53.

126. Abrams LS, Skee DM, Wong FA, Anderson NJ, Leese PT. Pharmacokinetics of norelgestromin and ethinyl estradiol from two consecutive contraceptive patches. *J Clin Pharmacol.* 2001;41:1232–7.

127. Minnis AM, Padian NS. Choice of female-controlled barrier methods among young women and their male sexual partners. *Fam Plann Perspect.* 2001;33:28–34.

128. Gupta N. Advances in hormonal contraception. *Adolesc Med Clin.* 2006;17:653–71, abstract xi.

129. Zacur HA, Hedon B, Mansour D et al. Integrated summary of Ortho Evra/Evra contraceptive patch adhesion in varied climates and conditions. *Fertil Steril.* 2002;77(2 Suppl 2):S32–5.

130. Lopez LM, Grimes DA, Gallo MF, Stockton LL, Schulz KF. Skin patch and vaginal ring versus combined oral contraceptives for contraception. *Cochrane Database Syst Rev.* 2013;(4):CD003552.

131. Sibai BM, Odlind V, Meador ML et al. A comparative and pooled analysis of the safety and tolerability of the contraceptive patch (Ortho Evra/Evra). *Fertil Steril.* 2002;77(2 Suppl 2):S19–26.

132. Zieman M, Guillebaud J, Weisberg E et al. Contraceptive efficacy and cycle control with the Ortho Evra/Evra transdermal system: The analysis of pooled data. *Fertil Steril.* 2002;77(2 Suppl 2):S13–8.

133. Cole JA, Norman H, Doherty M, Walker AM. Venous thromboembolism, myocardial infarction, and stroke among transdermal contraceptive system users. *Obstet Gynecol.* 2007;109:339–46.

134. Jick SS, Kaye JA, Russmann S, Jick H. Risk of nonfatal venous thromboembolism in women using a contraceptive transdermal patch and oral contraceptives containing norgestimate and 35 microg of ethinyl estradiol. *Contraception.* 2006;73:223–8.

135. Jick S, Kaye JA, Li L, Jick H. Further results on the risk of nonfatal venous thromboembolism in users of the contraceptive transdermal patch compared to users of oral contraceptives containing norgestimate and 35 microg of ethinyl estradiol. *Contraception.* 2007;76:4–7.

136. Dore DD, Norman H, Loughlin J, Seeger JD. Extended case-control study results on thromboembolic outcomes among transdermal contraceptive users. *Contraception.* 2010;81:408–13.

137. Archer DF, Bigrigg A, Smallwood GH et al. Assessment of compliance with a weekly contraceptive patch (Ortho Evra/Evra) among North American women. *Fertil Steril.* 2002;77(2 Suppl 2):S27–31.

138. Sarkar NN. The combined contraceptive vaginal device (NuvaRing): A comprehensive review. *Eur J Contracep Reprod Health Care.* 2005;10:73–8.

139. Novak A, de la Loge C, Abetz L, van der Meulen EA. The combined contraceptive vaginal ring, NuvaRing: An international study of user acceptability. *Contraception.* 2003;67:187–94.

140. Johansson ED, Sitruk-Ware R. New delivery systems in contraception: Vaginal rings. *Am J Obstet Gynecol.* 2004;190(2 Suppl 2):S54–9.

141. Haring T, Mulders TM. The combined contraceptive ring NuvaRing and spermicide co-medication. *Contraception.* 2003;67:271–2.

142. Verhoeven CH, Dieben TO. The combined contraceptive vaginal ring, NuvaRing, and tampon co-usage. *Contraception.* 2004;69:197–9.

143. Petrie KA, Torgal AH, Westhoff CL. Matched-pairs analysis of ovarian suppression during oral vs. vaginal hormonal contraceptive use. *Contraception.* 2011;84:e1–4.

144. Oddsson K, Leifels-Fischer B, de Melo NR et al. Efficacy and safety of a contraceptive vaginal ring (NuvaRing) compared with a combined oral contraceptive: A 1-year randomized trial. *Contraception.* 2005;71:176–82.

145. Ahrendt HJ, Nisand I, Bastianelli C et al. Efficacy, acceptability and tolerability of the combined contraceptive ring, NuvaRing, compared with an oral contraceptive containing 30 microg of ethinyl estradiol and 3 mg of drospirenone. *Contraception.* 2006;74:451–7.

146. Milsom I, Lete I, Bjertnaes A et al. Effects on cycle control and bodyweight of the combined contraceptive ring, NuvaRing, versus an oral contraceptive containing 30 microg ethinyl estradiol and 3 mg drospirenone. *Hum Reprod.* 2006;21:2304–11.

147. De Seta F, Restaino S, De Santo D, Stabile G, Banco R, Busetti M, Barbati G, Guaschino S. Effects of hormonal contraception on vaginal flora. *Contraception.* 2012;86:526–9.

148. Lete I, Cuesta MC, Marin JM, Guerra S. Vaginal health in contraceptive vaginal ring users 8 – A review. *Eur J Contracep Reprod Health Care.* 2013;18(4):234–41.

149. Connell EB. Contraception in the prepill era. *Contraception.* 1999;59(1 Suppl):7S–10S.

150. Thomas SL, Ellertson C. Nuisance or natural and healthy: Should monthly menstruation be optional for women? *Lancet.* 2000;355:922–4.

151. Glasier AF, Smith KB, van der Spuy ZM et al. Amenorrhea associated with contraception – An international study on acceptability. *Contraception.* 2003;67:1–8.

152. Andrist LC, Arias RD, Nucatola D, Kaunitz AM, Musselman BL, Reiter S, Boulanger J, Dominguez L, Emmert S. Women's and providers' attitudes toward menstrual suppression with extended use of oral contraceptives. *Contraception.* 2004;70:359–63.

153. Edelman A, Lew R, Cwiak C, Nichols M, Jensen J. Acceptability of contraceptive-induced amenorrhea in a racially diverse group of US women. *Contraception.* 2007;75:450–3.

154. Lakehomer H, Kaplan PF, Wozniak DG, Minson CT. Characteristics of scheduled bleeding manipulation with combined hormonal contraception in university students. *Contraception.* 2013;88:426–30.

155. Gerschultz KL, Sucato GS, Hennon TR, Murray PJ, Gold MA. Extended cycling of combined hormonal contraceptives in adolescents: Physician views and prescribing practices. *J Adolesc Health.* 2007;40:151–7.

156. Machado RB, de Melo N, Maia H. Bleeding patterns and menstrual-related symptoms with the continuous use of a contraceptive combination of ethinylestradiol and drospirenone: A randomized study. *Contraception.* 2010;81:215–22.

157. den Tonkelaar I, Oddens BJ. Preferred frequency and characteristics of menstrual bleeding in relation to reproductive status, oral contraceptive use, and hormone replacement therapy use. *Contraception.* 1999;59:357–62.

158. Wiegratz I, Hommel HH, Zimmermann T, Kuhl H. Attitude of German women and gynecologists towards long-cycle treatment with oral contraceptives. *Contraception.* 2004;69:37–42.

159. Shulman LP. The use of triphasic oral contraceptives in a continuous use regimen. *Contraception.* 2005;72:105–10.

160. Stewart FH, Kaunitz AM, Laguardia KD et al. Extended use of transdermal norelgestromin/ethinyl estradiol: A randomized trial. *Obstet Gynecol.* 2005;105:1389–96.

161. Miller L, Verhoeven CH, Hout J. Extended regimens of the contraceptive vaginal ring: A randomized trial. *Obstet Gynecol.* 2005;106:473–82.

162. Edelman AB, Gallo MF, Jensen JT et al. Continuous or extended cycle vs. cyclic use of combined oral contraceptives for contraception. *Cochrane Database Syst Rev.* 2005;3:CD004695.

163. Cachrimanidou AC, Hellberg D, Nilsson S et al. Long-interval treatment regimen with a desogestrel-containing oral contraceptive. *Contraception.* 1993;48:205–16.

164. Miller L. Continuous administration of 100 μ g levonorgestrel and 20 μg ethinyl estradiol: A randomized controlled trial. *Obstet Gynecol.* 2002;99:S25.

165. Klipping C, Duijkers I, Fortier MP, Marr J, Trummer D, Elliesen J. Contraceptive efficacy and tolerability of ethinylestradiol 20 μg/drospirenone 3 mg in a flexible extended regimen: An open-label, multicentre, randomized, control study. *J Fam Plann Reprod Health Care.* 2012;38:73–83.

166. Jensen JT, Garie SG, Trummer D, Elliesen J. Bleeding profile of a flexible extended regimen of ethinylestradiol/drospirenone in US women: An open-label, three-arm, active-controlled, multicenter study. *Contraception.* 2012;86:110–8.

167. Kaunitz AM, Portman DJ, Hait H, Reape KZ. Adding low-dose estrogen to the hormone-free interval: Impact on bleeding patterns in users of a 91-day extended regimen oral contraceptive. *Contraception.* 2009;79:350–5.

168. Sulak PJ, Kuehl TJ, Coffee A, Willis S. Prospective analysis of occurrence and management of breakthrough bleeding during an extended oral contraceptive regimen. *Am J Obstet Gynecol.* 2006;195:935–41.

169. Nanda K, Lendvay A, Kwok C, Tolley E, Dube K, Brache V. Continuous compared with cyclic use of oral contraceptive pills in the Domincan Republic: A randomized controlled trial. *Obstet Gynecol.* 2014;123:1012–22.

170. Coney P, DelConte A. The effects on ovarian activity of a monophasic oral contraceptive with 100 microg levonorgestrel and 20 microg ethinyl estradiol. *Am J Obstet Gynecol.* 1999;181:53–8.

171. Moghissi KS, Syner FN, McBride LC. Contraceptive mechanism of microdose norethindrone. *Obstet Gynecol.* 1973;41:585e94.

172. Moghissi KS, Marks C. Effects of microdose progestogens on endogenous gonadotrophic and steroid hormones, cervical mucus properties, vaginal cytology and endometrium. *Fertil Steril.* 1971;22:424e34.

173. Raymond E. Progestin-only pills. In: Hatcher RA, Trussell J, Nelson AL, Cates W, Kowal D, MS P,eds. *Contraceptive Technology.* 20th ed. New York, NY: Ardent Media; 2011:237e47.

174. Kesseru-Koos E. Influence of various hormonal contraceptives on sperm migration *in vivo. Fertil Steril.* 1971;22:584e603.

175. Cheng CY, Boettcher B. Effects of steroids on the vitro forward migration of human spermatozoa. *Contraception.* 1981;24:183e94.

176. Paltieli Y, Eibschitz I, Ziskind G, Ohel G, Silbermann M, Weichselbaum A. High progesterone levels and ciliary dysfunction—Possible cause of ectopic pregnancy. *J Assist Reprod Genet.* 2000; 17(2):103–6.

177. Landgren BM, Diczfalusy E. Hormonal effects of the 300 mcg norethisterone minipill. *Contraception.* 1980;21:87e113.

178. Gilliam ML, Derman RJ. Barrier methods of contraception. *Obstet Gynecol Clin North Am.* 2000;27:841–58.

179. Copen CE. Condom use during sexual intercourse among women and men aged 15–44 in the United States: 2011–2015 National Survey of Family Growth. *Natl Health Stat Report.* 2017;105:1–18.

180. Fihn SD, Boyko EJ, Normand EH et al. Association between use of spermicide-coated condoms and *Escherichia coli* urinary tract infection in young women. *Am J Epidemiol.* 1996;144:512–20.

181. Cromwell PF, Daley AM, Risser WL. Contraception for adolescents: Part two. *J Pediatr Health Care.* 2004;18:250–3.

182. Steiner MJ, Dominik R, Rountree RW, Nanda K, Dor inger LJ. Contraceptive effectiveness of a polyurethane condom and a latex condom: A randomized controlled trial. *Obstet Gynecol.* 2003;101:539–47.

183. Walsh TL, Frezieres RG, Peacock K, Nelson AL, Clark VA, Bernstein L. Evaluation of the efficacy of a nonlatex condom: Results from a randomized, controlled clinical trial. *Perspect Sex Reprod Health.* 2003;35:79–86.

184. Gallo MF, Grimes DA, Lopez LM, Schulz KF. Nonlatex versus latex male condoms for contraception. *Cochrane Database Syst Rev.* 2006;1:CD003550.

185. Federal Drug Administration. *Durex synthetic polyisoprene male condom: Pre-market notification 510(k) submission.* Silver Spring, MD: FDA; 2008. http://www.accessdata.fda.gov/cdrh_docs/pdf7/K072169.pdf.

186. Narrigan D. Women's barrier contraceptive methods: Poised for change. *J Midwifery Womens Health.* 2006;51:478–85.

187. Mauck C, Callahan M, Weiner DH, Dominik R. A comparative study of the safety and efficacy of FemCap, a new vaginal barrier contraceptive, and the Ortho All-Flex diaphragm. The FemCap Investigators' Group. *Contraception.* 1999;60:71–80.

188. Centers for Disease Control and Prevention. U.S. medical eligibility criteria for contraceptive use. *MMWR Recomm Rep.* 2010;59(RR-4):1–85.

189. Hatcher RA, Trussell J, Nelson A, Cates W, Kowal D, Policar M. *Contraceptive Technology.* 20th ed. New York, NY: Ardent Media; 2011.

190. Gallo MF, Kilbourne-Brook M, Coffey PS. A review of the effectiveness and acceptability of the female condom for dual protection. *Sex Health.* 2012;9:18–26.

191. Black A, Guilbert E. Canadian contraception consensus; Chapter 5: Barrier methods. *J Obstet Gynaecol Can.* 2015;37(11):S12–24.

192. Weismiller DG. Emergency contraception. *Am Fam Physician.* 2004;70:707–14.

193. Gemzell-Danielsson K, Berger C, Lalitkumar PGL. Emergency contraception – Mechanisms of action. *Contraception.* 2013;87:300–8.

194. [No Authors Listed]. Randomised controlled trial of levonorgestrel versus the Yuzpe regimen of combined oral contraceptives for emergency contraception. Task Force on Postovulatory Methods of Fertility Regulation. *Lancet.* 1998;352(9126):428–33.

195. Glasier AF, Cameron ST, Fine PM et al. Ulipristal acetate versus levonorgestrel for emergency contraception: A randomised non-inferiority trial and meta-analysis. *Lancet.* 2010;375:555–62.

196. Creinin MD, Schlaff W, Archer DF et al. Progesterone receptor modulator for emergency contraception: A randomized controlled trial. *Obstet Gynecol.* 2006;108:1089–97.

197. Cleland K, Zhu H, Goldstuck N, Cheng L, Trussell J. The efficacy of intrauterine devices for emergency contraception: A systematic review of 35 years of experience. *Hum Reprod.* 2012;27:1994–2000.

198. Glasier A. Emergency contraception: Clinical outcomes. *Contraception.* 2013;87:309–13.

199. Trussell J, Ellertson C, Stewart F, Raymond EG, Shochet T. The role of emergency contraception. *Am J Obstet Gynecol.* 2004;190(4 Suppl):S30–8.

200. Brunton J, Beal MW. Current issues in emergency contraception: An overview for providers. *J Midwifery Womens Health.* 2006;51:457–63.

201. Dada OA, Godfrey EM, Piaggio G, von Hertzen H. A randomized, double-blind noninferiority study to compare two regimens of levonorgestrel for emergency contraception in Nigeria. *Contraception.* 2010;82:373–8.

202. Piaggio G, Kapp N, von Hertzen H. Effect of pregnancy rates of the delay in the administration of levonorgestrel for emergency contraception: A combined analysis of four WHO trials. *Contraception.* 2011;84(1):35–9.

203. Salcedo J, Rodriguez MI, Curtis KM, Kapp N. When can a woman resume or initate contraception after taking emergency contraceptive pills? A systematic review. *Contraception.* 2013;87:602–4.

204. SOGC Committee Opinion. Injectable medroxyprogesterone acetate for contraception. Policy statement no. 94. *JSOGC.* 2000;22:616–20.

205. Glasier A, Cameron ST, Blithe D et al. Can we identify women at risk of pregnancy despite using emergency contraception? Data from randomized trials of ulipristal acetate and levonorgestrel. *Contraception.* 2011;84:363–7.

206. Kapp N, Abitbol JL, Mathe H, Scherrer B, Guillard H, Gainer E, Ulmann A. Effect of body weight and BMI on the efficacy of levonorgestrel emergency contraception. *Contraception.* 2015;91:97–104.

207. Moreau C, Trussell J. Results from pooled phased III studies of ulipristal acetate for emergency contraception. *Contraception.* 2012;86:673–80.

208. Brache V, Cochon L, Deniaud M, Croxatto HB. Ulipristal acetate prevents ovulation more effectively than levonorgestrel: Analysis of pooled data from three randomized trials of emergency contraception regimens. *Contraception.* 2013;88:611–8.

209. Jensen J. Emergency contraception. OB/GYN Clinical Alert 2014;30:81–4.

210. Wu S, Godfrey EM, Wojdyla D, Dong J, Wang C, von Hertzen H. Copper T380A intrauterine device for emergency contraception: A prospective, multicenter, cohort clinical trial. *BJOG.* 2010;117:1205–10.

211. Harper CC, Speidel JJ, Drey EA, Trussell J, Blum M, Darney PD. Copper intrauterine device for emergency contraception: Clinical practice among contraceptive providers. *Obstet Gynecol.* 2012;119:220–6.

212. Sitruk-Ware R, Nath A, Mischell DR. Contraception technology: Past, present and future. *Contraction.* 2013;87:319–30.

213. Halpern V, Stalter RM, Owen DH, Dorflinger LJ, Lendvay A, Rademacher KH. Towards the development of a longer-acting injectable contraception: Past research and current trends. *Contraception.* 2015;92:3–9.

Sexually transmitted infections in adolescents

17

CYNTHIA HOLLAND-HALL

EPIDEMIOLOGY

Over 41% of U.S. high school students report they have had sexual intercourse, including 21% of ninth grade girls and 57% of 12th grade girls.[1] By the 12th grade, 16% of girls state they have had four or more sexual partners. Only 52% of girls state they used a condom at the time of last intercourse. Students not enrolled in high school may engage in even riskier sexual behaviors than those reported in school-based surveys. Sexually transmitted infections (STIs) are one consequence of this behavior. It is estimated that one-half of all new STIs are diagnosed in young people 15–24 years of age[2] and that greater than one-third of sexually experienced 14- to 19-year-old girls are infected with a sexually transmitted pathogen.[3] On a global scale, young women similarly bear a disproportionate burden of these infections.[4]

Sexual activity at a young age and history of a prior STI are two of the largest risk factors for STI.[5,6] Multiple partners, concurrent partners, and unprotected sexual activity further increase the risk. Although condom use and careful sexual decision-making are important elements of risk reduction, it is important for providers to keep in mind that a patient's community and sexual network may play a greater role in determining her risk for STI than her individual behaviors. Complex racial, ethnic, and socioeconomic factors that contribute to many health disparities also impact STI prevalence, with non-Hispanic blacks demonstrating increased rates of several STIs.[7]

SCREENING AND PREVENTION

Taking the sexual history

Throughout the United States, adolescents have the right to consent to testing and treatment for STIs without parental involvement. This generally correlates with a right to confidentiality, even from the parent, regarding these services, although in some states, the provider retains the right to inform the parent. Providers need to be aware of the unique laws in their own state, for example, whether HIV services are included or considered separately and whether there is a minimum age limit required for minors to consent to testing (typically 12 or 14 years of age). State-specific guidelines are available through the Center for Adolescent Health and the Law or the Guttmacher Institute.[8,9] Providers also must understand their responsibilities as mandated reporters of childhood sexual abuse and must be familiar with their state's age-based limitations on consensual sexual activity.

Adolescents are more likely to disclose their sexual behaviors when they believe their confidentiality is ensured and they understand what the provider intends to do with the information obtained. Adults and others accompanying the adolescent should be asked to leave the room during this portion of the interview. Most parents are willing to comply with this request once they understand that they will be informed if their child's life or health is in immediate danger, as in the cases of abuse and risk of self-harm. The adolescent should further understand potential breaches to confidentiality, such as the explanation of benefits sent to the parents by a third-party payer (which may include laboratory tests performed) and the need to inform local health departments of reportable diseases in the event of a positive test result.

The provider needs to ask about specific sexual practices, using language the patient understands, in a matter-of-fact and nonjudgmental manner. The Centers for Disease Control and Prevention (CDC) encourages the use of "The Five Ps" to structure the sexual history; sample questions are included in Box 17.1.[10]

Box 17.1 "The Five Ps" structure for sexual history

- Partners
  - "Do you have sex with men, women, or both?"
  - "In the past 2 months, how many partners have you had sex with?"
- Practices
  - "To understand your risks for STDs, I need to understand the kind of sex you have had recently."
  - "Have you had vaginal sex, meaning 'penis in vagina' sex?" If yes, "Do you use condoms: never, sometimes, or always?" (Similarly for anal and oral intercourse)
- Prevention of pregnancy
  - "What are you doing to prevent pregnancy?"
- Protection from sexually transmitted diseases (STDs)
  - "What do you do to protect yourself from STDs and HIV?"
- Past history of STDs
  - "Have you ever had an STD?"
  - "Have any of your partners had an STD?"

Source: Adapted from Centers for Disease Control and Prevention. Sexually Transmitted Diseases Treatment Guidelines, 2015. *MMWR Recomm Rep.* 2015;64(RR-3):1–137.

Screening

Screening guidelines published by professional societies including the American College of Obstetricians and Gynecologists, the American Academy of Pediatrics, and the U.S. Preventive Services Task Force are largely consistent with one another.[10–12] All sexually active girls and young women should be screened for gonococcal and chlamydial infections at least once a year, regardless of the presence or absence of additional risk factors. A nucleic acid amplification test (NAAT) should be used for chlamydia screening, due to the superior sensitivity of this test; most commercial products pair this with a test for gonorrhea that can be run on the same specimen. Self-collected specimens such as vaginal swabs and urine are appropriate for screening asymptomatic persons and are preferred by adolescents.

Screening for *Trichomonas vaginalis* may be considered in populations in which the prevalence of this infection is high, and often is performed in adolescent health settings. Syphilis screening should be performed when risk factors, such as an adult sexual partner, a male partner who has sex with other males (MSM), high regional prevalence, or the diagnosis of another STI, are present. HIV testing should be performed by middle adolescence or with the onset of sexual activity in younger teens.[13] Specific age-based guidelines for HIV testing vary somewhat among professional organizations, and frequency of testing is not specified.

Prevention

Clinicians should provide developmentally appropriate counseling on reducing the risk of acquiring an STI. This may include a discussion of abstinence, monogamous relationships with uninfected partners, and reducing the number of sexual partners as possible risk reduction strategies. Specific instruction on the effective use of condoms is recommended (see Box 17.2).

Vaccination against human papillomavirus (HPV) is effective at reducing infection with and clinical sequelae of vaccine-type HPV.[14] Strong and unambiguous

---

Box 17.2 Counseling on male condom use

- Correct and consistent condom use greatly reduces (but does not eliminate) the risk of several sexually transmitted infections (STIs) and HIV.
- Latex or polyurethane condoms should be used consistently during vaginal, oral, or anal intercourse.
- A new condom should be used with each sexual act.
- Note the expiration date, but keep in mind that a recently expired condom is likely more effective than no condom.
- Avoid opening the package with a sharp object, and inspect the condom for holes or tears.
- Avoid oil-based lubricants with latex condoms (water- and silicone-based are acceptable).
- Pinch air out of the tip, and roll the condom down to the base of the penis.
- After intercourse, hold the condom at the base of the penis before withdrawal.

---

recommendation of this vaccine by trusted providers is associated with improved vaccine acceptance.[15] Vaccination is recommended at age 11–12 years, with catch-up vaccination recommended for older adolescents. The series may be initiated as early as 9 years of age for girls at elevated risk of infection, such as prior victims of sexual abuse. Adolescents who initiate the series prior to 15 years of age require two doses of the vaccine given 6–12 months apart; older adolescents require a three-dose series (0, 2, 6 months). Vaccination against hepatitis B virus in early childhood should be confirmed and the vaccine series completed if needed. Up-to-date information on adolescent vaccine schedules can be found on the CDC website (https://www.cdc.gov/vaccines/schedules/easy-to-read/adolescent-easyread.html).

BACTERIAL AND PARASITIC INFECTIONS
Chlamydia trachomatis

C trachomatis is the most common bacterial STI and the most common reportable infectious disease in the United States.[2] Adolescent and young adult females have the highest rates of infection, perhaps due to the presence of more columnar cells surrounding the external cervical os or a less robust immunologic response to infection. Infection typically is asymptomatic but may cause mucopurulent cervicitis, urethritis, or pelvic inflammatory disease (PID). All sexually active young women should be screened at least annually, using a NAAT. A vaginal swab collected by the clinician or the patient herself is the preferred specimen for screening.[10] Alternatively, first-catch urine may be utilized, although the sensitivity of this specimen is slightly lower.[16] Endocervical testing is appropriate if a speculum exam is performed. Culture of an endocervical specimen may be preferred when high specificity is required, such as in an evaluation for sexual assault, but the sensitivity is inferior to that of NAAT. At this time there are no point-of-care tests that demonstrate sufficiently high sensitivity to recommend their use in a clinical setting. Treatment options for uncomplicated lower urogenital tract chlamydial infections are presented in Table 17.1.

Neisseria gonorrhoeae

After declining for several decades and then plateauing, the rate of gonococcal infection is now increasing, with younger women and African Americans disproportionately affected (Figures 17.1 and 17.2). Although serious sequelae including PID, arthritis, and disseminated infection may occur, most young women with gonococcal infections are asymptomatic or present with evidence of cervicitis. Testing for *N. gonorrhoeae* may be performed on vaginal, cervical, or urine specimens using an approved NAAT. An endocervical or pharyngeal specimen may alternatively be tested using culture, with the advantages of high specificity and allowing antimicrobial susceptibility testing (AST).

N. gonorrhoeae continues to develop resistance to the antimicrobials used to treat it, and the most up-to-date

Table 17.1 Treatment of uncomplicated cervical, urethral, or vaginal infections caused by *C. trachomatis*, *N. gonorrhoeae*, and *T. vaginalis*.

	Recommended treatments	Possible alternatives
C. trachomatis	• Azithromycin 1 g orally, once • Doxycycline 100 mg orally twice daily × 7 days	• Erythromycin ethylsuccinate 800 mg orally four times a day × 7 days • Levofloxacin 500 mg orally once daily × 7 days
N. gonorrhoeae	• Ceftriaxone 250 mg intramuscular, once *and* • Azithromycin 1 g orally, once	If ceftriaxone is not available: • Cefixime 400 mg orally, once[a] *and* • Azithromycin 1 g orally
T. vaginalis	• Metronidazole 2 g orally, once • Tinidazole 2 g orally, once	• Metronidazole 500 mg orally twice daily × 7 days

Source: Adapted from Centers for Disease Control and Prevention. Sexually Transmitted Diseases Treatment Guidelines, 2015. *MMWR Recomm Rep.* 2015;64(RR-3):1–137.

[a] Oral cephalosporins do not reliably eradicate pharyngeal infections.

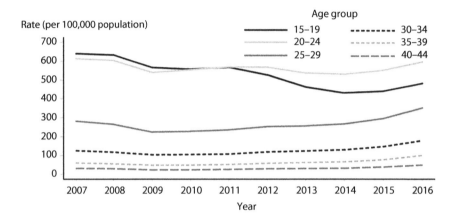

Figure 17.1 Gonorrhea. Rates of reported cases among women aged 15–44 years by age group, United States, 2007–2016. (From Centers for Disease Control and Prevention. *Sexually Transmitted Disease Surveillance 2016.* Atlanta, GA: U.S. Department of Health and Human Services; 2017.)

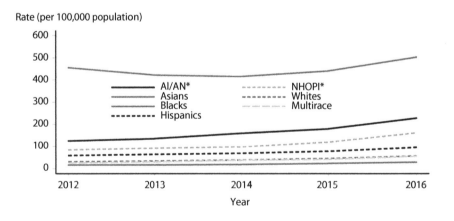

Figure 17.2 Gonorrhea. Rates of reported cases by race/ethnicity, United States, 2012–2016. *AI/AN = American Indian and Alaska Native; NHOPI = Native Hawaiians and Other Pacific Islanders. (From Centers for Disease Control and Prevention. *Sexually Transmitted Disease Surveillance 2016.* Atlanta, GA: U.S. Department of Health and Human Services; 2017.)

guidelines available should be used to determine therapy. Resistance to fluoroquinolones and tetracyclines is widespread, and resistance to cephalosporins (particularly oral agents) and macrolides appears to be emerging. Dual therapy with parenteral ceftriaxone and oral azithromycin is currently recommended to slow the emergence of resistance (Table 17.1). Limited clinical trials of azithromycin 2 g orally given in combination with oral gemifloxacin 320 mg or with intramuscular gentamicin 240 mg (all single doses) show promising results and may be considered as alternative treatment options for uncomplicated urogenital gonococcal infections.[17] Monotherapy with azithromycin is not recommended. Test-of-cure is not recommended for uncomplicated urogenital infections treated with recommended or alternative regimens but should be performed if an alternative regimen is used to treat a pharyngeal gonococcal infection. Suspected treatment failures should be reevaluated with culture, if possible, in order to perform AST.

Mycoplasma genitalium

Though often referred to as an emerging infection, many years of research demonstrate an association of *M. genitalium* with cervicitis and PID, as well as urethral infections in males.[18] Diagnostic challenges have limited the ability to fully understand its clinical significance as a genital pathogen. Culture is not clinically useful for the diagnosis of this slow-growing organism. In 2019, the U.S. Food and Drug Administration (FDA) approved a diagnostic test for this organism (Aptima, Hologic, San Diego, CA). A vaginal swab is the preferred specimen for this NAAT; endocervical and urine specimens are also approved but result in lower sensitivities. Testing or empiric treatment for *M. genitalium* may be considered for cases of persistent cervicitis or PID not responsive to treatment. Azithromycin given in a single dose (1 g) or a 5-day course (500 mg once, followed by 250 mg daily for 4 days) has been effective in some persons, but it is feared that macrolide resistance will rapidly emerge. Moxifloxacin 400 mg daily (7- to 14-day course) has also been used with apparent success in some women with cervicitis or PID, but more robust clinical trials are needed.[10]

Syphilis

Syphilis is relatively uncommon among adolescent girls, and a comprehensive discussion of this infection is beyond the scope of this chapter. Screening should be performed in high-risk adolescents, particularly those with adult sexual partners and sexual partners who are MSM, those with a history of substance abuse, and those diagnosed with an STI or HIV. Clinicians must be aware of regional outbreaks and prevalence of syphilis and adjust their screening practices accordingly. Screening may be performed using a nontreponemal test (rapid plasma reagin or the Venereal Disease Research Laboratory) and using a treponemal test (such as the florescent treponemal antibody absorbed test or *Treponema pallidum* particle agglutination) to confirm, since false-positive nontreponemal tests do occur.[10]

Primary infection is characterized by a painless ulcer (chancre) at the site of infection, 10–90 days after exposure. This lesion resolves spontaneously in 3–6 weeks. During primary infection, both treponemal and nontreponemal tests have a relatively low sensitivity (70%–85%). Darkfield microscopy or a direct florescent antibody test may identify *T. pallidum* in tissue or exudate from the lesion. Characteristics of secondary infection are many and varied, including a cutaneous rash that may involve the palms and soles, other mucocutaneous lesions, lymphadenopathy, alopecia, condyloma lata, and constitutional symptoms such as fever, malaise, and weight loss. Serologic tests have outstanding sensitivity during this stage of disease. Latent infection may persist for years without causing symptoms. Tertiary infection may result in devastating outcomes, including but not limited to degenerative neurologic changes and cardiac involvement. Central nervous system involvement can occur during any stage. Treatment is with parenteral penicillin G.[10] Duration of treatment varies with stage of infection; a single intramuscular dose is indicated for primary, secondary, or early latent syphilis. Management of syphilis should generally be performed under the guidance of an infectious disease specialist or other experienced provider. Syphilis is a reportable infection, and local health departments often can serve as a valuable resource in management.

Trichomonas vaginalis

Infections with the single-celled protozoan *T. vaginalis* are common among adolescent girls. Infection may be asymptomatic or may be characterized by a frothy, malodorous vaginal discharge and vulvar irritation. Trichomoniasis has been associated with increased risk of HIV transmission and adverse pregnancy outcomes.[19,20] The motile, flagellated organisms may be seen with light microscopy, but the sensitivity of this diagnostic modality is low. NAAT may be performed on urine or vaginal specimens with excellent sensitivity; culture and rapid testing also perform well.[21] Nonamplified DNA probe testing has poor sensitivity for this infection.[22] Treatment is with oral nitroimidazoles (Table 17.1); topical treatment will not reliably eradicate the infection. For patients with persistent symptoms, reinfection is believed to be the most likely cause, but antimicrobial resistance has been described. If true treatment failure is suspected following single-dose therapy, a course of metronidazole 500 mg twice daily should be used. CDC provides additional treatment options with high-dose nitroimidazoles and is available for consultation in the management of persistent infections.[10]

Bacterial vaginosis

Bacterial vaginosis (BV) is a common cause of vaginal discharge among sexually active adolescents and is occasionally seen in virginal women. It is caused by overgrowth of *Gardnerella vaginalis* and numerous other anaerobic and facultative bacteria, with an associated decrease of hydrogen peroxide–producing lactobacilli. It may cause a malodorous discharge and vaginal or urethral irritation. Frequent recurrences are common in some women. Clinical diagnosis can be made when three of the four criteria, known as the Amsel criteria, are present[1]: homogeneous white or gray vaginal discharge that is adherent to the vaginal walls[2]; vaginal pH greater than 4.5[3]; the presence of at least 20% "clue cells" (squamous epithelial cells stippled with bacteria) on saline microscopy[4]; and the presence of an amine ("fishy") odor released when 10% potassium hydroxide (KOH) is added to a sample of vaginal fluid. Rapid testing and nonamplified DNA probe testing for *G. vaginalis*

Table 17.2 Treatment of bacterial vaginosis.

	Recommended treatments	Possible alternatives
Systemic	• Metronidazole 500 mg orally twice daily × 7 days	• Tinidazole 2 g orally, once daily × 2 days • Tinidazole 1 g orally, once daily × 5 days • Clindamycin 300 mg orally twice a day × 7 days • Secnidazole oral granules, 2 g orally (sprinkled onto applesauce, yogurt, or pudding and consumed within 30 minutes), once[a]
Topical	• Metronidazole gel 0.75%, one applicator (5 g) intravaginally, once daily at bedtime × 5 days • Clindamycin cream 2%, one applicator (5 g) intravaginally, once daily at bedtime × 7 days	• Clindamycin ovules 100 mg intravaginally, once daily at bedtime × 3 days

Source: Adapted from Centers for Disease Control and Prevention. Sexually Transmitted Diseases Treatment Guidelines, 2015. *MMWR Recomm Rep.* 2015;64(RR-3):1–137.

[a] Kaufman MB. Pharmaceutical approval update. *P T.* 2017;42:733–55.

have demonstrated good performance and may be more convenient. Treatment can be applied topically or given systemically (Table 17.2).[10,23] Although some evidence for sexual transmissibility exists, there is currently no established role for partner treatment.[24]

VIRAL INFECTIONS

Herpes simplex virus (HSV)

Prevalence of HSV-2 infection has decreased or remained stable for nearly all demographics in the United States; HSV-1 prevalence has declined dramatically in adolescents as well.[2] Although HSV-1 positivity may represent genital, oral, or cutaneous infection, it is reasonable to assume that HSV-2 positivity is the result of a genital infection. Most infections are subclinical and remain undiagnosed. Most transmission occurs through subclinical shedding in asymptomatic infected persons, though the risk of transmission is higher when lesions are present. Both HSV-1 and HSV-2 can cause genital vesicular and ulcerative lesions; an estimated 30%–40% of genital infections in young people are caused by HSV-1. A primary HSV outbreak classically includes fever and flu-like symptoms in addition to genital lesions and inguinal lymphadenopathy. In practice, secondary outbreaks are much more commonly encountered and include fewer systemic symptoms. Although individual outbreaks are clinically indistinguishable between the two serotypes, HSV-2 is associated with more frequent recurrences. In both cases, the frequency of recurrence tends to decrease over time.

Diagnosis is made using NAAT or culture, the former offering superior sensitivity.[25] The sensitivity of culture decreases rapidly with the age of the lesion; freshly unroofed vesicles provide the highest yield. Although routine screening is not recommended, reliable type-specific HSV-2 antibody assays, based on the glycoprotein G2, are available, and may provide additional useful information when the diagnosis is in question. Antiviral therapy, when used, should be started as early as possible to reduce the severity and duration of symptoms (Table 17.3). Patients should have quick access to refills and should be counseled to begin treatment at the first signs of a new outbreak. Daily suppressive therapy may be considered in any patient who wishes to decrease her frequency of outbreaks and/or decrease the risk of transmission to a sexual partner, and decisions to prescribe suppressive therapy should not be based strictly on the number of outbreaks per year.

Table 17.3 Treatment regimens for genital herpes infections (all oral).

First clinical episode	Recurrent outbreaks	Daily suppressive therapy
Acyclovir 400 mg tid × 7–10 days	Acyclovir 400 mg three times a day × 5 days	Acyclovir 400 mg twice a day
Acyclovir 200 mg five times a day × 7–10 days	Acyclovir 800 mg twice a day × 5 days	Famciclovir 250 mg twice a day
Famciclovir 250 mg three times a day × 7–10 days	Acyclovir 800 mg twice a day × 2 days	Valacyclovir 500 mg daily
Valacyclovir 1 g twice a day × 7–10 days	Famciclovir 125 mg twice a day × 5 days	Valacyclovir 1 g daily
	Famciclovir 1 g twice a day × 1 day	
	Famciclovir 500 mg once, followed by 250 mg twice a day × 2 days	
	Valacyclovir 500 mg twice a day × 3 days	
	Valacyclovir 1 g daily × 5 days	

Source: Adapted from Centers for Disease Control and Prevention. Sexually Transmitted Diseases Treatment Guidelines, 2015. *MMWR Recomm Rep.* 2015;64(RR-3):1–137.

Human papillomavirus

HPV is by far the most prevalent STI in adolescents,[3] and it tends to be acquired rapidly after the onset of sexual activity.[26] Most remain asymptomatic; many appear to clear infection within a few years, whereas others have persistent infection. Of the approximately 40 HPV serotypes that are sexually transmissible, types 6 and 11 are associated with 90% of the cases of genital warts (condyloma acuminata). These lesions may be treated if they cause discomfort or are distressing to the patient. Untreated lesions may regress spontaneously or may persist and grow. A variety of treatments are available, including several patient-applied treatments (Table 17.4). Patients should be counseled that treatment does not eliminate the risk of sexual transmission.

Oncogenic HPV serotypes are strongly associated with cervical dysplasia and anogenital and oropharyngeal cancers. In adolescents, cervical cancer is extremely rare. Mild cervical dysplasia is common following HPV infection but resolves spontaneously in the vast majority of cases.[27] Cervical cancer screening therefore is not recommended until 21 years of age in immunocompetent women, nor is there a defined role for routine HPV testing. Screening should begin with the onset of sexual activity in HIV-infected or immunocompromised adolescents.

MANAGING CLINICAL SYNDROMES

Known exposure to an STI

Patients who report sexual contact with a partner known or believed to have a treatable STI such as gonorrhea, chlamydia, trichomonas, or syphilis, or a clinical STD syndrome such as nongonococcal urethritis, should be treated for that STI at the time of the visit. They should be evaluated clinically and tested for other STIs and HIV as well, but treatment for the exposure should not be delayed while awaiting test results, nor should treatment be terminated prematurely following a negative test result.

Cervicitis

Cervicitis may be diagnosed when a speculum examination reveals a mucopurulent cervical discharge and/or cervical friability when touched with a cotton swab. Patients may be asymptomatic or may complain of vaginal discharge or irregular vaginal bleeding, such as intermenstrual spotting or bleeding after vaginal intercourse. White blood cells typically are visible on microscopic evaluation of the discharge. N. gonorrhoeae and C. trachomatis are the most likely etiologic agents to be identified; endocervical or vaginal specimens should be tested for these organisms using NAAT. T. vaginalis testing should be performed as well, using an FDA approved test. M. genitalium, HSV, and BV also may be associated with cervicitis, and testing for these conditions may be indicated. Often no pathogen is identified. Adolescents with cervicitis should be evaluated for pelvic inflammatory disease, HIV, and syphilis. Presumptive treatment for N. gonorrhoeae and C. trachomatis should be strongly considered for adolescents with cervicitis, particularly if reliable follow up is not ensured or there are concerns about confidentiality when contacting an adolescent with test results.

Vaginal discharge

Bacterial vaginosis, vulvovaginal candidiasis, and trichomoniasis are the most common treatable causes of vaginal discharge in sexually active adolescents. Although each of these conditions is associated with characteristic clinical features, all may be associated with vulvar irritation and urinary discomfort as well as vaginal discharge and may not be easy to distinguish clinically. Mucopurulent cervicitis also may cause discharge from the vagina but is less likely to be associated with vulvar symptoms. It is therefore reasonable to evaluate symptomatic adolescents for the preceding three causes of vaginitis, as well as gonorrhea and chlamydia. Light microscopy, KOH evaluation, measurement of vaginal pH, rapid testing for BV and

Table 17.4 Medical therapies for external genital warts.

		Comments
Patient-applied treatments	• Imiquimod 5% cream, apply to lesions nightly, three nonconsecutive nights a week, up to 16 weeks	Wash area with soap and water in morning (6–10 hours after application).
	• Imiquimod 3.75% cream, apply to lesions every night, up to 8 weeks	
	• Podofilox 0.5% solution/gel, apply to lesions twice a day × 3 days, followed by 4 days of no therapy; repeat up to four cycles as needed	Total area treated not to exceed 10 cm²; total volume of product used not to exceed 0.5 mL daily. Allow to dry before dressing.
	• Sinecatechins 15% ointment, apply to lesions three times a day, up to 16 weeks	Do not wash off. Avoid sexual contact involving medicated area.
Clinician-administered treatments	• Trichloroacetic acid (TCA) or bichloroacetic acid (BCA) 80%–90%, apply small amount to lesions, let dry	May repeat every 1–2 weeks until lesions resolve; avoid surrounding skin.
	• Cryotherapy	For use by trained and experienced providers.
	• Surgical removal	

Source: Adapted from Centers for Disease Control and Prevention. Sexually Transmitted Diseases Treatment Guidelines, 2015. MMWR Recomm Rep. 2015;64(RR-3):1–137.

T. vaginalis, and molecular testing (NAAT or DNA probe, as previously described) may all be useful diagnostic tools. A vaginal swab is preferable to urine for molecular testing. If clinical findings suggest a specific diagnosis, it is appropriate to treat empirically for that condition. It is not unusual for an adolescent to present with a complaint of vaginal discharge, yet have a reassuring clinical and laboratory evaluation, consistent with a physiologic vaginal discharge or a nonspecific vaginitis. Reassurance and patient education are important interventions in this setting (see Chapter 8).

Genital ulcers

In a sexually experienced adolescent girl in the United States, HSV is the most likely cause of genital ulcers. Syphilis should be considered as well, particularly if lesions are singular and painless. Chancroid, caused by *Haemophilus ducreyi*, is uncommon in North America in recent years. Genital yeast infections or other causes of vulvar itching may lead to excoriations that appear to be shallow ulcers. More than one infectious agent may be present. Vulvovaginal aphthous ulcerations in virginal adolescents are sometimes associated with viral infections, but in most cases, an infectious etiology is not identified.

Evaluation should include culture or polymerase chain reaction (PCR) for HSV-1 and HSV-2 and syphilis serology. If there is a stronger suspicion of syphilis, darkfield microscopy or PCR should be considered. Serologic testing for type-specific HSV-2 antibody may assist with diagnosis and counseling in some patients. *H. ducreyi* testing may be considered in endemic regions; consultation with a microbiology laboratory or health department may facilitate testing. Sexually active adolescents should be tested for HIV, since the risk of both acquisition and transmission of HIV are increased in the presence of genital ulcers. If syphilis is suspected, presumptive treatment should be provided. Suspected genital herpes should be treated as well, since early treatment is associated with better outcomes.

Pelvic inflammatory disease

Sexually active adolescents with lower abdominal or pelvic pain must be evaluated for PID. This upper genital tract infection may involve the endometrium, fallopian tubes, ovaries, and/or the peritoneal cavity. Pathology may result from direct spread of infection from the lower genital tract or related immunologic and inflammatory processes. Although *N. gonorrhoeae* and *C. trachomatis* are the most likely organisms to be identified, they are detected in less than half of all cases. Laparoscopic evidence suggests that PID is often a polymicrobial infection, with anaerobic and facultative bacteria often isolated. *M. genitalium* has been detected in 15% of cases in the research setting.[28,29] In many cases, however, no organism is identified at the cervix, and this should not deter the provider from making the clinical diagnosis.

Presentation may vary greatly from mild pelvic discomfort to severe pain with peritoneal signs. Vaginal discharge, abnormal vaginal bleeding, and dyspareunia are variably present, but a more subtle presentation is common. Acute complications include tubo-ovarian abscess (TOA) and perihepatitis (Fitz-Hugh-Curtis syndrome). Long-term sequelae may include chronic pelvic pain, tubal infertility, and increased risk of ectopic pregnancy; the likelihood of these complications increases with the number of episodes of PID.[28]

Laparoscopy is the gold standard for PID diagnosis, but the diagnosis typically is made clinically. A speculum examination may reveal vaginal discharge, a mucopurulent discharge from the cervical os, or cervical friability; endocervical specimens may be obtained and tested for *N. gonorrhoeae* and *C. trachomatis*. Bimanual examination may reveal cervical, uterine, or adnexal tenderness or an adnexal mass or fullness, as well as evidence of peritoneal irritation. Criteria for diagnosis are listed in Table 17.5. The minimal clinical criteria favor high sensitivity over specificity, since undertreatment may lead to highly morbid sequelae. The presence of one or more supportive criteria increases the specificity for a diagnosis of PID. In the absence of *any* evidence of cervical infection (discharge, white blood cells [WBCs] on microscopy, or a positive STI test), the diagnosis of PID is unlikely. Other gynecologic, urologic, gastroenterologic, or musculoskeletal causes of pain should be considered.

Beyond STI testing, additional laboratory evaluation may not be necessary. If obtained, a patient may demonstrate an elevated WBC count, erythrocyte sedimentation rate (ESR), or C-reactive protein (CRP). Imaging is not required to make the diagnosis but may be obtained to evaluate for TOA or for other sources of pelvic pain such

Table 17.5 Criteria for treatment of pelvic inflammatory disease.

Minimal clinical criteria	Supportive criteria

• Lower abdominal or pelvic pain without another identifiable cause in a sexually active young woman
• One or more of the following:
  – Cervical motion tenderness
  – Uterine tenderness
  – Adnexal tenderness
	• Fever
	• Cervical discharge or friability
	• White blood cells prominent on microscopic evaluation of vaginal fluid
	• Elevated erythrocyte sedimentation rate or C-reactive protein
	• Positive test for *N gonorrhoeae* or *C trachomatis*

Source: Adapted from Centers for Disease Control and Prevention. Sexually Transmitted Diseases Treatment Guidelines, 2015. *MMWR Recomm Rep.* 2015;64(RR-3):1–137.

as appendicitis. Ultrasound may reveal an adnexal mass or free fluid in the pelvis.

Outpatient treatment is appropriate for most patients with mild-to-moderate severity of disease, with outcomes similar to those of hospitalized women.[28] Antibiotics must cover *N. gonorrhoeae* and *C. trachomatis*. Additional coverage for anaerobic organisms should be considered, particularly when history or findings suggest a more severe or prolonged infection. Recommended treatment regimens are included in Table 17.6. If an intrauterine device is in place, it does not need to be removed, provided the patient responds to antibiotic treatment.[30] Pain must be addressed and typically is manageable with nonsteroidal anti-inflammatory drugs. Follow-up should occur within 48–72 hours of initiation of therapy to assess response. If symptoms have worsened or failed to improve, the clinician may consider redosing with ceftriaxone, adding anaerobe coverage if this was not initially included in the antibiotic regimen, or hospitalizing for intravenous therapy. Imaging should

Table 17.6 Recommended antimicrobial regimens for pelvic inflammatory disease.

Outpatient regimens (intramuscular/oral):

- Ceftriaxone 250 mg intramuscular, single dose
  and
  Doxycycline 100 mg orally twice daily for 14 days
  with or without
  Metronidazole 500 mg orally twice daily for 14 days

- Cefoxitin 2 g intramuscular, single dose with Probenecid 1 g orally, single dose (given concurrently)
  and
  Doxycycline 100 mg orally twice daily for 14 days
  with or without
  Metronidazole 500 mg orally twice daily for 14 days

Inpatient regimens (parenteral/oral)[a]:

- Cefoxitin 2 g intravenous every 6 hours
  and
  Doxycycline 100 mg orally (preferred) or intravenous every 12 hours

- Cefotetan 2 g intravenous every 12 hours
  and
  Doxycycline 100 mg orally (preferred) or intravenous every 12 hours

- Clindamycin 900 mg intravenous every 8 hours
  and
  Gentamicin 2 mg/kg intravenous or intramuscular loading dose, then 1.5 mg/kg every 8 hours
  (Single daily dosing of gentamicin 3–5 mg/kg may be substituted)

Source: Adapted from Centers for Disease Control and Prevention. Sexually Transmitted Diseases Treatment Guidelines, 2015. *MMWR Recomm Rep.* 2015;64(RR-3):1–137.
[a] Patients treated parenterally should complete a 14-day (total) course of doxycycline 100 mg orally twice daily after discharge from hospital.

be considered at this time as well, if not already done. Alternative diagnoses should once again be considered.

Hospitalization may be appropriate for patients with one or more of the following: severe illness with the inability to rule out a surgical emergency, TOA, pregnancy, severe vomiting or other inability to tolerate oral medications, or lack of response to outpatient treatment. Young age alone is not an indication for hospitalization. Recommended parenteral antibiotic regimens for hospitalized patients are presented in Table 17.6. After 24–48 hours of clinical improvement, patients may be changed to oral doxycycline to complete 14 days of therapy. Patients with TOA should receive enhanced anaerobe coverage with metronidazole or clindamycin, and longer courses of therapy may be considered[31]; lesions larger than 8–10 cm are more likely to require surgical intervention. Alternative treatment regimens for special circumstances exist and may be found online at https://www.cdc.gov/std/treatment.[10]

Further management considerations

The diagnosis of an STI in an adolescent should prompt evaluation for other STIs and HIV, if this has not already been done. Education about the diagnosis should be provided, including a discussion of transmissibility to sexual partners, risk associated with untreated infection, and the expected course and prognosis. Counseling should include a discussion of safer sexual decision-making and risk reduction, as previously described. Concerns for sexual abuse or exploitation, transactional sex, and intimate partner violence should be addressed as well (Box 17.3).

When treating STIs, single-dose therapies are preferred whenever possible, in order to maximize adherence to treatment. Directly observed therapy (i.e., providing the actual medication to the adolescent in the office setting)

Box 17.3 Checklist for management of sexually transmitted infections (STIs)

- Counsel on diagnosis
- Provide antimicrobial or antiviral treatment, if appropriate
- Use single-dose, directly observed therapy when possible
- Encourage abstinence until completion of therapy (or 7 days after single-dose therapy)
- Test for other STIs and HIV
- Discuss partner treatment, and offer expedited partner therapy when appropriate
- Counsel on safer sex and risk reduction
- Confirm or complete vaccination against human papillomavirus and hepatitis
- Screen for sexual abuse, exploitation/trafficking, or intimate partner violence
- Assess contraceptive needs
- Schedule 3-month follow-up visit for test of reinfection (gonorrhea, chlamydia, trichomoniasis)
- Ensure that reportable infections are communicated to local health department

is ideal, since privacy concerns or financial barriers may deter an adolescent from filling a prescription. For curable infections, abstinence is recommended until the completion of therapy, or for 7 days following single-dose treatment. Gonorrhea, chlamydia, syphilis, chancroid, and HIV/AIDS are reportable diseases in every state in the United States; other reporting requirements may differ by state. Positive results may be reported to local health departments by the ordering provider or by the laboratory.

For treatable infections, partner therapy is an essential element of management. Sexual partners for at least the past 2 months should be informed that they have been exposed to an STI and treated appropriately. Providing simple, written information on the diagnosis and the necessary next steps may assist the adolescent patient with the difficult task of partner notification. Ideally, partners will receive comprehensive sexual health evaluation, counseling, testing, and treatment with their own provider or at a sexual health clinic. Unfortunately, this does not reliably occur. If it is felt that the sexual partner is unable or unlikely to seek such treatment, the diagnosing clinician may be able to provide the patient with a prescription for an additional dose of medication for the treatment of *C. trachomatis*, *N. gonorrhoeae*, or *T. vaginalis* infections, without examining the partner. This practice, known as Expedited Partner Therapy (EPT), is legal or potentially permissible in most states, but specific requirements and infections that may be treated vary. The CDC maintains an online resource to assist clinicians in determining the legality and implementation of this practice in their own state (https://www.cdc.gov/std/ept).[32] The patient should be encouraged to abstain from sexual activity until both partners have completed treatment.

When an approved therapy is used to treat gonorrhea, chlamydia, or trichomoniasis and the symptomatic patient improves clinically, test-of-cure is not required. If treatment failure is suspected, repeat testing and retreatment may be appropriate. For suspected treatment failure for a gonococcal infection, culture and sensitivity testing should be obtained. Due to high rates of reinfection following STI diagnosis and treatment, adolescents should be encouraged to return in 3 months for "test of reinfection." This testing should include all three of the aforementioned organisms, not only the one previously diagnosed.[10]

REFERENCES

1. Centers for Disease Control and Prevention. 1991–2015 High School Youth Risk Behavior Survey Data. https://nccd.cdc.gov/youthonline/. Accessed June 3, 2019.
2. Centers for Disease Control and Prevention. *Sexually Transmitted Disease Surveillance 2016*. Atlanta, GA: U.S. Department of Health and Human Services; 2017.
3. Forhan SE, Gottlieb SL, Sternberg MR et al. Prevalence of sexually transmitted infections among female adolescents aged 14 to 19 in the United States. *Pediatrics*. 2009;124(6):1505–12.
4. Dehne KL, Riedner G. *Sexually transmitted infections among adolescents: The need for adequate health services*. In: Berer M, ed. Geneva, Switzerland: World Health Organization; 2005.
5. Kaestle CE, Halpern CT, Miller WC, Ford CA. Young age at first sexual intercourse and sexually transmitted infections in adolescents and young adults. *Am J Epidemiol*. 2005;161(8):774–80.
6. Diclemente RJ, Wingood GM, Sionean C et al. Association of adolescents' history of sexually transmitted disease (STD) and their current high-risk behavior and STD status: A case for intensifying clinic-based prevention efforts. *Sex Transm Dis*. 2002;29(9):503–9.
7. Adimora AA, Schoenbach VJ. Social context, sexual networks, and racial disparities in rates of sexually transmitted infections. *J Infect Dis*. 2005;191(Suppl 1):S115–S22.
8. English A, Kenney KE. *State Minor Consent Laws: A Summary*. 3rd ed. Chapel Hill, NC: Center for Adolescent Health and the Law; 2010.
9. Guttmacher Institute. https://www.guttmacher.org. Accessed June 3, 2019.
10. Centers for Disease Control and Prevention. Sexually transmitted diseases treatment guidelines, 2015. *MMWR Recomm Rep*. 2015;64(RR-03):1–137.
11. Murray PJ, Braverman PK, Adelman WP, Breuner CC. Screening for nonviral sexually transmitted infections in adolescents and young adults. *Pediatrics*. 2014;134(1):e302–11.
12. Lee KC, Ngo-Metzger Q, Wolff T, Chowdhury J, LeFevre ML, Meyers DS. Sexually transmitted infections: Recommendations from the U.S. Preventive Services Task Force. *Am Fam Physician*. 2016;94(11):907–15.
13. Emmanuel PJ, Martinez J. Adolescents and HIV infection: The pediatrician's role in promoting routine testing. *Pediatrics*. 2011;128(5):1023–9.
14. Garland SM, Kjaer SK, Munoz N et al. Impact and effectiveness of the quadrivalent human papillomavirus vaccine: A systematic review of 10 years of real-world experience. *Clin Infect Dis*. 2016;63(4):519–27.
15. Brewer NT, Hall ME, Malo TL, Gilkey MB, Quinn B, Lathren C. Announcements versus conversations to improve HPV vaccination coverage: A randomized trial. *Pediatrics*. 2017;139(1).
16. Lunny C, Taylor D, Hoang L et al. Self-collected versus clinician-collected sampling for chlamydia and gonorrhea screening: A systemic review and meta-analysis. *PLOS ONE*. 2015;10(7):e0132776.
17. Kirkcaldy RD, Weinstock HS, Moore PC et al. The efficacy and safety of gentamicin plus azithromycin and gemifloxacin plus azithromycin as treatment of uncomplicated gonorrhea. *Clin Infect Dis*. 2014;59(8):1083–91.
18. Wiesenfeld HC, Manhart LE. *Mycoplasma genitalium* in women: Current knowledge and research priorities for this recently emerged pathogen. *J Infect Dis*. 2017;216(Suppl 2):S389–S95.

19. Kissinger P, Adamski A. Trichomoniasis and HIV interactions: A review. *Sex Transm Inf.* 2013;89(6): 426–33.

20. Cotch MF, Pastorek II JG, Nugent RP et al. *Trichomonas vaginalis* associated with low birth weight and preterm delivery. *Sex Transm Dis.* 1997;24(6):353–60.

21. Nathan B, Appiah J, Saunders P et al. Microscopy outperformed in a comparison of five methods for detecting *Trichomonas vaginalis* in symptomatic women. *Int J STD AIDS.* 2015;26(4):251–6.

22. Cartwright CP, Lembke BD, Ramachandran K et al. Comparison of nucleic acid amplification assays with BD affirm VPIII for diagnosis of vaginitis in symptomatic women. *J Clin Microbiol.* 2013;51(11):3694–9.

23. Kaufman MB. Pharmaceutical approval update. *P T.* 2017;42(12):733–55.

24. Unemo M, Bradshaw CS, Hocking JS et al. Sexually transmitted infections: Challenges ahead. *Lancet Infect Dis.* 2017;17(8):e235–79.

25. Van Der Pol B, Warren T, Taylor SN et al. Type-specific identification of anogenital herpes simplex virus infections by use of a commercially available nucleic acid amplification test. *J Clin Microbiol.* 2012;50(11):3466–71.

26. Winer RL, Feng Q, Hughes JP, O'Reilly S, Kiviat NB, Koutsky LA. Risk of female human papillomavirus acquisition associated with first male sex partner. *J Infect Dis.* 2008;197(2):279–82.

27. Ault KA. Epidemiology and natural history of human papillomavirus infections in the female genital tract. *Infect Dis Obstet Gynecol.* 2006;2006(Suppl):40470.

28. Ness RB, Soper DE, Holley RL et al. Effectiveness of inpatient and outpatient treatment strategies for women with pelvic inflammatory disease: Results from the Pelvic Inflammatory Disease Evaluation and Clinical Health (PEACH) Randomized Trial. *Am J Obstet Gynecol.* 2002;186(5):929–37.

29. Burnett AM, Anderson CP, Zwank MD. Laboratory-confirmed gonorrhea and/or chlamydia rates in clinically diagnosed pelvic inflammatory disease and cervicitis. *Am J Emerg Med.* 2012;30(7):1114–7.

30. Centers for Disease Control and Prevention. U.S. Selected Practice Recommendations for Contraceptive Use, 2016. *MMWR Recomm Rep.* 2016;65(4): 1–66.

31. Chappell CA, Wiesenfeld HC. Pathogenesis, diagnosis, and management of severe pelvic inflammatory disease and tuboovarian abscess. *Clin Obstet Gynecol.* 2012;55(4):893–903.

32. Centers for Disease Control and Prevention. Sexually Transmitted Diseases: Expedited Partner Therapy. https://www.cdc.gov/std/ept. Accessed June 3, 2019.

Chronic pelvic pain and endometriosis

18

JOSEPH S. SANFILIPPO, JESSICA PAPILLON SMITH, and M. JONATHON SOLNIK

INTRODUCTION

Notwithstanding recent bridges in our knowledge gap surrounding chronic pelvic pain in adolescent females, providers who care for this younger population continue to face challenges that ultimately result in a delay in care.[1] These include delays in the patient seeking care, an ongoing lack of knowledge from the provider in the pathogenesis of pain, and a relative uneasiness in managing younger patients. Furthermore, there may be a reluctance of gynecologists to proceed with an operative intervention for similar reasons. The most successful therapy stems from the ability to provide an accurate diagnosis in a short period of time, which is frequently difficult to achieve given the multiple interlocking causes of pelvic pain. This alone contributes to substantial delays in effective care.[1]

During clinical encounters, providers utilize historical intake to help characterize pain, but given the highly subjective nature of pain, the ability of researchers to provide reliable data has been weakened by historical publications that did not use consistent definitions of chronic pain. Chronic pelvic pain is defined as "non-cyclic pain of six or more months" in duration that localizes to the anatomic pelvis, anterior abdominal wall at or below the umbilicus, the lumbosacral region, or the buttocks and is of sufficient severity to cause functional disability or lead to medical care. A lack of physical findings does not negate the significance of a patient's pain, and normal examination results do not preclude the possibility of finding pelvic pathology."[2] In fact, this lack of objective findings maintains the diagnostic challenge. The International Association for the Study of Pain (IASP) defines chronic pelvic pain as an "unpleasant sensory and emotional experience associated with actual or potential tissue damage or described in terms of such damage," and while there is no standardized definition within the literature, chronic pelvic pain as described by IASP is that which "has a gynecological origin but for which no definitive lesion or cause is identified."[3] This lack of consistency creates challenges for both epidemiologists and clinicians who have an interest in evaluating women with chronic pain syndromes.

The incidence of pelvic pain has been reported to be 15% in women over the age of 18.[4] This translates to one in seven, or over 9 million women in the United States. Of interest, the management cost is equated with a healthcare expenditure of approximately $3 billion annually, including indirect costs. Analogy has been equated with the incidence of asthma or irritable bowel syndrome. Dysmenorrhea, or cyclic pain occurring with menses, is altogether more common than chronic pain, affecting up to 90% of adolescent females.[5] While these statistics reflect the prevalence of chronic pelvic pain in the United States, a World Health Organization (WHO) meta-analysis evaluated studies from across the globe, 51.2% of which were from developed countries. The authors concluded that there was actually a wide range of prevalence for dysmenorrhea (16.8%–81%), dyspareunia (8%–21.8%), and noncyclic pain (2.1%–24%).[6]

THE DIFFERENTIAL DIAGNOSIS

While endometriosis is one of the most common causes of chronic pelvic pain (CPP) in adolescents, as clinicians, we must approach CPP from a multisystem perspective, or we risk failing to appropriately evaluate this large group of patients. For a list of nongynecologic causes of pain, see Table 18.1. The most common gastrointestinal etiologies responsible for CPP include chronic constipation and irritable bowel syndrome (IBS). Disorders of the urinary tract should be routinely considered when evaluating young patients with chronic pain. The European Society for the Study of Interstitial Cystitis has worked to create a consensus regarding the diagnosis of interstitial cystitis (IC) given the lack of agreement among experts. They recommend changing the name to painful bladder syndrome (PBS): chronic pain, pressure, or discomfort related to urinary bladder, accompanied by one urinary symptom.[7] To facilitate discussion, the two may be grouped together as IC/PBS, whereby the definition of IC has been standardized by the National Institute of Diabetes and Digestive and Kidney Diseases (NIDDK). This definition of IC contains three inclusion criteria: bladder pain or urinary urgency, Hunner ulcer or glomerulations on cystoscopic examination, and hydrodistention under anesthesia showing diffuse glomerulations in at least four quadrants of the bladder (with at least 10 lesions per quadrant), and 18 exclusion criteria.[8]

The initial evaluation of any adolescent with either acute or chronic pelvic pain should be directed toward excluding organic pathology. In an older study, a group of investigators found that 73% of adolescents presenting with CPP symptoms had notable findings at laparoscopy, the most common of which was pelvic inflammatory disease (PID). Nineteen percent had documented endometriosis, a diagnosis that was more predictive if severe dysmenorrhea was a presenting complaint.[9] Despite the high prevalence of disease, approximately one-third of patients had no abnormal findings at time of laparoscopy, suggesting that disease was not recognized by the surgeon or that patients with chronic pain should be thoroughly assessed prior to surgical exploration. Refer to Table 18.2 for a list of pathologies found at the time of laparoscopy in adolescents with CPP.[10]

Table 18.1 Nongynecologic conditions that may cause or exacerbate chronic pelvic pain, by level of evidence.

Level of evidence	Urologic	Gastrointestinal	Musculoskeletal	Other
Level A[a]	Bladder malignancy	Carcinoma of the colon	Abdominal wall myofascial pain (trigger points)	Abdominal cutaneous nerve entrapment in surgical scar
	Interstitial cystitis[b]	Constipation	Chronic coccygeal or back pain[b]	Depression[b]
	Radiation cystitis	Inflammatory bowel disease	Faulty or poor posture	Somatization disorder
	Urethral syndrome	Irritable bowel syndrome[b]	Fibromyalgia	
			Neuralgia of iliohypogastric, ilioinguinal, and/or genitofemoral nerves	
			Pelvic floor myalgia (levator ani or piriformis syndrome)	
			Peripartum pelvic pain syndrome	
Level B[c]	Uninhibited bladder contractions (detrusor dyssynergia)	—	Herniated nucleus pulposus	Celiac disease
	Urethral diverticulum		Low back pain[b]	Neurologic dysfunction
			Neoplasia of spinal cord or sacral nerve	Porphyria
				Shingles
				Sleep disturbances
Level C[d]	Chronic urinary tract infection	Colitis	Compression of lumbar vertebrae	Abdominal epilepsy
	Recurrent, acute cystitis	Chronic intermittent bowel obstruction	Degenerative joint disease	Abdominal migraine
	Recurrent, acute urethritis	Diverticular disease	Hernias: ventral, inguinal, femoral, spigelian	Bipolar personality disorders
	Stone/urolithiasis		Muscular strains and sprains	Familial Mediterranean fever
	Urethral caruncle		Rectus tendon strain	
			Spondylosis	

Source: Reproduced with permission from Howard FM. *Obstet Gynecol.* 2003;101:594–611.
[a]   Level A: Good and consistent scientific evidence of causal relationship to chronic pelvic pain.
[b]   Diagnosis frequently reported in published series of women with chronic pelvic pain.
[c]   Level B: Limited or inconsistent scientific evidence of causal relationship to chronic pelvic pain.
[d]   Level C: Causal relationship to chronic pelvic pain based on expert opinions.

Table 18.2 Laparoscopic findings in adolescents with chronic pelvic pain.

Normal pelvis	25%–40%
Endometriosis	38%–45%
Ovarian cyst	2%–5%
Uterine malformations	5%–8%
Postoperative adhesions	4%–13%
Pelvic inflammation	5%–15%

Source: With permission from Proctor M et al. *Cochrane Database Syst Rev.* 2002;(1):CD002123.

HISTORY OF PRESENT ILLNESS

Details on the nature of the pain may be the most critical portion of the intake, as this may provide the greatest yield insofar as assessment and diagnosis. The relationship of pain to the menstrual cycle should be elicited, focusing on the specific description of pain and determining whether the cyclic pain, if present, bears any similarity with noncyclic pain. In adolescents, use of a printed diagram is especially helpful with their marking of areas of most intense pain. Likewise, the use of a simple visual analogue scale (VAS) with numeric or graphic symbols can be useful in establishing pain severity (Figure 18.1). Any associated changes in weight or symptoms such as fatigue, joint pain, and headache should be noted, as these may be indicative of a systemic disorder. The effect of the pain on activities of daily living, lifestyle changes, and the effect on the family are similarly important, as these may help determine the severity of symptoms and impact on function and performance. Prior to taking a complete history, however, the teen must understand the concept of confidentiality, which should be explained and acknowledged. More sensitive subjects, such as social or sexual history, should be discussed in the absence of parents or caregivers to minimize discomfort during the conversation and allow for a more honest discussion.

Her past medical history should include prior surgical procedures and chronic medical illnesses. Prior treatments and results as well as current medications should be noted. A thorough obstetric and gynecologic history

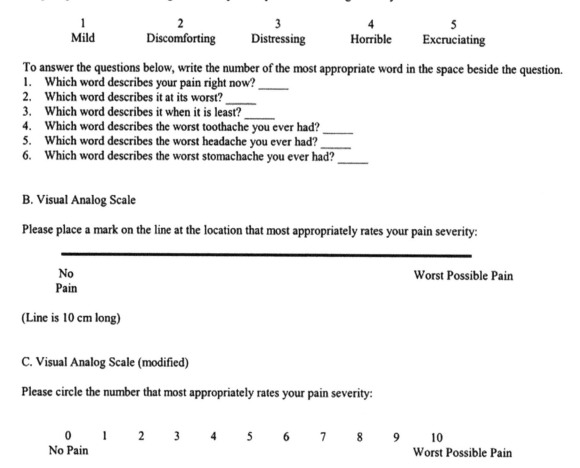

People agree that the following 5 words represent pain of increasing intensity.

1	2	3	4	5
Mild	Discomforting	Distressing	Horrible	Excruciating

To answer the questions below, write the number of the most appropriate word in the space beside the question.
1. Which word describes your pain right now? _____
2. Which word describes it at its worst? _____
3. Which word describes it when it is least? _____
4. Which word describes the worst toothache you ever had? _____
5. Which word describes the worst headache you ever had? _____
6. Which word describes the worst stomachache you ever had? _____

B. Visual Analog Scale

Please place a mark on the line at the location that most appropriately rates your pain severity:

No
Pain   Worst Possible Pain

(Line is 10 cm long)

C. Visual Analog Scale (modified)

Please circle the number that most appropriately rates your pain severity:

0   1   2   3   4   5   6   7   8   9   10
No Pain   Worst Possible Pain

Figure 18.1 McGill Present Pain Index. (Reproduced with permission from Howard F. *Obstet Gynecol.* 2003;101[3]:594–611.)

is also necessary, including risk factors such as previous pregnancy terminations, sexually transmitted infections (STIs), or Müllerian anomalies. Information about the characteristics of menses should be obtained no different from any adult patient, which includes intervals, flow, and quantification. A detailed history focused on the gastrointestinal system is considered standard of care, and a comprehensive assessment by a gastroenterologist familiar with pain syndromes may be necessary, as ancillary studies may better characterize organic causes of the intestinal tract. However, treatment for conditions such as IBS may be as simple as implementing dietary changes.

In addition, a family history to include suggestion or evidence for endometriosis, inflammatory bowel disease (IBD), fibromyalgia, depression, and other associated pain or autoimmune conditions should be elicited. A psychosocial history is equally important in the evaluation of adolescents with CPP. Patients with CPP will often have a history of comorbid depression, somatization, or symptomatology related to borderline personality disorder.[11] A psychological history includes demographic variables and current mental status such as ongoing depression, anxiety, and mood lability. Social history should include information regarding family dysfunction, parental divorce, grief, school difficulties, or issues with bullying and intimidation.[12] This may be

more relevant in recent years with popularization of virtual formats for provocation with social media. In addition, habits such as tobacco use, alcohol, and/or chemical dependency should be documented. A complete sexual history is necessary in all patients with CPP, and it is of paramount importance to inquire about prior sexual, physical, verbal, or emotional abuse in this population.

PHYSICAL EXAMINATION

Physical examination should include general appearance, gait, posture alterations, and facial expressions. Always begin with a detailed abdominal exam designed to identify points of maximum tenderness as well as trigger points. Evidence for incisional hernia or nerve entrapment from previous surgical exploration, neuropathic pain, and joint disease should also be assessed. This first step is noninvasive and often well accepted by young patients, but an awareness of muscle integrity and alignment and the distribution of dermatomes must be learned by the clinician. As indicated, pelvic exam should include inspection of the external genitalia, vulva, hymen/vestibule, and urethral meatus for any structural or congenital abnormalities. Following general inspection, vestibular hyperesthesia can then be determined with a Q-tip or gentle digital exam. A single-digit exam, rather than a full bimanual exam, may first be used to assess the pelvic floor musculature. The ability to perform such an exam may depend on her sexual history, since virginal girls may not tolerate any form of invasive examinations. Similarly, patients with vaginismus or pelvic floor myalgia may not tolerate even a single-digit examination. In many circumstances, bimanual exam may not even be necessary, but palpation or inspection of the anus may help elucidate the presence of pelvic floor spasm, and a rectal, rather than a rectovaginal, examination may be useful for patients with suspected deep infiltrating endometriosis. Fibrotic disease, which may involve the uterosacral ligaments or retrocervical areas, is not necessarily spared in younger patients and can be missed if a comprehensive examination is not performed. Assessment for vaginal discharge, cervical motion tenderness, uterine size, tenderness, mobility, and adnexal masses is equally useful. If not urgent, and it becomes apparent that the patient or parent is not comfortable proceeding with an exam on the initial visit, she should be offered a follow-up visit for this portion of the evaluation.

Dyspareunia, genitourinary symptoms, or gastrointestinal symptoms can be the presenting symptom of pelvic floor dysfunction in adolescents as well as in adults. The trigger points are distinctive, focal areas on physical examination. Referred pain, however, is often poorly localized and does not follow discrete dermatomes. A thorough physical exam is most important in identifying trigger points. The specific technique involves gently pinching the abdominal skin along each dermatome from T10 to L1; contralateral sides should be compared. Sharper sensation is indicative of areas of hypersensitivity and thus a trigger point. Assessing dermatomes for potential nerve entrapments

that would manifest as discrete regions of hyperesthesia, as well as checking for adequate reflexes, may be useful even in this young population. Adolescents with pelvic floor dysfunction may best be examined by palpation of the pelvic musculature to help identify trigger points.[13]

Levator spasms may also result in a sensation similar to that in those with prolapse, described as organs falling out. The pain radiates to the low-back area, and there is absence of a cyclic pattern to the pain. In the sexually active teen, there may also be an element of dyspareunia or bowel-related complaints such as dyschezia. This pain is often sacral area in location. On physical exam, tenderness on palpation is noted, and the pain increases with muscle contraction. Piriformis spasms are characterized by pain in the morning when the patient wakes up, and exacerbation with climbing stairs or driving a car. On physical exam, the pain is elicited on external rotation of the thigh. It may also be palpated over the involved muscle or may require a vaginal exam to elicit.

Table 18.3 presents a list of differential causes of chronic pain and tests to facilitate a more accurate diagnosis. Figure 18.2 offers an algorithm for the diagnosis of pelvic pain based on such information.

GENERAL TREATMENT STRATEGIES

Hormonal therapy remains the cornerstone of suppressive therapies for targeted causes of pelvic pain. Multiple regimens aimed at inducing a hypoestrogenic state exist and are discussed in detail later in this chapter.

Another important option that is often overlooked is pelvic floor physiotherapy, which is associated with 65%

Table 18.3 Differential diagnosis and diagnostic tests useful in the evaluation of pelvic pain in women.

Symptom, finding, or suspected diagnosis	Potentially useful diagnostic tests
Endometriosis-endosalpingosis	Pelvic ultrasound, magnetic resonance imaging, surgical diagnosis, tumor markers
Adenomyosis	Pelvic ultrasound, magnetic resonance imaging; histopathologic diagnosis
Pelvic floor tension myalgia	Assess posture, single-digit examination for trigger points
Constipation	Colonic transit time
Depression	Thyroid-stimulating hormone, thyroxine, tri-iodothyronine levels, antithyroid antibody, complete blood count, renal function tests, hepatic function tests, electrolytes, rapid plasma reagin, refer for analysis
Diarrhea	Stool specimen for ova and parasites, stool for polymorphonuclear leukocytes and erythrocytes, stool cultures, stool for *Clostridium difficile* toxin, stool guaiac testing, barium enema radiography, colonoscopy, upper gastrointestinal series with follow through, computed tomography
Dyspareunia	Urethral and cervical gonorrhea and *Chlamydia* cultures, vaginal cultures, urine cultures, vaginal wet preparations, vaginal pH, pelvic floor assessment
Cystitis	Urine culture
Interstitial cystitis	Cystourethroscopy, potassium chloride challenge test, urine culture, urine cytologies, urodynamic testing, bladder biopsy
Hernias	Abdominal wall ultrasound, computed tomography, herniography
Pelvic congestion syndrome	Pelvic venography, ultrasonography ± Doppler
Irritable bowel syndrome	Rome criteria
Müllerian anomaly	Magnetic resonance imaging

Source: With permission from Solnik MJ. *Curr Opin Obstet Gynecol.* 2006;18:511–8.

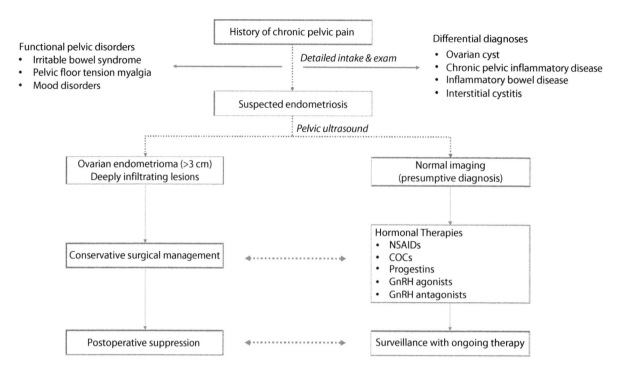

Figure 18.2 Algorithm for treatment of chronic pelvic pain in adolescents. (Modified with permission from Solnik MJ. *Curr Opin Obstet Gynecol.* 2006;18:511–8.)

improvement in pain, especially when pelvic floor myofascial trigger points are noted.[14] Other treatment options that have been described include magnetic field therapy, which involves placement of magnets at abdominal trigger points, and transcutaneous electrical nerve stimulation (TENS).[15,16] Acupuncture and acupressure have entered clinical trials, and current data are lacking to support the application for dysmenorrhea.[10]

Surgical intervention in the form of laparoscopy remains an option, especially when medical therapy fails or is not tolerated. Surgical exploration may represent first-line therapy for certain patients, including those who do not wish to trial hormonal options or those with a pelvic mass (which could include a larger endometrioma). Song and Advincula reported a high rate of abnormal findings at time of surgery, ranging from 60% to 75%, which supports the appropriateness of surgery in a select group of patients.[17]

The role of presacral neurectomy (PSN) remains controversial and has been proposed to be a potential option for patients with significant midline pelvic pain.[2] More recent findings from Italy, however, suggest that PSN may be offered as a surgical adjunct rather than a primary procedure in patients with endometriosis. These authors also recommended that surgeons who offer this procedure should be judicious in counseling patients about failure rates and the relatively high risk of postoperative bowel and bladder complaints that could further incapacitate this young cohort of women.[18] Any surgeon offering PSN should be skilled and familiar with the anatomy of the presacral space given the potential for significant intraoperative hemorrhage.

Appendectomy has been evaluated as another potential surgical therapy in women with CPP. A retrospective study evaluated the role of prophylactic appendectomy in 190 women with chronic pain. Incidentally, 154 appendices were abnormal, and pathologic findings included endometriosis, carcinoid, chronic appendicitis, periappendicitis, fibrous obliteration, and lymphoid hyperplasia. The authors concluded that prophylactic appendectomy in patients being evaluated for CPP is appropriate in light of the high incidence of abnormal findings, but this study was not limited to adolescents.[19] Other studies have found more conflicting results, and while appendectomy may be safe and feasible, lack of conclusive evidence in the setting of pain management limits the generalizability of appendectomy in this population.[20] Refer to Table 18.4 for a list of options available for the treatment of CPP.

MUSCULOSKELETAL CAUSES OF PELVIC PAIN

Quite frequently, adolescents who seek medical advice for chronic pain unfortunately are left with no conclusive diagnosis. As a result, treatment options often fail, since the first or second treatment offerings are often speculative. Herein lies the dilemma of organic versus functional pain, the latter being defined as pain with no identifiable or physical source. To provide patients with this diagnosis, a thorough evaluation as described in the preceding section must first be performed. These women may represent a group who demonstrate an exaggerated response to a normal stimulus, but otherwise do not suffer from significant physical morbidity. These patients are often diagnosed with associated pain syndromes such as IBS or

Table 18.4 Chronic pelvic pain management.

Analgesics (e.g., nonsteroidals, COX-2 inhibitors)
Hormonal therapy:
- Combined hormonal contraceptives (combined oral contraceptive, patch, ring)
- Progestin-only methods (LNG-IUS, Dienogest, DMPA)
- Gonadotropin-releasing hormone agonists

Nonhormonal therapy (e.g., neuroleptics)
Pelvic physical therapy
Psychotherapy
Acupuncture
Surgical intervention

Table 18.5 Features suggesting organic versus functional pain.

Organic pain	Functional Pain
Consistently localized	Periumbilical or diffuse
Awakens patient from sleep	Variable location
Precipitated by eating	Exacerbated by stress
Recent onset	Present for months before seeking medical treatment
Involuntary weight gain	Functional impairment out of proportion
Delayed puberty	No objective findings
Systemic symptoms consistent with single disease	

Source: With permission from Solnik MJ. Curr Opin Obstet Gynecol. 2006;18:511–8.

fibromyalgia. See Table 18.5 for a list of characteristics that help identify organic from functional pain.

To better refine the diagnosis of functional pain, the clinician should evaluate pelvic floor musculature, a component that must not be overlooked in the adolescent female. This has been frequently not emphasized by clinicians, simply because of the lack of consistent experience during training. One study identified a musculoskeletal (MSK) etiology in 26% of patients presenting with CPP.[21] Trigger points on physical exam provide the initial basis for a musculoskeletal origin to the CPP. Trigger points are areas of hyperirritability that are locally tender on compression and cause referred pain and tenderness; the myofascial pain syndrome occurs within taut bands of skeletal muscle that cause pain.[22] Currently, most of the theories related to development of trigger points implicate noxious stimuli to the affected fascia and muscles. Sustained muscle contractions, like those caused by poor posture or in response to an injury, may be a trigger. Cold or damp weather or a new physical activity in an unconditioned adolescent can also play a role in the etiology of pain.[23] Nevertheless, pelvic floor tension myalgia is common in patients with both organic and functional pelvic pain. In a cross-sectional analysis of 987 women being evaluated for CPP, investigators found 22% had levator ani tenderness and 14% had piriformis tenderness. Pain at these sites correlated with a greater number of pain sites, previous surgery for pelvic pain, and higher pain scores by validated surveys.[24]

Both acute and chronic pelvic pain can be associated with trigger points in the abdomen, vagina, or sacral area. The referred pain can also be visceral in nature, similar to and complicating the picture associated with dysmenorrhea. Treatment involves injection of local anesthetics, such as 0.25% bupivacaine or 1% procaine, into the trigger points. Pelvic floor physical therapy, with or without injections, provides exceptional relief for many patients with pain related to pelvic floor dysfunction.[25] Vasocoolants and stretching have also been advocated as well as chiropractic flexion-distraction in combination with trigger points.[26,27] Other drugs such as neuroleptics (e.g., tricyclic antidepressants or gabapentinoids) have been successfully used in adults to treat MSK-associated pain. Some of these have been tested in the treatment of pain disorders in pediatrics and can be considered to address CPP in this population.[28]

ENDOMETRIOSIS

Introduction and epidemiology

Endometriosis is a chronic inflammatory condition defined by endometrial stroma and glands found outside of the uterine cavity. This has long been known to affect adolescent girls.[29] Despite the initial series reported by Meigs over six decades ago, many young patients presenting with chronic pain experience significant delays in diagnosis or treatment due, in part, to the lack of awareness by clinicians. In recent years, this cohort has received more attention, and as a result, we should see improvement in therapeutic outcomes. Given the high prevalence of disease, we should not underestimate patient complaints, particularly among those who describe progressive dysmenorrhea that does not respond to first-line therapies.[30] Estimates reveal that almost 70% of adolescents with pelvic pain that is nonresponsive to combined oral contraceptives (COCs) have endometriosis.[30] Most referral centers will likely encounter higher rates due to self-selection. Another series noted a higher prevalence of endometriosis in older subsets of adolescents, suggesting that this disease may be progressive in certain groups of patients.[31,32] This raises the question as to whether early intervention in this susceptible group can prevent or minimize adverse outcomes later in life, that is, chronic pain and infertility.

Presentation

Although progressive dysmenorrhea remains one of the most common complaints among girls with endometriosis, symptomatology can vary significantly. Primary dysmenorrhea, or cyclic pain that occurs in the absence of pelvic pathology, is particularly common in adolescent females and may be difficult to separate from symptoms suggestive of endometriosis. Many with endometriosis, however, will eventually present with chronic, nonmenstrual pain that may differ in quality from the cyclic component. Often, the ability to distinguish one from the other becomes blurred.

These patients often miss school, have affected family lives, and may refrain from activities such as organized sports or social events because of pain.[33] Possibly the most worrisome area of concern is the long delay many patients experience from onset of symptoms to diagnosis and eventual treatment. Data from the Endometriosis Association confirmed this delay. Approximately 50% of patients who answered surveys reported seeking medical advice from at least five physicians prior to receiving acceptable care.[1] The average interval from onset of symptoms to diagnosis in adult patients was approximately 10 years. Failing to seek advice until symptoms are severe and physician reluctance to treat younger patients likely contribute to such a delay. Needless to say, educating those who care for adolescent patients may reduce this lengthy wait. Our ability to impact disease progression through early treatment is not established, but initiating treatment that could improve the quality of life in patients with pain is indispensable.

Pathophysiology and genetics

From a mechanistic perspective, Sampson's theory of retrograde menstruation remains one of the most widely accepted pathophysiologic models to explain the development of endometriosis.[34] As a stand-alone process, though, this theory fails to explain why only a minority of patients who demonstrate retrograde flow develop endometriosis. Certain patients must not be able to clear the menstrual debris, whereas others may have a structural lesion that increases the cellular burden on the peritoneal surface. The latter can be corroborated by the small group of patients with Müllerian anomalies that result in outflow obstruction of the reproductive tract.[35] Most of, if not all, menstrual effluent is unable to follow the path outward, resulting in consistent exposure of peritoneal surfaces to menstrual content. Once normal anatomy is restored and the obstruction relieved, these patients may experience a remarkable transformation and represent a group that can achieve a relative cure of their disease.

To help explain why retrograde menstruation may lead to the development of endometriosis in a subset of women, various investigators are attempting to establish a link between this disease and selectively deficient cell-mediated immune clearance pathways. Studies assessing circulating immunologic markers reveal that levels of serum interleukin-4, peritoneal interleukin-2, and peritoneal interleukin-4 can discriminate between patients with endometriosis and control groups, further lending support to an immunologic theory.[36]

Patients with more advanced stages of disease may have infiltrative lesions, resulting in peritoneal fibrosis and distortion of the anatomy. Some of these patients may even present prior to menarche. This supports the proposal of Müllerian rests, cells present in the female pelvis during embryogenesis. These primordial cells are stimulated by estrogen produced early in puberty with the activation of the hypothalamic-pituitary-ovarian (HPO) axis, leading to the development of deep ectopic endometrial implants. Since depth of invasion has been clearly associated with pain symptoms.[37] these patients may be more at risk for pain at a younger age.

Alternatively, new theories suggest that neonatal menstrual bleeding may lead to retrograde flow and seeding of the pelvic peritoneum with endometrial progenitor cells.[38] These highly angiogenic implants lead to recurrent ectopic bleeding and endometrioma formation under the influence of estrogen.[39] Rather than appearing as surface lesions from retrograde flow at menarche, these cells may invade into deeper tissues over time. Early life events may therefore play a role in identifying young women at higher risk of severe disease.

The role of oxidative stress and generation of free radicals in promoting endometriosis is another area of research, even at the gene level. Perhaps environmental exposures and toxins may facilitate progression in at-risk patients.[40]

Finally, large epidemiologic studies have identified some factors associated with the presence of endometriosis. These include early age at menarche, early onset dysmenorrhea, obstructive congenital malformations, asthma, exposure to secondhand smoke, a family history of endometriosis, a sedentary lifestyle, and neonatal exposure to soy-based formulas.[41-44] A larger body size appears to be a protective factor.[45]

Diagnostic workup

The initial historical intake often provides enough information to provide a diagnosis, although physical exam will clearly be useful in ruling out other or associated causes of pain. It is not unreasonable to have the patient return for a second consultation to perform an exam. This degree of patience may relieve stress associated with the much anticipated visit and may go a long way to help establish a positive and interactive relationship.

Imaging modalities such as ultrasound are useful for evaluating pelvic anatomy, and in the setting of endometriosis, may diagnose ovarian involvement (see Table 18.3). If she is unable to tolerate a vaginal probe, excellent imaging can often be obtained with an abdominal probe with a full bladder. However, the absence of pelvic disease on ultrasound does not rule out the potential for peritoneal disease. Magnetic resonance imaging may be useful for detecting infiltrating lesions and can help guide the clinician for surgical intervention but is not absolutely necessary. If the suspicion for endometriosis is high, and surgery is indicated, it can be offered at any point in the evaluation.[46] However, clinicians should take great care to avoid repetitive surgeries, since this paradigm results in increasing intraoperative risk and rarely yields therapeutic results.

Surgical characteristics

Direct visualization of implants at time of surgery and histopathology do not always correlate, since atypical lesions may be difficult to assess without biopsy, and there is no standardized method used by all pathologists.[47] Positive predictive values of peritoneal biopsies are between 40% and 50%, but surgeons with experience identifying adolescent-type lesions may reach a sensitivity of 97%.[48] Approximately 25% of peritoneal biopsies are unrevealing. Surgical characteristics of endometriosis in adolescents favor earlier-stage disease, based on the American Society for Reproductive Medicine (ASRM) revised classification system. These are often clear to colored, vesicular lesions superficially embedded on the peritoneal surface.[49–51] Historically, these were not recognized as endometriotic implants, affecting the true prevalence documented in years past. These lesions are active prostaglandin producers, an attribute that substantiates the high rate of dysmenorrhea.[5] Older adolescents are more likely to have fewer early stage (formerly considered atypical) implants and more resemble adults.[37] This suggests a progressive disorder, and unfortunately, deep and painful implants are not unique to adults (Figure 18.3).[50]

In a systematic review published in 2013, approximately two-thirds of adolescent girls with chronic pelvic pain or dysmenorrhea were found to have laparoscopic evidence of endometriosis. Nearly one-third of these were considered moderate to severe according to the ASRM classification.[52] Similarly, in a review of 86 patients less than 22 years of age who were undergoing laparoscopic surgery for endometriosis, 76% were found to have stage I–II disease, while 23% were found to have advanced-stage

Table 18.6 Comparison of adolescent versus adult endometriosis.

	Adolescent	**Adult**
Presenting symptoms	Primary dysmenorrhea, severe, refractory to first-line medical therapy	Secondary dysmenorrhea, moderate to severe, often accompanied by noncyclic chronic pelvic pain
Surgical findings	Red, clear and/or vesicular peritoneal implants; minimal fibrosis; smaller and less adhesiogenic ovarian endometrioma	Black peritoneal implants, white-appearing or nodular fibrosis, dense adhesions that may include rectosigmoid colon; ovarian endometrioma more common with dense adhesions to ovarian cortex
Deeply infiltrating endometriosis	Uncommon finding	Variable, but more common; may be difficult to identify if inexperienced
Other features	Association with outflow obstruction of reproductive tract	Rectovaginal or bladder lesions; adenomyosis

Source: See further Benagiano G et al. *Reprod Biomed Online.* 2018;36/1:102–14.

endometriosis, most commonly in the form of an endometrioma.[53] See Table 18.6 that describes the typical phenotype of an adolescent female with endometriosis, as compared to an adult.

Treatment options

Only after a comprehensive assessment that facilitates exclusion of other organic or functional causes of pain should the clinician provide endometriosis-targeted therapies. If empiric therapy is offered wantonly, therapy is more apt to fail, resulting in frustration and the possibility of distrust on behalf of the patient.

Whether the early diagnosis and treatment of adolescents with endometriosis prevent disease progression or merely increase the number of interventions without affecting long-term outcomes is debatable.[54] Nevertheless, effective treatment of endometriosis in this population may improve quality of life by reducing symptoms. No one therapy has been proven substantially superior to the other, and most experts would agree that if pain is the main complaint, then reducing it to an acceptable level should be the goal. Even if treatment is deemed successful, many patients are not cured of their pain, and many will experience recurrent symptoms. Being honest and realistic while

(a)
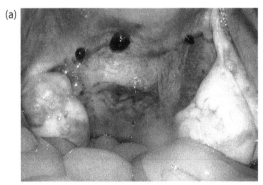

(b)
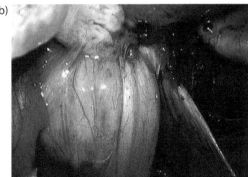

Figure 18.3 (a,b) Endometriosis implants in adolescents.

providing individualized care will ultimately facilitate a positive interaction and improvement in the patients' quality of life. Needless to say, the best management involves early evaluation and prompt intervention.

Most treatment paradigms used in adolescents have been based on research focusing on adults, with a smaller percentage of the literature centering on this group. Although medical management is frequently used as first-line therapy, surgical intervention can be offered at any point in the evaluation or if advanced disease is clinically suspected. Various experts in the field differ in opinion with regard to the timing of surgical intervention, with opponents offering that one surgery at a young age may lead to several others by the time the patient has reached adulthood. Proponents feel that long-term medical therapy, which is often necessary to suppress symptoms, should not be considered until a surgical diagnosis is confirmed.

Most nonsurgical remedies are composed of hormonal agents that suppress endometriotic growth, either directly or indirectly. Nonsteroidal anti-inflammatory drugs (NSAIDs), on the other hand, represent a nonhormonal pharmaceutical class that may reduce the inflammatory response produced by this disease process and limit symptoms.[55] There appears to be positive feedback between prostaglandin (PG) synthesis, aromatase activity, and estrogen production, mediated by abnormally high cyclooxygenase-2 (COX-2) activity in the setting of endometriosis.[56] Superficial, often atypical implants are active PG producers. As COX-2 inhibitors, NSAIDs may improve symptoms by interrupting receptor-mediated signaling pathways. *In vitro* studies suggest that COX-2 inhibitors reduce endometriosis implants through anti-angiogenic properties.[57] Variable responses may be seen with different medications in each patient. The only trials designed to assess the impact of NSAIDs studied groups of patients with primary dysmenorrhea, in the absence of endometriosis.[58] Nevertheless, NSAIDs remain a first-line adjunct to combined oral contraceptives (COCs), since they are relatively safe and have positive anecdotal therapeutic effect.

Along the same lines, COCs have traditionally been used as first-line agents for patients with presumed endometriosis, yet no study has consistently demonstrated a therapeutic response.[59] Despite this, if a patient has no contraindication to the use of COCs and needs contraceptive measures, these remain an ideal first-line therapy. COCs suppress the HPO axis and subsequent estrogen/progesterone secretion, thereby inducing atrophy of ectopic endometrial implants. If given continuously, patients may become amenorrheic and will experience less cyclic pain. ACOG supports the continuous use of CHCs in adolescents to induce amenorrhea, but states that "this modality can result in significant breakthrough bleeding." Side effects of COCs are generally mild and include irregular bleeding, nausea, bloating, headache, and breast tenderness. To reiterate, patients who have symptoms refractory to cyclic or continuous COCs have a relatively high probability of true disease.

Progestin-based medical treatments can also significantly reduce pain symptoms if used continuously.[60] Progesterone induces decidualization and eventual atrophy of endometrial implants. Certain formulations also suppress the HPO axis, resulting in decreased steroid hormone stimulation of implants. Many such patients will become amenorrheic. Depot medroxyprogesterone acetate (DMPA), a progestin administered intramuscularly or subcutaneously every 3 months, also serves as an effective form of contraception. DMPA suppresses the HPO axis, resulting in a hypoestrogenic state. Since progestins inhibit estrogen and progesterone receptor synthesis, patients experience long periods of low estrogen production at a time when bone mineralization is high. Although we lack long-term follow-up of adolescents being treated with prolonged DMPA, caution should be used when prescribing. Physicians are not required to monitor bone mineral density (BMD).

Dienogest is an oral progestin now used as a monotherapy at a dose of 2 mg daily in patients with endometriosis. This medication is highly selective for the progesterone receptor, leading to strong progestational effects, moderate antigonadotrophic effects, and minimal androgenic, glucocorticoid, or mineralocorticoid effects.[61] Multiple studies have shown dienogest to be both safe and effective in the treatment of adults with endometriosis.[62–64] However, studies in the pediatric adolescent population were lacking until recently. In 2017, Ebert et al. published the results of the VISanne Study to Assess Safety in ADOlescents (VISADO study). This prospective observational study evaluated the safety and efficacy of dienogest 2 mg daily in adolescents aged 12–18 with clinically suspected or laparoscopically confirmed endometriosis. Results demonstrated that endometriosis-associated pain was substantially reduced and that the drug was very well tolerated during the 52-week trial. However, there was an associated decrease in lumbar bone mineral density with only a partial recovery after 6 months of treatment discontinuation.[65] In light of these findings, it is necessary to adopt an individualized approach when prescribing dienogest, as with DMPA. One must balance the benefits of decreased pain with the potential risks to bone health in each patient, and provide counseling in this regard. Patients should also be informed that dienogest has not been tested or approved as a contraceptive, so the concomitant use of barrier contraception is necessary in sexually active teenagers.

The levonorgestrel intrauterine system (LNG-IUS) is a long-acting reversible contraceptive that has also been evaluated for the treatment of endometriosis. This IUS delivers levonorgestrel, a progestin, to the uterine cavity at a steady state, causing atrophy and pseudodecidualization of the endometrial lining and apoptosis of endometrial glands and stroma.[66] In a number of studies, the LNG-IUS showed improved CPP, dyspareunia, and improved dysmenorrhea related to rectovaginal endometriosis in adults.[67,68] In a review of the literature, the use of the LNG-IUS for the treatment of dysmenorrhea was found to be equal or superior to systemic progestins and oral contraceptives, even in adolescent populations.[69]

The use of LNG-IUS has been shown to be both safe and acceptable in adolescents, with ACOG endorsing it as a first-line method of contraception in this population.[70] While the LNG-IUS is frequently used for contraception, heavy menstrual bleeding, and dysmenorrhea in adolescents, there are minimal data assessing its role in the treatment of endometriosis in this population. A recent retrospective cohort study of 18 adolescents aged 14–22 with biopsy-proven endometriosis found the LNG-IUS to be effective in decreasing pain following surgical treatment.[66] However, prospective trials are needed to better understand the effectiveness and long-term outcomes of the LNG-IUS in adolescent patients with endometriosis.

Gonadotropin-releasing hormone (GnRH) agonists rapidly induce a hypoestrogenic state by downregulating the HPO axis. An initial rise in gonadotropins and estrogen (flare) occurs after administration, but chronic exposure to GnRH agonists disrupts the pulsatile secretion of GnRH and induces a hypogonadal state. Formulations of this drug vary, but most GnRH agonists are delivered via subcutaneous injections every 1–3 months. The majority of data on GnRH agonists is extrapolated from the adult literature, which shows that approximately 85% of patients with confirmed endometriosis will experience significant reduction in pain complaints.[71] Side effects of GnRH agonists are related to hypoestrogenism (vasomotor symptoms, vaginal dryness, mood swings, and sleep disturbance). Prolonged exposure (>6 months) without hormonal add-back therapy can lead to an irreversible decrease in BMD, but this loss does not correlate with the age at which therapy was initiated.[72] These side effects may contribute to a patient's or provider's reluctance in initiating this treatment. Since adolescence is a critical time for bone accretion, the use of GnRH agonists should be used with caution in this age group, as this hormonal regimen leads to hypoestrogenism.[73,74] The use of GnRH agonists is typically reserved for the treatment of teenagers with surgically confirmed endometriosis that is unresponsive to other medical therapies.[75] Although the U.S. Food and Drug Administration approves the use of GnRH agonists alone for 6–9 months, hormonal add-back therapy should be initiated at the onset of GnRH agonist treatment in adolescents to mitigate side effects and loss of BMD. This has no impact on the efficacy of the GnRH agonist and successfully limits the side-effect profile.[76] In a recent randomized trial of adolescents with surgically confirmed endometriosis, the use of norethindrone acetate (5 mg/d) plus conjugated equine estrogen (0.625 mg/d) for add-back therapy resulted in significantly improved quality of life and BMD scores compared to norethindrone acetate plus placebo.[77] When prescribed with adequate add-back therapy and with appropriate monitoring of BMD, the long-term use of GnRH agonists can be safe and highly effective for the treatment of endometriosis in the adolescent population.[75]

More recently, the safety and efficacy of oral GnRH antagonists have been evaluated for the treatment of endometriosis in the adult population. This drug acts by competitively inhibiting the GnRH receptors in the pituitary gland, resulting in a rapid decrease in circulating gonadotropins and estradiol. Recent randomized phase 2 and phase 3 trials have demonstrated the ability of GnRH antagonists to significantly reduce the symptoms related to moderate and severe endometriosis.[78] However, these agents were also found to result in hypoestrogenic side effects, including reduced BMD, increased lipid levels, and vasomotor symptoms.[78] The pharmaceutical name, Elagolix, is now approved in the United States and Canada under the trade name, Orlissa. Partial suppression can be achieved with a dose of 150 mg daily (for up to 24 months) and full suppression with a higher regimen of 200 mg twice daily (for up to 6 months). Addback therapy is recommended with use of the higher dosing to reduce the risk of bone loss. Elagolix should not be considered a contraceptive and estrogen-containing contraceptive options have been shown to reduce efficacy so consideration towards progestin-only options or barrier protection should be used if appropriate. Studies using this drug in the adolescent population are lacking.

Although androgens such as danazol have been shown to be equally effective in treating endometriosis-associated pain (and the only pharmacologic agents to show improvement in surgical scoring), the side effect profile that includes acne, hirsutism, and metabolic disturbances may be limiting in adolescent patients.[79]

Other investigational agents such as aromatase and progesterone inhibitors, as well as steroid-hormone receptor modulators, are emerging as options for adult protocols. These may prove beneficial as long-term options in that side effects are minimized while efficacy is spared. At this point, any patient offered such a drug should be done so under a formal study protocol.

Surgery

Surgical management of endometriosis is indicated for pain refractory to medical management, advanced disease with involvement of the bowel, ureters, or nerves, and associated subfertility (generally not a concern for this cohort). Conservative surgical management with laparoscopic excision or ablation of visible implants and restoration of pelvic anatomy can provide effective treatment of pain-related complaints. However, recurrence of disease is not uncommon, and there is no consensus as to when surgery should be offered.[80–82] Several randomized controlled trials have established a clear relationship between surgical intervention and reduction of pain in patients with endometriosis. One trial demonstrated a significant reduction in pain, lasting up to 6 months, when compared to controls who underwent diagnostic laparoscopy (sham surgery).[80] Another trial confirmed these results and included quality of life measures, which were also improved at 6-month follow-up. There was a 20% nonresponder rate with a 30% placebo effect.[83] In a recent review, approximately 50% of adolescents were noted to have severe disease at time of laparoscopy.[51] They demonstrated an excellent response to resection, which promotes the use of more aggressive surgical measures in order to limit recurrence.

Although laparoscopic findings do not always correlate with the degree of symptoms, pain seems to correlate well with the depth of peritoneal invasion.[37] Ablative therapy with electrosurgery or laser can effectively provide relief (for at least 6 months) in patients with minimal to moderate disease.[83] Radical excision of affected areas with restoration of normal anatomy is the preferred method of treating symptomatic patients with deep peritoneal disease, and may limit the risk of recurrent symptoms.[37,84,85] Improvement in pain may last up to 5 years after surgery (Video 18.1), but the risk of reintervention approaches 50% in patients with moderate to severe disease. Less aggressive surgical measures and younger age are predictive of recurrence.[86] Notwithstanding the noted improvement, surgery has its risks. Although a small percentage of patients will undergo reoperation due to recurrent symptoms and disease, adhesion formation and altered surgical planes may increase morbidity upon each return to the operating suite.

Ovarian endometriomas are a form of deep disease that originates from the encapsulation of endometrial tissue between the ovarian cortex and the posterior leaf of the parametrium.[87] Ectopic endometrial cells on the ovarian surface can result in mesenchymal cell metaplasia in the interstitial ovarian tissue, sclerosis, ovarian adhesions, follicle loss, and decreased fertility potential.[87] Although less common in the adolescent population, the presence of unilateral or bilateral ovarian masses should raise suspicion for endometriosis.[88] In adolescent girls, endometriomas are thought to be a sign of a more aggressive pathologic process with a tendency toward disease progression.[89] Recent evidence suggests that surgical treatment in the early stage may be beneficial, resulting in less ovarian damage caused by the disease itself and caused by a less invasive procedure.[87,90] The short-term recurrence rate of endometriomas in adolescents following laparoscopic cyst enucleation is low, with a median time to recurrence of 53 months.[91] However, the recurrence rate appears to increase with time, reaching 30% at 8 years. For this reason, some experts suggest using postoperative hormonal suppression to prevent the recurrence of endometriomas. A retrospective cohort study published in 2017 demonstrated that long-term treatment with cyclic oral contraceptives can be effective in this respect.[92] In light of this, long-term gynecologic follow-up is warranted in patients who undergo surgical treatment for endometriosis during adolescence (Video 18.2).

Video 18.1   https://youtu.be/ZogdSExNAY8
Surgery for deep infiltrating endometriosis.

Video 18.2   https://youtu.be/PS1oMonDBTI
Endometrioma.

Appendectomy should be considered in patients undergoing laparoscopic surgery for suspected endometriosis, especially if complaining of right-sided pain or if the appendix appears grossly involved. Up to 50% of appendiceal specimens will yield abnormal pathology, but the effect on pain and future adverse outcomes is difficult to assess.[93] In patients undergoing laparoscopy for pelvic pain or endometriosis, consideration should be made to place a hormonal IUD during the procedure and minimize pain of insertion.[74]

Nerve ablative techniques such as laparoscopic uterine nerve ablation (LUNA) and presacral neurectomy (PSN) are also not without risk and have not been effectively studied in the adolescent population.[19,94]

Recurrence

Pre- and postoperative hormonal suppression may improve revised ASRM scores at time of surgery[95]; however, experts disagree on the role of hormonal treatment in preventing disease recurrence or the need for future surgery. Young age appears to be a profound risk factor for recurrent disease, particularly for ovarian endometrioma formation.[96] The challenge in determining a relative rate of recurrence is the heterogeneity of disease and the assumption that symptom recurrence is equivalent to surgically confirmed recurrence. In clinical practice, symptomatology should be the driving force for offering therapy and is most appropriate from a care-pathway perspective. In prevalence studies targeting adolescent females, only a relatively small percentage of patients underwent repeat laparoscopy, but the majority of these patients had surgically confirmed recurrence. For example, Tandoi et al. documented recurrence in 11 of 57 (34%) young women who presented with symptoms suggestive of recurrence.[97] This is relevant since younger patients who develop pain-related complaints have a longer reproductive life and are at risk for repeat surgeries, and they may wish to have children in years to follow. In a study by Audebert et al., 55 young women with surgically confirmed endometriosis were followed over several years (mean follow-up of 125.5 months).[98] They found that 7 of 19 (36.8%) women with endometrioma demonstrated recurrence, but 5 (9%) were diagnosed with new ovarian lesions, confirming that the disease may progress. Approximately 50% of patients with deep infiltrating endometriosis (DIE) demonstrated recurrence over the study period. Long-term follow-up allowed for the capacity of some of these women to conceive, which included 13 successful pregnancies, a success rate of approximately 72%. Most of these women, however, had early stage disease.

CONCLUSION

- Although prevalence rates have been difficult to estimate because of the various definitions used, CPP in adolescents is a common disorder and may affect up to 15% of girls.
- All disciplines that provide care to young girls and teenagers should be aware of potential causes of pelvic pain in order to provide appropriate referrals and limit the

repercussions of delays that contribute to long-standing morbidity.

- Functional pelvic pain, or that which has no easily identified source, should be assessed for in any young patient presenting with chronic complaints.
- Musculoskeletal disorders of the pelvic floor are often overlooked and do not respond to most medical or surgical options, but they may be elicited in up to 20% of such patients.
- A multidisciplinary evaluation should be undertaken in any adolescent presenting with chronic pain, especially prior to initiating therapy. Avoiding delays in effective treatment and limiting undue risks are crucial to caring for this young cohort.
- Endometriosis should be suspected in any female complaining of progressively worsening dysmenorrhea that does not respond to NSAIDs and combined hormonal contraceptives.
- The diagnosis of endometriosis can typically be made by history and examination. Ancillary imaging studies may be useful for targeting therapy but are not absolutely indicated other than to rule out other pathology.
- Most diagnostic and treatment paradigms used to treat adolescents have been derived from those used in adults, but new and effective, mainly progestin-based therapies have come to market in recent years.
- Medical management of endometriosis focuses on suppressing the HPO axis and inducing atrophy of peritoneal implants. Side-effect profiles of any agents should be thoroughly addressed with the patient and her parents, especially those that may impact bone mineralization.
- Conservative surgery may be used to diagnose and treat endometriosis but is limited by recurrent disease that commonly affects young patients.
- Aggressive resection of endometriosis may provide more long-standing relief from pain and may reduce the need to perform repeat surgeries. This must be balanced with operator experience and surgical risk.

REFERENCES

1. Ballweg ML. Big picture of endometriosis helps provide guidance on approach to teens: Comparative historical data show endometriosis starting younger, is more severe. *J Pediatr Adolesc Gynecol.* 2003;16:S21–6.
2. Benagiano G, Guo SW, Puttemans P et al. Progress in the diagnosis and management of adolescent endometriosis: An opinion. *Reprod Biomed Online.* 2018;36/1:102–14.
3. Merskey H, Bogduk M, eds. Classification of chronic pain: Descriptions of chronic pain syndromes and definitions of pain terms. 2nd update. Seattle, WA: International Association for the Study of Pain (IASP) Press; 1994.
4. Mathias S, Kuppermann M, Lieberman R et al. Chronic pelvic pain: Prevalence, health-related quality of life an economic correlates. *Obstet Gynecol.* 1996;87:321–7.
5. Davis AR, Westhoff CL. Primary dysmenorrhea in adolescent girls and treatment with oral contraceptives. *J Pediatr Adolesc Gynecol.* 2001;14:3–8.
6. Latthe P, Latthe M, Say L, Gülmezoglu M, Khan KS. WHO systematic review of prevalence of chronic pelvic pain: A neglected reproductive health morbidity. *BMC Public Health.* 2006;1:177.
7. van de Merwe JP, Nordling J, Bouchelouche P et al. Diagnostic criteria, classification, and nomenclature for painful bladder syndrome/interstitial cystitis: An ESSIC proposal. *Eur Urol.* 2008;53:60–7.
8. National Institute of Diabetes and Digestive and Kidney Disease (NIDDK). Interstitial cystitis/painful bladder syndrome 2011. NIH Publication No. 11–3220. The National Kidney and Urologic Diseases Information Clearinghouse (NKUDIC). https://www.urologic.niddk.nih.gov. Accessed May 28, 2019.
9. Wolfman WL, Kreutner K. Laparoscopy in children and adolescents. *J Adolesc Health Care.* 1984;5:261–5.
10. Proctor M, Smith C, Farquhar C, Stones R. Transcutaneous electrical nerve stimulation and acupuncture for primary dysmenorrhoea. *Cochrane Database Syst Rev.* 2002;(1):CD002123.
11. Walker E, Katon W, Neras K, Jemelka R, Massoth D. Dissociation in women with chronic pelvic pain. *Am J Psychiatry.* 1992;149:534–7.
12. The Association of Professors of Gynecology and Obstetrics (APGO). Educational series on women's issues. *Chronic Pelvic Pain: An Integral Approach.* Crofton, MD: APGO; 2000:1–55.
13. Slocumb J. Neurological factors in chronic pelvic pain: Trigger points and the abdominal pelvic pain syndrome. *Am J Obstet Gynecol.* 1984;149:536.
14. Petros P, Skilling P. Pelvic floor rehabilitation in the female according to the integral theory of female urinary incontinence. First report. *Eur J Obstet Gynecol Reprod Biol.* 2001;94:264–9.
15. Aboseif S, Tamaddon C, Chalfin S, Freedman S, Kaptein J. Sacral neuromodulation as an effective treatment for refractory pelvic floor dysfunction. *Urology.* 2002;60:52–6.
16. Brown C, Ling F, Wan J, Phila A. Efficacy of static magnetic field therapy in chronic pelvic pain: Double-blind pilot study. *Am J Obstet Gynecol.* 2002;187:1581–7.
17. Song A, Advincula A. Adolescent chronic pelvic pain. *J Pediatr Adolesc Gynecol.* 2005;18:371–7.
18. Zullo F, Palomba S, Zupi E, Russo T, Morelli M, Sena T, Pellicano M, Mastrantonio P. Long-term effectiveness of presacral neurectomy for the treatment of severe dysmenorrhea due to endometriosis. *J Am Assoc Gynecol Laparosc.* 2004;11:23–8.
19. Lyons T, Winer W, Woo A. Appendectomy in patients undergoing laparoscopic surgery for pelvic pain. *J Am Assoc Gynecol Laparosc.* 2001;8:542–4.
20. Lal AK, Weaver AL, Hopkins MR, Famuyide AO. Laparoscopic appendectomy in women without identifiable pathology undergoing laparoscopy for chronic pelvic pain. *JSLS.* 2013;1:82.

21. Peters A, van Dorst E, Jellis B et al. A randomized clinical trial to compare two different approaches to women with chronic pelvic pain. *Obstet Gynecol.* 1991;77:740.

22. Ling F, Slocumb J. Use of trigger point injections in chronic pelvic pain. *Obstet Gynecol Clin North Am.* 1993;20:809.

23. Aftimos S. Myofacial pain in children. *NZ Med J.* 1989;102:440.

24. Tu FF, As-Sanie S, Steege JF. Prevalence of pelvic musculoskeletal disorders in a female chronic pain clinic. *J Reprod Med.* 2006;51:185–9.

25. Schroder B, Sanfilippo JS, Hertweck SP. Musculoskeletal pelvic pain in a pediatric and adolescent gynecology service. *J Pediatr Adolesc Gynecol.* 2004;17:23–7.

26. Gallegos N, Hobsley M. Recognition and treatment of abdominal wall pain. *J R Soc Med.* 1989;82:343.

27. Hawk C, Long C, Azad A. Chiropractic care for women with chronic pelvic pain: A prospective single-group intervention study. *J Manipulative Physiol Ther.* 1997;20:73.

28. Teitelbaum JE, Arora R. Long-term efficacy of low-dose tricyclic antidepressants for children with functional gastrointestinal disorders. *J Pediatr Gastroenterol Nutr.* 2011;53(3):260–4.

29. Meigs JV. Endometriosis. *Ann Surg.* 1948;127:795.

30. Laufer MR, Goitein BA, Bush M et al. Prevalence of endometriosis in adolescent girls with chronic pelvic pain not responding to conventional therapy. *J Pediatr Adolesc Gynecol.* 1997;10:199–202.

31. Wilson-Harris BM, Nutter B, Falcone T. Long-term fertility after laparoscopy for endometriosis-associated pelvic pain in young adult women. *J Minim Invasive Gynecol.* 2014;21(6):1061–6.

32. Wheeler J. Epidemiology of endometriosis-associated infertility. *J Reprod Med.* 1989;34:41–6.

33. Zannoni L, Giorgi M, Spagnolo E, Montanari G, Villa G, Seracchioli R. Dysmenorrhea, absenteeism from school, and symptoms suspicious for endometriosis in adolescents. *J Pediatr Adolesc Gynecol.* 2014;27(5):258–65.

34. Sampson JA. The development of the implantation theory for the origin of peritoneal endometriosis. *Am J Obstet Gynecol.* 1940;40:549–57.

35. Sanfilippo JS, Wakim NG, Schikler KN et al. Endometriosis in association with uterine anomaly. *Am J Obstet Gynecol.* 1986;154:39–43.

36. Drosdzol-Cop A, Skrzypulec-Plinta V, Stojko R. Serum and peritoneal fluid immunological markers in adolescent girls with chronic pelvic pain. *Obstet Gynecol Surv.* 2012;67(6):374–81.

37. Koninckx PR, Meuleman C, Demeyere S et al. Suggestive evidence that pelvic endometriosis is a progressive disease, whereas deeply infiltrating endometriosis is associated with pelvic pain. *Fertil Steril.* 1991;55:759–65.

38. Brosens I, Benagiano G. Progesterone response in neonatal endometrium is key to future reproductive health in adolescents. *Women's Health.* 2016;12(3):279–82.

39. Brosens I, Gargett CE, Guo SW, Puttemans P, Gordts S, Brosens JJ, Benagiano G. Origins and progression of adolescent endometriosis. *Reprod Sci.* 2016;23(10):1282–8.

40. Rier S, Foster WG. Environmental dioxins and endometriosis. *Semin Reprod Med.* 2003;21:145–54.

41. Matalliotakis M, Goulielmos GN, Matalliotaki C, Trivli A, Matalliotakis I, Arici A. Endometriosis in adolescent and young girls: Report on a series of 55 cases. *J Pediatr Adolesc Gynecol.* 2017;30(5):568–70.

42. Nnoaham KE, Webster P, Kumbang J, Kennedy SH, Zondervan KT. Is early age at menarche a risk factor for endometriosis? A systematic review and meta-analysis of case-control studies. *Fertil Steril.* 2012;98(3):702–12.

43. Kvaskoff M, Bijon A, Clavel-Chapelon F, Mesrine S, Boutron-Ruault MC. Childhood and adolescent exposures and the risk of endometriosis. *Epidemiology.* 2013;24(2):261–9.

44. Upson K, Sathyanarayana S, Scholes D, Holt VL. Early-life factors and endometriosis risk. *Fertil Steril.* 2015;104(4):964–71.

45. Vitonis AF, Baer HJ, Hankinson SE, Laufer MR, Missmer SA. A prospective study of body size during childhood and early adulthood and the incidence of endometriosis. *Hum Reprod.* 2010;25(5):1325–34.

46. Bazot M, Darai E, Hourani R et al. Deep pelvic endometriosis: MR imaging for diagnosis and prediction of extension of disease. *Radiology.* 2004;232:379–89.

47. Marchino GL, Gennarelli G, Enria R et al. Diagnosis of pelvic endometriosis with use of macroscopic versus histologic findings. *Fertil Steril.* 2005;84:12–5.

48. Walter AJ, Hentz JG, Magtibay PM et al. Endometriosis: Correlation between histologic and visual findings at laparoscopy. *Am J Obstet Gynecol.* 2001;184:1407–11.

49. Marsh EE, Laufer MR. Endometriosis in premenarcheal girls who do not have an associated obstructive anomaly. *Fertil Steril.* 2005;83:758–60.

50. Davis GD, Thillet E, Lindemann J. Clinical characteristics of adolescent endometriosis. *J Adolesc Health.* 1993;14:362–8.

51. Stavroulis AI, Saridogan E, Creighton SM et al. Laparoscopic treatment of endometriosis in teenagers. *Eur J Obstet Gynecol Reprod Biol.* 2006;125:248–50.

52. Janssen EB, Rijkers AC, Hoppenbrouwers K, Meuleman C, d'Hooghe TM. Prevalence of endometriosis diagnosed by laparoscopy in adolescents with dysmenorrhea or chronic pelvic pain: A systematic review. *Hum Reprod Update.* 2013;19(5):570–82.

53. Smorgick N, As-Sanie S, Marsh CA, Smith YR, Quint EH. Advanced stage endometriosis in adolescents and young women. *J Pediatr Adolesc Gynecol.* 2014;27(6):320–3.

54. Sarıdoğan E. Adolescent endometriosis. *Eur J Obstet Gynecol Reprod Biol.* 2017;209:46–9.

55. Brown J, Crawford TJ, Allen C, Hopewell S, Prentice A. Nonsteroidal anti-inflammatory drugs for pain in women with endometriosis. *Cochrane Database Syst Rev*. 2017;1:CD004753.

56. Bulun SE, Gurates B, Fang Z et al. Mechanisms of excessive estrogen formation in endometriosis. *J Reprod Immunol*. 2002;55:21–33.

57. Ozawa Y, Murakami T, Terada Y et al. A selective cyclooxygenase-2 inhibitor suppresses the growth of endometriosis xenografts via antiangiogenic activity in severe combined immunodeficiency mice. *Fertil Steril*. 2006;86(Suppl 4):1146–51.

58. Marjoribanks J, Proctor ML, Farquhar C. Nonsteroidal anti-inflammatory drugs for primary dysmenorrhoea. *Cochrane Database Syst Rev* 2003;(4):CD001751.

59. Moore J, Kennedy S, Prentice A. Modern combined oral contraceptives for pain associated with endometriosis. *Cochrane Database Syst Rev* 2007;(3):CD001019.

60. Prentice A, Deary AJ, Bland E. Progestagens and antiprogestagens for pain associated with endometriosis. *Cochrane Database Syst Rev* 2000;(2):CD002122.

61. Köhler G, Faustmann TA, Gerlinger C, Seitz C, Mueck AO. A dose-ranging study to determine the efficacy and safety of 1, 2, and 4 mg of dienogest daily for endometriosis. *Int J Gynecol Obstet*. 2010;108(1):21–5.

62. Momoeda M, Harada T, Terakawa N, Aso T, Fukunaga M, Hagino H, Taketani Y. Long-term use of dienogest for the treatment of endometriosis. *J Obstet Gynaecol Res*. 2009;35(6):1069–76.

63. Petraglia F, Hornung D, Seitz C, Faustmann T, Gerlinger C, Luisi S, Lazzeri L, Strowitzki T. Reduced pelvic pain in women with endometriosis: Efficacy of long-term dienogest treatment. *Arch Gynecol Obstet*. 2012;285(1):167–73.

64. Strowitzki T, Marr J, Gerlinger C, Faustmann T, Seitz C. Dienogest is as effective as leuprolide acetate in treating the painful symptoms of endometriosis: A 24-week, randomized, multicentre, open-label trial. *Hum Reprod*. 2010;25(3):633–41.

65. Ebert AD, Dong L, Merz M et al. Dienogest 2 mg daily in the treatment of adolescents with clinically suspected endometriosis: the VISanne Study to Assess Safety in ADOlescents. *J Pediatr Adolesc Gynecol*. 2017;30(5):560–7.

66. Yoost J, LaJoie AS, Hertweck P, Loveless M. Use of the levonorgestrel intrauterine system in adolescents with endometriosis. *J Pediatr Adolesc Gynecol*. 2013;26(2):120–4.

67. Vercellini P, Aimi G, Panazza S, De Giorgi O, Pesole A, Crosignani PG. A levonorgestrel-releasing intrauterine system for the treatment of dysmenorrhea associated with endometriosis: A pilot study. *Fertil Steril*. 1999;72(3):505–8.

68. Fedele L, Bianchi S, Zanconato G, Portuese A, Raffaelli R. Use of a levonorgestrel-releasing intrauterine device in the treatment of rectovaginal endometriosis. *Fertil Steril*. 2001;75(3):485–8.

69. Imai A, Matsunami K, Takagi H, Ichigo S. Levonorgestrel-releasing intrauterine device used for dysmenorrhea: Five-year literature review. *Clin Exp Obstet Gynecol*. 2014;41(5):495–8.

70. American College of Obstetricians and Gynecologists. Adolescents and long-acting reversible contraception: Implants and intrauterine devices. ACOG Committee Opinion No. 735. *Obstet Gynecol* 2018;131:e130–9.

71. Dlugi AM, Miller JD, Knittle J. Lupron depot (leuprolide acetate for depot suspension) in the treatment of endometriosis: A randomized, placebo-controlled, double-blind study. *Lupron Study Group. Fertil Steril*. 1990;54:419–27.

72. Agarwal, Shaw RW. A risk benefit assessment of drugs used in the treatment of endometriosis. *Drug Saf*. 1994;11:104–13.

73. Matkovic V, Jelic T, Wardlaw G et al. Timing of peak bone mass in Caucasian females and its implication for the prevention of osteoporosis: Inference from a cross-sectional model. *J Clin Invest*. 1994;93:799–808.

74. Dysmenorrhea and Endometriosis in the Adolescent. ACOG Committee Opinion No. 760. American College of Obstetricians and Gynecologists. *Obstet Gynecol*. 2018;132:e249–58.

75. DiVasta AD, Laufer MR. The use of gonadotropin releasing hormone analogues in adolescent and young patients with endometriosis. *Curr Opin Obstet Gynecol*. 2013;25(4):287–92.

76. Lubianca JN, Gordon CM, Laufer MR. "Add-back" therapy for endometriosis in adolescents. *J Reprod Med*. 1998;43:164–72.

77. DiVasta AD, Feldman HA, Gallagher JS, Stokes NA, Laufer MR, Hornstein MD, Gordon CM. Hormonal add-back therapy for females treated with gonadotropin-releasing hormone agonist for endometriosis: A randomized controlled trial. *Obstet Gynecol*. 2015; 126(3):617.

78. Taylor HS, Giudice LC, Lessey BA et al. Treatment of endometriosis-associated pain with elagolix, an oral GnRH antagonist. *N Engl J Med*. 2017;377(1): 28–40.

79. Selak V, Farquhar C, Prentice A et al. Danazol for pelvic pain associated with endometriosis. *Cochrane Database Syst Rev* 2007;(4):CD000068.

80. Sutton CJ, Pooley AS, Ewen SP et al. Follow-up report on a randomized controlled trial of laser laparoscopy in the treatment of pelvic pain associated with minimal to mild endometriosis. *Fertil Steril*. 1997;68:1–74.

81. Jacobson TZ, Duffy JM, Barlow D, Koninckx PR, Garry R. Laparoscopic surgery for pelvic pain associated with endometriosis. *Cochrane Database Syst Rev* 2009;(4):CD001300.

82. Busacca M, Chiaffarino F, Candiani M et al. Determinants of long-term clinically detected

recurrence rates of deep, ovarian, and pelvic endometriosis. *Am J Obstet Gynecol.* 2006;195:426–32.

83. Abbott JA, Hawe J, Clayton RD et al. The effects and effectiveness of laparoscopic excision of endometriosis: a prospective study with 2–5 year follow-up. *Hum Reprod.* 2003;18:1922–7.

84. Stratton P, Winkel CA, Sinaii N et al. Location, color, size, depth, and volume may predict endometriosis in lesions resected at surgery. *Fertil Steril.* 2002;78:743–9.

85. Chopin N, Vieira M, Borghese B et al. Operative management of deeply infiltrating endometriosis: Results on pelvic pain symptoms. *J Minim Invasive Gynecol.* 2005;12(2):106–12.

86. Fedele L, Bianci S, Zanconato G et al. Tailoring radicality in demolitive surgery for deeply infiltrating endometriosis. *Am J Obstet Gynecol.* 2005;193:114–7.

87. Gordts S, Puttemans P, Gordts S, Brosens I. Ovarian endometrioma in the adolescent: A plea for early-stage diagnosis and full surgical treatment. *Gynecol Surg.* 2015;12(1):21–30.

88. Wright KN, Laufer MR. Endometriomas in adolescents. *Fertil Steril.* 2010;94(4):1529–e7.

89. Benagiano G, Bianchi P, Brosens I. Ovarian endometriomas in adolescents often represent active angiogenic disease requiring early diagnosis and careful management. *Minerva Ginecol.* 2017;69(1):100–7.

90. Özyer Ş, Uzunlar Ö, Özcan N, Yeşilyurt H, Karayalçın R, Sargın A, Mollamahmutoğlu L. Endometriomas in adolescents and young women. *J Pediatr Adolesc Gynecol.* 2013;26(3):176–9.

91. Lee SY, Kim ML, Seong SJ, Bae JW, Cho YJ. Recurrence of ovarian endometrioma in adolescents after conservative, laparoscopic cyst enucleation. *J Pediatr Adolesc Gynecol.* 2017;30(2):228–33.

92. Seo JW, Lee DY, Yoon BK, Choi D. The efficacy of postoperative cyclic oral contraceptives after gonadotropin-releasing hormone agonist therapy to prevent endometrioma recurrence in adolescents. *J Pediatr Adolesc Gynecol.* 2017;30(2):223–7.

93. Berker B, Lashay N, Davarpana R et al. Laparoscopic appendectomy in patients with endometriosis. *J Minim Invasive Gynecol.* 2005;12:206–9.

94. Johnson NP, Farquhar CM, Crossley S et al. A double-blind randomised controlled trial of laparoscopic uterine nerve ablation for women with chronic pelvic pain. *BJOG.* 2004;111:950–9.

95. Yap C, Furness S, Farquhar C. Pre and postoperative medical therapy for endometriosis surgery. *Cochrane Database Syst Rev.* 2004;(3):CD003678.

96. Kikuchi I, Takeuchi H, Kitade M et al. Recurrence rate of endometriomas following a laparoscopic cystectomy. *Acta Obstet Gynecol Scand.* 2006;85:1120–24.

97. Tandoi I, Somigliana E, Riparini J et al. High rate of endometriosis recurrence in young women. *J Pediatr Adolesc Gynecol.* 2011;24:376–9.

98. Audebert A, Lecointre L, Afors K et al. Adolescent endometriosis: Report of a series of 55 cases with a focus on clinical presentation and long-term issues. *J Minim Invasive Gynecol.* 2015;22:834–40.

Perioperative care of the pediatric and adolescent gynecology patient

19

GERI D. HEWITT and MARY E. FALLAT

INTRODUCTION

Although there are many similarities to adults, this chapter describes perioperative considerations for infants, children, and adolescents who have a variety of conditions involving the reproductive tract and highlights areas of interest to health-care providers.

PREOPERATIVE DIET GUIDELINES

It is generally recognized that a full stomach can be associated with aspiration syndromes. In children, preoperative food restriction guidelines may vary locally. Table 19.1 provides guidelines for elective anesthesia or sedation that represent safe practice.[1,2] Regular medications for seizures, or cardiac or respiratory conditions, may be given before operation at the usual time with a small sip of water. Gum chewing before general anesthesia increases the amount of gastric residual and results in an increased risk for aspiration on induction.[3] Gum is treated like a clear liquid in some institutions, and the case will be delayed accordingly.

PREOPERATIVE LABORATORY EVALUATION

Regardless of sexual history, postpubertal patients should have a preoperative urine or serum qualitative human chorionic gonadotropin (HCG) evaluation to rule out pregnancy. Depending on the procedure and concern for anemia, patients may require a preoperative complete blood count. Coagulation studies are needed in girls who have a personal or family history of easy bruising or bleeding or a history of heavy menstrual bleeding.[4] Type and crossmatch should be drawn on patients who will have extensive procedures performed, who have large abdominal or pelvic masses, who are already anemic, or who are expected to lose more than 15% of their total blood volume.[5] If there is time (at least a month before operation), and the child is age-appropriate and can assent, depending on the procedure planned, autologous blood can be drawn and made available for the surgery date. Although directed donation is possible, blood from relatives, friends, and paid donors is not known to be safer than that from a blood bank, and associated processing costs may be higher.[6]

Evaluation of electrolytes and renal function is generally unnecessary unless the patient has been on intravenous (IV) fluids preoperatively, has other body fluid losses such as through a nasogastric tube, is undergoing mechanical bowel prep, or is on medications that may affect the values. Girls with an adnexal mass with features concerning for malignancy require serum tumor markers including lactate dehydrogenase (LDH), α-fetoprotein (AFP), quantitative HCG, CA-125, and possibly luteinizing hormone (LH), follicle-stimulating hormone (FSH), estradiol, progesterone, and/or free testosterone depending on the clinical presentation. Tumor markers are beneficial for both preoperative risk assessment of malignancy as well as long-term follow-up if a malignancy is diagnosed.

ANTIMICROBIAL PROPHYLAXIS

It has long been recognized that the risk of surgical site infection (SSI) can be reduced by the prophylactic administration of appropriate antibiotics within 60 minutes before making the first incision in clean contaminated and contaminated cases.[7] The antimicrobial agent should be (1) active against the pathogens most likely to contaminate the surgical site; (2) given in an appropriate dose and at a time that ensures adequate serum and tissue concentrations during the period of potential contamination; (3) safe; and (4) administered for the shortest effective time to minimize adverse effects, development of resistance, and cost (i.e., soon after the procedure and at least within 24 hours).[8] The use of a protocol that includes an automatic stop order for the prophylaxis achieves a reduction in postoperative wound infections and cost.[9]

Agents that are approved by the U.S. Food and Drug Administration (FDA) for use in surgical antimicrobial prophylaxis include cefazolin, cefuroxime, cefoxitin, cefotetan, ertapenem, and vancomycin. Alternatives are provided for patients who have β-lactam allergies. The most common gynecologic procedures that require antibiotic prophylaxis include hysterectomy and suction curettage. The American College of Obstetricians and Gynecologists (ACOG) does not recommend antibiotic prophylaxis for diagnostic laparoscopy or exploratory laparotomy.[10] For gynecologic procedures requiring prophylaxis, the drug of choice is cefazolin at a dose of 25 mg/kg (maximum dose of 2 g). Vancomycin is an alternative agent in patients with a

Table 19.1 Diet restriction guidelines before sedation or anesthesia.

Intake	Age (months)		
	0–5	6–36	>36
Clear liquids	2 hours	2 hours	2 hours
Breast milk	4 hours	6 hours	
Formula	4 hours	6 hours	
Solids/milk	4 hours	6 hours	8 hours

β-lactam allergy. For patients known to be colonized with methicillin-resistant *Staphylococcus aureus*, it is reasonable to add a single preoperative dose of vancomycin to the recommended agent(s). Pediatric patients weighing more than 40 kg should receive weight-based doses unless the dose or daily dose exceeds the recommended adult dose.[11] In obese patients, serum and tissue concentrations of some drugs may differ from those in normal-weight patients because of pharmacokinetic alterations, and these changes may increase the dosing needed to achieve effective levels.

Patients with obstructive anomalies causing hematometra may develop perioperative fever, but there is no evidence that prolonged antimicrobial treatment after surgical correction is helpful in prevention of postoperative infection. Fever could be associated with inadequate drainage. Regardless, if fever occurs, the patient should be evaluated in the routine manner for postoperative fever and treatment with broad-spectrum antibiotics considered until cultures return. Further research in this area is needed, as there is no literature to guide treatment.

Urologic procedures may be part of a major gynecologic procedure or reconstruction (such as division of a urogenital sinus). The two goals of antimicrobial prophylaxis after urologic procedures are prevention of bacteremia and SSIs and postoperative bacteriuria. After urologic procedures, postoperative urinary tract infections are a primary concern for morbidity. *Escherichia coli* is the most commonly isolated organism in patients with postoperative bacteriuria. Clean urologic cases with or without entry into the urinary tract should receive prophylaxis. Basic cystoscopy in the presence of clean urine does not require prophylaxis.[12]

In 2007, the recommendations for prevention of infective endocarditis (IE) were updated by the American Heart Association.[13] The administration of antibiotics solely to prevent endocarditis is not recommended for patients who undergo a genitourinary (GU) or gastrointestinal (GI) procedure. The risk of antibiotic-associated adverse events exceeds the benefit, if any, of the prophylactically administered antibiotics. Although a large number of diagnostic and therapeutic procedures that involve the GU or GI tracts may cause transient enterococcal bacteremia, no published data demonstrate a conclusive link between these procedures and the development of IE, and no studies exist to show that prophylactic administration of antibiotics in high-risk patients during these procedures reduces the incidence of IE. In a patient with an established GU or GI infection who must undergo an operative procedure, it may be reasonable to include in the antibiotic regimen an agent active against enterococci, such as penicillin, ampicillin, piperacillin, or vancomycin, or to delay the procedure if it is not urgent.

RESPIRATORY ILLNESS

A patient with an acute respiratory illness poses a morbidity risk and should have a preanesthetic consultation before surgery, with consideration given to procedure delay, if reasonable.

Table 19.2 Mechanical bowel preparation guidelines.

Age	Volume (mL)
Enema volume by age using normal saline until clear	
Newborn	100
1 year	150
2 years	200
3 years	250
4 years	280
6 years	350
8 years	450
10 years	500
12 years	600
14 years	700
16 years	800

Weight (kg)	Dose (mg)
Erythromycin and neomycin base by mouth at 1 p.m., 2 p.m., 11 p.m. (based on 8 a.m. start time)[a]	
0–7.5	62.5
7.6–15	125
15.1–30	250
>30	500

[a] These medications may be difficult to get from an outpatient pharmacy or cost may be prohibitive, and they might need to be excluded.

MECHANICAL BOWEL PREPARATION

Major procedures involving reconstruction of the vagina or surgery in proximity to the rectum or anus have a high risk of unintentional entry or planned operation on the GI tract, and should include a mechanical bowel prep and oral antibiotics the day before surgery.[14,15] A clear liquid diet is preferred for 24 hours before surgery. For infants, toddlers, or patients at higher risk of dehydration, an inpatient preparation is preferred so that IV fluids can be administered simultaneously. One example of a mechanical prep is polyethylene glycol given at a dose of 20 mL/kg administered orally (PO) or through a nasogastric tube in combination with age-appropriate enemas (Table 19.2). Oral erythromycin base and neomycin are given the day before at 1 p.m., 2 p.m., and 11 p.m. (based on 8 a.m. surgery cut time, or adjusted accordingly). Children and adolescents not at high risk for dehydration may prefer a bowel prep at home. One example includes drinking a 300 mL (10 ounce) bottle of magnesium citrate at noon, followed by 2–4 bisacodyl 5 mg tablets a few hours later (dose adjusted based on patient age/weight). A cleansing enema at the hospital on the morning of surgery will complete the prep.

DEEP VEIN THROMBOSIS PROPHYLAXIS

Risk of surgery-related deep vein thrombosis (DVT) is lower in children compared with adolescents and adults. There are limited data and no consensus guidelines regarding perioperative anticoagulation in children or adolescents.[16] Because sequential compression devices offer potential benefit with minimal exposure to side effect or risk, they should be considered in most prolonged surgical cases in adolescents. Chemical prophylaxis in children and adolescents is limited to a very small group of patients deemed high risk due to personal and/or hereditary factors.[17]

PREOPERATIVE COUNSELING AND DOCUMENTATION

Preoperative counseling begins with the provision of information, in understandable and developmentally appropriate language, of the nature of the condition or process, the proposed diagnostic steps and/or treatment and probability of success, what to expect during and after the tests and treatment, risks and potential benefits, and alternative strategies if they exist. This information must be presented by the physician without apparent coercion or manipulation or bias, and there must be an assessment of the parent/patient's understanding of the information and assessment of the capacity of the parent/patient to make the necessary decision. Counseling should include a discussion of the impact (if any) the proposed procedure may have on future fertility.

In December 2016, the FDA released a Drug Safety Communication raising concerns about the impact that general anesthesia or sedating drugs used for prolonged periods of time or on repeated episodes may have on the developing brain in patients less than 3 years of age. The Society for Pediatric Anesthesia has a statement on their website (https://pedsanesthesia.org) with links to the actual communication as well as a summary of the data surrounding this issue to aid surgeons in clinical decision-making and when counseling families. Surgeons should be prepared to discuss these important issues with families as part of the preoperative risk assessment. In light of these concerns, it is important to remember that regional anesthesia is being used successfully and safely for a wide range of procedures in the pediatric and adolescent population.

A preoperative note should be included in the chart before surgery documenting that the risks, benefits, alternatives, and potential side effects of the planned procedure have been discussed in detail with the parents or guardian of the child and with the age-appropriate patient. Laboratory and other test results specific to the procedure should be included in the documentation. An operative permission form should be signed and on the chart. The need for blood or blood products should be discussed as indicated by the procedure, and most hospitals will have a permission for transfusion form that needs to be signed separately. Operative site marking will be dictated by the procedure and should be done before transferring the patient to the operating room.

INFORMED CONSENT, PARENTAL PERMISSION, AND ASSENT

When a patient is a minor, permission for medical treatment must be obtained from a parent or legal guardian (discussion in this section covers U.S. law only).[18] Technically speaking, only patients who have decisional capacity and legal empowerment can give informed consent to medical care. Parents or other surrogates provide informed permission for their children. Most parents seek to safeguard the best interests of their children with regard to health care, and the "proxy" consent process works fairly well. However, pediatric and adolescent health-care providers have legal and ethical duties to their patients independent of parental desire or proxy consent. Therefore, patients should be included in and participate in decision-making commensurate with their development and provide assent when reasonable. Under some circumstances, a parent will not be custodial or available, and Table 19.3 gives guidance to gaining permission under special conditions. Appropriate documentation must be scanned into the chart.

Table 19.3 Obtaining permission for surgery or treatment for a minor child.

Circumstance	May give permission	Conditions to be met
Court-appointed guardian	Yes	Upon provision of the orders of appointment issued by a court
Committed to a state cabinet of health services	Family services case worker	Must be assigned to the child; if parental rights have not been terminated, parent must give permission
Foster parents	No, if under state supervision	Permission is required from the family services worker assigned to the child
Divorced parents	Conditional	Only custodial parent(s) may give permission
Stepparents	Conditional	Child must be legally adopted
Law enforcement while child is in police custody or under arrest	No	Parent or legal guardian must give permission
Adoptive parents	Yes	Possess full and unrestricted authority to make health-care decisions in the best interests of their minor children
Prospective parents in the process of adoption	Yes	Provided they have the appropriate documentation from the court or state that gives this authority

Given the number of children today who are in single-parent homes, blended households, adopted, in foster care, or emancipated, there are a number of potential challenges to obtaining consent. Two dictums are clear: (1) obtain a good social history as part of the initial encounter, and provide adequate documentation in the chart; and (2) work on any challenges before the procedure is actually scheduled, as obtaining last-minute consents may be awkward and delay the case. The age of majority is determined by an individual state, but in most states, this is 18 years old. The age of majority for children with disabilities may be different. Exceptions to authorization of medical treatment by the parent or legal guardian include (1) emergencies (when the risk to the minor's life or health is of a nature that treatment should not be delayed) and (2) emancipated minor status (is married, has delivered a child, is a parent, is financially self-supporting and living independently, is a member of the armed services, or was declared to be emancipated by a court). A mature minor exception is also recognized by some states for treatment of certain diseases, including sexually transmitted infections (STIs), pregnancy, contraception or childbirth, or alcohol and drug abuse, that allows diagnostic examination and treatment without the permission of or notification of the parent or guardian. State law may provide that the treating physician or health-care official may inform the parent or legal guardian of any treatment given or needed, where, in the judgment of the physician or health-care professional, informing the parent or legal guardian would benefit the health and treatment of the minor patient.

Special circumstances in the permission for surgery process may apply if the parents have religious objections to blood or blood product transfusion. In this case, the best practice is to have a special consent form that has been prepared with input from the religious denomination of record that details the process to be followed in these patients.

If a minor patient refuses to assent (i.e., dissents) to a procedure, this should carry considerable weight if the procedure or intervention is not essential to his or her welfare, the procedure can be deferred without substantial risk, or the patient needs more time to better understand the condition being treated or the intervention proposed or to seek another opinion.

There are many helpful resources available online, including information regarding minor emancipation laws by state (https://www.law.cornell.edu/wex/table_emancipation) and teen reproductive health and associated laws (https://www.guttmacher.org/state-policy/explore/overview-minors-consent-law).

PERIOPERATIVE POSITIONING

The patient's position during surgery should provide optimal exposure for the procedure as well as access to IV lines, tubes, and monitoring devices.[19,20] Attention should be given to the patient's overall safety and comfort, as well as to the circulatory, respiratory, neurologic, and musculoskeletal systems. Patient injury can occur due to the alteration of normal defense mechanisms as well as forced prolonged immobility during the procedure. The surgeon, anesthesiologist, and nursing staff should work as a team. This includes a preoperative assessment to determine the patient's tolerance of the planned position, including age, skin condition, height and weight, nutritional status, preexisting conditions, and physical/mobility limits. Intraoperative factors include type of anesthesia, length of surgery, and position(s) required.

Positioning devices including padding and pressure relief devices should be available, clean, and in working order. Properly functioning equipment and devices contribute to patient safety and provide adequate surgical site exposure. Studies suggest that positioning devices should maintain a normal capillary interface pressure of 32 mm Hg or less. Use of gel pads decreases pressure at any given point by redistributing overall pressure across a larger surface area, while pillows, blankets, and molded foam devices may produce only a minimum of pressure reduction. Table 19.4 lists injury risks and safety considerations for the most common positions used in gynecologic surgery.

Table 19.4 Injury risks and safety considerations for perioperative positioning.

	Position risks	Safety considerations
Supine	Pressure to occiput, scapulae, thoracic vertebrae, olecranon process, sacrum/coccyx, calcanei, knees Brachial plexus, ulnar and pudendal nerve injuries	Pad elbows, knees, spinal column, heels; align occiput with hips; legs parallel and uncrossed Arm boards at <90° angle, head in neutral position, arm and table pads level with each other
Lithotomy	Hip and knee joint injury Lumbar and sacral pressure Vascular congestion Obturator, saphenous, femoral, common peroneal, ulnar neuropathy Restricted diaphragm movement Compartment syndrome	Place stirrups at even height Elevate and lower legs slowly and simultaneously Minimize external rotation of hips Pad lateral/posterior knees and ankles Keep arms away from chest to facilitate respirations Arms on arm boards at <90° angles or over abdomen Minimize time in stirrups Use sequential compression devices and antiembolic hose

Special precautions must be taken when the patient is positioned in lithotomy, where the patient is supine with the legs raised and abducted to expose the perineum. Extreme thigh flexion may increase intraabdominal pressure and impair respiratory function by decreasing tidal volume. With the legs in stirrups, venous return from the lower extremities is enhanced, and blood pools in the splanchnic bed. Blood loss during the procedure may not immediately manifest until the legs are repositioned at the end of the procedure. The legs should be repositioned together (by two persons) and slowly to allow for physiologic adjustment to the extra volume circulating through the lower extremities again. Arms are best extended on arm boards or folded across the torso rather than positioned at the sides, where the hands will be at risk of getting caught in the lower table as it is raised at the end of the procedure.

There are three lithotomy positions described: high, medium, and low. The high lithotomy position is often used in the adult for vaginal hysterectomy or for patients with frozen joints. The low lithotomy position is used for surgical procedures that require excellent exposure of both the abdomen and perineum.

Stirrups are secured in holders on each side of the operating table at the level of the patient's upper thighs. They are adjusted at equal height so that symmetry will be achieved when the legs are raised. Each of two persons raises one leg by grasping the sole of a foot in one hand and supporting the calf at the knee with the other. The knees are flexed and the legs placed inside the posts of the stirrups. The use of loop stirrups is no longer recommended, as they provide inadequate support and may increase the risk of nerve injury. After the patient is positioned in the stirrups, the lower section of mattress is removed, and the bed is lowered. The buttocks must not extend beyond the end of the operating bed. For lengthy procedures, antiembolic stockings or sequential compression devices may be used to minimize the risk of venous stasis and DVT. Other potential risks include pressure sores and nerve damage or compartment syndrome from prolonged immobilization. When using universal stirrups with a boot, keep the toe, knee, and opposite shoulder in a relatively straight line and avoid knee abduction to gain exposure.

UNIVERSAL PROTOCOL

The World Health Organization was the first to recommend a universal protocol that has now been widely adopted by the Joint Commission and hospitals worldwide.[21,22] The optimal protocol involves a checklist composed of three parts: preoperative component, operative component, and sign out after the procedure is completed. The preoperative component includes site marking by the surgeon as appropriate and confirmation of a signed permission/consent for surgery. Anesthesia and nursing participate in patient identification and review of preoperative considerations, risks, need for blood, implants, and any special equipment before the patient is anesthetized. The in-room portion or "time out" should be surgeon initiated and led and includes patient identification, the procedure that will be performed, expected blood loss and anticipated need for transfusion, preoperative antibiotics, special equipment availability/readiness, specimens to be obtained and handling, patient comorbidities and allergies, and expected length of the procedure. The first case of the day will often include introductions of the entire team and their role in the procedure. The postprocedure component includes the procedure that was performed; patient disposition (home, inpatient, or intensive care); estimated blood loss; pain control needs, especially if anesthesia service will be involved; review of specimens and labeling; and any other postoperative considerations for the postoperative anesthesia care unit (PACU) or receiving unit. This portion may also include debriefing of any issues that came up that need to be addressed for future cases. If the patient is to be transported directly to intensive care, a process for a safe handoff should be in place that includes anesthesia, the surgeon, and the receiving physician.

LAPAROSCOPY

While many adolescent patients are adult sized, there are several technical considerations when performing laparoscopy on pediatric patients, including patient positioning, peritoneal access, intraabdominal pressure tolerance, incision sites, and port and instrument sizes. Patient positioning should mirror that of the adult patient, with access to the vagina for uterine manipulation. Uterine manipulation can be accomplished with a digit in the posterior vaginal fourchette or with a small cervical dilator attached to a single-tooth tenaculum secured in the anterior lip of the cervix. Patients that are large enough should be placed in dorsal lithotomy position with their legs in Allen stirrups; if patients are too small, they can be placed supine and frog legged for vaginal access. Tucking the arms (with thumb pointing anterior to avoid median nerve damage) as opposed to placing arms outstretched offers the advantage of more room for the surgeon. A pediatric-sized Foley catheter should be placed to drain the bladder if the patient cannot void just before the procedure or the procedure is likely to take more than 2 hours. For shorter cases, catheter use will be guided by surgeon judgement. Vaginal prep is accomplished with a sponge stick in prep solution, or if needed, a Toomey syringe filled with prep solution can be introduced through the hymenal opening allowing for vaginal irrigation.[23]

Similar to the adult patient, peritoneal access can be achieved by a wide range of methods, including Veress needle, direct trocar entry, direct visual entry using a laparoscopic trocar (there are several on the market), or open entry. Because it is the thinnest portion of the abdominal wall, entry through the midpoint of the umbilicus is generally recommended.[23] There is no evidence in the literature directly comparing complication rates among the various entry methods in pediatric patients, and individual surgeon experience and preference will influence the method chosen. Pediatric patients are proportionately smaller than adults, with a significantly shorter distance between umbilicus and pelvic brim. Care and understanding of these anatomic differences is key in avoiding entry-related injuries to large vessels or the bowel.[24]

Insufflation in the pediatric age group is based on size and age of the patient, body habitus, and abdominal wall compliance. The pediatric abdominal wall is less resistant and more compliant compared to adults, making trocar placement more difficult and increasing the risk for injury to other intraabdominal structures.[25] Recommended maximum intraabdominal pressures are 6–8 mm Hg in infants (0–2 years), 8–10 mm Hg in children (2–10 years), and 10–12 mm Hg in adolescents (>10 years).[25] If an open technique is used to place the camera port, transient increases up to 15 mm Hg to facilitate port placement are well tolerated but then can be decreased to a lower pressure in most patients.[23] Insufflation rates should start out at low flow to avoid a vagal response and then increase only as much as needed to overcome loss from leak or suction. Average flow rates to start are as follows: infants 1 L/min, all others 1–2 L/min. Most cases should not require a maximum of more than 5 L/min.

Placing lateral, accessory ports should be done under direct visualization. Because of smaller size and anatomic variation in pediatric patients, consideration for placing the ports relatively higher on the abdominal wall than what would be typical in adult patients allows for a more ergonomic approach to the pelvis and decreases the likelihood of injuring the bladder.[23] A surgeon should use the smallest ports necessary to complete the intended procedure. Unless extracting a large specimen that cannot be decompressed, most cases can be accomplished with 3 or 5 mm instruments. There are currently 2, 3, 5, and 10 mm ports available. The 3 or 5 mm ports are usually adequate and have a full range of instruments available, whereas 2 mm ports may not have all of the desired instruments. There are many obese adolescent patients in the United States, and extra-long trocars are commercially available. The 10 mm specimen entrapment sacs including the cannula require 10 mm ports, but there are also 5 mm specimen bags, and the 10 mm bag can be placed through a 5 mm incision by inserting just the bag and not the cannula it is loaded in. While optics vary, there is no loss of optical quality with the use of a 5 mm rather than 10 mm lens or telescope.[25]

POSTOPERATIVE NOTE

Immediately following the procedure, a postoperative note should be written in the chart to include the preoperative and postoperative diagnoses, operation performed, surgeon, any assistants, findings at surgery, estimated blood loss, drains, specimens, and complications. Any pictures taken during the procedure should be stored in the institution's digital warehouse or transferred electronically to the patient's chart.

POSTOPERATIVE MANAGEMENT

Evidence suggests that less than half of all patients who undergo surgery have adequate postoperative pain relief.

The American Pain Society has developed a multidisciplinary statement outlining best practices on the management of postoperative pain in both children and adults.[26] These guidelines focus on preoperative education, appropriate pain assessment tools, and the use of multimodal analgesia. When opioids are required, they should be administered orally if possible. If IV administration is necessary, patient-controlled analgesia (PCA) is preferred, and intramuscular narcotics should be avoided. Morphine sulfate, fentanyl, and hydromorphone are the drugs most amenable to PCA administration in children. The child must be age-appropriate in terms of ability to understand how to self-administer the medication, as parents are generally not allowed to participate in PCA administration. Acetaminophen and/or nonsteroidal anti-inflammatory drugs should be included as part of the multimodal regimen unless contraindicated. Additional recommendations include preincision surgical site–specific local anesthetic infiltration and peripheral regional anesthetic techniques.[26] Surgeons should work collaboratively with acute pain teams and/or anesthesiologists to minimize postoperative pain.[2]

IV fluid administration should be continued postoperatively at a maintenance rate in patients who will be admitted and have limited oral intake. An order can be written to saline lock the IV once the patient is tolerating oral liquids well. It has been recognized that postsurgical patients are at high risk of developing hyponatremia due to the presence of nonosmotic stimuli for antidiuretic hormone release. Administration of hypotonic maintenance fluids is associated with increased rates of hyponatremia, and the best available data demonstrate that administration of isotonic fluid reduces hyponatremia risk.[27] A patient with external losses such as through a nasogastric tube will need added potassium chloride. Volume deficits should be replaced with isotonic fluids before the initiation of maintenance fluids; fluids of an appropriate composition should be used to replace ongoing losses at a rate commensurate with the volume lost. For patients needing prolonged IV fluids, accurate daily weights should be obtained, blood pressures monitored, and fluid balance evaluated frequently throughout the day to allow for adjustments. If the child will need IV fluids for several days and will be on strict intake and output, IV fluid rate may be titrated to keep urine output greater than or equal to 1 mL/kg/h average up to a maximum of ≥30 mL/hr, which is the minimum urine output expected in an adult. Consideration should be given for supplemental peripheral or central total parenteral nutrition if the patient will be without oral intake (NPO) for several days or has a history of significant weight loss or poor nutritional status before surgery. Postoperatively, the safest way to resume oral intake after anesthesia is to initiate clear fluids and advance as tolerated. Patients who have had major intraabdominal procedures can probably safely start sips of clear liquids and/or ice chips soon after surgery. Patients tend to limit their intake to what is appealing to them. Those who have been NPO for several days should have diet advanced over a period of days and only as tolerated. If a patient required nasogastric suction, noncarbonated liquids are recommended.

Activity following a procedure will be dictated by the procedure and its extent as well as the extent of the incision required. In general, most closed surgical wounds will be sealed within 48 hours, allowing bathing and showering to resume. Laparoscopic procedures require a limited period of reduced activities to allow fascial healing of umbilical and larger access incisions, or approximately 2–3 weeks. In infants and thin patients, consideration should be given to closing the anterior fascia of even a small port site, as there is a higher rate of hernias. Major laparotomies require restriction from organized sports and physical education for approximately 4–6 weeks. School-age children who need to refrain from carrying heavy backpacks but are otherwise ready to resume attending school may request a second set of books for temporary use at home. "Quiet activities" or "limiting rough play" can be advised in toddlers and small children, but up to school age, it is doubtful that parents will have complete control over their children's behavior once they are feeling better, and a surgeon must have realistic expectations.

POSTOPERATIVE COMPLICATIONS

The most frequent postoperative complications in children and adolescents are similar to those seen in adults and include complications related to the respiratory tract, urinary tract, and wound. Patients should be encouraged to participate in their own care as soon as possible, including after major operations. Enhanced Recovery After Surgery (ERAS) protocols are being embraced in many disciplines.[28] These are multimodal perioperative care pathways designed to achieve early recovery after surgical procedures. The key elements of ERAS protocols include preoperative counseling, optimization of nutrition, standardized analgesic and anesthetic regimens, and early mobilization.

Coughing, deep breathing, incentive spirometry, and early mobilization are all maneuvers to aid with minimizing postoperative atelectasis. Early mobilization decreases the incidence of postoperative ileus. Constipation due to narcotics can be minimized with both early mobilization and a postoperative bowel regimen that might include stool softeners, laxatives, and/or package enemas depending on a patient's normal regularity. Foley catheters should be removed as soon as possible to minimize the risk of an acquired urinary tract infection. Wound infections occur with increasing incidence after clean contaminated, contaminated, and dirty procedures. The use of antimicrobial prophylaxis can minimize the risk but not completely prevent it. Postoperative DVT is unusual but can occur in adolescents who require prolonged bedrest. This risk can be minimized by using sequential compression devices, or with the use of temporary anticoagulation, if indicated.

DISCHARGE INSTRUCTIONS

Discharge instructions should include wound care and return to other than normal functions of daily living, which are generally permitted even after a major procedure. Instructions should include hygiene such as bathing and showering and return to school, sports, work, physical education, driving, and sexual intercourse (if age appropriate and sexually active). There is little evidence-based guidance regarding return to physical and sexual activities, and much of this is driven by conventional wisdom, practice patterns, and what is known about normal wound healing. Generally speaking, return to school and driving are permitted when the patient no longer needs narcotic pain medicine. Return to work and more exertional physical activities will be dependent on the type of procedure, incision(s), and underlying frailty of the patient, depending on the patient's age, weight, and preexisting comorbidities.

REFERENCES

1. Mesbah A, Thomas M. Preoperative fasting in children. *BJA Education*. 2017;17:346–50.
2. Cohen IT, Deutsch N, Motoyama EK. Induction, maintenance, and recovery. In: Davis PJ, Cladis FP, Motoyama EK, eds. *Smith's Anesthesia for Infants and Children*. 8th ed. Philadelphia, PA: Elsevier; 2011:365–94. https://doi.org/10.1016/B978-0-323-06612-9.00013-4
3. Schoenfelder RC, Ponnamma CM, Freyle D et al. Residual gastric fluid volume and chewing gum before surgery. *Anesth Analg*. 2006;102:415–17.
4. Seravalli V, Linari S, Peruzzi E et al. Prevalence of hemostatic disorders in adolescents with abnormal uterine bleeding. *J Ped Adol Gyn*. 2013;26:285–9.
5. Bharadwai A, Khandelwal M, Bhargava SK. Perioperative neonatal and paediatric blood transfusion. *Indian J Anaesth*. 2014;58:652–7.
6. Bekker L-G, Wood R. Blood safety – At what cost? *Lancet*. 2006;295:557–8.
7. Antimicrobial prophylaxis for surgery. *Treat Guide Med Lett* 2006;4:83–8.
8. Bratzler DW, Dellinger EP, Olsen KM et al. Clinical practice guidelines for antimicrobial prophylaxis in surgery. *Am J Health-Syst Pharm*. 2013;70:195–283.
9. Gomez MI, Acosta-Gnass SI, Mosqueda-Barboza L et al. Reduction in surgical antibiotic prophylaxis expenditure and the rate of surgical site infection by means of a protocol that controls the use of prophylaxis. *Infect Control Hosp Epidemiol*. 2006;27:1358–65.
10. Prevention of Infection After Gynecologic Procedures. ACOG Practice Bulletin No. 195. American College of Obstetricians and Gynecologists. *Obstet Gynecol*. 2018;131:e172–89.
11. Bratzler DW, Dellinger EP, Olsen KM et al. Clinical practice guidelines for antimicrobial prophylaxis in surgery. *Surg Infect*. 2013;14:73–156.

12. Garcia-Perdomo HA, Jimenez-Mejias E, Lopez-Ramos H. Efficacy of antibiotic prophylaxis in cystoscopy to prevent urinary tract infection: A systematic review and meta-analysis. *Int Braz J Urol.* 2015;41:412–24.

13. Wilson WW, Taubert KA, Gewitz M et al. Prevention of infective endocarditis: Guidelines from the American Heart Association. *Circulation.* 2007;116:1736–54.

14. Klinger AL, Green H, Monlezun DJ et al. The role of bowel preparation in colorectal surgery: Results of the 2012–2015 ACS-NSQIP data. *Ann Surg.* 2019;269(4):671–7.

15. Ohman KA, Wan L, Guthrie T et al. Combination of oral antibiotics and mechanical bowel preparation reduces surgical site infection in colorectal surgery. *J Am Coll Surg.* 2017;225:465–71.

16. Humes DJ, Nordenskjold A, Walker A et al. Risk of venous thromboembolism in children after general surgery. *J Ped Surg.* 2015;50:1870–3.

17. Casey J, Yunker A, Anderson T. Gynecologic surgery in the pediatric and adolescent populations: Review of perioperative and operative considerations. *J Minim Invasive Gynecol.* 2016;23:1033–9.

18. Katz AL, Webb SA, AAP Committee on Bioethics. Informed consent in decision-making in pediatric practice. *Pediatrics.* 2016;138(2):e20161485.

19. Patient Care. Recommended practices for positioning the patient in the perioperative practice setting. 2009 Perioperative Standards and Recommended Practices. AORN, Inc. 2009;525–48.

20. Fleisch MC, Bremerich D, Schulte-Mattler W et al. The prevention of positioning injuries during gynecologic operations. Guideline of DGGG (S1-Level, AWMF Registry No. 015/077), Geburtshilfe Frauenheilkd 2015; 75: 792–807.

21. Haynes AB, Weiser TG, Berry WR et al. A surgical safety checklist to reduce morbidity and mortality in a global population for the safe surgery saves lives study group. *N Engl J Med.* 2009;360:491–9.

22. The Joint Commission. https://www.jointcommission .org/assets/1/18/UP_Poster1.PDF. Accessed May 23, 2019.

23. Broach A, Mansuria S, Sanfilippo J. Pediatric and adolescent gynecologic laparoscopy. *Clin Obstet Gynecol.* 2009;52(3):380–9.

24. Biscette S, Yoost J, Hertweck P, Reinstine J. Laparoscopy in pregnancy and the pediatric patient. *Obstet Gynecol Clin N Am.* 2011;28:757–76.

25. Tomaszewski J, Casella D, Turner R, Casal P, Ost M. Pediatric laparoscopic and robot-assisted laparoscopic surgery: Technical considerations. *J Endourol.* 2012;26(6):602–13.

26. Chou R, Gordon D, de Leon-Casasola OA et al. Management of postoperative pain: A clinical practice guideline from the American Pain Society, the American Society of Regional Anesthesia and Pain Medicine, and the American Society of Anesthesiologists' Committee on Regional Anesthesia, Executive Committee, and Administrative Council. *J Pain.* 2016;17:131–57.

27. Oh GJ, Sutherland SM. Perioperative fluid management and postoperative hyponatremia in children. *Pediatr Nephrol.* 2016;31:53–60.

28. Ljungqvist O, Scott M, Fearon KC. Enhanced recovery after surgery: A review. *JAMA Surg.* 2017;152(3):292–8.

Adolescent pregnancy

20

SHIRLEY M. DONG, EMILY K. REDMAN, TIA M. MELTON, and JOSEPH S. SANFILIPPO

INTRODUCTION

The Centers for Disease Control and Prevention has focused on teen pregnancy prevention as one of its top six priorities.[12,13] While pregnancy rates have declined, it remains a problem in North America. There is considerable disparity among ethnic and racial groups with respect to teen pregnancy and birth rates.[2] Adolescent pregnancy continues to be a "significant public health concern" occurring in 13% of the population in the United States and approximately 25% of women worldwide.[3]

Adolescent mothers are at high risk for repeat pregnancies in 1–2 years following their initial conception.[3] According to the World Health Organization (WHO), approximately 16 million girls aged 15–19 years and 2.5 million girls under 16 years give birth each year in developing countries.[4] Adolescent pregnancies remain a global problem that does not have any clear-cut distinction among high-, middle-, and low-income countries. In fact, the teen pregnancy rate in the United States, in comparison to other industrialized nations, is significantly higher.[1] It is clear that for some adolescents, these pregnancies are planned. In developing countries, many girls face social pressure to marry young and bear children. Worldwide each year, approximately 15 million girls are married before the age of 18 years, and 90% of births to girls age 15–19 years occur within marriage.[5]

In the United States, "every minute of every day," one to two adolescents become pregnant. Of these pregnancies, 30%–35% are terminated, 15% end in spontaneous abortion (miscarriage, ectopic, or molar pregnancy) and the remaining result in live births.[6,7] There are limited data regarding the adoption rates resulting from adolescent pregnancies. Overall, the prevalence of adoptions in never-married women under the age of 45 years has declined over the past several decades, with rates lower than 1% in the mid-1990s.[8] When adoptions are arranged, it is estimated that approximately half of these infants are adopted by relatives or someone known to the birth mother.[8]

Teen pregnancy rates vary by age, race, and social-economic status. The overall teen birth rate in the U.S. population of adolescent girls age 10–14 reached a record low with a rate of 0.2 births per 1000 females in 2016 (Figure 20.1).[9-11] There is also large variance in rates of adolescent pregnancies between different states, with a range of rates between 8.2 per 1000 in Massachusetts to 32.8 in Arkansas.

Adolescents also have a high rate of rapid repeat pregnancies, with 25% becoming pregnant within 1 year of delivery and 35% within 2 years of delivery.[9] African American teens ages 15–19 years have experienced the steepest decline in birth rates.[10] Despite this trend, the overall birth rates for African American and Latina adolescents continues to be the highest among all ethnic groups (Figure 20.1).[10]

The U.S. adolescent birth rate overall decreased from 61.8/1000 in 1991 to 41.4/1000 in 2004. In 2017, the

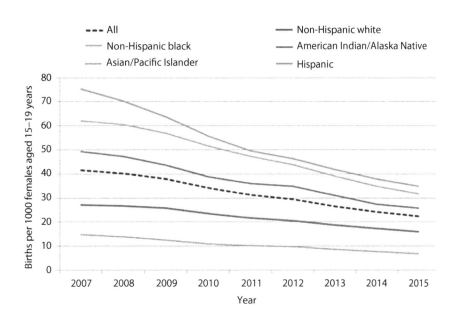

Figure 20.1 Births per 1000 females aged 15–19 years by race and Hispanic ethnicity, 2007–2015. (Adapted from Martin JA et al. *Natl Vital Stat Rep.* 2017;66[1]:1–70.)

Year and race and Hispanic origin	Total fertility rate	Age of mother (years)									
		10–14	15–19			20–24	25–29	30–34	35–39	40–44	45–49[1]
			Total	15–17	18–19						
All races and origins[2]											
2017	1765.5	0.2	18.8	7.9	35.1	71.0	98.0	100.3	52.3	11.6	0.9
2016	1820.5	0.2	20.3	8.8	37.5	73.8	102.1	102.7	52.7	11.4	0.9
2015	1843.5	0.2	22.3	9.9	40.7	76.8	104.3	101.5	51.8	11.0	0.8
2014	1862.5	0.3	24.2	10.9	43.8	79.0	105.8	100.8	51.0	10.6	0.8
2013	1857.5	0.3	26.5	12.3	47.1	80.7	105.5	98.0	49.3	10.4	0.8
2012	1880.5	0.4	29.4	14.1	51.4	83.1	106.5	97.3	48.3	10.4	0.7
2011	1894.5	0.4	31.3	15.4	54.1	85.3	107.2	96.5	47.2	10.3	0.7
2010	1931.0	0.4	34.2	17.3	58.2	90.0	108.3	96.5	45.9	10.2	0.7

Figure 20.2 Pregnancy and fertility rates, 2010–2017. [1] Birth rates computed by relating births to women aged 45 and over to women aged 45–49. [2] Includes births to race and origin groups not shown separately, such as Hispanic single-race white, Hispanic single-race black, and non-Hispanic multiple-race women, and births with origin not stated. (Adapted from Hamilton BE et al. *NVSS Vital Stat Rapid Release*. 2018;67[8]:1–23.)

adolescent birth rate in females age 15–19 years continued to decrease to 18.8/1000 (Figure 20.2). While the decrease in the adolescent birth rate is promising, the rate in the United States continues to be higher than other developed countries, including the United Kingdom and Canada.[11] The trend is a reflection of better education at all levels, access to contraception, and more recently, utilization of long-acting reversible contraception (LARC), including intrauterine devices and implants.[2,10] To date, a number of predictors for teen pregnancy exist. These include early pubertal development, sexual abuse history, poverty, lack of attentive and nurturing parents, and cultural and family patterns that include substance abuse, poor school performance, and dropping out of school (Table 20.1).[7,14,15]

While discussions on teen pregnancy tend to focus on girls, engaging boys in reproductive health is a major aim of the Centers for Disease Control and Prevention (CDC), as teen fatherhood occurs at a rate of 10.4 births per 1000 boys aged 15–19 years. Statistics indicate teen fathers are less likely to graduate from high school. Furthermore, young men's involvement in contraception has been shown to increase its use and also decrease rates of sexually transmitted infections (STIs).[1] In general, family planning services are not as often utilized for males as they are for females. Studies have shown that adolescent males often resort to the media or their peers for advice regarding sexual activity and contraception. Adolescent males may also be embarrassed to ask a medical professional about proper condom usage, which may result in improper use.[12] It should be emphasized to both adolescent males and females that, while using an oral form of contraception or LARC may prevent pregnancy, dual usage of a barrier form of contraception such as a condom is imperative in order to prevent transmission of STIs. It has been found that increased free access to condoms

Table 20.1 Risk factors for teen pregnancy.

Early puberty	Cultural or family patterns
History of sexual abuse	Personal or familial substance abuse
Poverty	Lack of parental involvement
Black or Hispanic	Poor school performance

Table 20.2 Key considerations in programming for men as family planning users.

- Provide information and services to men and boys where and when they need it
- Address gender norms that affect men's use of contraceptive methods
- Improve couple and community communication
- Meet men's needs while respecting women's autonomy
- Link men's family planning use with their desire to support their families
- Teach adolescent boys about pregnancy prevention and healthy sexual relationships
- Develop national policies and guidelines that include men as family planning users
- Scale up programs for men
- Fill the gaps through monitoring, evaluation, and implementation science
- Create more contraceptive options for men

Source: Reprinted from Hardee K et al. *Reprod Health.* 2017;14(1): 14–17, under Creative Commons license.

does increase usage, while interaction with a third party, such as a sales clerk, deters adolescents from buying condoms.[13] Thus, adolescent pregnancy remains a challenge for all clinicians to appropriately counsel for both males and females (Table 20.2).

DIAGNOSIS

The diagnosis of adolescent pregnancy is no different from diagnosis of pregnancy in adults. A higher index of suspicion is sometimes necessary in the younger adolescent with an immature hypothalamic-pituitary-ovarian axis. Irregular menstrual cycles are common in adolescents and may lead to a delay in diagnosis. In 2008, the CDC reported that 25% of teens in the United States had an STI. Undiagnosed STIs may have long-term repercussions such as pelvic inflammatory disease (PID) associated with fallopian tube damage leading to infertility, ectopic pregnancy, and chronic pelvic pain. Therefore, the possibility of ectopic pregnancy must be considered in the pregnant adolescent. While adolescents have been found to lower rates of ectopic pregnancies, risk factors that adolescents

Table 20.3 Physical exam findings in pregnancy.

Chadwick sign	Bluish discoloration of the cervix, vagina, and labia as a result of increased blood flow; evident approximately 6–8 weeks following conception
Hegar sign	Softening of the uterus upon bimanual physical exam; evident approximately 4–6 weeks following conception
Goodell sign	Softening of the vaginal portion of the cervix due to increased blood flow; evident approximately 4 weeks following conception

may have for ectopic pregnancy include history of sexually transmitted diseases and PID and smoking.[14]

The classic signs of an enlarging uterus coupled with the usual symptoms (nausea, breast tenderness, change in diet, change in weight, etc.) may be presenting signs of a pregnancy. Historically, several physical exam findings described in Table 20.3 may also suggest pregnancy but are not always specific. It is paramount to perform a pregnancy test in teenagers in the right clinical scenario, even when the teen may deny sexual activity. Having a good relationship with adolescent patients creates a more trusting patient–physician relationship, and adolescents may therefore be more forthcoming regarding their social and sexual history.

RATES OF CONTRACEPTIVE USE

The National Youth Risk Behavior Survey from 2017 found that 13.8% of U.S. high school students did not use any form of contraception during their last sexual intercourse.[15] There are varying estimates regarding the use of contraception, with estimates ranging from 23% to 33% of adolescent females using some form of oral contraception. Overall, the most common form of contraception utilized by both males and females is condoms.[16] More effective forms of contraception are less commonly chosen, with an estimated 2% of sexually active adolescent females utilizing LARCs.[17] A comprehensive review of contraception in adolescents is found in Chapter 16.

CASE PRESENTATIONS

Case 1: Shauna is a 15-year-old African American female. She presents to the emergency department with nausea and worsening pelvic pain. Physical exam reveals diffuse lower abdominal tenderness and significant cervical tenderness. Wet mount demonstrates an abundance of white blood cells. She reports one lifetime male sexual partner for the past 6 months; last sexual intercourse was a few days ago and was consensual. She was brought to the hospital by a friend because her single mother works multiple jobs and is rarely home, and the patient has not told her that she is sexually active.

When asked about contraception, Shauna reports she has been prescribed oral contraceptive pills to regulate her heavy periods but forgets to take them frequently. She and her partner do not use condoms, because he does not like how they make intercourse feel, and she is afraid her mother might find them. She has never considered LARC methods, because she is uncomfortable with "a device being placed inside my body," and friends have voiced concerns over possible side effects like pain, irregular bleeding, and infertility. The pregnancy test is negative, but she tests positive for *Chlamydia trachomatis* and is diagnosed with PID. She is treated with antibiotics.

Case 1 highlights several risk factors for adolescent pregnancy, including race, being raised in a single-parent household, and low socioeconomic status. Research suggests that having a two-parent family decreases the risk of adolescent pregnancy. Compared with two-parent families, children of single-parent families have greater reported difficulties (i.e., poverty, greater high school dropout rates, etc.).[18]

Furthermore, it also displays some misconception barriers teens face regarding use of contraception, and it highlights possible complications of STI transmission. These misconceptions showcase the importance of obtaining an accurate and thorough sexual and gynecologic history from adolescent females. Appropriate education about different forms of contraception may also allow patients to voice their concerns about methods such as intrauterine devices or implants.

Case 2: Megan is a 17-year-old non-Hispanic white female. She presents with her mother to her pediatrician's office with reported positive home pregnancy test. She has a history of polycystic ovarian syndrome (PCOS) and has never had regular periods. She is obese and has a significant family history of diabetes and hypertension. She had not disclosed to her doctor or her mother that she is sexually active. Given her irregular periods, she has never considered being on birth control, as she did not believe that she could become pregnant.

Of note, Megan also carries a diagnosis of post-traumatic stress disorder (PTSD) due to a history of sexual abuse that occurred when she was raped by her stepfather at 10 years old. A detailed history reveals that while her partner is overall supportive, he sometimes forces her to have sexual intercourse when she does not want to. Pregnancy is confirmed in the office. She is upset by the news and repeatedly blames herself for this unplanned pregnancy.

Case 2 provides an example of sexual abuse in adolescents. The majority of first intercourse experiences prior to age 15 are nonvoluntary.[19] Younger teens are vulnerable to coercive and nonconsensual sex. Involuntary sexual activity is reported by 74% of adolescents aged less than 14 years and 60% of adolescents less than 15 years.[16] In the United States and in countries around the world, teens who are in abusive relationships are believed to be at greater risk of pregnancy secondary to emotional damage, birth control sabotage, self-medication with alcohol or drugs, and increased sexual contact. Victims of abuse are at increased risk of being involved with violent or coercive partners. Their use of drugs or alcohol to blunt emotions may expose them to unprotected sexual activity.[20] In the developing world, forced prostitution is another form of violence that places adolescents at great risk. Sex workers are exposed to STIs and pregnancy and often have limited access to reproductive health care.[21] There are limited data available about the effect of emotional abuse and neglect on adolescent pregnancy rates.[22] A direct cause and effect between abuse and teenage pregnancy is still being debated and explored. However, many studies suggest a link. Fear of infertility or a desire to be loved and give love is sometimes the motivation for adolescents who plan a pregnancy. The prevalence of sexual abuse and coercion in modern society therefore highlights a gap in education for our adolescents.

ABORTION

While the rate of adolescent pregnancies has decreased over the past several decades, the United States continues to have the highest rate of adolescent pregnancies (57 pregnancies per 1000 adolescents in 2010) when compared to other developed and industrialized countries.[23] It is estimated that 80% of these adolescent pregnancies are unplanned, and one-third of these pregnancies will end in abortion.[24] Worldwide, out of 21 countries with liberal abortion laws, countries were found to have varying adolescent abortion rates, with a range from 11 to 44 abortions per 1000 females age 15–19 years old.[23] Countries with higher adolescent birth rates had lower adolescent abortion rates. While adolescents in the United States account for approximately 10% of all abortions conducted in the United States, the number has decreased in the past several decades. From 2005 to 2014, the percentage of abortions accounted for by adolescents decreased 38%.[25] This trend may account for better forms of birth control that may be available, most importantly including LARCs.

However, recent legislation has also increased the number of abortion restrictions that may hinder adolescents from seeking care. Between 2008 and 2011, 24 states enacted a total of 106 abortion restrictions.[26] Worldwide, it is estimated that 4.5 million adolescents have abortions yearly. Approximately 40% of these abortions may be unsafe, with the most occurring in Africa.[27] While the term is broad, an unsafe abortion is any abortion that is performed by someone who lacks the skills to perform the procedure with safe techniques in sanitary conditions. While these unsafe procedures may be catastrophic and lead to death, they may also cause cervical tearing, perforation of the uterus or bowel, sepsis, chronic pelvic disease, and infertility.[27]

Providing adolescents with adequate care when patients seek abortions requires a multidisciplinary approach. These patients may present in a variety of settings, including the primary care setting at their pediatrician's office, the emergency department, or an independent women's health clinic, such as Planned Parenthood. A study has shown that these providers may often be unprepared to discuss management of a pregnancy with adolescents.[28] It is also possible that adolescents may present to a variety of different providers depending on their medical care, including personnel such as pediatricians, school nurses, or family planning providers, such as Planned Parenthood.

Counseling adolescents regarding pregnancy management

Providers should therefore be prepared to discuss options such as medical abortion, surgical abortion, and alternatives such as adoption. On a broader scope, physicians and other health-care providers play a vital role in adolescent sexual health and should be comfortable regularly providing comprehensive sexual and reproductive health counseling to all adolescents, including contraceptive and pregnancy options. It is also important to properly identify any biases a provider may have regarding abortions in order to provide future counseling in an impartial manner.

The availability of additional support staff including social workers and mental health specialists is also important. This is particularly true given the risk factors for adolescent pregnancy, which were previously discussed, that may include poverty, history of sexual or substance abuse, and lack of proper education.

Counseling patients should include the fact that abortions are not associated with decreased future fertility. If patients are interested in surgical abortions, it is notable that 87% of counties in the United States do not have an abortion provider. Other aspects of care that may vary on a state-by-state basis also include whether the state offers open abortion, the locations and gestational age limits of abortions, and parental notification laws. Organizations such as the National Abortion Federation Hotline may assist in providing adolescents with travel arrangements as well as estimates of the cost of abortions.[29]

OBSTETRIC COMPLICATIONS ASSOCIATED WITH ADOLESCENT PREGNANCIES
Preterm birth and low birth weight

By definition, preterm birth involves delivery before 37 weeks' gestation, and a low birth weight infant is one weighing less than 2500 g at birth. Studies have found that adolescent pregnancies have a higher incidence of preterm birth and low birth weight. Theories regarding this trend may be related to teenage biology (such as the immaturity of adolescent organ systems) and higher incidences of smoking in adolescents versus adults, as smoking is a known risk factor for preterm birth.[30] Other risk factors for preterm birth in the general female population include low maternal body mass index (BMI), low maternal socioeconomic status, and black maternal race. Other obstetric risk factors include prior history of preterm birth and short cervical length.[31]

An additional contributing factor may be a lack of appropriate prenatal care in adolescents, including delayed interventions or limited education regarding standard of care. Other adolescents may have no form of health insurance prior to pregnancy and may therefore have financial constraints when initially considering prenatal care. Studies have found that adolescents have lower rates of taking folic acid compliantly during their pregnancy as well as lower hemoglobin levels during their third trimester.[32] These factors may be due to poor diet and nutritional deficiencies, both of which may be attributed to concerns for bodily appearance, low socioeconomic status, or lack of access to a balanced diet.

Hypertensive disorders

Preeclampsia and eclampsia are prevalent in pregnancy, with the WHO estimating that approximately 5% of pregnancies are complicated by some form of hypertensive disorder worldwide.[33] Risk factors for development of these disorders include chronic hypertension, multiple pregnancy, gestational diabetes, obesity, and family history of preeclampsia or eclampsia. Further studies have estimated that adolescents are at a two- to sixfold increased risk for developing some sort of hypertensive disorder during their pregnancy.[34] Preeclampsia is defined by a patient's blood pressure of at least 140 mm Hg systolic or 90 mm Hg diastolic blood pressure. When considering any possible link between adolescent pregnancy and hypertensive disorders, a majority of adolescents are nulliparous. Nulliparity has been linked to increased rates of hypertensive disorders and preterm delivery in pregnancy. Current data suggest that nulliparity rather than age is the primary etiology of the higher rate of preeclampsia and hypertensive disorders seen in adolescent pregnancy.[35] Studies have also shown that adolescent patients may present with eclampsia with seizures and other end-organ failure without the formal diagnosis of preeclampsia.[34]

Racial disparities

Studies have found conflicting data regarding the effects of race on obstetric outcomes. Notably, a study conducted found that non-white adolescents (including African American, Asian, and Latina adolescents) had lower odds of severe obstetric complications such as cesarean delivery, gestational diabetes, and Apgar scores less than 7.[36] These trends may be related to gynecologic maturity. Caucasian females may experience menarche and puberty at later ages than other races and therefore may have less physically matured bodies. These physiologic differences may provide non-Caucasian adolescents a foundation to have fewer obstetric complications due to earlier menarche.

In contrast, racial and ethnic obstetric disparities are present with respect to several complications in the adult population. Studies have found that severe postpartum hemorrhage and peripartum infection are least common in non-Hispanic white women; these results also adjusted for parity, age, and BMI.[37] The difference in the odds of obstetric complications in adolescents versus adults in these studies highlights how racial and ethnic disparities in health care may change throughout a woman's life span. Investigation regarding differences in the care of adolescents versus adults may therefore be warranted in the future.

Delivery trends

Studies have found that adolescents have lower rates of cesarean delivery when compared to adults.[30] This trend may be related to the lower incidence of macrosomic neonates and gestational diabetes in adolescent pregnancies. Others have hypothesized that the connective tissue elasticity may be greater in younger women, also favoring higher rates of vaginal deliveries.[38] Studies have also shown that adolescents statistically undergo higher rates of vaginal birth after cesarean (VBAC) attempts but may have similar VBAC success rates when compared to all women of all ages.[39] The same study also found that VBAC success was associated with delivering at an academic or teaching facility, highlighting a disparity in obstetric care; given the success rate, VBACs should be attempted whenever possible in order to reduce the number of repeat cesarean sections and their associated complications.

PSYCHOSOCIAL OUTCOMES

Great debate continues about the psychological and social outcomes of teenage pregnancy. Increased rates of developmental delay, academic difficulty, substance abuse, depression, and early sexual activity have all been reported in the children of adolescents.[16] Furthermore, children of adolescent pregnancies have been shown to have decreased scores in language and communication skills, decreased emotional and physical well-being, and diminished approaches to learning. Once socioeconomic status and background characteristics have been eliminated, many of these adverse outcomes are decreased.[40,41] Children of adolescent pregnancies are themselves more likely to become teenage mothers and fathers.[42] Siblings of adolescent mothers are also at increased risk of teenage pregnancy.

Studies have also found that adolescent mothers hold a high amount of reliance on public assistance for financial support.[43] Reliance on public assistance has been found to vary by race as well, with Latina adolescents requiring more support than their non-Latina counterparts. Financial and emotional support from the father of the baby is more likely to be present when the adolescent mother is ages 16–18 years, rather than younger. Theories regarding this trend may be correlated to educational attainment or emotional maturity.[44]

Are such problems related to teenage pregnancy? Or are such adverse psychological outcomes related to disadvantages and problems that antedate and are exacerbated by the adolescent pregnancy? Many teen mothers are single (80% of fathers do not marry teen mothers) and depend on public assistance during or shortly after pregnancy.[42] In the United States, children of single-parent families may face increased life challenges.[18] Studies that demonstrate increased psychosocial and developmental problems in children of adolescents must therefore be evaluated with caution.

Mental health risks

The period of adolescence is signified by a variety of transitions in life that may increase the risk for psychiatric and mood disorders. Additionally, mood disorders such as depression are known to increase adverse outcomes in pregnancy, such as preterm birth, low birth weight, and attachment difficulties during the postpartum period.[45] In a meta-analysis involving 40 publications, it was found that the prevalence of depressive symptoms was higher in pregnant adolescents when compared to adults during pregnancy. The presence of depression during an adolescent's pregnancy is also correlated to higher rates of poor school performance, criminal activity, and substance use in the offspring.[46] These findings highlight the importance of screening for maternal depression and postpartum depression in patients regardless of their age or presentation, as these mood disorders have both short- and long-term repercussions for the mother and the child.

SUBSTANCE USE

Overall, women who use substances have higher rates of unplanned pregnancies, with rates upward of 80%–90%. While adolescents who use substances are also at an increased risk of unplanned pregnancies, this association may be confounded by the association of increased sexual activity with substance use.[47]

During pregnancy, 18.3% of pregnant teens surveyed in 2011 were found to have used a substance at one point in their pregnancy.[47] Rates of using substances such as marijuana, cocaine, and prescription medications were also the highest in pregnant women ages 15–17 in comparison to pregnant women of varying ages up to age 44. In contrast, alcohol use was significantly lower in pregnant adolescents when compared to nonpregnant age-matched peers. Last, approximately one in five pregnant adolescents reported using tobacco during their pregnancy; these studies did not take into account secondhand exposure to possibly teratogenic chemicals that are in cigarettes.[47] Pregnant adolescents were also found to have a 1.5- to 2-fold increased risk of meeting the *Diagnostic and Statistical Manual of Mental Disorders, Fourth Edition* (*DSM-IV*) criteria for a substance use disorder.[48]

OBSTETRIC CARE

When caring for pregnant adolescent patients, some additional measures should be taken that are not as applicable in the adult population.[49] Pregnant adolescents may have high risks of poor mental health outcomes and may face negative social stigmas. Additional multidisciplinary care is also pivotal when caring for adolescents. Resources such as social workers, teen parent support groups, and lactation specialists should be utilized, if possible.

During the initial presentation, the physician should also take time to discuss all options regarding management of the pregnancy, including termination, adoption, and parenthood. Adolescents should also be started on appropriate supplements as soon as possible, as it is likely that the teens were not knowledgeable about or compliant with prenatal vitamins.

Additionally, the postnatal period should have increased emphasis on maternal education on proper care

Table 20.4 Tiers of intervention for adolescent pregnancy prevention.

Counseling and education	Effective on an individual's behavior
Clinical interventions	Allowing better access to family planning services; reducing stigma regarding contraception and different age groups; implementing the Affordable Care Act
Long-lasting protection	Increasing the use of LARCs in adolescents
Changing the context	Encouraging healthy life decisions by promoting parent–child communication; educating adolescents regarding sexual behavior
Socioeconomic factors	Promoting family and community wellness in addition to educational achievement

of her newborn baby with assistance from social workers and midwives. Adequate contraception should also be encouraged with adolescents to prevent rapid repeat pregnancies.

PREVENTION

As the adolescent pregnancy rate has continued to decline over the past two decades, we have seen more and more policies geared toward prevention from both national and state levels of government. Most recently, the federal Teen Pregnancy Prevention Program, implemented in 2010, provides services for adolescent expecting mothers to assist them to find housing and also complete their high school or postsecondary education.[50]

Prevention may occur at a variety of different levels, with the broadest interventions involving socioeconomic factors that impact populations as a whole. Individually, prevention may occur at the physician–patient level, with counseling and education being key in preventing teen pregnancy on a case-by-case basis (Table 20.4).

SUMMARY

There is a continued and urgent need to make adolescent pregnancy a health-care priority. The negative outcomes that have been ascribed to teenage pregnancy have long-term repercussions for both the mother and the child, most notably with respect to a variety of socioeconomic factors. Poverty, violence, lack of knowledge, and access to reproductive health options are challenges that many teens encounter and must overcome during their pregnancy. While we have seen declines in the adolescent pregnancy rate over the past several decades, the United States continues to see a higher risk in adolescent pregnancy in patients with low socioeconomic status as well as in certain races. These teens face higher rates of preterm birth, low birth weight infants, and neonatal morbidity and mortality. Furthermore, there is evidence that the recent declines in adolescent pregnancy and birth may be slowing. While many societies have implemented some form of contraception education for adolescents, there is still much room for improvement in systems worldwide. Future considerations may include more heavy involvement of males in their own sexual health as well as increased education about more reliable forms of contraception such as LARCs for adolescent females. Additionally, legal aspects of obstetrical and gynecologic care must be taken into consideration regarding patient confidentiality for minors, as well as whether adolescents are able to pursue medical or surgical abortions in their local area. Teens must be supported both emotionally and financially but may not always have adequate health care. Adolescent health-care advocates must support policies and laws that improve teens' reproductive health-care rights and their safety. Only by considering these aspects of their care will we then be able to provide holistic care for adolescents.

REFERENCES

1. Centers for Disease Control and Prevention (CDC). About teen pregnancy. https://www.cdc.gov/teenpregnancy/about/. Accessed June 5, 2019.
2. McCracken KA, Loveless M. Teen pregnancy: An update. *Curr Opin Obstet Gynecol.* 2014;26(5):355–9.
3. Leftwich HK, Alves MVO. Adolescent pregnancy. *Pediatr Clin North Am.* 2017;64(2):381–8.
4. Neal S, Matthews Z, Frost M et al. Childbearing in adolescents aged 12–15 years in low resource countries: A neglected issue. New estimates from demographic and household surveys in 42 countries. *Acta Obstet Gynecol Scand.* 2012;91(9):1114–8.
5. United Nations Children's Fund. *Ending Child Marriage; Progress and prospects.* New York, NY: UNICEF; 2014. https://www.unicef.org/media/files/Child_Marriage_Report_7_17_LR..pdf.
6. Guttmacher Institute. *Fact Sheet: American Teens' Sexual and Reproductive Health.* 2014. https://www.guttmacher.org/sites/default/files/pdfs/pubs/FB-ATSRH.pdf.
7. Power to Decide, the campaign to prevent unplanned pregnancy. *Fast Facts: Teen Pregnancy in the United States.* http://powertodecide.org
8. Hornberger LL. Options counseling for the pregnant adolescent patient. *Pediatrics.* 2017;140(3):e20172274.
9. Baldwin MK, Edelman AB. The effect of long-acting reversible contraception on rapid repeat pregnancy in adolescents: A review. *J Adolesc Heal.* 2013;52(4 Suppl):S47–53.
10. Henshaw SK, Feivelson DJ. Teenage abortion and pregnancy statistics by state, 1996. *Fam Plann Perspect.* 2010;32(6):272–80.
11. Office of Adolescent Health. Trends in Teen Pregnancy and Childbearing. June 2, 2016.
12. Hardee K, Croce-Galis M, Gay J. Are men well served by family planning programs? *Reprod Health.* 2017;14(1):14–17.
13. Adolescent Pregnancy, Contraception, and Sexual Activity. Committee Opinion No. 699. American College of Obstetricians and Gynecologists. *Obstet Gynecol.* 2017;129:e142–9.
14. Vichnin M. Ectopic pregnancy in adolescents. *Curr Opin Obstet Gynecol.* 2008;20(5):475–8.
15. Kann L, McManus T, Harris WA et al. Youth Risk Behavior Surveillance—United States, 2017. *MMWR Surveill Summ.* 2018. https://www.cdc.gov/healthyyouth/data/yrbs/results.htm. Accessed June 5, 2019.
16. Klein JD. Adolescent pregnancy: Current trends and issues. *Pediatrics.* 2005;116(1):281–6.
17. Dodson NA, Gray SH, Burke PJ. Teen pregnancy prevention on a LARC: An update on long-acting reversible contraception for the primary care provider. *Curr Opin Pediatr.* 2012;24(4):439–45.
18. National Campaign to Prevent Teen Pregnancy. One in three: The case for wanted and welcomed pregnancy. *Teen Pregnancy.* 2007.
19. Moore K, Miller B, Sugland B. Beginning Too Soon: Adolescent Sexual Behavior, Pregnancy and Parenthood. 1995. https://aspe.hhs.gov/report/beginning-too-soon-adolescent-sexual-behavior-pregnancy-and-parenthood-review-research-and-interventions.
20. Leiderman S, Almo C. *Interpersonal Violence and Adolescent Pregnancy: Prevalence and Implications for Practice and Policy.* Washington, DC; 2006. https://www.healthyteennetwork.org/wp-content/uploads/2014/10/Interpersonal-Violence-and-Teen-Pregnancy.pdf.
21. Bearinger LH, Sieving RE, Ferguson J, Sharma V. Global perspectives on the sexual and reproductive health of adolescents: Patterns, prevention, and potential. *Lancet.* 2007;369(9568):1220–31.
22. Blinn-Pike L, Berger T, Dixon D, Kuschel D, Kaplan M. Is there a causal link between maltreatment and adolescent pregnancy? A literature review. *Perspect Sex Reprod Health.* 2002;34(2):68–75.
23. Sedgh G, Finer LB, Bankole A, Eilers MA, Singh S. Adolescent pregnancy, birth, and abortion rates across countries: Levels and recent trends. *J Adolesc Heal.* 2015;56(2):223–30.
24. Finer LB, Henshaw SK. Disparities in rates of unintended pregnancy in the United States, 1994 and 2001. *Perspect Sex Reprod Health.* 2006;38(2):90–6.
25. Jatlaoui TC, Shah J, Mandel MG et al. Abortion surveillance—United States, 2014. *MMWR Surveill Summ.* 2017;66(24):1–48.
26. Jones RK, Jerman J. Abortion incidence and service availability in the United States, 2014. *Perspect Sex Reprod Health.* 2017;49(1):17–27.
27. Morris JL, Rushwan H. Adolescent sexual and reproductive health: The global challenges. *Int J Gynecol Obstet.* 2015;131(Suppl):S40–2.
28. Coles MS, Makino KK, Phelps R. Knowledge of medication abortion among adolescent medicine providers. *J Adolesc Heal.* 2012;50(4):383–8.

29. Dobkin LM, Perrucci AC, Dehlendorf C. Pregnancy options counseling for adolescents: Overcoming barriers to care and preserving preference. *Curr Probl Pediatr Adolesc Health Care*. 2013;43(4):96–102.

30. Ozdemirci S, Kasapoglu T, Cirik DA, Yerebasmaz N, Kayikcioglu F, Salgur F. Is late adolescence a real risk factor for an adverse outcome of pregnancy? *J Matern Neonatal Med*. 2016;29(20):3391–4.

31. Prediction and prevention of preterm birth. Practice Bulletin No. 130. American College of Obstetricians and Gynecologists. *Obstet Gynecol*. 2012;120:964–73.

32. Kirbas A, Gulerman HC, Daglar K. Pregnancy in adolescence: Is it an obstetrical risk? *J Pediatr Adolesc Gynecol*. 2016;29(4):367–71.

33. Bakwa-Kanyinga F, Valério EG, Bosa VL et al. Adolescent pregnancy: Maternal and fetal outcomes in patients with and without preeclampsia. *Pregnancy Hypertens*. 2017;10:96–100.

34. Olaya-Garay SX, Velásquez-Trujillo PA, Vigil-De Gracia P. Blood pressure in adolescent patients with pre-eclampsia and eclampsia. *Int J Gynecol Obstet*. 2017;138(3):335–9.

35. World Health Organization. Contraception: Issues in adolescent health and development. WHO discussion papers on adolescence. 2004.

36. Penfield CA, Cheng YW, Caughey AB. Obstetric outcomes in adolescent pregnancies: A racial/ethnic comparison. *J Matern Neonatal Med*. 2013;26(14):1430–4.

37. Grobman WA, Bailit JL, Rice MM et al. Racial and ethnic disparities in maternal morbidity and obstetric care. *Obstet Gynecol*. 2015;125(6):1460–7.

38. Conde-Agudelo A, Belizán JM, Lammers C. Maternal-perinatal morbidity and mortality associated with adolescent pregnancy in Latin America: Cross-sectional study. *Am J Obstet Gynecol*. 2005;192(2):342–9.

39. Damle LF, Wilson K, Huang CC, Landy HJ, Gomez-Lobo V. Do they stand a chance? Vaginal birth after cesarean section in adolescents compared to adult women. *J Pediatr Adolesc Gynecol*. 2015;28(4):219–23.

40. Makinson C. The health consequences of teenage fertility. *Fam Plann Perspect*. 1985;17(3):132–9.

41. Terry-Humen E, Manlove J, Moore K. *Playing Catch-Up: How Children Born to Teen Mothers Fare*. Washington, DC: National Campaign to Prevent Teen Pregnancy; 2005.

42. National Campaign to Prevent Teen Pregnancy. *Not Just Another Single Issue: Teen Pregnancy Preventions Link to Other Critical Social Issues*. Washington, DC: National Campaign to Prevent Teen Pregnancy; 2006.

43. Kumar NR, Raker CA, Ware CF, Phipps MG. Characterizing social determinants of health for adolescent mothers during the prenatal and postpartum periods. *Women's Health Issues*. 2017;27(5):565–72.

44. Roye CF, Balk SJ. Evaluation of an intergenerational program for pregnant and parenting adolescents. *Matern Child Nurs J*. 1996;24(1):32–40.

45. Siegel RS, Brandon AR. Adolescents, pregnancy, and mental health. *J Pediatr Adolesc Gynecol*. 2014;27(3):138–50.

46. Shaw M, Lawlor DA, Najman JM. Teenage children of teenage mothers: Psychological, behavioural and health outcomes from an Australian prospective longitudinal study. *Soc Sci Med*. 2006;62(10):2526–39.

47. Connery HS, Albright BB, Rodolico JM. Adolescent substance use and unplanned pregnancy: Strategies for risk reduction. *Obstet Gynecol Clin North Am*. 2014;41(2):191–203.

48. Salas-Wright CP, Vaughn MG, Ugalde J, Todic J. Substance use and teen pregnancy in the United States: Evidence from the NSDUH 2002–2012. *Addict Behav*. 2015;45:218–25.

49. McCarthy FP, O'Brien U, Kenny LC. The management of teenage pregnancy. *BMJ*. 2014;349.

50. Kappeler EM, Farb AF. Historical context for the creation of the Office of Adolescent Health and the Teen Pregnancy Prevention Program. *J Adolesc Health*. 2014;54(3 Suppl):S3–9.

51. Martin JA, Hamilton BE, Osterman MJK et al. Birth: Final data for 2015, *Natl Vital Stat Rep*. 2017;66(1):1–70.

52. Hamilton BE, Martin JA, Osterman MJK et al. Births: Provisional data for 2017, *NVSS Vital Stat Rapid Release*. 2018;67(8):1–23.

Nutrition and eating disorders

21

ERIN H. SIEKE and ELLEN S. ROME

INTRODUCTION

Adolescence is a critical period of development in which rapid biological, social, psychological, and environmental changes occur. Balanced nutrition is essential for appropriate physical and cognitive development, with dietary requirements increasing to meet the rapid growth during this period. This critical time of development creates a window of vulnerability during which eating disorders (EDs) may develop. Clinicians caring for adolescents should use each contact as an opportunity to assess nutritional status, encourage healthy habits, and screen for potential disordered eating behaviors.

NUTRITION

Nutrition in adolescence: Important factors

Growth

The adolescent years are characterized by the second highest rate of growth during the life cycle, second only to the rapid growth of infancy. This rapid physical growth depends on adequate nutrition, which requires increased intake of energy, protein, fat, and micronutrients.

Sound nutrition is not only important for growth and development, but also for the prevention of chronic disease. Nutrition in adolescence has been show to influence rates of obesity, coronary heart disease, certain types of cancer, and type 2 diabetes.[1–5] Thus, it is important that healthy eating behaviors are established in childhood and maintained during adolescence and adulthood.

Puberty

The sequence of puberty is generally consistent for adolescents, although there can be significant variability in the age of onset and the pace of each stage of puberty. In females, the first sign of puberty is thelarche, or the development of breast buds, which usually occurs between 8 and 13 years of age.[6,7] Thelarche is followed by adrenarche, the stage in which the adrenal gland increases hormone production and leads to increased axillary hair and sebaceous secretions, and pubarche, or pubic hair development.[8] In 25% of youth, adrenarche precedes thelarche, but in a majority of youth, breast buds come before pubic hair. Peak height velocity occurs in Sexual Maturity Rating (SMR) 2 for girls, usually between 9 and 14 years of age. For boys, peak height velocity occurs at SMR 4, which makes middle school an awkward time for girls with early puberty and boys with late development. For girls, menarche generally occurs at SMR 4, on average, 2 years after the start of puberty. Nutritional intake affects age at menarche, height, weight, and peak bone mass and density,

highlighting the importance of appropriate nutrition to promote health and achieve full growth potential.

Bone development

In addition to the immense social changes that occur during adolescence, this period is also characterized by rapid bone formation and skeletal development. Skeletal mass approximately doubles between the onset of puberty and young adulthood, and this bone mass accrual is a major determinant of peak bone mass. Thus, adequate nutrition during this period is extremely critical to ensure adequate peak bone mass is achieved. Key factors that promote normal skeletal development include adequate energy intake; sufficient intake of minerals such as vitamin D, calcium, and phosphorus; and regular physical activity.[9]

Common nutritional challenges for adolescents

Multiple population-based studies have demonstrated that adolescents often fail to meet dietary recommendations, both for overall energy intake and for specific nutrients. Factors that contribute to inadequate dietary intake include increased activity with sports and other endeavors, greater time spent at school and elsewhere, work, extracurricular activities, increasing autonomy with decreased parental influence over food, preoccupation with body image, and an increasingly erratic eating schedule.[9–14] With busy schedules, adolescents frequently eat outside of the home and opt for fast foods or snack on foods that are high in calories but low in nutrients.[15,16] In addition, adolescents are more likely to engage in experimentation in multiple realms, including food choices, and are at high risk of engaging in dangerous dieting behaviors that may put them at increased risk for nutritional deficiencies and eating disorders.[17] Family meals have been shown to be protective for adolescents and are associated with lower rates of eating disorders, mental health problems, risky behaviors including drug and alcohol use, and adolescent obesity, and they should be encouraged whenever possible.[18,19]

NUTRITIONAL NEEDS

Prior to the onset of puberty, nutritional requirements are similar for males and females. During puberty, however, changes in body composition lead to increased adiposity in female relative to male adolescents. These changes as well as other biologic changes such as menarche lead to gender-specific nutrient needs. In addition, the differing timelines of puberty for males and females lead to variation in when adolescents may require the highest intake. During the peak growth velocity stage of puberty

(11–14 years for most girls), nutrient needs are highest, with intake needs that are double that of the remainder of the adolescent period.[15]

The Food and Nutrition Board of the Institute of Medicine publishes recommendations for daily intake as the Dietary Reference Intakes (DRIs) Tables.[16] However, it is important to note that these tables are based on chronological age categories, not individual biological development and pubertal stage, so clinicians must evaluate nutritional needs for each given adolescent on an individual basis.

Multiple population-based surveys have found that adolescents often fail to achieve recommended intake levels, both for overall macronutrient intake as well as for specific nutrients. Commonly, adolescents receive an outsized proportion of energy from saturated fat and added sugar intake, while intake of nutrients such as vitamin A, vitamin E, folic acid, fiber, iron, calcium, and zinc is limited.[12,20] The following sections summarize estimated intake needs and highlight the importance of these common nutrients that are often deficient in the adolescent diet, as well as food sources and signs of deficiency.

Energy and macronutrients

Energy

Energy requirements are multifactorial, and estimates of calorie needs must take into account basal metabolic rate, calorie needs for adequate growth, and each adolescent's individual activity level. Basal metabolic rate varies with lean body mass, so as lean body mass is deposited during growth, basal metabolic rate increases rapidly. The World Health Organization (WHO) recommends the Schofield equations for the estimation of basal metabolic rate. The equation for female adolescents age 10–18 years is as follows[21,22]:

$$BMR \ (kcal/day) = (13.38 \times Body \ weight \ [kg]) + 693$$

This basal metabolic rate estimate, however, does not take into account intake necessary for growth and energy expenditures from daily activities. Prediction equations for total energy requirements of female children and adolescents ages 9 through 18 years are shown in Table 21.1.

In this equation, the physical activity (PA) factor takes into account the activity level of the adolescent, and the factor of 25 is included to account for the energy cost of growth.[25]

These equations were used to create estimates of calorie needs for adolescents of varying activity levels, which can be found in the Dietary Guidelines for Americans 2015–2020 and are summarized in Table 21.2. However, keep in mind that these are averages based on chronological age; each individual patient's pubertal status, activity level, and specific growth needs should be taken into account when recommending intake goals. An adolescent during recovery from an eating disorder may have caloric needs in excess of 3500 calories per day to help with catch-up growth.

Table 21.1 Calculation for estimated energy requirements.

Energy Needs (kcal/d) = 135.3 − (30.8 × Age [y]) + PA × (10.0 × Weight [kg] + 934 × Height [m]) + 25		
Physical activity factor (PA)	**Daily physical activity level**	**Approximate daily exercise level**
1.00	Sedentary	None
1.16	Low active	30 Minutes of moderately intense exercise
1.31	Active	60 Minutes of moderately intense exercise
1.56	Very active	90 Minutes of moderately intense exercise

Source: Trumbo P et al. *J Am Diet Assoc.* 2002;102:1621–30; Brooks GA et al. *Am J Clin Nutr.* 2004;79:921S–30S.

Note: The equation here is the energy requirement for girls. For boys, there is a different equation. Each are based on the DRI (Dietary Reference Intake) developed by the Institute of Medicine.

Table 21.2 Estimated energy needs based on activity level for ages 9–18 years.

	Estimated calorie needs based on activity level (kcal)		
Age (years)	**Sedentary**	**Moderately active**	**Active**
9	1400	1600	1800
10	1400	1800	2000
11	1600	1800	2000
12–13	1600	2000	2200
14–18	1800	2000	2400

Source: 2015–2020 Dietary Guidelines, health.gov. https://health.gov/dietaryguidelines/2015/guidelines/. Accessed April 23, 2018.

Providers, families, and adolescents can reference the Choose My Plate website (https://www.choosemyplate.gov/), which allows a user to see how nutritional guidelines and requirements fit into an individual's daily food choices. This tool has replaced the Food Guide Pyramid and has more individualized curriculums available for special populations, such as individuals who follow a vegetarian diet.[27,28]

Protein

Protein requirements are determined by the amount of protein required for maintenance of lean body mass and accrual of additional lean body mass during the adolescent growth spurt. Thus, protein needs are highest during peak growth velocity, generally between 11 and 14 years of age for female adolescents. When protein intake is consistently inadequate, pubertal progression may be delayed with corresponding reductions in linear growth, delays in sexual maturation, and reduced accumulation of lean body mass. While most U.S. adolescents consume adequate or more than adequate amounts of protein, some subgroups of adolescents are at higher risk for insufficient protein intake. These groups include adolescents from food-insecure households, adolescents who severely restrict calories, and adolescents following a vegan diet.[29,30]

Carbohydrates

Carbohydrates provide the primary source of dietary energy, and dietary recommendations suggest that 45%–65% of total daily calories should come from carbohydrates. Whole-grain products should be an important part of carbohydrate intake, making up at least half of grain intake. Adolescents should also seek to take in a variety of fruits and vegetables and can be taught to select vegetables of all colors to encourage diverse nutrient intake. Alternatively, providers can recommend that individuals select from all five vegetable subgroups (dark green, orange, legumes, starchy vegetables, and other vegetables) several times per week.

No more than 10% of daily calorie intake should come from added sugars.[26] Sugar-sweetened beverages often contribute significantly to caloric intake in children and adolescents, with one study demonstrating that 10%–15% of total daily calorie intake in adolescents comes from sugar-sweetened beverages alone.[18] Intake of sugar-sweetened beverages has been shown to have a negative impact on diet quality,[31] be associated with weight gain,[32,33] and be an important predictor of cardiometabolic risk independent of weight status.[34] Choosing foods that limit the intake of added sugars is recommended.

Fat

Fat intake is crucial for normal growth and development as well as adequate absorption of the fat-soluble vitamins A, D, E, and K. Fat intake should make up approximately 20%–35% of calories (Table 21.3; Figure 21.1), with the vast majority of fat calories coming from sources of polyunsaturated and monounsaturated fatty acids, such as fish, nuts, avocado, and vegetable oils. All dietary fats are composed of a mix of polyunsaturated, monounsaturated, and saturated fatty acids. Fats that are higher in unsaturated and lower in saturated fats should be prioritized in order to restrict intake of saturated fats to less than 10% of calories per day. Solid fats such as butter and shortening have higher proportions of saturated fats and are less preferable to liquid fats such as olive oil, sesame oil, or canola oil. Trans fats are found primarily in partially hydrogenated vegetable oils and should be avoided in the diet, as they are associated with significant increases in cardiometabolic risk.

Vitamins, minerals, and micronutrients

Vitamin A

Vitamin A is important not only for normal vision, but also for normal growth, immune function, and reproductive health. The Recommended Dietary Allowance for vitamin A for female adolescents is 600 micrograms for ages 9–13 years and 700 micrograms for ages 14 and above (Table 21.4). Common dietary sources of vitamin A include fortified breakfast cereal, milk, carrots, and cheese. Beta-carotene is a precursor of vitamin A and is found in high concentrations in carrots, tomatoes, and green leafy vegetables. However, because adolescents frequently do

Table 21.3 Recommendations for macronutrient intake.

	Protein		Fat		Carbohydrate	
Age (years)	g	% kcal	g	% kcal	g	% kcal
9–13	34	10–30	n/aª	25–35	130	45–65
14–18	46	10–30	n/aª	25–35	130	45–65
19–30	46	10–35	n/aª	20–35	130	45–65

ª Recommended Dietary Allowances are not established for total fat intake.

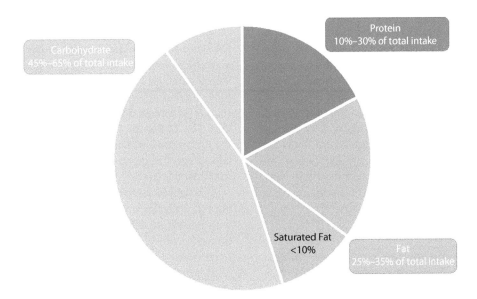

Figure 21.1 Recommended dietary macronutrient composition.

Table 21.4　Recommended Dietary Allowances for fat-soluble vitamins.

Age group (years)	Vitamin A	Vitamin D	Vitamin E	Vitamin K
9–13	600 mcg	600 IU	11 mg	60 mcg
14–18	700 mcg		15 mg	75 mcg
18+				90 mcg

Source:　2015–2020 Dietary Guidelines, health.gov. https://health.gov/dietaryguidelines/2015/guidelines/. Accessed April 23, 2018; Institute of Medicine. *Dietary reference intakes for vitamin C, vitamin E, selenium, and carotenoids.* Washington, DC: The National Academies Press; 2000.

Table 21.5　Recommended Dietary Allowances of selected water-soluble vitamins.

Age group (years)	Vitamin B1 (thiamine)	Vitamin B9 (folate)	Vitamin B12 (cobalamin)	Vitamin C (ascorbic acid)
9–13	0.9 mg	300 mcg	1.8 mcg	45 mg
14–18	1 mg	400 mcg	2.4 mcg	65 mg
19–30	1.1 mg			75 mg

Source:　2015–2020 Dietary Guidelines, health.gov. https://health.gov/dietaryguidelines/2015/guidelines/. Accessed April 23, 2018.

not meet recommended intake levels of fruits, vegetables, and dairy products, they may be at risk for deficiency of vitamin A.[35] Vitamin A deficiency commonly manifests with night blindness and vision impairment, which occurs after vitamin A stores have been depleted within the body. Vision impairment secondary to vitamin A is uncommon in the developed world since the advent of fortified food sources, but it is commonly seen in developing countries.[36]

Vitamin E

Vitamin E is an important antioxidant and also functions as an inhibitor of cell proliferation, platelet aggregation, and monocyte adhesion. The Recommended Dietary Allowance of vitamin E for adolescents is 11 milligrams for ages 9–13 years and 15 milligrams for ages 14 and above (Table 21.4).[26,37] Like the other fat-soluble vitamins A, D, and K, the bioavailability of vitamin E depends on physiologic mechanisms for fat digestion and absorption and requires the presence of lipases, bile salts, and pancreatic enzymes for appropriate absorption. Common sources of vitamin E include margarine; sweets such as cakes, cookies, and donuts; salad dressings; mayonnaise; and nuts and seeds. As many foods that are high in vitamin E are high fat, high added-sugar foods, it may be helpful to recommend fortified breakfast cereals and nuts as good sources of vitamin E that provide other nutritional benefits without trans fats, excess saturated fat, or added sugar. Low vitamin E status has been associated with several adverse health outcomes, including impaired immune responses and increased risk of atherosclerosis and cardiovascular disease, cancer, and vision deficits.[38] Vitamin E deficiency is rare in the developed world, although serum levels are noted to be lowest during adolescence.[38] Deficiency can occur in patients with fat malabsorption or those with very restricted fat intake, such as in adolescents with anorexia nervosa or other restrictive eating disorders.[39,40]

Vitamin C

Vitamin C is necessary for the synthesis of collagen and other connective tissues, making it critical for normal growth and development during puberty. The Recommended Dietary Allowance for vitamin C is 45 mg for females aged 9–13 years, 65 mg for females 14–18 years,

and 75 mg for ages 19–30 years (Table 21.5). Vitamin C is found in high concentrations in fruits and vegetables, with citrus fruits, tomatoes, and potatoes major contributors to dietary intake of vitamin C among adolescents. In addition, fortified breakfast cereals provide another source of vitamin C. Adolescents who smoke cigarettes have increased vitamin C requirements as compared to nonsmokers, as smoking increases oxidative stress and metabolic turnover of vitamin C.[41] In addition, adolescents who use tobacco and other substances have poorer quality diets and are less likely to consume adequate amounts of fruits and vegetables, so they may be at even higher risk of vitamin C deficiency.

Folate

Folate is essential for DNA, RNA, and protein synthesis and is necessary in increased amounts during puberty as growth accelerates. The Recommended Dietary Allowance for folate is 300 mcg/day for adolescents ages 9–13 years and 400 mcg/day for adolescents 14 years and older (Table 21.5). Common dietary sources of folate include fortified breakfast cereals, orange juice, bread, milk, and dried beans or lentils. Adolescents who routinely skip breakfast or avoid orange juice and cereal may be at increased risk for low folate intake. Folate deficiency can lead to macrocytic, megaloblastic anemia, which must be distinguished from B12 deficiency using serum levels of MMA (methylmalonic acid) and homocysteine. MMA levels are a sensitive marker of B12 deficiency and are not elevated in folate deficiency, while homocysteine will be elevated in both vitamin B12 and folate deficiency.[42] Mean folate intake among female adolescents is substantially less than recommended intake, with one study demonstrating that 42% of female adolescents had folate intakes below the Recommended Dietary Allowance, with 40% of female adolescents having low red cell folate levels indicative of subclinical folate deficiency.[43]

Adequate intakes of folate in women of childbearing age are especially important, as low folate levels are associated with neural tube defects and other congenital anomalies. The protective effects of folate intake occur early in pregnancy, often before the adolescent may be aware of a pregnancy. Thus, any female adolescent who is sexually active should consume 400 mcg/day of folate from supplements or fortified cereals in addition to a varied diet containing folate from food sources such as fruits, vegetables, and whole grains.

Calcium

Calcium is a crucial component of the diet in order to ensure bone health and attainment of peak bone mass during puberty. Skeletal growth peaks during adolescence, with 45% of peak bone mass attained during this period. As a result of this dramatic increase in skeletal growth, calcium needs correspondingly reach a peak. Adequate calcium and vitamin D are necessary not only for the development of peak bone mass, but also the reduction of lifetime risk of fractures and osteoporosis.[44,45] Dietary studies have demonstrated that mean calcium intake among adolescent females is significantly lower than the DRIs recommend, with only 19% of adolescent females meeting their calcium intake requirements.[46] Calcium can be obtained through dairy products such as milk, cheese, yogurt, or ice cream. In addition, calcium-fortified foods such as orange juice, fortified cereals, and breakfast bars are widely available with similar amounts of calcium per serving to milk and may be a good alternative for lactose-intolerant individuals. Nondairy beverages (i.e., soy, almond, coconut, and flax milk) fortified with calcium are also useful options for those with lactose intolerance or a milk protein allergy. Of note, these beverages are often lower in total energy, fat, and protein and should be used complementary to a balanced diet. Soft drink consumption has been associated with decreased intake of calcium-containing foods and beverages, so it is important to screen adolescents for soft drink intake and provide recommendations for how calcium can be incorporated in the diet.[47,48]

Iron

Iron is needed in increasing amounts during puberty due to rapid growth and the expansion of blood volume and muscle mass. In female adolescents, the onset of menstruation leads to additional iron needs. Iron is necessary for transporting oxygen in the bloodstream. Iron deficiency can lead to anemia with associated symptoms of weakness, fatigue, and shortness of breath, among others. Studies have suggested that almost half of female adolescents did not meet recommended dietary intake guidelines for iron.[20] Iron can be found in many foods, but the availability of dietary iron for absorption varies by form. Heme iron, found in meat, fish, and poultry, is much more easily absorbed than nonheme iron, which is found in grains and plant-based foods. Thus, adolescents following a vegetarian diet will need to consume significantly more iron to meet their daily requirement.[49]

Zinc

Zinc has many roles within the body, including catalytic, structural, and regulatory functions. Zinc is naturally abundant in red meats, shellfish, and whole grains, and is often fortified in breakfast cereals. Zinc is important during adolescence for growth and sexual maturation, and female adolescents commonly do not meet recommended intake levels of zinc in their diets. In one study, approximately half of adolescent females took in less than 75% of recommended levels of zinc.[20] Similarly to iron, plant-based sources of zinc are less easily absorbed, so vegans, and to a lesser degree vegetarians, are at higher risk for zinc deficiency.[50] In addition, zinc and iron compete for absorption binding sites, so increased intake (or supplementation) of iron may put adolescents at increased risk for zinc deficiency. Given the high rates of iron deficiency anemia and iron supplementation among adolescent females, zinc intake should be monitored, and clinicians should have a high index of suspicion for zinc deficiency.[51] Such deficiencies can easily be corrected with daily use of a multivitamin containing zinc.

Dietary fiber

Carbohydrate-rich foods, such as fruit, vegetables, whole grains, and legumes, provide the main source of dietary fiber. Dietary fiber is categorized into soluble and insoluble fiber. Insoluble fiber helps to recruit water, improve transit through the intestines, and treat constipation. Food sources of insoluble fiber include green leafy vegetables, whole wheat products, seeds, and nuts.[52] Soluble fiber, in contrast, has a lesser impact on intestinal transit but has been associated with decreased total and LDL cholesterol.[53] In addition, soluble fiber helps to regulate blood sugar levels and insulin secretion in individuals with diabetes.[54] Soluble fiber is found in oat, oat bran, nuts, barley, flax seed, and some fruits and vegetables. Mean adolescent fiber intake is well below the recommendations, likely secondary to the low intake of fruit, vegetables, and whole grains among adolescents. Adolescents who skip breakfast may be at higher risk of having an inadequate consumption of fiber, so recommending regularly scheduled meals with a balanced diet may help to increase fiber intake.[55] However, rapid increases in fiber in the diet can lead to diarrhea and abdominal cramping, so dietary changes should be made gradually to increase fiber intake as tolerated. It is also important to meet fluid recommendations when increasing fiber in the diet.

Physical activity

The 2015–2020 Dietary Guidelines for Americans recommends that children and adolescents should do 60 minutes or more of physical activity daily, with this activity consisting primarily of moderate or vigorous intensity aerobic physical activity.[26] Muscle-strengthening activities, such as strength training, resistance training, and muscular strength and endurance exercises, as well as bone-strengthening activities, including running, jumping rope, and weight lifting, should be included in the 60 minutes on at least 3 days of the week. Adolescents should be encouraged to participate in physical activities that are appropriate for their age and enjoyable, such as participating in team sports and engaging in fun free play outside with family and friends. Repetitive, compulsive activity should be discouraged and may be a first sign of an eating disorder.

EATING DISORDERS

Eating disorders (EDs) are the third most common chronic illness among adolescents, with the prevalence rate for anorexia nervosa (AN) estimated at 1%–4% of female adolescents.[56-59] AN carries the highest mortality rate of all psychiatric disorders at 5%–6%.[60,61] In addition to this high mortality rate, AN is also associated with serious medical sequelae secondary to malnutrition and disordered behaviors, including, but not limited to, disturbances of the cardiovascular, reproductive, gastrointestinal, and skeletal systems.[62,63] With increased attention within the community, recognition of eating disorders among previously unrecognized groups, and the release of the *Diagnostic and Statistical Manual of Mental Disorders, Fifth Edition* (*DSM-5*), the epidemiology of EDs is changing, with increases in the diagnosis of eating disorders among males, minorities, and individuals of all age groups.[64-66]

Etiology

Although the pathophysiology of eating disorders is not clearly delineated, both biologic and psychosocial factors contribute to their development. Significant evidence supports a genetic component to eating disorders, with multiple epidemiologic studies supporting the heritability of eating disorders. Estimates of the heritability range between 33% and 84% for AN and between 28% and 83% for bulimia nervosa (BN).[67,68] A recent genome-wide association study of AN identified the first genome-wide significant locus, located on chromosome 12 in a region harboring a previously reported type 1 diabetes and autoimmune disorder locus.[69] Research is ongoing into the consequences of this candidate gene locus as well as neurobiologic factors that may contribute to the development of or maintenance of EDs.

Clinical presentation

Any patient, regardless of BMI class, who presents with weight loss, unexplained growth stunting or pubertal delay, restrictive or abnormal eating behaviors, excessive or compulsive exercise, or recurrent vomiting, should prompt concern for an eating disorder. Younger patients and male patients may be more likely to have atypical presentations and delayed presentation to care and often will not vocalize the body image concerns that many individuals (and providers) associate with EDs.[67] Adolescents with chronic illness, such as insulin-dependent diabetes mellitus, are also at higher risk of developing disordered eating behaviors due to the ease of manipulating insulin use and/or other medications that may alter weight or body composition, such as diuretics. Adolescents may present with cognitions including obsession over dietary intake, significant increase in exercise, repeated body checking behaviors, and new dietary restrictions of food they previously enjoyed. Parents and caregivers may be the first to notice these changes, and their concerns should be carefully considered, as they know their child best. If a parent voices concern over a child or adolescent's disordered eating, that young person needs to be carefully evaluated for an eating disorder and followed closely over time. Many parents bring their concern to the pediatrician or other clinician, with early diagnosis associated with improved outcomes.

Screening and diagnosis

Providers should routinely monitor growth trajectories and BMI and assess for the presence of high-risk behaviors such as dieting or excessive exercise. The SCOFF questionnaire is a brief screening tool that is commonly used in the primary care setting for ED screening, although its use has only been validated in adults (Table 21.6). Positive answers to these questions should certainly prompt further investigation and referral.

Diagnostic criteria were updated in 2013 with the release of the *DSM-5*. This update sought to improve the applicability and precision of ED diagnoses. The revised criteria for AN take into account expected weight and growth for children and adolescents and eliminated the amenorrhea criteria that excluded males, premenarchal females, and adolescents who remain eumenorrheic despite low body weight. In addition, although body image distortion remains a diagnostic criterion, AN can still be diagnosed if a patient persistently fails to recognize the seriousness of his or her low body weight even if he or she verbally acknowledges that he or she is too skinny. BN, which is characterized by recurrent episodes of binge eating accompanied by inappropriate compensatory behaviors, was updated to reduce the requirement of the frequency of these behaviors from three times per week to once per week for 3 months. In addition to updating the diagnostic criteria for AN and BN to better reflect patient presentations, several new eating disorder diagnoses were introduced. Binge eating disorder (BED) was formalized as an eating disorder, and avoidant/restrictive food intake disorder (ARFID) is a new diagnosis that represents a variety of restrictive eating behaviors, including swallowing phobias and aversions to specific textures that lead to impaired growth and significant social impairment. Other specified feeding and eating disorders (OSFED) is a group of other

Table 21.6 The SCOFF questionnaire.

1. Do you make yourself Sick because you feel uncomfortably full?
2. Do you worry you have lost Control over how much you eat?
3. Have you recently lost more than One stone (14 lb/6.3 kg) in a 3-month period?
4. Do you believe yourself to be Fat when others say you are too thin?
5. Would you say that Food dominates your life?

Scoring: One point is given for every "yes" answer.

A score of 2 or greater indicates a likely diagnosis of an eating disorder.

diagnoses, which includes atypical AN (in which patients have lost a significant amount of weight through restrictive and/or maladaptive eating patterns but remain within a normal or overweight BMI category), subthreshold bulimia nervosa, purging disorder, and night eating syndrome. The final category, unspecified feeding and eating disorder (UFED), comprises any other clinically significant EDs that do not fit into other specific eating disorders. Table 21.7 outlines the various diagnostic criteria for these disorders found in *DSM-5*.

Medical complications

In addition to a high mortality rate, eating disorders are associated with serious medical sequelae secondary to malnutrition and disordered eating behaviors. Eating disorders impact every organ system, including the cardiovascular, neurologic, gastrointestinal, reproductive, and skeletal systems. Common medical complications of eating disorders are summarized in Figure 21.2.

Treatment

Early referral or treatment is associated with improved outcomes, and delayed access to care can lead to potentially irreversible impacts on growth and development. Thus, any signs of disordered eating behaviors should warrant prompt referral to an eating disorder specialist for treatment. Historically, treatment for eating disorders focused on individual therapy and removed eating disorder patients from their families and caregivers. However, more recent evidence has led to a paradigm shift, in which nutritional rehabilitation is the primary focus early in treatment, and parents and caregivers are critical allies and major determinants of treatment success. Treatments that have been investigated in the treatment of children and adolescents with eating disorders include individual therapy, cognitive behavioral therapy (CBT), dialectical behavioral therapy (DBT), and family-based treatment (FBT).

FBT has the largest evidence base of any treatment and has shown high efficacy in the treatment of adolescents and young adults with AN, with studies demonstrating improved rates of weight restoration and lower relapse rates relative to alternative treatment methods.[70–76] In addition, there is an increasing body of evidence supporting FBT for the treatment of young children with AN and adolescents with BN and other eating disorders.[70,77] FBT utilizes a three-phase intensive outpatient model in which clinicians partner with parents to achieve recovery. The first phase of treatment has the parents take control over meals in order to achieve weight restoration. Phase II begins when the patient accepts the parental prescription for increased food intake and achieves steady weight gain, and in this phase, control is gradually returned to the children in an age-appropriate manner. In phase III, the treatment focus shifts from medical treatment of starvation to focusing on the psychological impact of the disorder. In phase III, adolescents work with a therapist to establish a healthy identity.[74] CBT has demonstrated efficacy in other eating disorders, including BN and BED.[78]

Pharmacologic agents are commonly used in patients with eating disorders, despite minimal evidence supporting their efficacy. Selective serotonin reuptake inhibitors (SSRIs) and tricyclic antidepressants (TCAs) have not been shown to be better than placebo in either weight gain or improvement in eating disorder symptomatology in studies of adults with AN.[79] In addition, no large randomized controlled trials of atypical antipsychotics in the treatment of AN are available, although limited evidence suggests that these medications may be useful in reducing anxiety and rigidity and improving early weight gain.[80,81] Pharmacotherapy in AN should not be first line given the limited evidence available, but may be useful in individual patients resistant to treatment, with high anxiety or debilitating depression. Short-term use of an antianxiety medication such as lorazepam (0.5–1 mg) given 15–30 minutes before meals can help reduce "meal panic" but rarely is required chronically. Such use can act as a cycle breaker for the young person who is relearning to eat.

Outcomes

Early diagnosis and effective treatment with FBT has led to improved outcomes in adolescents with eating disorders. Studies suggest that more than three-quarters of youth with AN recover, developing normal eating and weight control habits and returning to activities including school, work, and social relationships. However, a subset of patients goes on to develop chronic disease, as evidenced by high estimates of relapse rates, with 35%–65% of AN patients and 42% of BN patients requiring repeat hospitalization.[61,82,83] Clinicians should focus on early diagnosis and treatment as modifiable risk factors for poor prognosis.

Special concerns for the obstetrician-gynecologist caring for patients with eating disorders

Amenorrhea and pubertal development

Delayed puberty and amenorrhea can occur due to suppression of gonadotropin-releasing hormone (GnRH) by the hypothalamus in a starvation state. Although pubertal development occurs across a spectrum, delayed puberty is defined as no onset of secondary sexual characteristics at an age that is 2–2.5 standard deviations beyond the population mean, generally accepted as a chronological age of 13 years in girls and 14 years in boys.[84] Sexual dysfunction is common in women with eating disorders, including decreased libido, higher sexual anxiety, and decreased self-focused sexual activity. Adequate iron and protein consumptions must be encouraged, especially in patients who avoid red meat or follow a vegan or vegetarian diet. After refeeding has begun, menses typically resume around the same weight that menses ceased in patients with secondary amenorrhea. Current research suggests that most patients with amenorrhea secondary to eating disorders do not benefit from hormonal therapy in the form of oral contraceptives to regulate periods, and its use is not recommended.[85] In fact, return of

Table 21.7 Diagnostic criteria for eating disorders.

Anorexia nervosa

- Restriction of energy intake relative to requirements leading to a significantly low body weight in the context of age, sex, developmental trajectory, and physical health. Significantly low weight is defined as a weight that is less than minimally normal, or, for children and adolescents, less than that minimally expected.
- Intense fear of gaining weight or becoming fat, or persistent behavior that interferes with weight gain, even though at a significantly low weight.
- Disturbance in the way in which one's body weight or shape is experienced, undue influence of body weight or shape on self-evaluation, or persistent lack of recognition of the seriousness of the current low body weight.
  - *Restricting type*: No recurrent episodes of binges or purging in the last 3 months.
  - *Binge-eating/purging type*: In last 3 months, the person has engaged in recurrent episodes of binge eating or purging behavior (i.e., self-induced vomiting or the misuse of laxatives, diuretics, or enemas).

Bulimia nervosa

- Recurrent episodes of binge eating, characterized by BOTH:
  - Eating, in a discrete period of time (e.g., within any 2-hour period) an amount of food that is definitely larger than most people would eat during a similar period of time and under similar circumstances.
  - A sense of lack of control over eating during the episode.
  - Recurrent inappropriate compensatory behavior in order to prevent weight gain, such as self-induced vomiting; misuse of laxatives, diuretics, or other medications; fasting; or excessive exercise.
  - The binge eating and inappropriate compensatory behaviors both occur, on average, at least once a week for 3 months.
  - Self-evaluation is unduly influenced by body shape and weight.
  - The disturbance does not occur exclusively during episodes of anorexia nervosa.

Binge-eating disorder

- Recurrent episodes of binge eating, defined by eating an amount of food larger than what most people would eat in the same discrete period of time, plus a sense of lack of control during episodes.
- Binges associated with three or more of the following:
  - Eating much more rapidly than normal.
  - Eating until feeling uncomfortably full.
  - Eating large amounts of food when not feeling physically hungry.
  - Eating alone because of feeling embarrassed by how much one is eating.
  - Feeling disgusted with oneself, depressed, or very guilty afterward.
- Other characteristics:
  - Marked distress regarding binge eating.
  - Binges at least once a week for 3 months.
  - Binges not associated with the recurrent use of inappropriate compensatory behavior (e.g., purging) and no evidence of anorexia nervosa, bulimia nervosa, or avoidant/restrictive food intake disorder.

Avoidant/restrictive food intake disorder

- Eating or feeding disturbance (including but not limited to apparent lack of interest in eating or food; avoidance due to sensory characteristics of food; or concern about aversive consequences of eating) as manifested by persistent failure to meet appropriate nutritional and/or energy needs associated with one or more of the following:
  - Significant weight loss (or failure to gain weight or faltering growth in children).
  - Significant nutritional deficiency.
  - Dependence on enteral feeding.
  - Marked interference with psychosocial functioning.
- No evidence of lack of available food or an associated culturally sanctioned practice.

Other specified feeding or eating disorder (OSFED)

Atypical anorexia nervosa: All of the criteria for anorexia nervosa are met, except that, despite significant weight loss, the individual's weight is within or above the normal range.

Subthreshold bulimia nervosa (low frequency or limited duration): All of the criteria for Bulimia Nervosa are met, except that the binge eating and inappropriate compensatory behaviors occur, on average, less than once a week and/or for less than for 3 months.

Purging disorder: Recurrent purging behavior to influence weight or shape, sucas self-induced vomiting, misuse of laxatives, diuretics, or other medications, in the absence of binge eating. Self-evaluation is unduly influenced by body shape or weight or there is an intense fear of gaining weight or becoming fat.

Night eating syndrome: Recurrent episodes of night eating, as manifested by eating after awakening from sleep or excessive food consumption after the evening meal, with awareness and recall of the eating. The night eating is not better accounted for by external influences such as changes in the individual's sleep/wake cycle or by local social norms. Accompanied by significant distress and/or impairment in functioning.

Other feeding or eating condition not elsewhere classified: This is a residual category for clinically significant problems meeting the definition of a Feeding or Eating Disorder but not satisfying the criteria for any other Disorder or Condition.

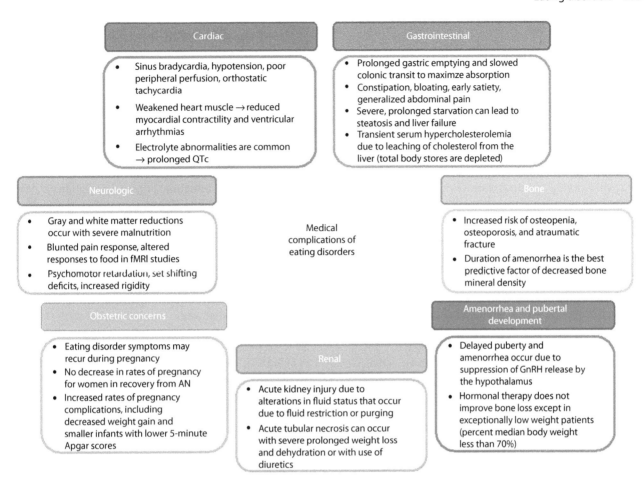

Figure 21.2 Medical complications of eating disorders.

menses without hormonal help can be a useful indicator of a healthy weight in patients recovering from eating disorders that is masked by hormonal therapy. However, there may be a role for hormonal therapy in exceptionally low weight patients (percent median body weight less than 70%).[86] Although hormonal therapy may prevent further bone loss in exceptionally low weight patients, the best treatment for amenorrhea and reduced bone mineral density is weight gain with resumption of normal endogenous hormonal cycles.[87]

Contraception in adolescents with eating disorders

Although many patients with restrictive eating disorders may have amenorrhea secondary to hypogonadotropic hypogonadism and anovulation, it is important to encourage responsible contraceptive practices in all sexually active adolescents. Impact on bone health is an important consideration when comparing contraceptive methods in adolescents with eating disorders. However, other important factors to consider include ease of compliance, reliability of method, and potential side effects. Research suggests that low estrogen containing combined oral contraceptives (oral contraceptives containing ≤20 µg of ethinyl estradiol) reduce peak bone mineral density in adolescent and young adult females.[88] Early initiation of oral contraceptives, lower dosages of ethinyl estradiol, and longer duration of use are all factors known to

contribute to reductions in peak bone mass in this population. Similarly to low-dose ethinyl estradiol–containing oral contraceptives, depot medroxyprogesterone acetate is also thought to interfere with peak bone mass deposition and may not be the best first-line choice in adolescents with eating disorders.[89] The American College of Obstetricians and Gynecologists as well as the American Academy of Pediatrics recommend that long-acting reversible contraceptives (LARCs), including intrauterine devices (IUDs) and contraceptive implants, should be considered a first-line method for pregnancy prevention in adolescents.[90,91]

Obstetric concerns

Adolescents and young adults with active eating disorders may have difficulty becoming pregnant due to hypogonadotropic hypogonadism leading to anovulation. However, women in recovery from AN have no differences in rates of pregnancy or reported infertility when compared with the general population.[92,93] In fact, multiple large observational studies have demonstrated that women in recovery from eating disorders have significantly higher rates of unplanned pregnancy than women in the general population.[92–94] However, women with BN and BED may have difficulties with fertility and have greater risks of miscarriage.[95–97] Pregnancy complications may be higher among women in recovery from eating disorders as compared to healthy women. In one study, patients in ED recovery gained less weight, had smaller babies with lower 5-minute Apgar scores, and had higher rates of difficulty with breastfeeding and postpartum depression.[98]

CONCLUSIONS

Adolescence is a rapid period of biological, social, and psychological development in which young girls undergo significant physical changes while experimenting with autonomy. Dietary changes are common during this period and are often chosen due to ease of access or peer influence. Adolescents frequently eat a diet that is high in saturated fat and added sugars while lacking in many critical nutrients to promote growth and cognitive development. Adolescents are vulnerable to developing eating disorders and require close monitoring by parents, caregivers, and health-care providers to promote healthy habits and catch disordered behaviors early. Eating disorders are common biopsychosocial illnesses that can present in adolescence and are associated with high rates of morbidity and mortality. Early diagnosis and treatment are key for optimal outcomes, so all providers caring for young women should engage in conversations about balanced eating habits and screen for early signs of disordered eating cognitions and behaviors.

REFERENCES

1. Thompson DR, Obarzanek E, Franko DL et al. Childhood overweight and cardiovascular disease risk factors: The National Heart, Lung, and Blood Institute Growth and Health Study. *J Pediatr.* 2007;150:18–25.
2. Pan Y, Pratt CA. Metabolic syndrome and its association with diet and physical activity in US adolescents. *J Am Diet Assoc.* 2008;108:276–86; discussion 286.
3. Van Horn L, McCoin M, Kris-Etherton PM et al. The evidence for dietary prevention and treatment of cardiovascular disease. *J Am Diet Assoc.* 2008;108:287–331.
4. Dauchet L, Amouyel P, Dallongeville J. Fruits, vegetables and coronary heart disease. *Nat Rev Cardiol.* 2009;6:599–608.
5. Steinberger J, Daniels SR, Hagberg N et al. Cardiovascular health promotion in children: Challenges and opportunities for 2020 and beyond: A scientific statement from the American Heart Association. *Circulation.* 2016;134:e236–55.
6. Rosenfield RL. Puberty and its disorders in girls. *Endocrinol Metab Clin North Am.* 1991;20:15–42.
7. Rosenfield RL, Bachrach LK, Chernausek SD et al. Current age of onset of puberty. *Pediatrics.* 2000;106:622–3.
8. Campbell B. Adrenarche in comparative perspective. *Am J Hum Biol.* 2011;23:44–52.
9. Bonnet N, Ferrari SL. Exercise and the skeleton: How it works and what it really does. *IBMS BoneKEy.* 2010;7:235–48.
10. Neumark-Sztainer D, Story M, Hannan PJ, Croll J. Overweight status and eating patterns among adolescents: Where do youths stand in comparison with the Healthy People 2010 objectives? *Am J Public Health.* 2002;92:844–51.
11. Larson NI, Neumark-Sztainer D, Hannan PJ, Story M. Trends in adolescent fruit and vegetable consumption, 1999-2004: Project EAT. *Am J Prev Med.* 2007;32:147–50.
12. Banfield EC, Liu Y, Davis JS, Chang S, Frazier-Wood AC. Poor adherence to US dietary guidelines for children and adolescents in the National Health and Nutrition Examination Survey Population. *J Acad Nutr Diet.* 2016;116:21–7.
13. Kann L. McManus T, Harris WA et al. Youth risk behavior surveillance – United States, 2015. *MMWR Surveill Summ.* 2016;65:1–74.
14. Moore LV, Thompson FE, Demissie Z. Percentage of youth meeting federal fruit and vegetable intake recommendations, Youth Risk Behavior Surveillance System, United States and 33 States, 2013. *J Acad Nutr Diet.* 2017;117:545–53.e3.
15. Cusatis DC, Shannon BM. Influences on adolescent eating behavior. *J Adolesc Health Off Publ Soc Adolesc Med.* 1996;18:27–34.
16. French SA, Story M, Neumark-Sztainer D, Fulkerson JA, Hannan P. Fast food restaurant use among adolescents: Associations with nutrient intake, food choices and behavioral and psychosocial variables. *Int J Obes Relat Metab Disord.* 2001;25:1823–33.
17. Gu X, Tucker KL. Dietary quality of the US child and adolescent population: Trends from 1999 to 2012 and associations with the use of federal nutrition assistance programs. *Am J Clin Nutr.* 2017;105:194–202.
18. Berge JM, Wall M, Hsueh T-F et al. The protective role of family meals for youth obesity: 10-year longitudinal associations. *J Pediatr.* 2015;166:296–301.
19. Skeer MR, Ballard EL. Are family meals as good for youth as we think they are? A review of the literature on family meals as they pertain to adolescent risk prevention. *J Youth Adolesc.* 2013;42:943–63.
20. Stang J, Story MT, Harnack L, Neumark-Sztainer D. Relationships between vitamin and mineral supplement use, dietary intake, and dietary adequacy among adolescents. *J Am Diet Assoc.* 2000;100:905–10.
21. Schofield WN. Predicting basal metabolic rate, new standards and review of previous work. *Hum Nutr Clin Nutr.* 1985;39(Suppl 1):5–41.
22. Schofield C. An annotated bibliography of source material for basal metabolic rate data. *Hum Nutr Clin Nutr.* 1985;39(Suppl 1):42–91.
23. Trumbo P, Schlicker S, Yates AA, Poos M, Food and Nutrition Board of the Institute of Medicine, The National Academies. Dietary reference intakes for energy, carbohydrate, fiber, fat, fatty acids, cholesterol, protein and amino acids. *J Am Diet Assoc.* 2002;102:1621–30.

24. Brooks GA, Butte NF, Rand WM, Flatt J.-P, Caballero B. Chronicle of the Institute of Medicine physical activity recommendation: How a physical activity recommendation came to be among dietary recommendations. *Am J Clin Nutr.* 2004;79:921S–30S.

25. Baumgartner RN, Roche AF, Himes JH. Incremental growth tables: Supplementary to previously published charts. *Am J Clin Nutr.* 1986;43:711–22.

26. 2015–2020 Dietary Guidelines, health.gov. https://health.gov/dietaryguidelines/2015/guidelines/. Accessed April 23, 2018.

27. Choose MyPlate. *Choose MyPlate.* https://www.choosemyplate.gov/. Accessed April 23, 2018.

28. Haddad EH, Sabaté J, Whitten CG. Vegetarian food guide pyramid: A conceptual framework. *Am J Clin Nutr.* 1999;70:615S–9S.

29. Messina V, Mangels AR. Considerations in planning vegan diets: Children. *J Am Diet Assoc.* 2001;101:661–9.

30. Soliman A, De Sanctis V, Elalaily R. Nutrition and pubertal development. *Indian J Endocrinol Metab.* 2014;18:S39–47.

31. Frary CD, Johnson RK, Wang MQ. Children and adolescents' choices of foods and beverages high in added sugars are associated with intakes of key nutrients and food groups. *J Adolesc Health Off Publ Soc Adolesc Med.* 2004;34:56–63.

32. Ebbeling CB, Feldman HA, Osganian SK et al. Effects of decreasing sugar-sweetened beverage consumption on body weight in adolescents: A randomized, controlled pilot study. *Pediatrics.* 2006;117:673–80.

33. Malik VS, Schulze MB, Hu FB. Intake of sugar-sweetened beverages and weight gain: A systematic review. *Am J Clin Nutr.* 2006;84:274–88.

34. Ambrosini GL, Oddy WH, Huang RC et al. Prospective associations between sugar-sweetened beverage intakes and cardiometabolic risk factors in adolescents. *Am J Clin Nutr.* 2013;98:327–34.

35. Ribeiro-Silva R de C, Nunes IL, Assis AMO. Prevalence and factors associated with vitamin A deficiency in children and adolescents. *J Pediatr (Rio J).* 2014;90:486–92.

36. McLaren DS, Kraemer K. Vitamin A in health. *World Rev Nutr Diet.* 2012;103:33–51.

37. Institute of Medicine. *Dietary reference intakes for vitamin C, vitamin E, selenium, and carotenoids.* Washington, DC: The National Academies Press; 2000.

38. Bendich A. Vitamin E status of US children. *J Am Coll Nutr.* 1992;11:441–4.

39. Moyano D, Sierra C, Brandi N et al. Antioxidant status in anorexia nervosa. *Int J Eat Disord.* 1999;25:99–103.

40. Pfeiffer RF. Neurologic manifestations of malabsorption syndromes. *Handb Clin Neurol.* 2014;120:621–32.

41. Strauss RS. Environmental tobacco smoke and serum vitamin C levels in children. *Pediatrics.* 2001;107:540–2.

42. Allen LH. Causes of vitamin B12 and folate deficiency. *Food Nutr Bull.* 2008;29:S20–34; discussion S35–37.

43. Tsui JC, Nordstrom JW. Folate status of adolescents: Effects of folic acid supplementation. *J Am Diet Assoc.* 1990;90:1551–6.

44. Stang J, Story MT, University of Minnesota. Center for Leadership, Education and Training in Maternal and Child Nutrition, 2005. Guidelines for Adolescent Nutrition Services.

45. Baker SS, Flores CA, Georgieff MK et al. American Academy of Pediatrics. Committee on Nutrition. Calcium requirements of infants, children, and adolescents. *Pediatrics.* 1999;104:1152–7.

46. Alaimo K, McDowell MA, Briefel RR et al. Dietary intake of vitamins, minerals, and fiber of persons ages 2 months and over in the United States: Third National Health and Nutrition Examination Survey, Phase 1, 1988–91. *Adv Data.* 1994;(258):1–28.

47. Harnack L, Stang J, Story M. Soft drink consumption among US children and adolescents: Nutritional consequences. *J Am Diet Assoc.* 1999;99:436–41.

48. de Oliveira CF, da Silveira CR, Beghetto M, de Mello PD, de Mello ED. Assessment of calcium intake by adolescents. *Rev Paul Pediatr Orgao of Soc Pediatr Sao Paulo.* 2014;32:216–20.

49. Pawlak R. Vegetarian diets in the prevention and management of diabetes and its complications. *Diabetes Spectr Publ Am Diabetes Assoc.* 2017;30:82–8.

50. Donovan UM, Gibson RS. Iron and zinc status of young women aged 14 to 19 years consuming vegetarian and omnivorous diets. *J Am Coll Nutr.* 1995;14:463–72.

51. Roohani N, Hurrell R, Kelishadi R, Schulin R. Zinc and its importance for human health: An integrative review. *J Res Med Sci Off J Isfahan Univ Med Sci.* 2013;18:144–57.

52. Williams LA, Wilson DP. Nutritional management of pediatric dyslipidemia. In: Feingold KR et al. eds. *Endotext.* Dartmouth, MA: MDText.com; 2000.

53. Lattimer JM, Haub MD. Effects of dietary fiber and its components on metabolic health. *Nutrients.* 2010;2:1266–89.

54. White J, Jago R, Thompson JL. Dietary risk factors for the development of insulin resistance in adolescent girls: A 3-year prospective study. *Public Health Nutr.* 2014;17:361–8.

55. Zakrzewski-Fruer JK, Plekhanova T, Mandila D, Lekatis Y, Tolfrey K. Effect of breakfast omission and consumption on energy intake and physical activity in adolescent girls: A randomised controlled trial. *Br J Nutr.* 2017;118:392–400.

56. Rosen DS, American Academy of Pediatrics Committee on Adolescence. Identification and management of eating disorders in children and adolescents. *Pediatrics.* 2010;126:1240–53.

57. Ornstein RM, Rosen DS, Mammel KA et al. Distribution of eating disorders in children and adolescents using the proposed DSM-5 criteria for feeding and eating disorders. *J Adolesc Health.* 2013;53:303–5.

58. Herpertz-Dahlmann B. Adolescent eating disorders: Update on definitions, symptomatology, epidemiology, and comorbidity. *Child Adolesc Psychiatr Clin N Am.* 2015;24:177–96.

59. Gonzalez A, Kohn MR, Clarke SD. Eating disorders in adolescents. *Aust Fam Physician.* 2007;36:614–9.

60. Arcelus J, Mitchell AJ, Wales J, Nielsen S. Mortality rates in patients with anorexia nervosa and other eating disorders. A meta-analysis of 36 studies. *Arch Gen Psychiatry.* 2011;68:724–31.

61. Steinhausen H.-C. Outcome of eating disorders. *Child Adolesc Psychiatr Clin N Am.* 2009;18:225–42.

62. Mitchell JE, Crow S. Medical complications of anorexia nervosa and bulimia nervosa. *Curr Opin Psychiatry.* 2006;19:438–43.

63. Meczekalski B, Podfigurna-Stopa A, Katulski K. Long-term consequences of anorexia nervosa. *Maturitas.* 2013;75:215–20.

64. Smink FRE, van Hoeken D, Oldehinkel AJ, Hoek HW. Prevalence and severity of DSM-5 eating disorders in a community cohort of adolescents. *Int J Eat Disord.* 2014;47:610–9.

65. Mangweth-Matzek B, Hoek HW, Rupp CI et al. Prevalence of eating disorders in middle-aged women. *Int J Eat Disord.* 2014;47:320–4.

66. Dominé F, Berchtold A, Akré C, Michaud P-A, Suris J-C. Disordered eating behaviors: What about boys? *J Adolesc Health Off Publ Soc Adolesc Med.* 2009;44:111–7.

67. Campbell K, Peebles R. Eating disorders in children and adolescents: State of the art review. *Pediatrics.* 2014;134:582–92.

68. Trace SE, Baker JH, Peñas-Lledó E, Bulik CM. The genetics of eating disorders. *Annu Rev Clin Psychol.* 2013;9:589–620.

69. Duncan L, Yilmaz Z, Gaspar H et al. Significant locus and metabolic genetic correlations revealed in genome-wide association study of anorexia nervosa. *Am J Psychiatry.* 2017;174:850–8.

70. Lock J, Le Grange D, Agras WS et al. Randomized clinical trial comparing family-based treatment with adolescent-focused individual therapy for adolescents with anorexia nervosa. *Arch Gen Psychiatry.* 2010;67:1025–32.

71. Blessitt E, Voulgari S, Eisler I. Family therapy for adolescent anorexia nervosa. *Curr Opin Psychiatry.* 2015;28:455–60.

72. Couturier J, Kimber M, Szatmari P. Efficacy of family-based treatment for adolescents with eating disorders: A systematic review and meta-analysis. *Int J Eat Disord.* 2013;46:3–11.

73. Lock J. Evaluation of family treatment models for eating disorders. *Curr Opin Psychiatry.* 2011;24:274–9.

74. Katzman DK, Peebles R, Sawyer SM, Lock J, Le Grange D. The role of the pediatrician in family-based treatment for adolescent eating disorders:

Opportunities and challenges. *J Adolesc Health Off Publ Soc Adolesc Med.* 2013;53:433–40.

75. Le Grange D. Examining refeeding protocols for adolescents with anorexia nervosa (again): Challenges to current practices. *J Adolesc Health Off Publ Soc Adolesc Med.* 2013;53:555–6.

76. Doyle PM, Le Grange D, Loeb K, Doyle AC, Crosby RD. Early response to family-based treatment for adolescent anorexia nervosa. *Int J Eat Disord.* 2010;43:659–62.

77. Le Grange D, Lock J, Agras WS, Bryson SW, Jo B. Randomized clinical trial of family-based treatment and cognitive-behavioral therapy for adolescent bulimia nervosa. *J Am Acad Child Adolesc Psychiatry.* 2015;54:886–94.e2.

78. Berkman ND, Bulik CM, Brownley KA et al. Management of eating disorders. *Evid Report Technol Assess.* 2006;(135):1–166.

79. Holtkamp K, Konrad K, Kaiser N et al. A retrospective study of SSRI treatment in adolescent anorexia nervosa: Insufficient evidence for efficacy. *J Psychiatr Res.* 2005;39:303–10.

80. Kafantaris V, Leigh E, Hertz S et al. A placebo-controlled pilot study of adjunctive olanzapine for adolescents with anorexia nervosa. *J Child Adolesc Psychopharmacol.* 2011;21:207–12.

81. Kishi T, Kafantaris V, Sunday S, Sheridan EM, Correll CU. Are antipsychotics effective for the treatment of anorexia nervosa? Results from a systematic review and meta-analysis. *J Clin Psychiatry.* 2012;73:e757–66.

82. Carter JC, Mercer-Lynn KB, Norwood SJ et al. A prospective study of predictors of relapse in anorexia nervosa: Implications for relapse prevention. *Psychiatry Res.* 2012;200:518–23.

83. Grilo CM, Pagano ME, Stout RL et al. Stressful life events predict eating disorder relapse following remission: Six-year prospective outcomes. *Int J Eat Disord.* 2012;45:185–92.

84. Abitbol L, Zborovski S, Palmert MR. Evaluation of delayed puberty: What diagnostic tests should be performed in the seemingly otherwise well adolescent? *Arch Dis Child.* 2016;101(8):767–71.

85. ACOG Committee Opinion No. 740. American College of Obstetricians and Gynecologists. *Obstet Gynecol.* 2018;131:e205–13.

86. Klibanski A, Biller BM, Schoenfeld DA, Herzog DB, Saxe VC. The effects of estrogen administration on trabecular bone loss in young women with anorexia nervosa. *J Clin Endocrinol Metab.* 1995;80:898–904.

87. Bialo SR, Gordon CM. Underweight, overweight, and pediatric bone fragility: Impact and management. *Curr Osteoporos Rep.* 2014;12:319–28.

88. Ziglar S, Hunter TS. The effect of hormonal oral contraception on acquisition of peak bone mineral density of adolescents and young women. *J Pharm Pract.* 2012;25:331–40.

89. Cromer BA, Stager M, Bonny A et al. Depot medroxyprogesterone acetate, oral contraceptives and bone mineral density in a cohort of adolescent girls. *J Adolesc Health Off Publ Soc Adolesc Med.* 2004;35:434–41.

90. Committee on Adolescence. Contraception for adolescents. *Pediatrics.* 2014;134:e1244–56.

91. Committee on Adolescent Health Care Long-Acting Reversible Contraception Working Group, The American College of Obstetricians and Gynecologists. Committee opinion no. 539: Adolescents and long-acting reversible contraception: Implants and intrauterine devices. *Obstet Gynecol.* 2012;120:983–8.

92. Easter A, Treasure J, Micali N. Fertility and prenatal attitudes towards pregnancy in women with eating disorders: Results from the Avon Longitudinal Study of Parents and Children. *BJOG Int J Obstet Gynaecol.* 2011;118:1491–8.

93. Micali N, dos-Santos-Silva I, De Stavola B et al. Fertility treatment, twin births, and unplanned pregnancies in women with eating disorders: Findings from a population-based birth cohort. *BJOG Int J Obstet Gynaecol.* 2014;121:408–16.

94. Bulik CM, Hoffman ER, Von Holle A et al. Unplanned pregnancy in women with anorexia nervosa. *Obstet Gynecol.* 2010;116:1136–40.

95. Micali N, Simonoff E, Treasure J. Risk of major adverse perinatal outcomes in women with eating disorders. *Br J Psychiatry J Ment Sci.* 2007;190:255–9.

96. Linna MS, Raevuori A, Haukka J et al. Reproductive health outcomes in eating disorders. *Int J Eat Disord.* 2013;46:826–33.

97. Morgan JF, Lacey JH, Chung E. Risk of postnatal depression, miscarriage, and preterm birth in bulimia nervosa: Retrospective controlled study. *Psychosom Med.* 2006;68:487–92.

98. Kimmel MC, Ferguson EH, Zerwas S, Bulik CM, Meltzer-Brody S. Obstetric and gynecologic problems associated with eating disorders. *Int J Eat Disord.* 2016;49:260–75.

Reproductive effects of obesity in adolescents

22

WHITNEY WELLENSTEIN and NICHOLE TYSON

INTRODUCTION

It is currently estimated that 30% of children in North America are overweight or obese.[1,2] There are concerning disparities in obesity rates among population subgroups, with minority and low-income children and adolescents showing the highest rates of obesity.[1] Childhood obesity routinely translates into adult obesity, particularly for those children and teens with severe obesity and in older age groups.[3]

Childhood obesity is a risk factor for numerous health diseases such as cancer, cardiovascular disease, and diabetes.[1,4] In addition, obese females, specifically, can experience unique detrimental effects on their reproductive health, including menstrual dysfunction, polycystic ovarian syndrome, endometrial cancer, subfertility/infertility, and poor obstetric outcomes. They can also be at risk for unhealthy sexual behaviors and decreased contraception use.

Children and adolescents should be consistently screened for obesity. Once identified as obese or overweight, the patients and their parents should be educated about consequences of their children's condition and early interventions should be initiated to avoid the long-term effects of childhood obesity. Obesity management interventions should begin at the earliest age possible.[5] There is increasing evidence that childhood weight management strategies and education should begin even as early as managing weight gain in the pregnant mother.[3,6]

Providers should also provide education on normal versus abnormal pubertal stages as well as regularly assess development, menstrual cycles, body image, and warning signs for risky sexual behaviors. Specific considerations should be taken when starting treatment for various gynecologic conditions in obese adolescents to maximize efficacy and minimize side effects.

PUBERTY

Many factors, including race, genetics, body mass index (BMI), and environmental variations, play a role in the age of onset of puberty. Obese girls can fall on both ends of the spectrum, having been shown to experience either earlier menarche (before age 10 years) or late/absent menstruation, the latter being secondary to chronic anovulation.[7] One study showed that girls with high BMI had a higher prevalence of thelarche from ages 8 to 9, pubarche from 8 to 10, and menarche in preteen years than their normal weight counterparts.[8] It must be noted, however, that excess chest wall adiposity can mimic breast buds, and so palpation is the preferred method for assessing breast Tanner stage.

It has been debated whether increased body weight causes earlier onset of puberty or the onset of puberty triggers weight gain. Studies have shown that high BMI at ages as young as 5 years old and greater percentages of weight gain in the prepubertal years are associated with earlier onset of puberty. These studies suggest that it is a higher BMI in childhood and prepubertal years that serves as a risk factor for early puberty.[9,10]

MENSTRUAL CYCLE DYSFUNCTION

Menstrual irregularities are common in adolescents, often due to immaturity of the hypothalamic-pituitary-ovarian axis. However, obese girls may be at higher risk for menstrual irregularities due to abnormal hormonal fluctuations. With increasing adipose tissue, there are increased circulating estrogens secondary to peripheral aromatization. As a result, the follicle-stimulating hormone (FSH)/luteinizing hormone (LH) feedback system is disrupted, ovarian follicular development and endometrial proliferative/secretory cycles are altered and out of sync, and menstrual cycles become irregular and unpredictable.

Little research has addressed menstrual disturbances specifically in obese adolescents, so most data have been extrapolated from obese adult women. One study in Mexico looking at obese women without the diagnosis of polycystic ovarian syndrome (PCOS) showed that with increasing obesity, women had a higher probability of experiencing oligomenorrhea and amenorrhea.[11] This likely translates into the pediatric population as well.

Both the American Academy of Pediatrics and American College of Obstetricians and Gynecologists recommend annual evaluation of puberty development and menstrual cycles, when indicated, as a vital sign of overall health. A major piece of this evaluation is educating patients and families on what is "normal" puberty and what warrants further evaluation. Specific concerns in obese patients that require evaluation are not starting menses within 3 years of thelarche, not starting menses by age 14, with or without signs of hirsutism, having cycles that occur more frequently than 21 days or less frequently than every 45 days, and cycles more than 90 days apart.[12]

Polycystic ovarian syndrome

PCOS in adolescence is controversial, and the role of obesity in the development of PCOS is not fully understood, though it is thought to be a strong risk factor. Studies have shown that the prevalence of obesity in PCOS adolescent patients is higher than those without PCOS (63% versus 16%) and that the prevalence of PCOS in obese girls increases from a threefold elevation in overweight girls up to a 14-fold elevation in extremely obese girls.[13] In addition, obesity in adolescence is associated with development of PCOS and infertility later in life.[14,15]

Treatment mainstays primarily target ovulatory dysfunction. In addition, dietary and lifestyle modifications, which are discussed in the following, should also be encouraged. Weight reduction should be considered a primary therapy, as studies have shown that a 5%–10% weight loss can result in return of menstrual cycles and improve metabolic syndrome parameters.[16] All obese adolescents should be screened for signs and symptoms of PCOS, and those with PCOS and/or obesity should be screened for potential comorbid conditions. For a more comprehensive review of diagnosis and treatment, refer to Chapter 15.

Endometrial hyperplasia/cancer

Chronic anovulation and obesity are both risk factors for developing endometrial hyperplasia and endometrial cancer. Hyperplasia and cancer result from unopposed estrogen persistently stimulating the endometrial lining. While endometrial cancer is typically considered a disease of adult women (mean age at diagnosis is 61 years), there are case reports of endometrial cancer occurring in obese adolescents without hereditary malignancies as young as age 14, presenting with irregular menses and/or heavy bleeding.[17,18]

It is prudent to refer obese teens with oligomenorrhea and/or heavy menstrual bleeding for a gynecology consult for management and long-term follow-up. Treatment mainstay is to add progestins in the form of oral contraceptives (progestin-only or combined), cyclic progesterone, or levonorgestrel intrauterine device (IUD) to balance estrogen effects on the endometrium and prevent subsequent hyperplasia or cancer.

SEXUAL ACTIVITY

Beyond detrimental effects on physical health, pediatric obesity can also have negative consequences on psychosocial health. Depression, low self-esteem, and bullying are commonly reported in overweight and obese adolescents.[19–21] One's state of emotional well-being is important when establishing healthy behaviors and relationships, both friendly and sexual.

While several factors, such as low socioeconomic status and substance use, are known to contribute to high-risk sexual behaviors, obesity may be a less obvious but important aspect as well. There have been mixed results when looking at obese adolescents and their likelihood of engaging in risky sexual behaviors, with some studies showing a negative effect and some a positive effect. Higher rates of obesity in lower socioeconomic groups confound this research. However, when looking specifically at contraception use, a study looking at 18- to 19-year-old females showed that sexually active obese girls were less likely to use contraception, and if they did, were less likely to use

it regularly, than normal weight girls.[22] The underlying reason for less contraceptive use was not evaluated in this study, but possible hypotheses include low self-confidence to approach health-care providers and poorer access to health care in general. In addition, studies investigating generalized risky sexual behavior (i.e., young age at first intercourse, use of contraception, number of partners, substance use with intercourse) among adolescents show that girls who *perceived* themselves as overweight were more likely to engage in risky sexual behaviors than those who perceived themselves as normal weight.[23]

Understanding obesity as a risk factor for high-risk sexual behaviors is important when performing mental and sexual health screenings. While weight is a simple vital sign to assess, body perception requires more investigation. It is crucial to evaluate all adolescents' body image with each visit, whether overweight or not, to identify those potentially at risk for high-risk sexual behaviors. Whatever the cause—lack of education, poor access to health care, or low self-confidence that deters obese girls from using contraception—all adolescents, and particularly these patients, would benefit from regular discussions about contraception and healthy sexual behaviors.

REPRODUCTIVE TRACT INFECTIONS

Sexually transmitted infections (STIs) are difficult to study, in general, because they often go undetected, and rates are underreported. Along with sexual behaviors, one should inquire about risk of STIs in this population. A study looking specifically at obese 16- to 24-year-olds found no difference in STI rate compared to their normal weight counterparts.[24] As far as nonsexually transmitted reproductive tract infections, there are no studies looking at obese adolescents and rates of vaginitis infections, such as bacterial vaginosis or yeast.

Human papillomavirus (HPV)

The HPV vaccine is recommended in girls as young as 9 years up to age 45 to decrease the risk of cervical cancer later in life.[25] While the uptake of the HPV vaccine in the obese adolescent population is equivalent to that of normal weight adolescents, it is equally suboptimal in both groups.[26] In addition, obese women have been shown to have similar rates of HPV as normal weight women.[27] Therefore, all girls should receive equal counseling on vaccination and HPV transmission, with the goal of increasing HPV vaccination across the BMI spectrum.

CONTRACEPTIVE CONCERNS

As previously mentioned, hormonal contraceptives are indicated for the management of various conditions in obese adolescents, in addition to pregnancy prevention.

This section focuses on specific considerations when recommending contraceptive options to obese adolescents. The Centers for Disease Control and Prevention has published Criteria for Contraceptive use, which include

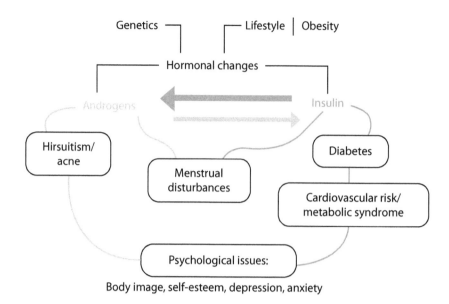

Figure 22.1 CDC medical eligibility criteria for contraceptive use. (From https://www.cdc.gov/reproductivehealth/contraception/pdf/summary-chart-us-medical-eligibility-criteria_508tagged.pdf, with permission.)

the condition of obesity. While no form of contraception is contraindicated in this group (Figure 22.1), some may be preferred over others to maximize efficacy and minimize side effects and risks (Table 22.1).

In summary, the implant and IUD remain the most effective forms of birth control across the BMI spectrum, with pregnancy rates less than 1%. If possible, depot medroxyprogesterone acetate (DMPA) should not be considered a top-tier option in these patients to avoid additional weight gain. Oral contraceptive pills and the vaginal ring have the same efficacy in obese and nonobese patients, with the transdermal patch possibly less effective with increasing body weight greater than 90 kg.[28] All combined hormonal options may pose an increased risk of venous thromboembolism, given that obesity and estrogen are both independent risk factors, and so patients should be assessed for risk and counseled accordingly.[41] If emergency contraception is needed in an obese patient, consider ulipristal acetate (UA) or the copper IUD as first-line agents.[39,40]

FERTILITY AND PREGNANCY OUTCOMES

Obesity and PCOS not only may have a detrimental effect on one's ability to get pregnant, but also increase the risk of complications once pregnancy is achieved. The etiology of obesity-related infertility is related to anovulation and the hyperandrogenic/insulin-resistant state discussed previously (see "Polycystic ovarian syndrome"). While not all obese women are infertile, those with a BMI greater than or equal to 32 at age 18 years have a relative risk of 2.7 of developing subsequent anovulatory infertility.[42] In addition, obese women may also require increased doses and more cycles of assisted reproductive technology (ART) to achieve pregnancy. Once pregnant, obese women, especially those with BMI greater than 40,

are at increased risk for miscarriage, birth defects, pre-eclampsia, gestational diabetes, and cesarean section.[42]

TREATMENT/PREVENTION OF OBESITY

Weight management in the child and adolescent includes strategies to both reduce obesity and promote sustained change. The key to weight loss in the child and adolescent is making changes in both diet and exercise. Most weight loss programs are based on promoting behavioral changes in the child and family. Bariatric surgery is also becoming more common in morbidly obese adolescents.

As previously mentioned, weight loss is considered a primary therapy for menstrual irregularities caused by anovulation and obesity. Even weight loss as small as 5%–10% of one's body weight can result in return of menstrual cycles and improve metabolic syndrome parameters.[16]

Diet

Treatment regimens for obesity in children and adolescents include modification of both the quantity and the quality of food consumed. Specific dietary modifications that have been associated with successful weight loss include decreasing sugary beverages, consuming fewer low-nutrient foods, and increasing consumption of high-nutrient foods such as fruits and vegetables.[43–47]

Activity

Strategies to promote weight loss in the child and adolescent include both increasing physical activity and reducing sedentary activity. Numerous studies have shown that when exercise is used as a primary intervention, significant improvements were demonstrated in numerous parameters, such as decreased fasting insulin, increased HDL,

Table 22.1 Contraceptive considerations in obese adolescents.

Contraceptive	Increased risk of pregnancy in obese patients?	Other considerations	Recommendations
Combined (estrogen/progesterone) hormonal options			
Combined oral contraceptive pills (COCs)	Data are mixed, but obese women do *not* seem to be at higher risk for pregnancy;[28,29] however, more research is needed on females with body mass index (BMI) >35	None	Can consider this method if no other medical contraindications
Transdermal patch	Higher body weight, >90 kg, possibly associated with higher rates of pregnancy[28]	Possible increased venous thromboembolism (VTE) risk compared with COCs[30,31]	Consider alternative options prior to starting this method in obese women
Vaginal ring	No[32]	High approval and acceptability compared with oral contraceptive pills in adolescent population[33]	Good first-line option
Progesterone-only options			
Progestin-only pills	No[34]	Unpredictable breakthrough bleeding	An option in girls with contraindication to estrogen
Depot medroxyprogesterone acetate (DMPA)	No	Baseline obesity associated with increased weight gain compared with nonobese patients (9 kg versus 4 kg after 18 months)[35]	Consider alternative options to avoid worsening obesity
Levonorgestrel intrauterine device (IUD)	No	Shown to be effective up to 7 years[36]	Good first-line option
Etonogestrel implant	No[37]	Has been shown to be effective up to 5 years, though more studies needed on 5-year use in obese women[38]	Good first-line option
Emergency contraception (EC)			
Levonorgestrel (LNG) pill	• BMI 25–29: Pregnancy odds ratio (OR) 2.09 versus normal weight patients • BMI >30: OR 4.41 versus normal weight patients[39]	None	Consider other EC options in overweight and obese patients
Ulipristal acetate	• BMI 25–29: No increased risk • BMI >30: OR 2.6 versus normal weight patients[39]	None	Preferred over LNG in patients with BMI >25
Copper IUD	No	• Most effective EC method • Requires insertion procedure • Provides up to 12 years of contraception[40]	Good first-line option

reduced body fat, and decreased insulin sensitivity.[48] The consensus for general exercise recommendations to promote weight loss for a child 5 years or older is to incorporate 60 minutes of moderate to vigorous physical activity daily and 180 minutes of any intensity physical activity daily for children under 4 years.[44–47]

Behavior

While dietary and physical activity changes are the key components of weight loss in children and adolescents, behavioral strategies are routinely employed as well.

Promoting small, successive changes in behavior, such as self-monitoring, goal setting, reinforcement for goal achievement, social support, and motivational techniques have all been shown to be successful.[43] Other strategies that have been found beneficial include eating out less, increasing frequency of family meals eaten together in the home, and discouraging using food as a reward.[44–47]

Family involvement

Childhood obesity treatments are most successful if they include family members (i.e., parents/caregivers) who are specifically involved in treatment and help facilitate and maintain these weight changes.[49] Interventions involving the family that center on promoting healthy diets, increasing exercise, and modifying eating behaviors can lead to improvements in weight-related illness, even with minor weight losses of 5%–10%.[50]

Prevention

It is imperative that preventative initiatives are implemented to promote healthy eating and physical activity. Preventing obesity in children and adolescents can be complex, as research has shown that rigid restriction or control of diet can trigger eating disorders in this vulnerable population.[51–53] Prevention programs that involve changes for the whole family that promote healthier food choices and increases in exercise are most likely to lead to positive and enduring change.[54]

Bariatric surgery

Bariatric surgery in adolescents will likely increase as the prevalence and severity of childhood obesity rises. The specific indications and patient criteria for bariatric surgery in adolescents are still being developed. However, it is generally agreed that those with severe obesity (BMI >40) with obesity-related health conditions who have unsuccessfully attempted weight loss with nonsurgical options are good candidates.[55] Surgery timing is ideally delayed until mid to late teen years, when skeletal maturity is reached. The risks of bariatric surgery vary depending on which procedure is used. Laparoscopic sleeve gastrectomy and adjustable gastric band are both restrictive procedures. The sleeve gastrectomy carries risks of bleeding, ulcers, gastroesophageal reflux disease, and staple disruption, while the adjustable band can have band slippage and/or erosion.[55] The Roux-en-Y gastric bypass surgery is a restrictive and malabsorptive procedure. It is the most effective for weight loss but carries more risks. Short-term risks include anastomotic leak and bowel obstruction, while long-term risks include nutritional deficiencies, dumping syndrome, and complications of the caliber of the bowel anastomosis.[55]

Early bariatric surgery could potentially alleviate several gynecologic and obstetric complications. Some studies have shown that fertility drastically improves following dramatic weight loss; therefore, having a contraceptive plan in place until optimal weight goal is achieved is recommended. Contraception would be advised for at least 12–18 months postoperatively and continued longer until the patient is ready to conceive. The gastric band and sleeve gastrectomy are both restrictive procedures, and so all contraceptives can be considered. However, in the Roux-en-Y gastric bypass, malabsorption is a key component of the rapid weight loss after bariatric surgery. Nonoral contraceptives, such as the IUD, implant, vaginal ring, or patch, may be preferred in this population for increased efficacy, with consideration of placing an IUD at the time of surgery if desired.[56,57]

CONCLUSIONS

In summary, childhood obesity can lead to numerous reproductive health conditions in adolescence and into adulthood. It is an important stage of development where lifelong habits are formed. There is enormous potential for prevention and treatment of lifestyle disease in the youth to prevent future issues with infertility, endometrial cancer, and metabolic syndrome. Weight loss programs should include the whole family and focus on health and growth, not just weight. Parents, communities, and the health-care system all need to be involved in both treatment and prevention programs. Positive education and prevention programs that focus on health promotion are the ideal models of reducing childhood obesity.

REFERENCES

1. Ogden CL, Carroll MD, Kit BK et al. Prevalence of childhood and adult obesity in the United States, 2011–2012. *JAMA.* 2014;311:806–14.
2. Roberts KC, Shields M, de Groh M et al. Overweight and obesity in children and adolescents: Results from the 2009 to 2011 Canadian Health Measures Survey. *Health Rep.* 2012;23:37–41.
3. Tyson N, Frank M. Childhood and adolescent obesity definitions as related to BMI, evaluation and management options. *Best Pract Res Clin Obstet Gynaecol.* 2017;48:158–64.
4. Boyer BP, Nelson JA, Holub SC. Childhood body mass index trajectories predicting cardiovascular risk in adolescence. *J Adolesc Health.* 2015;56:599–605.
5. Serdula MK, Ivery D, Coates RJ et al. Do obese children become obese adults? A review of the literature. *Prev Med.* 1993;22:167–77.
6. Lau EY, Liu J, Archer E et al. Maternal weight gain in pregnancy and risk of obesity among offspring a systematic review. *J Obes.* 2014;2014:524939.
7. Must A, Strauss RS. Risks and consequences of childhood and adolescent obesity. *Int J Obes Relat Metab Disord.* 1999;23(Suppl 2):S2–11.
8. Rosenfield RL, Lipton RB, Drum ML. Thelarche, pubarche, and menarche attainment in children with normal and elevated body mass index. *Pediatrics.* 2009;123:84–8.
9. Davison KK, Susman EJ, Birch LL. Percent body fat at age 5 predicts earlier pubertal development among girls at age 9. *Pediatrics.* 2003;111:815–21.
10. Lee JM, Appugliese D, Kaciroti N, Corwyn RF, Bradley RH, Lumeng JC. Weight status in young girls and the onset of puberty. *Pediatrics.* 2007;119:e624–30.
11. Castillo-Martínez L, López-Alvarenga JC, Villa AR et al. Menstrual cycle length disorders in 18- to 40-y-old obese women. *Nutrition.* 2003;19:317–20.
12. Menstruation in girls and adolescents: Using the menstrual cycle as a vital sign. Committee Opinion No. 651. American College of Obstetricians and Gynecologists. *Obstet Gynecol.* 2015;126:e143–6.

13. Christensen SB, Black MH, Smith N, Martinez MM, Jacobsen SJ, Porter AH, Koebnick C. Prevalence of polycystic ovary syndrome in adolescents. *Fertil Steril*. 2013;100:470-7.

14. Laitinen J, Taponen S, Martikainen H et al. Body size from birth to adulthood as a predictor of self-reported polycystic ovary syndrome symptoms. *Int J Obes*. 2003;27:710.

15. Rich-Edwards JW, Goldman MB, Willett WC, Hunter DJ, Stampfer MJ, Colditz GA, Manson JE. Adolescent body mass index and infertility caused by ovulatory disorder. *Am J Obstet Gynecol*. 1994;171:171-7.

16. Moran LJ, Pasquali R, Teede HJ, Hoeger KM, Norman RJ. Treatment of obesity in polycystic ovary syndrome: A position statement of the Androgen Excess and Polycystic Ovary Syndrome Society. *Fertil Steril*. 2009;92:1966-82.

17. Mitamura T, Warari H, Todo Y et al. A 14-year-old female patient with FIGO stage 1B endometrial carcinoma: A case report. *Int J Gynecol Cancer*. 2009;19:896-7.

18. Farhi DC, Nosanchuk J, Silverberg SG. Endometrial adenocarcinoma in women under 25 years of age. *Obstet Gynecol*. 1986;68:741-5.

19. Puhl R, Suh Y. Health consequences of weight stigma: Implications for obesity prevention and treatment. *Curr Obes Rep*. 2015;4:182-90.

20. Lunde C, Frisen A, Hwang CP. Is peer victimization related to body esteem in 10 year old girls and boys? *Body Image*. 2006;3:25-33.

21. Danielsen YS, Stormark KM, Nordhus IH et al. Factors associated with low self-esteem in child with overweight. *Obes Fact*. 2012;5:722-33.

22. Chang T, Davis M, Kusunoki Y et al. Sexual behavior and contraceptive use among 18- to 19-year-old adolescent women by weight status: A longitudinal analysis. *J Pediatr*. 2015;167:586-92.

23. Akers A, Cohen ED, Marshal MP et al. Objective and perceived weight: Associations with risky adolescent sexual behavior. *Perspect Sex Reprod Health*. 2016;48:129-37.

24. DeMaria AL, Lugo JM, Rahman M et al. Association between body mass index, sexually transmitted infections, and contraceptive compliance. *J Women's Health*. 2013;22:1062-8.

25. Meites E, Kempe A, Markowitz LE. Use of a 2-dose schedule for human papillomavirus vaccination–updated recommendations of the advisory committee on immunization practices. *MMWR*. 2016;65:1405-8.

26. Sundaram ME, Mason SM, Basta NE. HPV vaccine uptake among overweight and obese US adolescents: An analysis of the National Health and Nutrition Examination Survey (NHANES) 2009-2014. *Vaccine*. 2016;34:2501-6.

27. Wee CC, Huang A, Huskey KW et al. Obesity and the likelihood of sexual behavioral risk factors for HPV and cervical cancer. *Obesity*. 2008;16:2552-5.

28. Lopez LM, Bernholc A, Chen M et al. Hormonal contraceptives for contraception in overweight or obese women. *Cochrane Database Syst Rev*. 2013;4:7-8.

29. Brunner Huber LR, Toth JL. Obesity and oral contraceptive failure: Findings from the 2002 National Survey of Family Growth. *Am J Epidemiol*. 2007;166:1306-11.

30. Dore DD, Norman H, Loughlin J, Seeger JD. Extended case-control study results on thromboembolic outcomes among transdermal contraceptive users. *Contraception*. 2010;81(5):408-13.

31. Tepper NK, Dragoman MV, Gaffield ME, Curtis KM. Nonoral combined hormonal contraceptives and thromboembolism: A systematic review. *Contraception*. 2017;95:130-9.

32. Westhoff C. Higher body weight does not affect NuvaRing's efficacy. *Obstet Gynecol*. 2005;105:56S.

33. Stewart FH, Brown BA, Raine TR et al. Adolescent and young women's experience with the vaginal ring and oral contraceptive pills. *J Pediatr Adolesc Gynecol*. 2007;20:345-51.

34. Dinger JC, Cronin M, Möhner S et al. Oral contraceptive effectiveness according to body mass index, weight, age, and other factors. *Am J Obstet Gynecol*. 2009;201:263-e1.

35. Bonny AE, Ziegler J, Harvey R et al. Weight gain in obese and nonobese adolescent girls initiating depot medroxyprogesterone, oral contraceptive pills, or no hormonal contraceptive method. *Arch Pediatr Adolesc Med*. 2006;160:40-5.

36. Rowe P, Farley T, Peregoudov A, Piaggio G, Boccard S, Landoulsi S, Meirik O. Safety and efficacy in parous women of a 52-mg levonorgestrel-medicated intrauterine device: A 7-year randomized comparative study with the TCu380A. *Contraception*. 2016;93:498-506.

37. Hanna X, Wade JA, Peipert JF et al. Contraceptive failure rates of etonogestrel subdermal implants in overweight and obese women. *Obstet Gynecol*. 2012;120:21-6.

38. Ali M, Akin A, Bahamondes L et al. WHO study group on subdermal contraceptive implants for women. Extended use up to 5 years of the etonogestrel-releasing subdermal contraceptive implant: Comparison to levonorgestrel-releasing subdermal implant. *Hum Reprod*. 2016;31:2491-8.

39. Kapp N, Abitbol JL, Mathé H et al. Effect of body weight and BMI on the efficacy of levonorgestrel emergency contraception. *Contraception*. 2015;91:97-104.

40. United Nations Development Programme/ United Nations Population Fund/World Health Organization. Long-term reversible contraception; twelve years of experience with the TCu380A and TCu220C. *Contraception*. 1997;56:341-52.

41. Horton LG, Simmons KB, Kurtis KM. Combined hormonal contraceptive use among obese women and risk for cardiovascular events: A systematic review. *Contraception*. 2016;94:590-604.

42. Practice Committee of the American Society for Reproductive Medicine. Obesity and reproduction: An educational bulletin. *Fertil Steril*. 2008;90:S21–9.

43. TODAY Study Group. Design of a family-based lifestyle intervention for youth with type 2 diabetes: The TODAY study. *Int J Obes*. 2010;34:217–26.

44. Gurmani M, Birken C, Hamilton J. Childhood obesity. Causes, consequences and management. *Pediatr Clin North Am*. 2015;62:821–40.

45. Lau DCW, Douketis JD, Morrison KM et al. 2006 Canadian clinical practice guidelines on the management and prevention of obesity in adults and children (summary). *CMAJ*. 2007;176:S1–13.

46. Birken C, Hamilton J. Obesity in a young child. *CMAJ*. 2014;186:443.

47. Tremblay MS, Warburton DE, Janssen I et al. New Canadian physical activity guidelines. *Appl Physiol Nutr Metab*. 2011;36:36–46.

48. Davis CL, Pollock NK, Waller JL et al. Exercise dose and diabetes risk in overweight and obese children: A randomized control trial. *JAMA*. 2012;308:1103–12.

49. Boutelle KN, Cafri G, Crow SJ. Parent predictors of child weight change in family based behavioral obesity treatment. *Obesity*. 2012;20:1539–43.

50. Freedman DS, Sherry B. The validity of BMI as an indicator of body fatness and risk among children. *Pediatrics*. 2009;124(Suppl 1):S23–34.

51. Batch JA, Baur LA. Management and prevention of obesity and its complications in children and adolescents. *MJA*. 2005;182:130–5.

52. Fisher JO, Birch LL. Parents' restrictive feeding practices are associated with young girls' negative self-evaluation of eating. *J Am Diet Assoc*. 2000;100:1341–6.

53. Birch LL, Fisher JO. Development of eating behaviors among children and adolescents. *Pediatrics*. 1998;101(Suppl 2):539–49.

54. Strauss RS. Childhood obesity and self-esteem. *Pediatrics*. 2000;105:e15.

55. Greydanus DE, Agana M, Kamboj MK, Shebrain S, Soares N, Eke R, Patel DR. Pediatric obesity: Current concepts. *Dis Mon*. 2018;64(4):98–156.

56. Hillman JB, Miller RJ, Inge TH. Menstrual concerns and intrauterine contraception among adolescent bariatric surgery patients. *J Women's Health*. 2011;20:533–8.

57. Murthy AS. Obesity and contraception: Emerging issues. *Semin Reprod Med*. 2010;28:156–63.

Transgender care in adolescents

23

STEPHANIE CIZEK and GYLYNTHIA TROTMAN

OVERVIEW

Gender identity is a person's innermost concept of self as male, female, a blend of both, or neither.[1] One's self-awareness as male or female evolves gradually during infant life and childhood.[2] Gender variant or nonconforming children and adolescents experience and express gender in ways that often do not follow societal expectations and cultural norms.[3] For transgender children, their gender identity does not match with the gender they were assigned at birth.[4] One's identification as transgender or gender nonconforming (TGN) itself is not considered a pathologic diagnosis; however, gender dysphoria (GD), which has replaced the previous diagnosis of gender identity disorder, refers to the discomfort or distress that may occur when one's self-identified gender is not aligned with the sex assigned at birth and is defined in the *Diagnostic and Statistical Manual of Mental Disorders, Fifth Edition (DSM-5)*.[5] It is important to note that not every TGN individual will have gender dysphoria, as distressing symptoms may improve with treatment, such as social transitioning, social and family support, hormonal therapy, or surgical intervention.[1]

The concepts of gender identity and gender expression, as well as the etiology of gender dysphoria, likely reflect a complex interplay of biological, environmental, and cultural factors.[2] Although the term *transgender* is commonly used, it is considered a blanket term encompassing many gender identities, and terminology and its use continue to evolve. Table 23.1 shows common current definitions, albeit not an exhaustive list.[2,6–8] For our discussion, we use the terms *transgender girls/females/women* in reference to individuals who are assigned male at birth (AMAB) and *transgender boys/males/men* for individuals who are assigned female at birth (AFAB).

HEALTH AND SOCIAL RISKS

Recently there has been heightened public awareness and an increase in the number of TGN youth presenting for care.[4,6] However, there continues to be significant gaps in knowledge and lack of robust scientifically validated information on which to guide care.[1] Transgender youth are an underserved population confronted with numerous health and social hardships. This population often faces bullying and harassment at home, in schools, and in their communities and reports the highest rates of sexual harassment.[3,6] Given the rates of discrimination, victimization, and family rejection, they are at increased risk of homelessness and entering the foster care system.[6] This, in turn, can lead to increased risk-taking behaviors, such as exchanging sex for money and drug use with higher rates of substance abuse, HIV, and other sexually transmitted infections (STIs).[4,6,9] Transgender girls have among the highest rates of HIV reported.[3,9] Research also shows a significant mental health burden with higher rates of depression and anxiety among TGN youth. One of the most alarming statistics is the risk of suicidality and self-harm among this vulnerable group. The attempted suicide rate has been reported to be as high as 41%, compared to 1.6% in the general population.[3,4,6,9] Unfortunately, access to health care also remains a challenge, and many postpone medical care or are unable to afford it.[6] Familial acceptance and support is one key factor to counteracting the increased risks, as it is shown to improve psychological outcomes and decreases suicide attempts, homelessness, and involvement with sex work.[1]

PREVALENCE AND NATURAL HISTORY

The number of youth who identify as TGN is difficult to determine. Current best estimates are derived from the Youth Risk Behavior Survey of 2011, which surveyed 2730 students in 22 public schools, and found that 1.3% of those students identified as TGN.[10]

It is known that not all TGN children will persistently identify as transgender into adolescence, and the likelihood of persistence from childhood into adolescence and adulthood is difficult to predict for any specific child.[1,2] Reported rates of persistence or continued gender variance versus desistance or reversion to alignment with their gender assigned at birth range from 2.2%–30% among transgender females and 12%–50% among transgender males.[6] However, these estimates are extremely flawed, largely due to high variability in definitions, and it is likely that the proportion of patients who persist from childhood into adulthood is much higher.[2] Among children whose gender-variant identity persists into adolescence, it has been shown that the overwhelming majority will indeed maintain transgender identity as adults.[1]

DIAGNOSIS

When a child's or adolescent's gender nonconforming behavior and associated dysphoria remain persistent, support and intervention is indicated. The *DSM-5* outlines the criteria for diagnosis of GD, which includes at least 6 months of marked incongruence with one's experienced gender and the gender assigned at birth and significant distress and/or impairment in social, school, or other important areas of functioning.[2,5] While there is no proven optimal approach for any individual person, the World Professional Association for Transgender Health (WPATH), Endocrine Society (ES),

Table 23.1 Definitions.

Term	Definition
Cisgender/Cis	Someone who exclusively identifies as their sex assigned at birth.
Transgender/Trans	An umbrella term of many gender identities describing those who do not identify or exclusively identify with their sex assigned at birth.
Gender nonconforming	A term used to describe some people whose gender expression is different from conventional expectations of masculinity and femininity. Not all gender nonconforming people identify as transgender, nor are all transgender individuals gender nonconforming.
Gender expression	The physical/external manifestation of one's gender identity through clothing, hairstyle, voice, pronouns, body characteristics, etc.
Gender identity	One's internal, deeply held sense of gender.
Gender incongruence	This is an umbrella term used when the gender identity and/or gender expression differ from what is typically associated with the designated gender. Gender incongruence is also the proposed name of the gender identity–related diagnoses in *International Classification of Diseases, Eleventh Revision* (ICD-11).
Sex	Attributes that typically characterize biological maleness or femaleness, such as sex chromosomes, gonads, internal and external genitalia, etc.
Sexual orientation	This term describes an individual's enduring physical and emotional attraction to another person.
Transition	A person's process of developing and assuming a gender expression to match their gender identity.
Gender fluid	A changing or "fluid" gender identity.
Transgender female	This refers to individuals assigned male at birth (AMAB) but who identify and live as a woman or girl.
Transgender male	This refers to individuals assigned female at birth (AFAB) but who identify and live as a man or boy.

Source: Hembree W et al. J Clin Endocrinol Metab. 2017;102:3869–903; Conard L. J Pediatr Urol. 2017;13:300–4; LGBTQ+ Definitions. Trans student educational resources. http://www.transstudent.org/definitions. Accessed November 30, 2017; GLAAD Media Reference Guide-Transgender. Glossary of terms. https://www.glaad.org/reference/ transgender. Accessed November 30, 2017.

and American Psychological Association (APA) all support the following:

1. Diagnosis of gender dysphoria by a trained mental health provider (MHP)
2. Treatment of coexisting psychiatric conditions in both the child and the caregivers
3. Education and counseling regarding treatment options, including age-appropriate information given to the child
4. Safety assessment

All three organizations discourage the use of punishment for gender-variant behaviors.[2,9,11] The ES and WPATH provide detailed clinical practice guidelines for diagnosis and management and support the initiation of medical management for adolescents who fulfill eligibility criteria and have undergone appropriate psychological assessment.[1,2,11] In addition, standardized questionnaires that assess gender identity and dysphoria in children and adolescents have been developed, which can be used as a guide for clinicians in the office[3,12–14]; however, clinicians should be aware that all currently available versions have been criticized as overly binary.

MANAGEMENT

Management for transgender youth includes social transitioning or externally presenting in one's authentic/affirmed gender, use of puberty blockers, gender-affirming hormonal management with estrogen or testosterone, and gender-affirming surgical management.[6] In addition to the role of the MHP in aiding with diagnosis, an array of providers including endocrinologists, adolescent medicine specialists, gynecologists, urologists, and other surgeons and family practitioners may manage hormonal, surgical, and general medical care as appropriate.[3] Treatment is patient centered: some TGN youth do not require complete phenotypic transition and experience improvement or significant relief of gender dysphoria with social transition alone, while some youth will proceed with hormonal and/or surgical management.[3] Ultimately, the management of patients seeking gender-affirming therapy is best undertaken with a multidisciplinary team, with providers skilled in caring for gender diverse youth. Incorporating social workers and nursing into the care of TGN youth is essential, as they can often aid in the process of educating the patients and families while offering support and addressing parental consent, insurance, and social and financial concerns.

Hormone management: Puberty suppression

Hormonal management of the adolescent may be considered in two phases. The first phase involves the use of pubertal suppression with the use of gonadotropin-releasing hormone agonists (GnRHas), which prevents progression of secondary sexual characteristics incongruent with the affirmed gender and allows time for further exploration of gender identity (Table 23.2).[3,4,15] Alternate medications to suppress puberty, such as oral/depot progestins or antiestrogens, are not as effective as GnRHas in suppressing puberty; however, these may be considered

Table 23.2 Pubertal suppression.

Care goals	Management	Adverse effects	Monitoring as clinically indicated
• Decrease the psychologic distress caused by puberty • Prevent development of secondary sex characteristics that are difficult to reverse • May induce some pubertal regression (atrophy of breast tissue and cessation of menses in girls, decreases in testicular volume in boys) • Allow time for patients to explore gender identity and their desired degree of social transition before initiating irreversible therapies	• GnRH agonists • Injection: depot-leuprolide acetate, typically 3.75 mg monthly, or 11.25 mg every 10–12 weeks • Histrelin implant	Hot flashes, fatigue, mood changes, decreased bone mineral density/decreased bone mineral accrual, changes in growth velocity. Limiting growth of penis and scrotum may impact ability to use native genital tissue in future genital surgeries	Anthropometry • Blood pressure • Height/weight • Tanner stage Laboratory evaluation • Luteinizing hormone/follicle-stimulating hormone • Estradiol/testosterone • 25OH vitamin D Dual-energy x-ray absorptiometry scan every 1–2 years Bone age (if clinically indicated)

Source: Hembree W et al. *J Clin Endocrinol Metab.* 2017;102:3869–903; Coleman E et al. *Int J Transgend.* 2011;13:165–232.

if GnRHas are not available or are cost prohibitive.[2] For some, the experience of full endogenous puberty may seriously interfere with healthy psychological functioning and well-being. Suppression prior to the onset of puberty is not recommended.[2] Eligibility and readiness criteria to support initiation of puberty suppression are as follows[2,4]:

1. Diagnosis of gender dysphoria established by qualified MHP
2. Physical examination reveals Tanner stage II or greater
3. Pubertal changes worsen gender dysphoria
4. Exclusion of psychiatric diagnosis that prevents proper diagnosis
5. No psychiatric or medical contraindications to treatment
6. Adequate support
7. Patient understands treatment plan and risks and is able to give informed consent

Puberty suppression is considered fully reversible with resumption of isosexual pubertal development upon discontinuation.[3,4] The benefits of pubertal suppression have been demonstrated, with increased psychologic functioning and positive body image, in addition to high rates of satisfaction after hormone therapy and surgery.[16] This is likely attributed to the prevention of irreversible secondary sexual characteristics. Appropriate patient counseling should include both a review of known risks, as well as risks that are still unknown (such as long-term impact on bone health, growth, and cognitive development). The patients, families, and providers should then balance the reasonable risks of nontreatment. Nontreatment should not be viewed as a neutral option, given the potential distressing effects of irreversible secondary sexual characteristics.[6]

Gender-affirming hormone management

The second phase for some patients is pubertal induction with gender-affirming hormone therapy.[3] Unlike with pubertal suppression, changes induced by gender-affirming

hormone management may not be fully reversible.[2,4] The readiness criteria for gender-affirming hormone therapy include all criteria for GnRHa, plus a persistence of gender dysphoria. Although 16 years has traditionally been recommended as the lower age limit for initiating hormone treatment, it is now recognized that it is appropriate to initiate treatment earlier than age 16 years in some patients to avoid the potential psychological and physiologically adverse effects of prolonged delay of puberty.[2,3] In addition, for those patients who did not undergo pubertal suppression, continued dysphoria with secondary sexual characteristics not in alignment with their identity may be too distressing. Transgender girls may undergo feminizing therapy with estrogen to develop female secondary sexual characteristics, and transgender boys may undergo masculinizing therapy with testosterone to develop male secondary sexual characteristics.[17] Close follow-up and monitoring of laboratory and anthropomorphic measurements are required, especially initially, for patients on gender-affirming hormone therapy, as it is associated with several known risks.[4,17] Treatment guidelines are found in Table 23.3. All patients should be screened for contraindications to testosterone or estrogen use and counseled on risks.[2]

Transgender male: Methyltestosterone injections

Testosterone is given with low initial doses that are gradually increased, and maintained at the lowest level possible to achieve the desired masculinizing effects, while remaining within male physiologic levels (320–1000 ng/dL).[18]

Transgender female: Estrogen

Estrogen is also given in a slowly escalating regimen. Ideally, serum estradiol levels should be maintained in the premenopausal range ($<$200 pg/mL), and testosterone in the physiologic female range ($<$25–55 ng/dL).[2,18,19]

Table 23.3 Gender-affirming hormone management.

	Care goals	Pubertal induction regimen	Adverse effects	Monitoring as clinically indicated
Trans-male	Decrease psychologic distress, suppress menses, induce masculine secondary sex characteristics	• Testosterone esters (intramuscular or subcutaneous) • 25 mg/m² every 2 weeks initially • Increase dose by 25 mg/m² every 6 months to adult dose of 100–200 mg/m² every 2 weeks[a]	Erythrocytosis, hyperlipidemia, hypertension, mood changes, sleep apnea, weight gain, acne, salt retention	Anthropometry: • Blood pressure • Height/weight • Tanner stage Laboratory testing: • Hemoglobin/hematocrit, lipids, testosterone, 25–OH vitamin D
Trans-female	Decrease psychologic distress, induce breast enlargement and body fat redistribution, reduce testicular volume, reduce hair growth	• Oral 17β-estradiol • 5 ug/kg/d initially • Increase dose by 5 ug/kg/d every 6 months to adult dose 2–6 mg/day[a] • Transdermal 17β-estradiol (patches changed 2×/week) • 6.25–12.5 ug/24 hours initially • Increase by 12.5 ug/24 hours every 6 months to adult dose 50–200 ug/24 hours	Thromboembolism, hypertension, liver dysfunction, prolactinoma development	Anthropometry: • Blood pressure • Height/weight • Tanner stage Laboratory testing: • Estradiol, 25–OH vitamin D Prolactinoma screen (prolactin level, visual field screen) yearly during induction, then every 2 years

Source: Hembree W et al. *J Clin Endocrinol Metab.* 2017;102:3869–903; Care for Transgender Adolescents. Committee Opinion No. 685. American College of Obstetricians and Gynecologists. *Obstet Gynecol.* 2017;129:e11–6.

[a] Postpubertal patients may increase testosterone or estrogen dosing more rapidly. Alternate testosterone and estrogen regimens may include other routes of medication delivery or depot formulations.

Oral preparations of estrogen have increased risk of VTE compared with transdermal or parenteral regimens.[18,19] Additionally, conjugated and synthetic estrogens may also pose greater risk compared to 17β-estradiol administration due to the inability to regulate doses by measuring serum levels. It is recommended that ethinyl estradiol specifically not be used for any transgender treatment plan.[2]

For transgender girls who have not undergone puberty suppression, antiandrogens such as spironolactone or GnRH agonists are added concurrently to the hormone regimen as needed. These individuals may also require high doses of estrogen (2–6 mg/d) to achieve the desired results, and treatment with physiologic estrogen alone may be insufficient to adequately suppress testosterone.[2,18]

Surgical management

A variety of surgical options are available for transgender men and women (Table 23.4).

While mastectomy for transgender males may be considered and performed before the age of 18, the WPATH and ES recommend avoiding genital surgery until the adolescent reaches the legal age of majority, typically reserved for patients 18 years or older.[2,4,11] However, gender-affirming surgeries have been reported in adolescents under the age of 18 years, and discussion as to appropriate timing

remains very controversial.[3,20] Although every case should be considered individually, there are significant concerns associated with performing irreversible surgeries on minors. Variance from the current guidelines as established by ES and WPATH must be taken with extreme caution and involve a thorough discussion of ethical principles.[2,3,11,20]

Transgender males

For the transgender male patient, the gynecologist and the patient should discuss the benefits of salpingectomy compared with salpingo-oophorectomy at the time of hysterectomy.[4] In the perioperative period, there is a

Table 23.4 Gender-affirming surgeries.

Trans-female	• *Chest*: Breast augmentation • *Genital*: Vaginoplasty/creation of neovagina (may require vaginal dilation), labiaplasty, orchiectomy; in future, possible uterine/ovarian transplant • *Other*: Tracheal shave, facial feminization, voice therapy, facial hair removal
Trans-male	• *Chest*: Mastectomy • *Genital*: Hysterectomy ± salpingo-oophorectomy, metoidioplasty, phalloplasty

theoretical concern for increased risk of venous thrombo-embolism and some reports of increased risk of bleeding at the vaginal cuff for patients on testosterone; however, current evidence does not support increased perioperative risks associated with continuation of testosterone.[21] Temporary discontinuation of testosterone may only likely serve to increase patient psychologic stress.[21] Therefore, unless recommended for specific patient-driven indication, in general, mastectomy and genital surgery do not require interruption of testosterone. Vaginal hysterectomy is the recommended route of hysterectomy, followed by laparoscopic/robotic hysterectomy whenever possible over abdominal hysterectomy.[22] Studies have shown that vaginal hysterectomy is both feasible and safe among transgender men, including those on testosterone.[21,23]

Transgender females

Vaginoplasty procedures and orchiectomy for transgender women should be performed by specialists with surgical training in genital reconstructive surgeries. However, gynecologists can care for patients postoperatively with vaginal dilation and care of the neovagina.[4]

ROUTINE GYNECOLOGIC CARE

Gynecologists have an essential role in providing care for TGN youth, including preventive health care with essential counseling, screening exams and testing, fertility preservation counseling, and menstrual management.

Providers should refrain from assumptions regarding sexual partnership of transgender patients. Just as cis-gender persons can be heterosexual, homosexual, or bisexual, the same is true for transgender individuals.[1] As such, patients should be counseled and offered age- and risk-appropriate health screenings and contraception as indicated. All TGN patients should be counseled on safe sex practices and undergo regular STI screening for gonorrhea, chlamydial infection, hepatitis B, syphilis, and HIV based on local prevalence rate and individual sexual activity.[4,24] As transgender male adolescents most often have natal internal sex organs, providers should continue routine evaluation for menstrual and other gynecologic concerns, including but not limited to the use of ultrasonography, bleeding disorder workup, and pregnancy testing, as indicated. It is important that a provider does not ignore common presenting problems and does not miss diagnosing a serious underlying concern due to lack of knowledge regarding a patient's present sex organs.[4]

Contraception

Although gender-affirming hormone management may negatively impact fertility, the effects may be partially reversible. Transgender females on estrogen may still produce sperm and may have the ability to impregnate partners. As such, they should be counseled on barrier methods for themselves and contraception for their partners. In addition, transgender men on testosterone who retain reproductive organs also remain at risk for pregnancy.[4] Testosterone is a known teratogen, and patients at risk for pregnancy should have reliable contraception when using this medication. Many patients and even some providers believe, erroneously, that effective contraception is provided via the use of testosterone, especially in patients who develop amenorrhea. However, in one study of 41 pregnant transgender men, 25 were on testosterone at the time of pregnancy.[25] In another study of transgender men on testosterone who were at risk for pregnancy, most expressed a desire to avoid pregnancy, but few used condoms or contraception.[26] Although there is little information on contraceptive use among transgender women, patients should be counseled on all contraceptive options based on the Centers for Disease Control and Prevention (CDC) U.S. Medical Eligibility Criteria for Contraceptive Use (US MEC) and the U.S. Selected Practice Recommendations for Contraceptive Use.[27,28] Due to the concern or desire to limit exogenous estrogen, progestin-only methods are commonly used.[4] The progestin-containing intrauterine system (IUD) has become particularly useful for contraception, given the typically favorable bleeding profile and ease of use. However, providers should be aware that a number of TGN youth use combined hormonal contraceptive options and are happy with that method.

Menstrual management/suppression

Menses may be associated with significant anxiety in transgender men, and menstrual suppression should be offered for those who desire it. Dysmenorrhea or premenstrual syndrome may be the presenting symptoms of gender dysphoria.[4] Discussing the psychologic and physical impact of menstruation is important to guide treatment. As with any patient undergoing menstrual suppression, realistic goals and expectations should be discussed; particularly, complete amenorrhea should not be guaranteed, as it may be difficult to achieve.[6,29] Similar to contraceptive counseling, data on menstrual suppression for this population are lacking, and progestin-only options including progestin-only pills, medroxyprogesterone acetate injections, or IUD are often used. However, extended cycling or continuous-use combined hormonal contraceptives are also acceptable based on the desires of the patient.[4] The use of GnRH agonists in transgender patients for the indication of menstrual suppression is discouraged, given its adverse effect profile, associated costs, and safe hormonal alternatives. Patients on testosterone generally experience cessation of menses within 6 months and have an amenorrhea rate of greater than 90% by 1 year.[30]

Surgical methods of menstrual suppression include endometrial ablation and hysterectomy. However, endometrial ablation is not recommended in adolescents, due to the high failure rate, the overall lack of data in adolescents, and the increased risks if subsequent pregnancy occurs. Hysterectomy is discussed separately as part of surgical management for gender dysphoria; however, if considered solely for the purpose of menstrual suppression, it is not recommended due to the comparatively high risk of morbidity and mortality compared to other available methods.[29]

Cervical cancer screening/prevention

The HPV vaccine should be administered according to age-appropriate guidelines to both transgender male and female patients. Cervical cancer screening should follow current guidelines for patients who retain a cervix.[31] Patients with a neocervix that is created from the glans penis may consider cervical cancer screening with cytology, although this is controversial.[19] Screening guidelines for patients with a neovagina are not well established. Pap smears have an increased likelihood of insufficient tissue in transgender men, which is likely related to testosterone use.[32,33] In addition, they are also less likely to be up to date on their Pap smears, and, if Pap is inadequate, less likely to return for a repeat Pap smear within the recommended time period.[32,33] As a pelvic exam may be associated with significant distress in some patients, special consideration should be made for the patient's comfort. Pelvic exams should move at a pace that is appropriate for the patient. The patient should be counseled on the indications and reassured as to their control over the exam.

FERTILITY

Transgender youth face potential infertility as a result of medical treatments intended to facilitate transition to their affirmed gender.[15] Treatment guidelines recommend a discussion regarding fertility prior to the initiation of puberty blockers, gender-affirming hormones, and surgical management.[2,6] Currently, sperm banking and embryo/oocyte cryopreservation are established methods for fertility preservation. Ovarian tissue and testicular tissue cryopreservation are experimental options that are currently being investigated under research protocols.[15]

Although puberty blockers are reversible, they prevent maturation of primary oocytes and spermatogonia to mature oocytes and sperm. Transgender females who use estrogen may have impairment of spermatogenesis and an absence of Leydig cells in the testis. Testosterone use may result in ovarian stromal hyperplasia and follicular atresia. Although some of the effects of gender-affirming hormone therapy appear partially reversible, the threshold for which fertility is impaired is unknown, and duration of use will likely be an important factor.[2,15] Further research is needed to establish effects of hormone treatment on natal gonads. As TGN youth are presenting and initiating treatment at younger ages, a discussion on the limited currently available information and the potential for irreversible effects of hormone treatment on fertility is particularly important. However, adolescents may not feel qualified to make decisions on fertility or may not be able to consider the true impact.[2]

The majority of transgender adults believe that fertility preservation should be discussed and offered and express desire for biological children and fertility preservation, had it been offered.[34–36] However, rates of fertility preservation utilization among transgender youth are low.[37] In one survey, although many TGN youth reported knowledge of fertility-associated risks with treatment, few expressed the desire to have biological children.[38] In addition, there remains a paucity of literature on fertility desires and parenthood goals for TGN youth and whether these youth may change their perspectives about fertility preservation later in life, particularly after transitioning to their affirmed gender.[36]

Unfortunately, to date there are no formally evaluated decision aids. Although early discussion is desirable, it is not always possible to proceed with fertility preservation prior to initiating hormonal management.[15] Considerations for transgender males include the possibility of increased distress due to delays in treatment to allow for oocyte retrieval, increased circulating estrogen from ovarian stimulation, and invasive techniques required for harvesting oocytes, which may exacerbate dysphoria. For transgender females, the act of sperm extraction or masturbation may also be distressing.[15]

If fertility preservation was not accomplished prior to initiating treatment, patients can temporarily stop gender-affirming hormones or puberty suppression to allow for sperm banking or oocyte cryopreservation; however, the undesirable effects of development of isosexual secondary sexual characteristics may be distressing, and the length of time required off treatment to allow for maturation of gametes is unknown.[2,15] Alternatively, preservation of ovarian or testicular tissue using protocols approved by the Institutional Review Board (IRB) could be pursued prior to the use of gender-affirming hormones. However, the use of tissue cryopreservation in transgender minors is controversial and is not available at many institutions, unless specifically accounted for in current IRB protocols. Finally, the cost associated with available fertility preservation options may be prohibitive.

CREATING A SAFE SPACE FOR PATIENTS

The clinician providing care for transgender patients should be prepared to assist or refer transgender individuals as indicated.[19] Providers should work to create a safe and supportive environment for TGN youth. This includes inquiring about gender identity or variance as part of routine clinical care.[19] When a youth identifies as TGN, the use of the patient's preferred name and pronouns while communicating verbally and in medical records is critical. In addition, providing neutral intake forms, labeling restrooms as gender neutral, training office staff on knowledge and sensitivity toward TGN patients, and using gender-affirming language are a few things that can be done to encourage a welcoming environment.[4,19]

REFERENCES

1. Lopez X, Marinkovic M, Eimicke T et al. Statement on gender affirmative approach to care from the Pediatric Endocrine Society Special Interest Group on Transgender Health. *Curr Opin Pediatr.* 2017;29:475–80.

2. Hembree W, Cohen-Kettenis P, Gooren L et al. Endocrine treatment of gender dysphoric/incongruent persons: An Endocrine Society clinical practice guideline. *J Clin Endocrinol Metab.* 2017;102:3869–903.

3. Unger C. Gynecologic care for transgender youth. *Curr Opin Obstet Gynecol.* 2014;26:347–54.

4. Care for Transgender Adolescents. Committee Opinion No. 685. American College of Obstetricians and Gynecologists. *Obstet Gynecol.* 2017;129:e11–6.

5. American Psychiatric Association (APA). *Fact Sheet: Gender Dysphoria.* Washington, DC: APA; 2012. http://www.dsm5.org/Documents/Gender%20 Dysphoria%20Fact%20Sheet.pdf. Accessed December 28, 2017.

6. Conard L. Supporting and caring for transgender and gender nonconforming youth in the urology practice. *J Pediatr Urol.* 2017;13:300–4.

7. LGBTQ+ Definitions. Trans student educational resources. http://www.transstudent.org/definitions. Accessed November 30, 2017.

8. GLAAD Media Reference Guide-Transgender. Glossary of terms. https://www.glaad.org/reference/ transgender. Accessed November 30, 2017.

9. Grant J, Mottet L, Tanis J et al. *Injustice at Every Turn: A Report of the National Transgender Discrimination Survey.* Washington, DC: National Center for Transgender Equality and National Gay and Lesbian Task Force; 2011.

10. Shields J, Cohen R, Glassman J. Estimating population size and demographic characteristics of lesbian, gay, bisexual and transgender youth in middle school. *J Adoelsc Health.* 2013;52:248–50.

11. Coleman E, Bockting W, Botzer M et al. Standards of care for the health of transsexual, transgender and nonconforming people, version 7. *Int J Transgend.* 2011;13:165–232.

12. Deogracias J, Johnson L, Meyer-Bahlburg H et al. The gender identity/gender dysphoria questionnaire for adolescents and adults. *J Sex Res.* 2007;44:370–9.

13. Adelson S, Bockting W. *Caring for Gender Dysphoric Children and Adolescents.* Boston, MA: National LGBT Health Education Center; 2014. https://www. lgbthealtheducation.org/webinar/gender-dysphoric-youth/. Accessed June 5, 2019.

14. Johnson L, Bradley S, Birkenfeld-Adams A et al. A parent-report gender identity questionnaire for children. *Arch Sex Behav.* 2004;33:105–16.

15. Finlayson C, Johnson E, Chen D et al. Proceedings of the Working Group Session on Fertility Preservation for Individuals with Gender and Sex Diversity. *Transgender Health.* 2016;1:99–107.

16. De Vries A, McGuire J, Steensma T et al. Young adult psychological outcome after puberty suppression and gender reassignment. *Pediatrics.* 2014;134:696–704.

17. Jarin J, Pine-Twaddell E, Trotman G et al. Cross-sex hormones and metabolic parameters in adolescents with gender dysphoria. *Pediatrics.* 2017;139(5). doi: 10.1542/peds.2016-3173.

18. Jarin J, Johnson E, Gomez-Lobo V. Fertility preservation in patients with gender dysphoria. In: Woodruff T, Gosiengfiao Y, eds. *Pediatric and Adolescent Oncofertility: Best Practices and Emerging Technologies.* Philadelphia, PA: Springer; 2017, 179–192.

19. Health Care for Transgender Individuals. Committee Opinion No. 512. American College of Obstetricians and Gynecologists. *Obstet Gynecol.* 2011;118:1454–8.

20. Milrod C. How young is too young: Ethical concerns in genital surgery of the transgender MTF adolescent. *J Sex Med.* 2014;11:338–46.

21. Cizek S, Nguyen N, Lyon L et al. Combined hysterectomy and mastectomy surgery for transgender patients in an integrated health care setting. *Int J Transgend.* 2017;18:382–8.

22. Choosing the Route of Hysterectomy for Benign Disease. Committee Opinion No. 701. American College of Obstetricians and Gynecologists. *Obstet Gynecol.* 2017;129:e155–9.

23. Obedin-Maliver J, Light A, de Haan G, Jackson R. Feasibility of vaginal hysterectomy for female to male transgender men. *Obstet Gynecol.* 2017;129:457–63.

24. Centers for Disease Control and Prevention. STD and HIV screening recommendations. http://www. cdc.gov/std. Accessed August 20, 2017.

25. Light A, Obedin-Maliver J, Sevelius J et al. Transgender men who experienced pregnancy after female-to-male gender transitioning. *Obstet Gynecol.* 2014;124:1120–27.

26. Cipres D, Seidman D, Cloniger C et al. Contraceptive use and pregnancy intentions among transgender men presenting to a clinic for sex workers and their families in San Francisco. *Contraception.* 2017;95:186–9.

27. Curtis KM, Jatlaoui TC, Tepper NK et al. U.S. Selected practice recommendations for contraceptive use, 2016. *MMWR Recomm Rep.* 2016;65:1–66.

28. Curtis KM, Tepper NK, Jatlaoui TC et al. U.S. medical eligibility criteria for contraceptive use, 2016. *MMWR Recomm Rep.* 2016;65:1–104.

29. Menstrual Manipulation for Adolescents with Physical and Developmental Disabilities. Committee Opinion No. 668. American College of Obstetricians and Gynecologists. *Obstet Gynecol.* 2016;128:e20–5.

30. Ahmad S, Leinung M. The response of the menstrual cycle to initiaton of hormonal therapy in transgender men. *Transgend Health.* 2017;2:176–9.

31. Saslow D, Solomon D, Lawson HW et al. American Cancer Society, American Society for Colposcopy and Cervical Pathology, and American Society for Clinical Pathology screening guidelines for the prevention and early detection of cervical cancer. *CA Cancer J Clin.* 2012;62:147–72.

32. Peitzmeier S, Reisner S, Harigopal P, Potter J. Female-to-male patients have high prevalence of unsatisfactory paps compared to non-transgender females: Implications for cervical cancer screening. *J Gen Intern Med.* 2014;29:778–84.

33. Peitzmeier S, Khullar K, Reisner S, Potter J. Pap test use is lower among female-to-male patients than non-transgender women. *Am J Prev Med.* 2014;47: 808–12.

34. Wierckx K, Caenegem E, Pennings G. Reproductive wish in transsexual. *Human Reproduction.* 2012;27:483–7.

35. De Roo C, Tilleman K, T'Sjoen G, De Sutter P. Fertility options in transgender people. *Int Rev Psychiatry.* 2016;28:112–9.

36. Nahata L, Tishelman A, Caltabellotta N et al. Low fertility preservation utilization among transgender youth. *J Adolesc Health.* 2017;61:40–4.

37. Chen D, Simons L, Johnson E et al. Fertility preservation for transgender adolescents. *J Adolesc Health.* 2017;6:120–3.

38. Strang J, Jarin J, Call D et al. Transgender youth fertility attitudes questionnaire: Measure development in nonautistic and autistic transgender youth and their parents. *J Adolesc Health.* 2018;62(2):128–35.

Reproductive health care for adolescents with developmental delay

24

ELISABETH H. QUINT and SUSAN D. ERNST

INTRODUCTION

The pubertal changes, with the onset of hormonal fluctuations, menstrual cycles, and reproductive potential, are challenging for any teenager. For adolescents with developmental delay (DD) and their families, these changes can present an even more complicated transition, due to physical, psychological, or behavioral issues. Care providers have the unique opportunity to assist the teens and their families through this change. This chapter focuses on reproductive health in teenagers with special needs and addresses menstrual and hygiene issues, as well as specific concerns about sexual education, contraception, mood disorders, seizures, and abuse. The principle of any intervention is to provide the optimal and least harmful form of care and be evidence based where possible. The patient's level of participation should be based on her abilities, and her decisional capacity always addressed and respected.

HISTORY

The degree of disability will determine how much the patient can be involved in providing her own history, concerns, and the reason for her visit. Using basic language when asking the initial questions will help to assess how much the patient understands. Whether the patient should be offered a confidential part of the interview, as is customary in adolescent encounters, is dependent on the degree of intellectual disability.

Obtain a thorough menstrual history specifically asking how the cycles are influencing the teen's life. Ask about home and school situations, and inquire about issues with menstrual hygiene, behaviors, mood changes, concerns about sexual activity, potential for coercion, abuse, or depression (common in all teens, around 11%).[1]

If the teen is accompanied by a parent, there will be historical and family information available that may affect her care. However, if the patient is adopted or lives in a group home, this information may be unknown. Menstrual and behavioral calendars can be very helpful to get written information on menstrual cycles and accompanying symptoms and behaviors. This makes it easier to establish a diagnosis and to aid in judging treatment efficacy.

Common reasons for a reproductive health visit include anticipatory pubertal guidance, education, menstrual problems, including pain management, hygiene and menstrual control, cyclical behavioral concerns, or an evaluation for possible abuse or pregnancy.

EDUCATION

Clinical guidelines suggest sexual education as part of every preventive health visit for adolescents. Despite this, there is a lack of sexual education for teens with DD. Although it is challenging to try to teach all of these concepts in the setting of a brief office visit, it is suggested that providers attempt to assess the current knowledge base of each patient, then help the family and caregivers with information to continue educational efforts in the home setting, in conjunction with community-based resources.[2]

Just as with teaching other subjects to adolescents with learning difficulties, use simple terms and repetition of the topics, visual aids, pictures, signs, symbols, and anatomically correct dolls or models to enhance comprehension.

Education focuses on several areas:

1. Pubertal changes, including menstrual cycles and hygiene
2. Sex education, including gender roles, social boundaries, and healthy sexual behaviors
3. Sexual abuse and prevention

Development, puberty, and menstrual cycles

Many parents and caregivers of adolescents with DD seek anticipatory guidance and education regarding gynecologic issues before menarche even occurs. In one study about women with DD, concern over sequence and timing of pubertal events as well as menstrual control prompted frequent premenarchal referrals.[3] Pubertal timing and sequence vary in girls with DD depending on the underlying diagnosis, but those studies that look at age at menarche for all girls with DD suggest no change from typically developing girls.[4] However, girls with DD are more likely to have other medical conditions or take medications that can affect pubertal events. Once menarche starts, girls with DD may have physical challenges that may make menstrual hygiene difficult. These girls may have cognitive impairment and speech delays that would predictably make it hard for them to understand or communicate about the changes that occur with puberty and the menstrual cycle. Recommended content for education regarding puberty and menstrual hygiene is in Table 24.1.[5]

Sexual education

Sexual education should ideally be taught in multiple settings, including the home, school, and in the health-care provider's office.[6] However, it is clear that many girls with DD receive only minimal information.[7] At the most basic

Table 24.1 Basic puberty education.

1. Basic anatomy and reproductive function
2. General hygiene, mood changes, sexual feelings
3. Explain menstrual flow
4. Review hygiene—washing, changing pads, changing clothes and underwear
5. Handwashing after toileting
6. Family member models hygiene techniques

level, sex education should include an explanation of the differences between boys and girls and the proper labeling of body parts. Emphasis is placed on the concept of "public and private" to reinforce acceptable patterns of conduct. We distinguish between public and private body parts, as well as public and private places. If the teen has a lot of self-stimulation in public places, it can be taught that in private places that same behavior can be acceptable. Persons with DD often may not understand social norms and societal rules of behavior, leading to the common myth that they are hypersexual. Explain about good touch in contrast to bad or inappropriate touch, and in this context, introduce the issues of personal space and boundaries. Try to outline very specifically appropriate behaviors and appropriate responses to interactions with other people. Discuss sexual activity and potential consequences of sexual activity, including pregnancy and sexually transmitted infections (STIs), and outline contraceptive options as indicated[20] (Table 24.2).

It can be difficult to assess the ability of the patient to consent to sexual activity. While no single legal definition of consent exists for persons with disabilities, the following definition is accepted from the Sexuality Information and Education Counsel of the United States (SIECUS rep 1995): To be judged capable of giving consent, one must be the age of majority (age 16), must be able to indicate yes or no verbally or through gesture, must be free of coercion or intimidation, and must understand the potential risks and consequences of their behavior. Discuss with caregivers and patient, alone if possible, if there are any active issues related to sexual activity or consent.

A concept that is difficult for adolescents with DD, particularly those with autism, is appropriate social boundaries.[8] In teaching young women with DD about

Table 24.2 Elements of sexual education.

1. Simple accurate anatomy
2. Appropriate social boundaries
3. Public and private body parts and behaviors
4. Sexual identity—gender roles and socialization
5. Sexual activities—intercourse, masturbation, and alternative sensual activities
6. Reproductive health—protection against infection and pregnancy
7. Healthy relationships, abuse, and protective measures from exploitation

self-protection skills and appropriate social boundaries, the content of the education needs to be modified to their level. One basic strategy used to teach impaired individuals appropriate social boundaries is the "circles technique" described by Champagne and Walker-Hirsch.[9] This concept places individuals with disabilities in the center of the circle and teaches them that different people in their lives occupy various circles around them. Family is in the closest circle and strangers the farthest away, helping them understand social boundaries, distance, and touch. These boundaries may seem somewhat obvious to usually developing children but must be specifically reinforced for children and teens with cognitive impairment.

Sexual abuse

Unfortunately, many characteristics associated with developmental disability predispose individuals to sexual abuse: physical challenges, reliance on adults or caregivers for assistance with many activities of daily living, learned compliance, affectionate or loving nature, and decreased communication skills. Estimates of sexual abuse range from 25% to nearly 83% in national statistics, but clearly rates of sexual assault are higher among persons with disabilities.[10-12] Perpetrators are often known to their victims.[13] It may be difficult to obtain a history of sexual assault because of lack of verbal skills and the fact that the perpetrator is often someone in a position of authority over the victim. For this reason, the rates of abuse and assault may be even higher than reported.

A few studies demonstrate that women with mild to moderate mental delay can acquire skills for sexual abuse prevention.[14] Unfortunately, as previously stated, young people with DD often fail to receive even the needed sexual education, let alone abuse prevention. One study of sexually abused women with intellectual disability found that greater than 50% had not received any sexual education.[7] Most agree that a sexual abuse prevention program should include education on how to recognize an inappropriate advance or unwanted touch, how to verbally refuse or physically remove oneself from the unwanted situation, and how to report the incident to a trusted adult. One common theme in abuse prevention education is the

- NO, GO, TELL

model described by Krents and Adkins.[15] While these words and actions seem simple, they may be extremely difficult or complicated for an individual with impairments. Saying no to an authority figure who may be threatening the child, leaving the area physically, and being able to verbally communicate about assault are all real challenges for children with DD. Teaching this concept requires repetition, modeling, and generalization to use the technique in a variety of settings.

Clinicians should recognize that children with disabilities are at increased risk of sexual abuse and should advocate for appropriate sex education.[6] Care providers also need to provide necessary education in clinical encounters, alert the family and caregivers to risks of abuse, and provide the adolescent with tools to prevent abuse. In addition, we need to be vigilant in looking for physical signs, like unexplained bruising and symptoms or changes in behavior that may be indications of sexual abuse in those patients who may not be able to communicate details of their abuse.

PHYSICAL EXAMINATION

The gynecologic and vulvar examination of a patient with DD may cause anxiety due to previous examinations, invasive procedures like enemas, or an unknown history of abuse. Fortunately, these examinations are only indicated for specific circumstances, like vaginal discharge, vulvar pain, or concern about trauma. STI screening can be done by urine testing or vaginal swab. Cervical screening is recommended to start at age 21, unless the patient is immunocompromised, according to the most recent guidelines from the American College of Obstetricians and Gynecologists (ACOG) and the American Cancer Society.[16,17] There are some data to suggest that there is a decreased incidence of abnormal Pap smears among women with DD.[18] However, there is not enough evidence to suggest different guidelines for this population. Increased rates of sexual assault and difficulty obtaining an accurate sexual history make continued cervical screening recommended in the adult population. If a vulvar/pelvic examination is necessary, there are some specific aspects to address (Table 24.3). Positioning the legs for an internal exam may require extra assistance, due to physical handicaps. Use a Huffman speculum (narrow, but long) as opposed to a pediatric speculum, which is narrow, but often too short to visualize the cervix of a postmenarchal girl. Bimanual exam, if indicated, with one finger in the vagina, can be difficult due to cooperation of the client,

Table 24.3 Special aspects of a pelvic exam in teens with developmental disabilities.

1. Allow a trusted caregiver or family member to be present, if the patient desires.
2. Usually wear a white coat to clearly establish the professional nature of the caregiver.
3. Patience, slow down the exam.
4. It may require several visits to a caregiver before the patient is comfortable.
5. Practice may help: gowns, instruments, and the examining table.
6. Allow the patient as much control over the exam as possible by having her touch the instruments and assist, if possible.
7. Patients may have multiple handicaps (neurologic or orthopedic).
8. Adjust the positions:
   Frog-leg position
   V-position
   Elevate legs without abduction of the hips
   Side position.

body position like scoliosis, and very tight rectus muscles. A rectoabdominal exam can be helpful. Occasionally, emptying of the rectum before the exam is needed. Sedation for exams has been used in some clinic settings, but if a thorough evaluation is strongly indicated to rule out suspected pathology, an ultrasound or an exam under anesthesia is much more helpful and less traumatizing.

Quadrivalent and 9-valent HPV vaccines (4vHPV and 9vHPV, Gardasil and Gardasil 9, Merck and Co, Inc., Whitehouse Station, New Jersey) are licensed for use in females and males aged 9 through 45 years in the United States, but since 2016 only the 9-valent vaccine has been used. The most recent recommendations are two injections 6–12 months apart in children 9–14 years old; after the 15th birthday, a total of three injections is currently recommended.[19] There is a paucity of literature on the use of the HPV vaccine in girls with DD; however, the vaccination rates in the United Kingdom are reportedly lower than in the general population.[20] One study in the United States found decreased parental acceptability in this group.[21] All patients and families should be educated and counseled about this vaccine because of the increased risk for sexual assault and the long-term difficulty encountered in performing cervical cancer screening.

BLEEDING ISSUES AND CONTRACEPTION

When a teenager with DD comes in with a concern about her periods, the care provider addresses several components: Is the bleeding abnormal or medically unhealthy? Does it negatively affect the patient and her daily activities? Are there concerns regarding sexuality, abuse, and pregnancy risk?[22]

Is the bleeding abnormal or medically unhealthy?

Bleeding irregularities are common in all teens, with 85% of all cycles anovulatory during the first year after menarche.[23] This irregularity is not necessarily an indication of a problem; however, abnormal bleeding (irregular or heavy) is often more difficult to manage for girls with DD. There are several common issues in girls with DD that can contribute to irregular bleeding. Women with epilepsy have an increased incidence of reproductive endocrine disorders, including irregular menstrual cycles, anovulatory cycles, amenorrhea, and oligomenorrhea.[24] Polycystic ovarian syndrome occurs in 10%–20% of women with epilepsy compared with 5%–6% in the general population, and women on valproic acid may have an even higher incidence.[25] Neuroleptics and metoclopramide can cause hyperprolactinemia that can lead to abnormal bleeding and ultimately to amenorrhea due to a hypoestrogenic state. Thyroid disease, which can lead to subsequent disturbance of the cycle, is more prevalent in women with Down syndrome.[26] Poor food intake, swallowing problems, and gastric problems can lead to low weight and menstrual disturbances. Bleeding is only considered medically unhealthy if it leads to anemia or if it is very sparse. For heavy bleeding, leading to anemia, consider anovulation, poor food intake (leading to iron deficiency), or bleeding disorders like von Willebrand disease or platelet disorders (see Chapter 14). Very sparse cycles, due to anovulation, can lead to endometrial concerns long term.

Does the bleeding negatively affect the patient and her daily activities or her family and caregivers?

The families of children with disabilities can have a very delicate balance of caring for their girls, and menstrual cycles may disturb that. The issues may include menstrual hygiene, like accidents with bleeding due to removal of pads out of the underwear by the teens or getting menstrual blood on their hands. Menstrual cramping, heavy bleeding, and behavioral changes with the cycles can also impact the teen' life.[27] The care provider or care team can decide with the patients and their families whether an intervention like menstrual suppression is warranted.

Are there concerns regarding sexuality, abuse, and pregnancy?

If there is a concern for abuse, either within the surroundings or because the patient cannot be monitored closely enough or is unable to understand appropriate boundaries, the care provider should assist with evaluation of a potentially unsafe situation and also address contraception needs.

Treatment

Once the decision is made to treat the patient's cycles, based on the previously outlined principles, a treatment goal is decided. This can be to decrease heaviness of flow, relieve pain or symptoms, provide contraception, or achieve amenorrhea. A method causing unpredictable bleeding may be less desirable than infrequent but predictable withdrawal bleeding. Obtaining complete amenorrhea by any method is difficult.

Nonsteroidal anti-inflammatory drugs (NSAIDs): These medications, in appropriate dosages, can treat dysmenorrhea and decrease the menstrual flow by up to 20%–30%.[28]

Combined hormonal contraceptives (CHCs): CHCs can be used to regulate the cycles, decrease the flow, and treat dysmenorrhea. Extended cycling can be used if desired, especially if amenorrhea is a goal. Studies show high partial or complete amenorrhea rates after several months of combined oral contraceptives (COCs). There may be some troublesome spotting that can be addressed by taking two pills for several days or allowing periodic withdrawal bleeds.[29,30] In patients for whom swallowing is an issue, there is an option for a chewable COC, as well as the transdermal patch. The patch can cause some issues with patients with DD pulling it off, due to skin irritation or in those women with heightened tactile sensitivities. Placing it out of range on the lower or upper back may be helpful. Using CHC via the vaginal ring is usually not a good option for girls with DD, due to the difficulty and privacy issues with intravaginal placement.

The contraindications for CHC are the same as in the general population. Venous thromboembolism (VTE) is a multifactorial disease with risk factors including immobilization, estrogen-containing hormones, and familial clotting disorders like factor V Leiden.[31] VTE warrants special mention due to immobilization in many of our teens with DD. Because venous stasis is part of the Virchow triad,[31] immobilization is thought to increase the risk of VTE; however, no studies are available specifically on teenagers in wheelchairs. One recent study on patients with advanced multiple sclerosis (MS) and decreased mobility found a high rate of VTE (average age 58 years, men and women), leading the CDC to add MS with prolonged immobility as a category 3 for CHC to their most recent contraceptive recommendations.[32,33] A case of VTE was reported on a 36-year-old on oral contraceptive pills (OCP) with tetraparesis and wheelchair use.[34] In a review on how to screen for thrombophilic tendencies, recommendations were made to obtain a detailed family history before starting the OCP.[35] Some research suggests that the risk for VTE may be slightly higher in oral preparations with third-generation progestins.[36] Recommendations for starting COCs would then be a lower dose (35 μg or less) of ethinyl estradiol in combination with a first- or second-generation progestin. Although studies show mixed results, the risk of developing VTE is about twice as high with the patch as with COCs; however, the absolute risk of VTE remains low.[37] If the patient has more risk factors for VTE such as obesity and immobilization, one may consider not using the patch.

Progestin-only methods

Oral progestins include the progestin-only pill (POP): a low dose of norethindrone that can cause significant spotting, which may be an undesired side effect. Higher doses of oral norethindrone, medroxyprogesterone acetate, and megestrol have been used with complete suppression of the cycles. Side effects of these medications include mild weight gain and mood changes, with megestrol increasing appetite as well.[38] The majority of evidence does not suggest an increase in odds for VTE with the use of most POCs.[39]

The *levonorgestrel intrauterine device system (LNG-IUD)* decreases flow, can cause amenorrhea in 20% of women, and is now recommended as safe and appropriate for adolescents by ACOG. Expulsion may be slightly higher in nulliparous women.[40] Several case series in women with DD have been published describing its success in this population.[3,41,42] The 52 mg LNG-IUD is good for 5–7 years and has a better bleeding profile than the somewhat smaller 13.5 mg LNG-IUD and is therefore favored in this population. Dependent on the level of disability, the IUD insertion may have to be done under anesthesia, possibly combined with other procedures, like dental work. An ultrasound for uterine size is not recommended preoperatively.[43]

The *etonogestrel implant* provides excellent contraception, and although some women experience amenorrhea, it causes significant irregular bleeding for most, which makes it less desirable for young women with DD.[44]

Intramuscular (IM) depot medroxyprogesterone acetate (DMPA; Depo-Provera, Pfizer, Carlisle, Pennsylvania) has been used extensively in women with DD due to its high rate of amenorrhea (around 70%), ease of use, and birth control rates. Weight gain is often a concern from providers. Although the studies have mixed results, there appears to be some weight gain noted with Depo-Provera, especially in overweight girls, but with large individual variations. If a teenager gains significantly in the first year of use, the method of menstrual suppression may need to be revised.[38] Weight increases for adolescents who rely on wheelchair transfers, by themselves or others, may significantly affect their lives. Bone loss is also associated with DMPA use, due to its suppression of endogenous estrogen. Longitudinal studies report bone mineral density (BMD) losses of 0.5%–3.5% at the hip and spine after 1 year of DMPA use, 5.7%–7.5% loss in BMD after 2 years of use, and 5.2%–5.4% loss after 5 years of use.[45] There may be a small increase in fracture risk with DMPA, but the data are mostly from observational studies.[46] In trials that included both adults and adolescents, with a duration of DMPA use of 2–5 years and follow-up of up to 5 years after discontinuation, losses in BMD appeared to be substantially or fully reversible; however, recovery at the hip and femoral neck generally took longer compared with recovery at the spine; other studies did not confirm complete reversibility in adolescents.[45] Other bone health risk factors in teens with DD include antiepileptic medication and decreased mobility. Although the issue of wheelchair use and bone density has not been researched extensively, decreased bone density has been found in several small subpopulations.[47] There is good evidence that lifestyle choices affect peak bone density in teenagers, so adequate intake of calcium and vitamin D and as much adapted activity as possible are recommended.[48] The potential health risks associated with the effects of DMPA on weight and bone density must be balanced against excessive menstruation and the likelihood of unintended pregnancy.

Surgery, like hysterectomy or endometrial ablation, for cessation of normal menses is usually not recommended.[41,49]

Contraception

For contraceptive purposes, after abuse or coercion has been ruled out, hormonal methods are used most frequently in this population, as the barrier methods may be difficult to use. Long-acting reversible methods are preferred with the caveats outlined in the previous section. Discuss emergency contraception with adolescents, as they may have an unplanned sexual encounter. Sterilization of women who cannot give consent is a controversial and complicated ethical issue.

Use of anticonvulsant medications and hormones

Antiepileptic drugs (AEDs) are used commonly in teens with DD. AEDs that induce the hepatic cytochrome P450 system (EI-AED) can decrease serum concentrations of estrogen and progestin in combined OCPs and lead to decreased contraceptive efficacy and irregular bleeding (Table 24.4).[50] In addition, women taking combined OCPs and lamotrigine have been shown to have decreased serum concentrations of

Table 24.4 Interaction of antiepileptic medications with combined oral contraceptive pills (OCPs).

Decrease OCP efficacy	Do not affect OCP efficacy
Carbamazepine (Tegretol)	Ethosuximide (Zarontin)
Clobazam (Onfi)	Gabapentin (Neurontin)
Felbamate (Felbatol)	Levetiracetam (Keppra)
Eslicarbazepine acetate (Aptiom)	
Phenytoin (Dilantin)	Lamotrigine (Lamictal)
Phenobarbital	Tiagabine (Gabitril)
Primidone (Mysoline)	Valproate (Depakote)
Oxcarbazepine (Trileptal)	Zonisamide (Zonegran)
Rufinamide (Banzel)	
Topiramate (Topamax)	

lamotrigine and may need dose adjustments of lamotrigine when the medications are prescribed together or in combination with other anticonvulsants.[51] The American Academy of Neurology recommends that if a woman on EI-AED chooses to use an oral contraceptive pill, then a higher-dose pill with 50 micrograms of estrogen should be recommended with backup barrier methods.[52] The Centers for Disease Control and Prevention recommends U.S. Medical Eligibility Criteria for Contraceptive Use that show that all combined hormonal contraceptives (CHCs) are a category 3 (relative contraindication), and risks of contraceptive failure with CHCs and EI-AED may outweigh benefits.[34] Drug interactions are also reported with the implant.[50] IUDs are thought to be the optimal choice for contraception.

Table 24.5 reviews advantages and disadvantages of common methods for contraception in this population.

MOOD DISORDERS

Premenstrual symptoms (PMS), a menstrual-related disorder with both behavioral and physical symptoms that occur cyclically, are described in up to 90% of women of childbearing age, with less than 10% having a more severe form, premenstrual dysphoric disorder (PMDD). Cyclical behavior changes are a fairly common complaint in women with DD. In one study, 18% of women with DD were found to present with cyclical behavior changes.[53] In women with DD, these may include symptoms of temper tantrums, crying spells, autistic behavior, or self-abusive behavior. The diagnosis of cyclical behavior changes is made by documentation. ACOG recommends that one of the described symptoms in the affective and somatic categories has to be present in the 5 days before menses in two consecutive cycles.[54] For women with DD, it is more practical to track the most bothersome behavior on a daily symptom chart. The purpose of the documentation is to determine the cyclic nature, to rule out other behavioral or psychiatric disorders, and to help document treatment outcomes. Multiple studies suggest that adolescents with autism have a higher incidence of cyclic behavioral problems than girls with other types of disabilities and typically developing peers.[55,56]

Table 24.5 Contraceptive methods.

Barrier methods (i.e., foam and condoms, cervical caps, sponges, and diaphragms)
- Advantages:
  1. Protect against sexually transmitted infections
- Concerns:
  1. Require high degree of personal initiative and intellectual understanding
  2. Require physical dexterity

Levonorgestrel intrauterine device (system)
- Advantages:
  1. Decrease flow and cramping
  2. Long term
- Concerns:
  1. Inability to report pain or discomfort (complications)
  2. May require anesthesia for insertion

Combined oral contraceptives
- Advantages:
  1. Decrease flow and cramping, extended cycling
- Concerns:
  1. Requires supervisor to administer pills
  2. Use of antiseizure medication may necessitate higher estrogen content
  3. Unclear: immobilization and risk of deep vein thrombosis (DVT)

Contraceptive patch
- Advantages:
  1. Easy to use
  2. Decreases flow and cramping, extended cycling
- Concerns:
  1. Patient may pull it off (place on back)
  2. Skin irritation
  3. Weight limitations
  4. Higher risk for DVT

Contraceptive ring
- Advantages:
  1. Decrease flow and cramping, extended cycling
- Concerns:
  1. Difficult to place (privacy issues)

Intramuscular and subcutaneous medroxyprogesterone (i.e., Depo-Provera)
- Advantages:
  1. Amenorrhea rates high, easy to use
- Concerns:
  1. Weight gain (may make transfers more difficult)
  2. Long-term use and bone loss

Progestin-only pills
- Advantages:
  1. Can be used in women with estrogen contraindications
- Concerns:
  1. More breakthrough bleeding
  2. Lower pregnancy prevention

(Continued)

Table 24.5 (Continued)   Contraceptive methods.

Etonogestrel implant
- Advantages:
  1. Good for 3 years
- Concerns:
  1. Not studied in women with developmental delay
  2. More irregular bleeding

Sterilization/hysterectomy
- Ethically complex situation
  1. Consider use of ethics or advisory committee to review sterilization requests
  2. Be aware of state laws

No single therapy has been found to be always successful in treating cyclical behavior disorders.[57] The usual first-line treatments, such as dietary and lifestyle changes, can be difficult to administer to teens with DD. In women who may not be able to communicate their feelings, behaviors may be an outlet for pain. The first line of treatment for women with DD is an NSAID in adequate doses to start on the day of start of the behavior, which was found to be successful in 65% of 45 adult patients with cyclical behavior changes.[53] If that approach is unsuccessful, ovulation suppression may be tried. Several studies suggest that an oral contraceptive with drospirenone may be helpful.[58] Selective serotonin reuptake inhibitors (SSRIs) have not been used for this indication in teens with DD but are among the first-line therapy in the general population with severe PMS and PMDD.[59]

CATAMENIAL SEIZURES

Epilepsy is a common comorbidity in young women with DD. Overall, approximately 20% of women with DD have epilepsy; however, this rate is up to 50% in women with severe developmental delay.[60] Women with epilepsy may have variability in seizure frequency secondary to hormonal fluctuations throughout the menstrual cycle, a condition known as catamenial epilepsy. Estimates vary but may be as high as 70%.[61]

Varying definitions of catamenial epilepsy exist. Three different patterns of increased seizure frequency have

Table 24.6 Medication effect on catamenial seizures.

Author	Year	Medication	Percentage (%) decrease in seizures
Ross, IP	1958	Acetazolamide	40%
Feely, M	1982	Clobazam	78%
Herzog, AG	2012	Progesterone	71%
Mattson, RH	1984	Medroxyprogesterone acetate	39%
Herzog, AG	1988	Clomiphene citrate	87%
Bauer, J	1992	GnRH agonist—triptorelin	50%

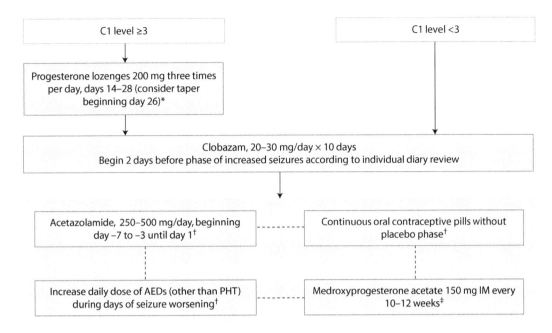

Figure 24.1 Treatment algorithm for catamenial C1 pattern of seizures. Most treatments are for focal-onset seizures in women with regular menses. C1 level 3 = three times more seizures on day 25, as compared with other days of the month. Abbreviations: AEDs, antiepileptic drugs; IM, intramuscular; PHT, phenytoin. Note: *If menses start before day 26, start dose tapering on that day according to the same pattern of decreases. †Widely undertaken but not supported by data from randomized, controlled trials. ‡Increased risk of osteoporosis and slow return to normal fertility. (From Harden CL, Pennell PB. *Lancet Neurol.* 2013;12[1]:72–83, with permission.)

been described, including perimenstrual (C1), periovulatory (C2), and inadequate luteal phase (C3).[62] The perimenstrual form, with increased seizure frequency 3 days before the onset of menstruation and ending 4 days after the onset, is the most common form of catamenial epilepsy, with day 1 of the menstrual cycle having the most seizure activity. One basic theory states that seizure frequency is altered secondary to fluctuations in endogenous hormone levels. Estrogen is known to increase neuronal excitability, decrease seizure threshold, and act as a proconvulsant. Progesterone increases seizure threshold and acts as an anticonvulsant. Other mechanisms may be involved in altering seizure frequency, including changes in adrenal hormones, androgens, fluctuations in antiepilepsy drug (AED) levels, and changes in water and electrolyte balance.[58] Regardless of the mechanism, these women with catamenial epilepsy experience a twofold or greater increase in seizure frequency at one of these times during their menstrual cycle, and approximately 30% may have refractory seizures.[63]

Despite the high incidence of catamenial epilepsy, there are few studies investigating treatment for this disorder. Acetazolamide, Clobazam, progesterones, and GnRH agonists have all shown some benefit in small studies (Table 24.6).[64-66] Oral contraceptive pills are often used in a continuous fashion to suppress endogenous hormonal fluctuations and treat catamenial epilepsy; however, no studies have been done to determine their efficacy. Harden and Pennell published a treatment algorithm (Figure 24.1) for catamenial epilepsy that suggests progesterone lozenges for C1 perimenstrual seizures or cyclic use of Clobazam as first-line therapy for catamenial seizures.[67,68]

SUMMARY

Teens with DDs pose a diagnostic and treatment challenge for their reproductive health care, with regard to menstrual function, medical comorbidities, social situation, and behavioral concerns. Working with the teen and the family usually results in a satisfying resolution of the issues through education, counseling, and medical treatment, as indicated.

REFERENCES

1. Mojtabai R, Olfson M, Han B. National trends in the prevalence and treatment of depression in adolescents and young adults. *Pediatrics.* 2016;138:e20161878.
2. Breuner CC, Mattson G, AAP Committee on Adolescence, AAP Committee on Psychosocial Aspects of Child and Family Health. Sexuality education for children and adolescents. *Pediatrics.* 2016;138:e20161348.
3. Kirkham YA, Allen L, Kives S et al. Trends in menstrual concerns and suppression in adolescents with developmental disabilities. *J Adolesc Health.* 2013;53:407–12.
4. Abells D, Kirkham YA, Ornstein MP. Review of gynecologic and reproductive care for women with developmental disabilities. *Curr Opin Obstet Gynecol.* 2016;28:350–8.

5. Healthy Bodies. http://vkc.mc.vanderbilt.edu/healthybodies/. Accessed February 23, 2018.

6. Murphy NA, Elias ER. Sexuality of children and adolescents with developmental disabilities. *Pediatrics*. 2006;118:398–403.

7. Barnard-Brak L, Schmidt M, Chesnut S et al. Predictors of access to sex education for children with intellectual disabilities in public schools. *Intellect Dev Disabil*. 2014;52:85–97.

8. Beddows N, Brooks R. Inappropriate sexual behaviour in adolescents with autism spectrum disorder: What education is recommended and why. *Early Interv Psychiatry*. 2016;10:282–9.

9. Champagne MP, Walker-Hirsch LW. *Circles I: Intimacy and Relationships*. Santa Barbara, CA: James Stanfield; 1993.

10. Jones L, Bellis MA, Wood S et al. Prevalence and risk of violence against children with disabilities: A review and meta-analysis. *Lancet*. 2012;380(9845):899–907.

11. Harrell E. *Crime Against Persons with Disabilities, 2009–2012-Statistical Tables*. Washington, DC: Bureau of Justice Statistics, U.S. Department of Justice; 2014.

12. Wissink IB, van Vugt E, Moonen X et al. Sexual abuse involving children with an intellectual disability (ID): A narrative review. *Res Dev Disabil*. 2015;36:20–35.

13. Bowen E, Swift C. The prevalence and correlates of partner violence used and experienced by adults with intellectual disabilities: A systematic review and call to action. *Trauma Violence Abuse*. 2017;1524838017728707.

14. Doughty AH, Kane LM. Teaching abuse prevention skills to people with intellectual disabilities: A review of the literature. *Res Dev Disabil*. 2010;31:331–7.

15. Krents E, Adkins D. *No – Go – Tell! A child protection curriculum for very young disabled children*. New York: Lexington Center; 1985.

16. Cervical cancer screening and prevention. Practice Bulletin 168. American College of Obstetricians and Gynecologists. *Obstet Gynecol*. 2016;128:e111–30.

17. Saslow D, Solomon D, Lawson H et al. American Cancer Society, American Society for Colposcopy and Cervical Pathology, and American Society for Clinical Pathology screening guidelines for the prevention and early detection of cervical cancer. *CA Cancer J Clin*. 2012;62:147–72.

18. Kavoussi SK, Smith YR, Ernst SD, Quint EH. Cervical cancer screening with liquid cytology in women with developmental disabilities. *J Womens Health (Larchmt)*. 2009;18:115–8.

19. Meites E, Kempe A, Markowitz LE. Use of a 2-dose schedule for human papillomavirus vaccination—Updated recommendations of the Advisory Committee on Immunization Practices. *MMWR*. 2016;65:1405–8.

20. MacLeod R, Tuffrey C. Immunisation against HPV in girls with intellectual disabilities. *Arch Dis Child*. 2014;99:1068–70.

21. Cody PJ, Lerand SJ. HPV vaccination in female children with special health care needs. *J Pediatr Adolesc Gynecol*. 2013;26:219–23.

22. Quint EH. Menstrual and reproductive issues in adolescents with physical and developmental disabilities. *Obstet Gynecol*. 2014;124:367–75.

23. Menstruation in girls and adolescents: Using the menstrual cycle as a vital sign. Committee Opinion No. 651. American College of Obstetricians and Gynecologists. *Obstet Gynecol*. 2015;126:e143–6.

24. Vélez-Ruiz NJ, Pennell PB. Issues for women with epilepsy. *Neurol Clin*. 2016;34:411–2.

25. Gotlib D, Ramaswamy R, Kurlander JE et al. Valproic acid in women and girls of childbearing age. *Curr Psychiatry Rep*. 2017;19:58.

26. Whooten R, Schmitt J, Schwartz A. Endocrine manifestations of Down syndrome. *Curr Opin Endocrinol Diabetes Obes*. 2018;25:61–6.

27. Kaskowitz AP, Dendrinos M, Murray PJ et al. The effect of menstrual issues on young women with Angelman syndrome. *J Pediatr Adolesc Gynecol*. 2016;29:348–52.

28. Lethaby A, Duckitt K, Farquhar C. Non-steroidal anti-inflammatory drugs for heavy menstrual bleeding. *Cochrane Database Syst Rev*. 2013;(1):CD000400.

29. Jacobson JC, Likis FE, Murphy PA. Extended and continuous combined contraceptive regimens for menstrual suppression. *J Midwifery Womens Health*. 2012;57:585–9.

30. Gold MA, Duffy K. Extended cycling or continuous use of hormonal contraceptives for female adolescents. *Curr Opin Obstet Gynecol*. 2009;21:407–11.

31. Stone J, Hangge P, Albadawi H et al. Deep vein thrombosis: Pathogenesis, diagnosis, and medical management. *Cardiovasc Diagn Ther*. 2017;7(Suppl 3):S276–84.

32. Arpaia G, Bavera PM, Caputo D et al. Risk of deep venous thrombosis (DVT) in bedridden or wheelchair-bound multiple sclerosis patients: A prospective study. *Thromb Res*. 2010;125:315–7.

33. Curtis KM, Tepper NK, Jatlaoui TC et al. U.S. Medical Eligibility Criteria for Contraceptive Use, 2016. *MMWR Recomm Rep*. 2016;65:1–103.

34. Lohiya GS, Crinella FM, Tan-Figueroa L et al. Deep vein thrombosis in a tetraparesic patient with mental retardation: Case report and review of the literature. *Brain Inj*. 2005;19:739–42.

35. Savelli SL, Kerlin BA, Springer MA et al. Recommendations for screening for thrombophilic tendencies in teenage females prior to contraceptive initiation. *J Pediatr Adolesc Gynecol*. 2006;19:313–16.

36. Dragoman MV, Tepper NK, Fu R et al. A systematic review and meta-analysis of venous thrombosis risk among users of combined oral contraception. *Int J Gynaecol Obstet*. 2018;141(3):287–94.

37. Galzote RM, Rafie S, Teal R, Mody SK. Transdermal delivery of combined hormonal contraception: A review of the current literature. *Int J Womens Health*. 2017;9:315–32.

38. Lopez LM, Ramesh S, Chen M et al. Progestin-only contraceptives: Effects on weight. *Cochrane Database Syst Rev*. 2016;28(8):CD00881.

39. Tepper NK, Whiteman MK, Marchbanks PA et al. Progestin-only contraception and thromboembolism: A systematic review. *Contraception*. 2016;94:678–700.

40. Adolescents and long-acting reversible contraception: Implants and intrauterine devices. ACOG Committee Opinion No. 735. American College of Obstetricians and Gynecologists. *Obstet Gynecol*. 2018;131:e130–9.

41. Menstrual manipulation for adolescents with physical and developmental disabilities. Committee Opinion No. 668. American College of Obstetricians and Gynecologists. *Obstet Gynecol*. 2016;128:e20–5.

42. Savasi I, Jayasinghe K, Moore P et al. Complication rates associated with levonorgestrel intrauterine system use in adolescents with developmental disabilities. *J Pediatr Adolesc Gynecol*. 2014;27:25–8.

43. Whyte H, Pecchioli Y, Oyewumi L et al. Uterine length in adolescents with developmental disability: Are ultrasound examinations necessary before insertion of the levonorgestrel intrauterine system? *J Pediatr Adolesc Gynecol*. 2016;29:648–52.

44. Zigler RE, McNicholas C. Unscheduled vaginal bleeding with progestin-only contraceptive use. *Am J Obstet Gynecol*. 2017;216:443–50.

45. Depot Medroxyprogesterone Acetate and Bone Effects. Committee Opinion No. 602. Americal College of Obstetricians and Gynecologists. *Obstet Gynecol*. 2014;123:1398–402.

46. Lopez LM, Chen M, Mullins Long S et al. Steroidal contraceptives and bone fractures in women: Evidence from observational studies. *Cochrane Database Syst Rev*. 2015;(7):CD009849.

47. Martinelli V, Dell'Atti C, Ausili E et al. Risk of fracture prevention in spina bifida patients: Correlation between bone mineral density, vitamin D, and electrolyte values. *Childs Nerv Syst*. 2015;31:1361–5.

48. Weaver CM, Gordon CM, Janz KF et al. The National Osteoporosis Foundation's position statement on peak bone mass development and lifestyle factors: A systematic review and implementation recommendations. *Osteoporos Int*. 2016;27:1281–386.

49. Quint EH, O'Brien RF, Committee on Adolescence. North American Society for Pediatric and Adolescent Gynecology. Menstrual management for adolescents with disabilities. *Pediatrics*. 2016;138(1):e20160295.

50. Gaffield ME, Culwell KR, Lee CR. The use of hormonal contraception among women taking anticonvulsant therapy. *Contraception*. 2011;83:16–29.

51. Wegner I, Wilhelm AJ, Lambrechts DA et al. Effect of oral contraceptives on lamotrigine levels depends on comedication. *Acta Neurol Scand*. 2014;129:393–8.

52. American Academy of Neurology. Counseling for Women of Childbearing Potential with Epilepsy. 2014. https://www.aan.com/siteassets/home-page/policy-and-guidelines/quality/quality-measures/17emchildberingpotential_pg.pdf. Accessed February 11, 2018.

53. Quint EH, Elkins TE, Sorg CA, Kope S. The treatment of cyclical behavioral changes in women with mental disabilities. *J Pediatr Adolesc Gynecol*. 1999;12:139–42.

54. American College of Obstetricians and Gynecologists. *Guidelines for Women's Health Care: A Resource Manual*. 4th ed. Washington, DC: American College of Obstetricians and Gynecologists; 2014:607–13.

55. Obaydi H, Puri BK. Prevalence of premenstrual syndrome in autism: A prospective observer-rated study. *J Int Med Res*. 2008;36:268–72.

56. Burke LM, Kalpakjian CZ, Smith YR, Quint EH. Gynecologic issues of adolescents with Down syndrome, autism, and cerebral palsy. *J Pediatr Adolesc Gynecol*. 2010;23:11–5.

57. Braverman PK. Premenstrual syndrome and premenstrual dysphoric disorder. *J Pediatr Adolesc Gynecol*. 2007;20:3–12.

58. Verma RK, Chellappan DK, Pandey AK. Review on treatment of premenstrual syndrome: From conventional to alternative approach. *J Basic Clin Physiol Pharmacol*. 2014;25:319–27.

59. Marjoribanks J, Brown J, O'Brien PM, Wyatt K. Selective serotonin reuptake inhibitors for premenstrual syndrome. *Cochrane Database Syst Rev*. 2013;(6):CD00139.

60. Camfield C, Camfield P. Preventable and unpreventable causes of childhood-onset epilepsy plus mental retardation. *Pediatrics*. 2007;120:e52–5.

61. Reddy DS. The role of neurosteroids in the pathophysiology and treatment of catamenial epilepsy. *Epilepsy Res*. 2009;85:1–30.

62. Herzog AG, Fowler KM, Sperling MR et al. Distribution of seizures across the menstrual cycle in women with epilepsy. *Epilepsia*. 2015;56:e58–62.

63. Reddy D. Role of neurosteroids in catamenial epilepsy. *Epilepsy Res*. 2004;62:99–118.

64. Lim LL, Feldvary N, Mascha E et al. Acetazolamide in women with catamenial epilepsy. *Epilepsia*. 2001;42:746–9.

65. Herzog AG, Fowler KM, Smithson SD et al. Progesterone vs placebo therapy for women with epilepsy. *Neurology*. 2012;78:1959–66.

66. Reddy DS. Do oral contraceptives increase epileptic seizures? *Expert Rev Neurother*. 2017;17:129–34.

67. Navis A, Harden C. A treatment approach to catamenial epilepsy. *Curr Treat Options Neurol*. 2016;18:30.

68. Harden CL, Pennell PB. Neuroendeocrine considerations in the treatment of men and women with epilepsy. *Lancet Neurol*. 2013;12(1):72–83.

Sexual abuse

MARCELLA DONARUMA-KWOH

25

INTRODUCTION

Sexual abuse is recognized both in state- and nationwide definitions of child maltreatment. In the United States, some states refer in general terms to sexual abuse, while others specify various acts as abusive in nature. Similarly, in Canada, definitions are province-specific. Some jurisdictions also include sexual exploitation as a component of sexual abuse.[1] The Child Abuse Prevention and Treatment Act (CAPTA), first signed into law in 1974, is one of the key pieces of legislation that guides child protection.[2] Statute information for any particular U.S. state or Canadian province is available online.[3]

There are many types of sexual violence, including child sexual abuse and sexual assault. Sexual assault can include fondling or unwanted sexual touching, forcing a victim to perform sexual acts, such as oral sex or penetrating the perpetrator's body, or penetration of the victim's body, also known as rape. For the purposes of this discussion, sexual abuse is defined as inclusion of a child in sexual activities that the child cannot comprehend, for which the child is developmentally unprepared and cannot give consent, and/or that violate the law or social taboos of society. In a recent American survey of children's exposure to violence, 14.3% of the older girls and 6% of the older boys said they had experienced a sexual assault during childhood.[4] Sexual violence in older children and teens was included in the U.S. National Crime Victimization study data from 2016, in which over 300,000 rapes were reported to law enforcement by U.S. citizens aged 12 years and older. To further add to the picture of this social burden, the survey publishing this data concedes that only 42% of victimizations from violent crimes of all types are actually reported to the police.[5]

As in a multitude of other pediatric and adolescent diagnoses, the first step to the diagnosis of child sexual abuse is being aware of and acknowledging the problem that patients face. Recognition of sexual abuse requires both a reasonable index of suspicion for its occurrence and familiarity with its physical and behavioral indicators, as well as facility in interpreting the historical clues to sexual abuse.

Clinical assessment

History

Shonkoff stated, "a competent pediatrician must be a skilled listener and a sensitive conveyor of both information and affect."[6] Clinicians occupy a unique and trusted space in the lives of their pediatric and adolescent patients, and a positive regard—even when hearing an often disturbing history of abusive events—can open a door for a child to share his or her experiences.[7] Disclosure of sexual abuse victimization is a slowly progressing, iterative process in most cases, yet there is evidence that thoughtful, direct questions may help elicit that first outcry of an unsafe environment.[8] Patient age is also a factor influencing disclosure. In 2002, Heger found a positive association between age and likelihood of disclosure: in the 2384 children referred for evaluation, the group of children who disclosed abuse was older than the group who had not made such a disclosure. In this study of children presenting for care at a children's assessment center, those who disclosed were 7.8 years old, compared to 4.5 years in the nondisclosing group.[9]

If the clinician has an evolving concern for abuse, discussion of the history of present illness should occur with the caregiver and the patient separately. Open-ended questions are recommended, which most smoothly facilitate a full history and explanation. For example, ask, "Has anyone ever touched you in a way you didn't like or didn't want?" Respond calmly and without strong emotions if the answer is affirmative.

History-taking also should include the nature of the abusive contact, when the last incident occurred, any signs or symptoms of sexually transmitted infections (STIs), and date of menarche, as well as a thorough review of systems, including questions about abdominal pain, dysuria, enuresis, encopresis, bleeding, and discharge. Specific, though rare, symptoms of sexual abuse include rectal or genital bleeding.[10] Additionally, a behavioral review can offer insight; endorsement of anxiety, difficulty sleeping, self-injury, social withdrawal, or appetite changes may be among the manifestations of an increased level of stress. Developmentally atypical sexually reactive behaviors may be reported by the caregiver or the child. Normal exploratory behavior surrounding genitalia is typically playful, driven by curiosity, and can involve other children within the same age range. Sexually reactive behaviors highly suspicious for exposure to inappropriate contact may include a child who engages in forceful, coercive, or painful interactions with a younger child or an age mate; a child who performs insertive acts on herself, toys, or playmates; or a child exhibiting frank mimicry of penetrative sexual behaviors.

It is also prudent to ask about suicidal or homicidal ideation and to have an action plan in place for mental health evaluation if that item is endorsed by patients.

If sufficient information is elicited to raise a concern that inappropriate contact has occurred, arrange a separate interview by a trained professional. The number of children's advocacy centers (CACs) in the United States is approaching 800 at the time of this writing. These centers function as centralized locations for victims of child maltreatment and sexual abuse and facilitate coordination among community agencies and professionals, including children's protective services, law enforcement, the judicial system, victim's advocacy, medical partners, and mental health services. Local CACs may be found online.[11]

If there is no available specialty clinic or hospital social worker, then a referral to the community partner agency for child safety and protection is warranted as the best next step. Rarely, it may be appropriate to delay the interview until the child can be seen at an advocacy center if follow-up can be arranged within a short period of time. This would be a reasonable choice if the patient is safe from the perpetrator after leaving the office (i.e., perpetrator does not share the home), the disclosure is of remote contact, and the child is without physical complaints.

Commercial sexual exploitation of children (CSEC) is closely related to sex trafficking and involves "crimes of a sexual nature committed against juvenile victims for financial or other economic reasons.... These crimes include trafficking for sexual purposes, prostitution, sex tourism, mail-order-bride trade, early marriage, pornography, stripping, and performing in sexual venues such as peep shows or clubs."[12] Many also include "survival sex" in this definition (exchange of sexual activity for basic necessities such as shelter, food, or money), a practice commonly seen among homeless/runaway youth.[13] This population presents further challenges both in history-taking and medical management and is beyond the focus of this chapter.

If there is a suspicion that a patient is a victim of human trafficking, ensure that she is not left alone. Separate the patient from her companion (call security if needed). Consult social work, and call a local community partner child protection agency. Additional resources include the following:

- National Human Trafficking Resource Center (NHTRC): 888-3737-888.
- The Homeland Security Investigations Tip Line is available at 1-866-347-2423 (24 hours a day, 7 days a week, >300 languages and dialects spoken), or submit a tip online at https://www.ice.gov/tips.

Physical exam

While lithotomy position is effective for most children at grade school age or above, the genital exam of a prepubertal girl is typically performed using the "frog leg" position and applying the technique of labial traction.

Gloved thumb and forefinger are used to gently grasp the distal third of the labia majora bilaterally and exert steady traction in the sagittal plane toward the examiner until the hymenal rim can be seen (see Chapter 3). Urethral dilation is an indicator that maximum traction has been achieved.

In prone knee-chest position, head, shoulders, and pectorals all lie in the same plane on the examination table with head rotated 90° toward the shoulder. Lordotic curve should be emphasized, and knees at least shoulder width apart. Examiner uses gloved hands with thumbs facing inward over ischial tuberosities to rotate 90° cranially and elevate buttocks for visualization of inferior hymenal rim.

Younger children may be reassured by examination in a caretaker's lap. The clothed adult is seated upright with their feet in the stirrups, and the child is arranged in the adult's lap with each leg overlapping the outside of the adult's at the knee in order to achieve a sufficient field of view. Apply traction subsequent to positioning. This position allows the adult to provide more contact to both embrace the child for reassurance and simultaneously aid in maintaining her in the exam position.

The overwhelming majority of children and adolescents with a history of sexual abuse present for an informed medical exam at a time remote from the event (or events) of their abuse. As a result, the anogenital exams of these patients most often demonstrate normal and uninjured anatomy.[9,14–19] However, it is critically important to understand that the absence of injury does not rule out the occurrence of abuse as a patient has described. Multiple factors effect this state of resilience: the anatomic purpose of a vagina, which is to tolerate penetrative contact and friction regardless of the individual's psychosocial readiness for such contact; the distensible nature of the hymenal and vaginal tissue at baseline that increases with estrogenization; and the rapid healing time of vaginal mucosa if any injury were to be inflicted. These factors are compounded by the typical time delay in disclosure of the abusive event to yield an overwhelming majority of normal anogenital exams in abuse and assault victims. This affords the opportunity for the clinician to provide a "therapeutic encounter" to the patient—in a position of respected authority, the physician can provide the child victim reassurance of a normal and healthy body or encourage her by assuring the child that her body can heal. Since many children report a feeling of being physically and emotionally different from their nonabused peers, that positive valuation alone can be deeply meaningful for child or adolescent abuse victims.[20–22]

Important points to document during the exam include the sexual maturity assessment of the child, the configuration of the hymen, the degree of estrogenization of the hymen, and the presence or absence of injury to the vestibule, perihymenal and hymenal tissue, and the vaginal fossa and fourchette. Figures 25.1 through 25.3 illustrate normal and suspicious finding encountered during a genital exam.

In the rare event that genital injury is present, an abnormal finding can be verified either via delineation with a cotton swab in pubertal young women or in an alternative position such as prone knee-chest in prepubertal girls whose unestrogenized tissue does not tolerate manipulation. Alternatively, application of a few drops of saline can be applied to the vestibule to allow adhered unestrogenized hymenal leaflets to "float" freely and provide a view of the hymenal rim and base. Traumatic findings that may be encountered include abrasions or bruising of the mucosa; tears or scars of the labia minora, fossa

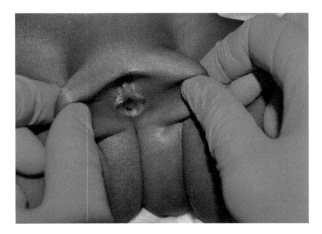

Figure 25.1 Labial traction technique in a prepubertal girl allows a clear view of an unestrogenized and uninterrupted annular hymen.

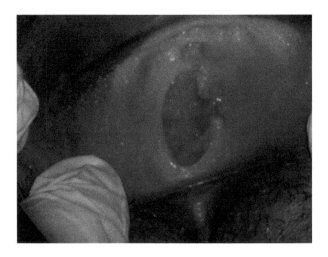

Figure 25.3 This postpubertal hymen has an avulsion of the hymen at 2 o'clock, clearly indicative of penetrating vaginal trauma. A longitudinal vaginal ridge inserts just inferior to the area of injury at 3 o'clock, creating a hymenal mound, which is a normal variant.

navicularis, posterior fourchette, or posterior hymen; tears interrupting the posterior hymen; or absent hymenal tissue. Table 25.1 reviews the findings associated with cases suspicious of sexual abuse.

Anal examination is typically accomplished with buttock separation to evaluate anal symmetry, tone, and integrity of the skin of the verge and rugae. This can be accomplished in any of the previously discussed positions or in the lateral decubitus position. It should be noted that prone knee-chest is a particularly vulnerable pose due to both the degree of exposure it creates as well as the patient's inability to observe the examiner's approach, and so it may not be the best choice for examining a child who reports anal assault. Definitive anal injury, such as bruising, laceration, or scarring, is vanishingly rare—even more so than genital injury—in the sexually abused child, described in 1% or fewer of various study populations.[9,24]

Documentation of the exam findings should reflect the care and complexity of the exam, whether the results show abnormality or not, with the goal of being as specific to the individual patient as possible. It is, therefore, recommended by Trotman[25] to avoid general terms as "normal genitalia," which fails to reflect the great variety of normal exam findings. "Virgo intacta," "virginal introitus," "marital hymen," "gaping vulva," or "enlarged vaginal opening" are imprecise and uninformative terms. These phrases should be strictly avoided.[22,26,27]

Forensic evidence collection

Most children and adolescents presenting in clinic will not have indications for a sexual assault evidence collection kit. Collection of forensic evidence is warranted when the last episode of abuse occurred within 96 hours, if the child is acutely injured, and if the history includes the potential for exposure to bodily fluids.[28] The examination should be conducted in accordance with institutional and local protocols for sexual assault victims in order to collect the evidence properly. To aid the child during exam, the presence of a nonoffending and supportive family member is also advised. Many hospitals have a pediatric sexual assault nurse examiner (SANE-P), child protection team, or child abuse pediatrician available as a resource or to assist in anogenital examination with colposcopy and photography, and with documentation. It is also worth noting that victim reactions to sexual assault are unpredictable; there is no standard emotional or social response to the violence. A patient may be minimally interactive, appear sad or withdrawn, or could engage with the medical team without outward signs of upset. Unless there are concerns for drug or alcohol intoxication, the patient's postassault demeanor should not influence the care provider's acceptance of the assault history.

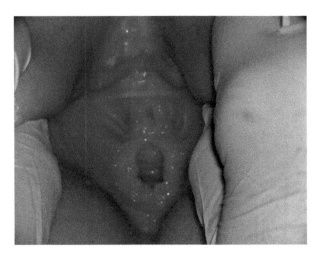

Figure 25.2 This Tanner stage 3 patient has an uninterrupted annular hymen with mucosal thickening, characteristic of estrogenization, as well as prominent periurethral bands.

Table 25.1 2018 updated approach to interpretation of medical findings in suspected child sexual abuse.

Section 1: Physical findings

A. *Findings documented in newborns or commonly seen in nonabused children. These findings are normal and are unrelated to a child's disclosure of sexual abuse.*

   1. Normal variations in appearance of the hymen:
      a. *Annular*: Hymenal tissue present all around the vaginal opening including at the 12 o'clock location.
      b. *Crescentic hymen*: Hymenal tissue is absent at some point above the 3–9 o'clock locations.
      c. *Imperforate hymen*: Hymen with no opening.
      d. *Microperforate hymen*: Hymen with one or more small openings.
      e. *Septate hymen*: Hymen with one or more septae across the opening.
      f. *Redundant hymen*: Hymen with multiple flaps, folding over each other.
      g. Hymen with tag of tissue on the rim.
      h. Hymen with mounds or bumps on the rim at any location.
      i. Any notch or cleft of the hymen (regardless of depth) above the 3 and 9 o'clock locations.
      j. A notch or cleft in the hymen, at or below the 3 o'clock or 9 o'clock location, that does not extend nearly to the base of the hymen.
      k. Smooth posterior rim of hymen that appears to be relatively narrow along the entire rim; may give the appearance of an "enlarged" vaginal opening.
   2. Periurethral or vestibular band(s).
   3. Intravaginal ridge(s) or column(s).
   4. External ridge on the hymen.
   5. Diastasis ani (smooth area).
   6. Perianal skin tag(s).
   7. Hyperpigmentation of the skin of labia minora or perianal tissues in children of color.
   8. Dilation of the urethral opening.
   9. Normal midline anatomic features:
      a. Groove in the fossa, seen in early adolescence.
      b. Failure of midline fusion (also called perineal groove).
      c. Median raphe (has been mistaken for a scar).
      d. Linea vestibularis (midline avascular area).
   10. Visualization of the pectinate/dentate line at the juncture of the anoderm and rectal mucosa, seen when the anus is fully dilated.
   11. Partial dilatation of the external anal sphincter, with the internal sphincter closed, causing visualization of some of the anal mucosa beyond the pectinate line, which may be mistaken for anal laceration.

B. *Findings commonly caused by medical conditions other than trauma or sexual contact. These findings require that a differential diagnosis be considered, as each may have several different causes.*

   12. Erythema of the anal or genital tissues.
   13. Increased vascularity of vestibule and hymen.
   14. Labial adhesion.
   15. Friability of the posterior fourchette.
   16. Vaginal discharge that is not associated with a sexually transmitted infection.
   17. Anal fissures.
   18. Venous congestion or venous pooling in the perianal area.
   19. Anal dilatation in children with predisposing conditions, such as current symptoms or history of constipation and/or encopresis, or children who are sedated, under anesthesia, or with impaired neuromuscular tone for other reasons, such as postmortem.

C. *Findings due to other conditions, which can be mistaken for abuse.*

   20. Urethral prolapse.
   21. Lichen sclerosus et atrophicus.
   22. Vulvar ulcer(s), such as aphthous ulcers or those seen in Behcet disease.
   23. Erythema, inflammation, and fissuring of the perianal or vulvar tissues due to infection with bacteria, fungus, viruses, parasites, or other infections that are not sexually transmitted.

(Continued)

Table 25.1 (Continued) 2018 updated approach to interpretation of medical findings in suspected child sexual abuse.

24. Rectal prolapse.

25. Red/purple discoloration of the genital structures (including the hymen) from lividity postmortem, if confirmed by histological analysis.

D. *No expert consensus regarding degree of significance. These physical findings have been associated with a history of sexual abuse in some studies, but at present, there is no expert consensus as to how much weight they should be given with respect to abuse. Findings 27 and 28 should be confirmed using additional examination positions and/or techniques, to ensure they are not normal variants (findings 1i, 1j) or a finding of residual traumatic injury (finding 37).*

26. Complete anal dilatation with relaxation of both the internal and external anal sphincters, in the absence of other predisposing factors, such as constipation, encopresis, sedation, anesthesia, and neuromuscular conditions.

27. Notch or cleft in the hymen rim, at or below the 3 o'clock or 9 o'clock location, which extends nearly to the base of the hymen but is not a complete transection. (This is a very rare finding that should be interpreted with caution unless an acute injury was documented at the same location.)

28. Complete cleft to the base of the hymen at the 3 or 9 o'clock location.

E. *Findings caused by trauma. These findings are highly suggestive of abuse, even in the absence of a disclosure from the child, unless the child and/or caretaker provides a timely and plausible description of accidental anogenital straddle, crush or impalement injury, or past surgical interventions that are confirmed from a review of the medical records. Findings that may represent residual/healing injuries should be confirmed using additional examination positions and/or techniques.*

Acute trauma to genital/anal tissues:

29. Acute laceration(s) or bruising of labia, penis, scrotum, or perineum.

30. Acute laceration of the posterior fourchette or vestibule, not involving the hymen.

31. Bruising, petechiae, or abrasions on the hymen.

32. Acute laceration of the hymen, of any depth, partial or complete.

33. Vaginal laceration.

34. Perianal laceration with exposure of tissues below the dermis.

Residual (healing) injuries to genital/anal tissues:

35. Perianal scar (a very rare finding that is difficult to diagnose unless an acute injury was previously documented at the same location).

36. Scar of posterior fourchette or fossa (a very rare finding that is difficult to diagnose unless an acute injury was previously documented at the same location).

37. Healed hymenal transection/complete hymen cleft—a defect in the hymen below the 3–9 o'clock location that extends to or through the base of the hymen, with no hymenal tissue discernible at that location.

38. Signs of female genital mutilation (FGM) or cutting, such as loss of part or all of the prepuce (clitoral hood), clitoris, labia minora or labia majora, or vertical linear scar adjacent to the clitoris (type 4 FGM).

Section 2: Infections

A. *Infections not related to sexual contact.*

39. Vaginitis caused by fungal infections such as *Candida albicans* or bacterial infections transmitted by nonsexual means, such as *Streptococcus* sp., *Staphylococcus* sp., *E. coli*, *Shigella*, or other gram-negative organisms.

40. Genital ulcers caused by viral infections such as Epstein–Barr virus or other respiratory viruses.

B. *Infections that can be spread by both nonsexual and sexual transmission; interpretation of these infections may require additional information, such as mother's gynecologic history (HPV) or child's history of oral lesions (HSV), or presence of lesions elsewhere on the body (Molluscum), which may clarify likelihood of sexual transmission. After complete assessment, a report to Child Protective Services may be indicated in some cases. Photographs or video recordings of these findings should be taken, then evaluated and confirmed by an expert in sexual abuse evaluation to ensure accurate diagnosis.*

41. *Molluscum contagiosum* in the genital or anal area. In young children, transmission is most likely nonsexual. Transmission from intimate skin-to-skin contact in the adolescent population has been described.

42. *Condyloma acuminatum* (HPV) in the genital or anal area. Warts appearing for the first time after age 5 years may be more likely to have been transmitted by sexual contact.

43. Herpes simplex type 1 or 2 infections in the oral, genital, or anal area.

C. *Infections caused by sexual contact, if confirmed by appropriate testing, and perinatal transmission has been ruled out.*

44. Genital, rectal, or pharyngeal *Neisseria gonorrhea* infection.

45. Syphilis.

(Continued)

Table 25.1 (Continued) 2018 updated approach to interpretation of medical findings in suspected child sexual abuse.

46. Genital or rectal *Chlamydia trachomatis* infection.

47. *Trichomonas vaginalis* infection.

48. HIV, if transmission by blood or contaminated needles has been ruled out.

Section 3: Findings diagnostic of sexual contact

49. Pregnancy.

50. Semen identified in forensic specimens taken directly from a child's body.

Source: With permission from Adams JA et al. *J Pediatr Adolesc Gynecol.* 2018;31:225–31.

Note: This table lists medical and laboratory findings; however, most children who are evaluated for suspected sexual abuse will not have physical signs of injury or infection. The child's description of what happened and report of specific symptoms in relationship to the events described are both essential parts of a full medical evaluation.

Diagnostic evaluation

If the abuse has occurred in the last 96 hours, complete or facilitate the collection of a forensic evidence kit.

Testing for STIs is dictated by exposure to potentially infected bodily secretions. Testing can be indicated by history, trauma on anogenital exam, positive genitourinary symptoms on review, or a shared environment with an STI-positive victim or perpetrator. Digital-genital contact alone is unlikely to transmit infection. On rare occasions, the presence of an STI is the only "evidence" that inappropriate contact occurred; the presence of an STI in a sample from a prepubertal patient outside the neonatal period suggests inappropriate contact. In the adolescent assault victim population, STI screening is recommended, not only for detecting potentially prevalent infections, but also for managing potential consensual sexual partners and monitoring reportable conditions (Table 25.2).[29] Gavril and colleagues reported on a group of over 700 prepubertal and adolescent patients in which 17.9% of those sexual abuse/assault victims were diagnosed with an STI; the authors note that most of these patients had normal or nonspecific exams, data that encourage a clinician to have a low threshold for STI evaluation.[30]

It is key to recognize that negative screening test results cannot exclude sexual abuse.

HIV prophylaxis

Prescription of a 28-day course of often costly postexposure prophylaxis, bearing a strong side effect profile, should be carefully considered. The decision to proceed with HIV postexposure prophylaxis (PEP) should be made in consultation with a pediatric specialist in infectious disease.[35] An additional useful resource is the PEPline (888/448–4911; http://nccc.ucsf.edu/clinician-consultation/pep-post-exposure-prophylaxis/).

Pregnancy

Remember to obtain a pregnancy test in a postmenarchal girl. Pregnancy or the detection of sperm/semen is diagnostic of sexual contact. Emergency contraception should be offered to those postmenarchal girls who present up to 5–7 days after their assault. Available options and initiation intervals are reviewed in Chapter 16.

Agency referral for child safety and protection

A report of a reasonable suspicion for a case of suspected child maltreatment to the state child protective services (CPS) agency is a mandate of medical care providers in order to address the child's safety and protection. Be aware that only a reasonable suspicion that abuse has occurred is necessary to warrant referring a child to an investigative agency; it is not the role or responsibility of the clinician to confirm the child's report. In addition, the Health Insurance Portability and Accountability Act does not apply to mandated reports because communication to appropriate child protection agencies is necessary to protect children. State laws can be found on the U.S. Department of Health and Human Services website.[36]

The provider's role in court

The clinician may be involved as one of several witnesses in the courtroom process in those cases of abuse or assault that are criminally prosecuted. Many children and young women who have been sexually victimized have undergone an evaluation by community partners who may include law enforcement, forensic interviewers, community protective agency social workers, mental health services, as well as medical providers from the emergency room to the outpatient office setting. Providers are unique because they obtain and record a history for the purposes of medical diagnosis and treatment as well as for patient safety and protection. Well-documented histories and exams are part and parcel of every clinician's training and are sufficient for courtroom purposes. (Forensic evidence collection kits are typically accompanied by paperwork that is a summary of the history and physical findings as well.) A provider can offer unique insight into how a girl's history can be found credible enough to rely on in creating a treatment plan, particularly because there are so rarely findings apparent on physical exam.[9,37,38]

A clinician who is an expert in the treatment of girls and young women may be subpoenaed to court in order to educate the jury. Dress professionally, and bring (and be familiar with) a current curriculum vitae with personal information such as home address and phone number removed. Be familiar with the child's name and birth date,

Table 25.2 Evaluation and management of sexually transmitted infections.

Organism	Method for testing	Interpretation	Treatment	Action recommended
Neisseria gonorrhoeae	NAATs should be collected from urine or the vagina as well as from other mucous membranes that may have had contact with bodily fluids (pharynx, rectum). An *N. gonorrhoeae* NAAT that does not react with nongonococcal commensal *Neisseria* species is recommended when testing oropharyngeal specimens.	*Indicative of child abuse* through contact with infected bodily secretions that is most likely sexual in nature [vertical transmission should be excluded]	Ceftriaxone 250 mg IM plus Azithromycin 1 g PO[a]	Referral to community partner agency for safety assessment. STI follow-up testing also recommended.
Chlamydia trachomatis	NAAT should be collected from urine or the vagina as well as from other mucous membranes that may have had contact with bodily fluids (pharynx, rectum).	*Indicative of child abuse* through contact with infected bodily secretions that is most likely sexual in nature [vertical transmission should be excluded]	Azithromycin 1 g PO	
Trichomonas vaginalis	NAATs for detection of *T. vaginalis* from vaginal swabs are recommended for adolescent assault victims over the more traditional wet mount microscopy. NAAT methods are not currently recommended for screening in prepubertal gir s.	*Indicative of child abuse* through contact with infected bodily secretions that is most likely sexual in nature [vertical transmission should be excluded]	Metronidazole or Tinidazole 2 g PO	Referral to community partner agency for safety assessment.
Syphilis	Serological testing: Nontreponemal studies such as RPR or VDRL, followed by treponeme-specific test such as FTA-ABS or TP-PA assay or various EIAs.	*Indicative of child abuse* through contact with infected bodily secretions that is most likely sexual in nature [vertical transmission should be excluded]	Treatment with benzathine penicillin G depending on stage of syphilis infection	Referral to community partner agency for safety assessment.
Human papillomavirus	Visual diagnosis typically suffices.	In the absence of an explanation, HPV in a prepubertal child *is indeterminate for abuse.* Human papillomavirus infection can derive from environmental contact, vertical transmission, or autoinoculation in addition to sexual contact.	HPV vaccination recommended for those child victims of sexual assault who are 9 years of age or older and have not already received the series; HPV vaccination at the time of initial assessment postassault serve to provide protection against vaccine types not yet acquired	Notify child protective agency of concern for potential sexual abuse.
Human herpesvirus-1 and 2	Vesicles, if present, should be unroofed and the sampled fluid collected and sent for viral culture. Antibody levels (IgM,IgG) rarely helpful.	In the absence of an explanation such as environmental or autoinoculation, HPV in a prepubertal child *is indeterminate for abuse.*	Acyclovir, valacyclovir, or famciclovir for acute outbreak; suppressive therapy may be needed depending on symptoms and number of repeat occurrences in a year	Notify child protective agency of concern for potential sexual abuse.

Source: Data from Sena AC et al. *Clin Infect Dis.* 2015;61:S856–64; Centers for Disease Control and Prevention. *MMWR Recomm Rep.* 2014;63(RR-02):1–19; Girardet RG et al. *Child Abuse Negl.* 2009;33:173–8; Olshen E et al. *Arch Pediatr Adolesc Med.* 2006;160:674–80; Adams JA et al. *J Pediatr Adolesc Gynecol.* 2017;31(3):225–31.

Abbreviations: EIA, enzyme immunoassay; FTA-ABS, fluorescent treponemal antibody absorption test; HPV, human papillomavirus; IM, intramuscularly; NAAT, nucleic acid amplification test; PO, orally; RPR, rapid plasma reagin; STI, sexually transmitted infection; TP-PA, *Treponema pallidum* particle agglutination assay; VDRL, Venereal Disease Research Laboratory.

[a] The potentially diminished efficacy of cephalosporins as solitary agents against *N. gonorrhoeae* organisms with increasing antimicrobial resistance is the basis for recommended dual empiric therapy with both an injectable cephalosporin as well as a macrolide.

as well as the date of your exam(s), and the general idea of the history and physical findings, especially if there were pertinent positives. The attorney can provide a copy of the record that is obtained from the health information management/medical records department of the treating facility. The role of the expert witness is to inform the jury about the meaning of what is contained in the medical records and how the medical impression was reached. When addressing the court, remove any personal or emotional attachments you may have to the case, and focus on delivering your findings truthfully.

Other considerations

Acquaintance rape/date rape

Terms such as "date rape" or "acquaintance rape" refer to sexual violence between people who encounter each other socially—this may be in the context of a relationship, a peer group, or just a shared event. It is important to be aware that simple miscommunication and sexual experimentation do not cause sexual violence. A perpetrator of date rape is not interested in romance or relationships, but rather in dominance and power. The idea of "dating" is used to gain first the trust of, and then access to, a potential victim, and alcohol and drugs may also be introduced in order to gain control over the other person. Rape myths can create confusion about acquaintance rape. Rape myths are culturally endorsed beliefs that exert a negative influence on disclosure of assault by proposing the victim perhaps invited the assault (i.e., "she was asking for it") or that a victim is lying and has ulterior motives (i.e., after contact occurs, changes her mind about consent). They can be invoked to trivialize an assault or to deny an assault occurred.[39,40]

Reproductive coercion

In some circumstances, the perpetrator of the sexual assault is someone with whom the victim has had a previous or ongoing physical relationship. In addition, reproductive coercion, which can manifest as threats of impregnation, impedance of access to contraception, or active interference with contraceptive methods such as throwing out birth control pills or condom manipulation, presents another form of "abuse."[41]

Among women surveyed by the Centers for Disease Control and Prevention (CDC), 10% reported reproductive coercion (RC) by a former partner. RC is more common among women with less education and is more prevalent among non-Hispanic African American, Latina, and multiracial women.[41-44] Women who experienced reproductive coercion were significantly more likely to have visited a clinician for more multiple pregnancy tests, STIs, or for emergency contraception in one study.[45] Although RC can occur in isolation or in conjunction with overt physical or sexual violence, these girls and women also benefit from simply being offered the opportunity to disclose their experiences in private. A recently published validation of a reproductive autonomy scale tool to assess a woman's feeling of autonomy in regard to her use of contraception and choice to pursue pregnancy and childbearing may be valuable to clinicians.[43]

Prevention

It is a challenge to consider reasonable options for prevention. Children are ideal victims given their dependence on their abusers and their inability to protect themselves.

Young children can be given the tools to enlist help from trusted adults by teaching them recognizable terms to discuss any problem with their anogenital region. Fanciful ("pouf-pouf") or opaque ("pocketbook") terms may confuse or complicate a discussion about inappropriate contact. A range of sexual abuse prevention programs have been provided to children, adolescents, or young adults through an array of venues, with varying efficacy in risk reduction. A curriculum that engages a community in a multilevel, multidisciplinary discussion and is provided in more than a single session is most effective, particularly when tailored to the needs of a specific community.[46,47] More information on primary prevention programs can be found at the Child Welfare Information Gateway (https://www.childwelfare.gov/topics/preventing/prevention-programs/schoolbased/) or via the National Sexual Violence Resource Center (https://www.nsvrc.org/).

Older girls can benefit from guidance regarding bystander behavior.[48] Encouraging supportive behaviors in groups of girls can take the form of agreements to arrive at and leave social events together and the identification of a "watcher" for companions at events when alcohol is involved. Moreover, young people should be encouraged to "see something, say something" and to question circumstances when consent to separate from the group or to engage in sexual contact is unclear.

Long-term effects

Adverse childhood experiences (ACEs), among which sexual abuse figures largely, have consistently been linked with poor mental and physical health in adulthood.[49-51] Sexual abuse is typically comorbid with other ACEs, and these experiences disrupt neurodevelopment. Subsequently, social, emotional, and cognitive regulation is impaired, leading adult victims of ACEs to adopt high-risk behaviors. Such a lifestyle can, in turn, result in disease, disability, and social difficulty, culminating in early death.[49] In particular, sexual abuse victims experience higher rates of Axis I disorders, such as anxiety, as well as suicideality.[48] This sobering progression emphasizes the importance of early recognition and intervention for abuse victims. Fostering resilience in these children and adolescents is key to their success as they process their experiences with sexual violence. Resilience is enhanced by a supportive and consistent adult in their lives and naturally is augmented by native intelligence. In addition to focused health services, there are several categories of interventions to which practitioners can refer their patients that appear to be effective: psychoeducational therapy groups offer some benefit for patients, specifically those that address single gender groups. Also, intensive case management and residential programs can foster healing among sexually exploited children and adolescents.[52]

CONCLUSIONS

Disclosure of sexual abuse or assault can be difficult for a pediatric patient. The clinician can assist in this challenging process by providing supportive listening, identifying the type of contact that occurred, and establishing the need for further medical and forensic evaluation. There are often medical and community partners available to collaborate with in order to ensure the child's safety and protection. The needs of child and adolescent victims of sexual abuse are not addressed by a single clinician visit, although there can be an enormous therapeutic value in a medical assessment where a trusted provider reassures a child of her good health and normal body after an assault. The repercussions of a sexual assault demand ongoing monitoring, not only for anogenital healing in response to rare trauma and surveillance for STIs, but also for the psychological effects that resonate long after medical interventions have taken effect.

REFERENCES

1. Child Welfare Information Gateway. *Definitions of Child Abuse and Neglect*. Washington, DC: U.S. Department of Health and Human Services, Children's Bureau; 2016.
2. U.S.C. 5101 et seq; 42 U.S.C. 5116 et seq.
3. Child Welfare Information Gateway. https://www.childwelfare.gov/topics/systemwide/laws-policies/state/; or Canadian Child Welfare Research Portal. http://cwrp.ca/legislation Accessed June 15, 2019.
4. Finkelhor D, Turner HA, Shattuck A, Hamby SL. Prevalence of childhood exposure to violence, crime, and abuse results from the national survey of children's exposure to violence. *JAMA Pediatr*. 2015;169(8):746–54.
5. Bureau of Justice Statistics, National Crime Victimization Survey (NCVS). 2016. https://www.bjs.gov/content/pub/pdf/cv16.pdf. Accessed December 21, 2017.
6. Shonkoff CJ. Reactions to the threatened loss of a child: A vulnerable child syndrome, by Morris Green, MD, and Albert A. Solnit, MD, *Pediatrics*, 1964;34:58–66. *Pediatrics*. 1998;102:239–41.
7. Finkel MA. I can tell you because you're a doctor. *Pediatrics*. 2008;122(2):442.
8. Ungar M, Tutty LM, McConnell S, Barter K, Fairholm J. What Canadian youth tell us about disclosing abuse. *Child Abuse Negl*. 2009;33:399–708.
9. Heger A, Ticson L, Velasquez O, Bernier R. Children referred for possible sexual abuse: Medical findings in 2384 children. *Child Abuse Negl*. 2002;26:645–59.
10. DeLago C, Deblinger E, Schroeder C, Finkel MA. Girls who disclose sexual abuse: Urogenital symptoms and signs after genital contact. *Pediatrics*. 2008;122(2):1.

11. National Children's Alliance. https://www.nationalchildrensalliance.org/ Accessed June 15, 2019.
12. Institute of Medicine and National Research Council. *Confronting Commercial Sexual Exploitation and Sex Trafficking of Minors in the United States*. Washington, DC: National Academies Press; 2013.
13. Greenbaum J, Crawford-Jakubiak JE. Child sex trafficking and commercial sexual exploitation: Health care needs of victims. *Pediatrics*. 2015;135:566.
14. Kellogg ND, Menard SW, Santos A. Genital anatomy in pregnant adolescents: "Normal" does not mean "nothing happened". *Pediatrics*. 2004;113(1):e67–9.
15. Anderst J, Kellogg N, Jung I. Reports of repetitive penile-genital penetration often have no definitive evidence of penetration. *Pediatrics*. 2009;124(3):e403–9.
16. Al-Jilaihawi S, Borg K, Jamieson K, Maguire S, Hodes D. Clinical characteristics of children presenting with a suspicion or allegation of historic sexual abuse. *Arch Dis Child*. 2018;103:533–9.
17. Kelly P, Koh J, Thompson JM. Diagnostic findings in alleged sexual abuse: Symptoms have no predictive value. *J Pediatr Child Health*. 2006;42:112–7.
18. Berenson AB, Chacko MR, Wiemann CM, Mishaw CO, Friedrich WN, Grady JJ. A case-control study of anatomic changes resulting from sexual abuse. *Am J Obstet Gynecol*. 2000;182(4):820–31.
19. Gallion HR, Milam LI, Littrell LL. Genital findings in cases of child sexual abuse. *J Pediatr Adolesc Gynecol*. 2016;29:604–11.
20. Hornor G, Scribano P, Curran S, Stevens J. Emotional response to the ano-genital examination of suspected sexual abuse. *J Forensic Nurs*. 2009;5:124–30.
21. De San Lazaro C. Making paediatric assessment in suspected sexual abuse a therapeutic experience. *Arch Dis Child*. 1995;73:174–6.
22. Hermann B, Navratil F. Sexual abuse in prepubertal children and adolescents. In: Sultan C, ed. *Pediatric and Adolescent Gynecology. Evidence-Based Clinical Practice*. 2nd revised and extended ed. Basel, Switzerland: Karger; 2012;22:112–37.
23. Adams JA, Farst KJ, Kellogg ND et al. Interpretation of medical findings in suspected child sexual abuse: An update for 2018. *J Pediatr Adolesc Gynecol*. 2018;31:225–31.
24. Myhre AK, Adams JA, Kaufhold M, Davis JL, Suresh P, Kuelbs CL. Anal findings in children with and without probable anal penetration: A retrospective study of 1115 children referred for suspected abuse. *Child Abuse Negl*. 2013;17(7):465–74.
25. Trotman G, Young-Anderson C, Deye KP. Acute sexual assault in the pediatric and adolescent population. *J Pediatr Adolesc Gynecol*. 29(6):518–26.
26. Finkel MA. Medical aspects of prepubertal sexual abuse. In: Reece RM, Christian CW, eds. *Child Abuse: Medical Diagnosis and Management*. 3rd ed. Elk Grove Village, IL: American Academy of Pediatrics; 2009:S269–320.

27. Kaplan R, Adams JA, Starling SP, Giardino AP. *Medical Response to Child Sexual Abuse: A Resource for Professionals Working with Children and Families.* St. Louis, MO: STM Learning; 2011.

28. Girardet R, Bolton K, Lahoti S, Mowbray H, Giardino A, Isaac R, Mead B, Paes N. Collection of forensic evidence from pediatric victims of sexual assault. *Pediatrics.* 2011;128(2):233–38.

29. Sena AC, Hsu KK, Kellogg N, Girardet R, Christian CW, Linden J, Griffith W, Jenny C, Hammerschlag MR. Sexual assault and sexually transmitted infections in adults, adolescents, and children. *Clin Infect Dis.* 2015;61:S856–64.

30. Gavril AR, Kellogg ND, Nair P. Value of follow-up examination of children evaluated for sexual abuse and assault. *Pediatrics.* 2012;129(2):282–9.

31. Centers for Disease Control and Prevention. Recommendations for the laboratory-based detection of *Chlamydia trachomatis* and *Neisseria gonorrhoeae*—2014. *MMWR Recomm Rep.* 2014;63 (RR-02):1–19.

32. Girardet RG, Lemme S, Biason TA, Bolton K, Lahoti S. HIV post-exposure prophylaxis in children and adolescents presenting for reported sexual assault. *Child Abuse Negl.* 2009;33:173–8.

33. Olshen E, Hsu K, Woods ER, Harper M, Harnisch B, Samples CL. Use of human immunodeficiency virus postexposure prophylaxis in adolescent sexual assault victims. *Arch Pediatr Adolesc Med.* 2006;160:674–80.

34. Adams JA, Farst KJ, Kellogg ND. Interpretation of medical findings in suspected child sexual abuse: An update for 2018. *J Pediatr Adolesc Gynecol.* 2017;31(3):225–31.

35. Centers for Disease Control and Prevention, U.S. Department of Health and Human Services. Updated Guidelines for Antiretroviral Postexposure Prophylaxis After Sexual, Injection Drug Use, or Other Nonoccupational Exposure to HIV. http://stacks.cdc.gov/view/cdc/38856 Accessed June 15, 2019.

36. Child Welfare Information Gateway. www.childwelfare.gov/systemwide/laws-policies/state/ Accessed June 15, 2019.

37. Kellogg ND, American Academy of Pediatrics Committee on Child Abuse and Neglect. Clinical report—The evaluation of sexual behaviors in children. *Pediatrics.* 2009;124(3):992–8.

38. Smith TD, Raman SR, Madigan S, Waldman J, Shouldice M. Anogenital findings in 3569 pediatric examinations for sexual abuse/assault. *J Pediatr Adolesc Gynecol.* 2018;31(2):79–83.

39. Franiuk R, Seefelt JL, Vandello JA. Prevalence of rape myths in headlines and their effects on attitudes toward rape. *Sex Roles.* 2008;58(11–12):790–801.

40. Burt MR. Cultural myths and supports for rape. *J Pers Soc Psychol.* 1980;38(2):217.

41. Miller E, Decker MR, McCauley HL et al. Pregnancy coercion, intimate partner violence and unintended pregnancy. *Contraception.* 2010;81:316.

42. Miller E, McCauley HL, Tancredi DJ, Decker MR, Anderson H, Silverman JG. Recent reproductive coercion and unintended pregnancy among female family planning clients. *Contraception.* 2014;89(2):122–8.

43. Upadhyay UD, Dworkin SL, Weitz TA, Foster DG. Development and validation of a reproductive autonomy scale. *Stud Fam Plann.* 2014;45(1):19–41.

44. Grace KT, Anderson JC. Reproductive coercion: A systematic review. *Trauma Violence Abuse.* 2016;1524838016663935.

45. Kazmerski T, McCauley HL, Jones K et al. Use of reproductive and sexual health services among female family planning clinic clients exposed to partner violence and reproductive coercion. *Matern Child Health J.* 2015;19(7):1490–6.

46. DeGue S, Valle LA, Holt MK, Massetti GM, Matjasko JL, Tharp AT. A systematic review of primary prevention strategies for sexual violence perpetration. *Aggress Violent Behav.* 2014;19(4):346–62.

47. Martyniuk H, Dworkin E. Child sexual abuse prevention: Programs for children. *National Sexual Violence Resource Center.* 2011;1–5.

48. Gable SC, Lamb S, Brodt M, Atwell L. Intervening in a "Sketchy Situation": Exploring the moral motivations of college bystanders of sexual assault. *J Interpers Violence.* 2017;0886260517730027.

49. Felitti VJ, Anda RF, Nordenberg D et al. Relationship of childhood abuse and household dysfunction to many of the leading causes of death in adults: The Adverse Childhood Experiences (ACE) Study. *Am J Prev Med.* 1998;14(4):245–58.

50. Lindert J, von Ehrenstein OS, Grashow R, Gal G, Braehler E, Weisskopf MG. Sexual and physical abuse in childhood is associated with depression and anxiety over the life course: Systematic review and meta-analysis. *Int J Public Health.* 2014;59(2):359–72.

51. Pérez-Fuentes G, Olfson M, Villegas L, Morcillo C, Wang S, Blanco C. Prevalence and correlates of child sexual abuse: A national study. *Compr Psychiatry.* 2013;54(1):16–27.

52. Moynihan M, Pitcher C, Saewyc E. Interventions that foster healing among sexually exploited children and adolescents: A systematic review. *J Child Sex Abus.* 2018;1–21.

Fertility preservation in pediatric and adolescent girls

26

MOLLY MORAVEK

INTRODUCTION

Due to significant advancements in treatment, more and more children are surviving cancer,[1] with the mortality rate in the United States dropping to 2.1 per 100,000 children between 2010 and 2014.[2] There were an estimated 93,478 female survivors of childhood cancer in the United States as of 2011,[3] but unfortunately, many of these girls and women have been rendered infertile from their lifesaving treatment. There are several studies that show that fertility, or lack thereof, is a pervasive concern for childhood cancer survivors.[4] Accordingly, multiple national societies, including the American Academy of Pediatrics, American Society for Reproductive Medicine, and American Society for Clinical Oncology, have published guidelines recommending fertility preservation counseling and/or care prior to cancer treatment.[5–7] There is also increasing recognition of other, nononcologic treatments and conditions that can threaten fertility, and these populations should be offered the same options as cancer patients. Access to a fertility specialist or a formal fertility preservation program has been shown to increase fertility counseling by oncologists and utilization of fertility preservation services.[8,9] Established in 2007, the Oncofertility Consortium is a global, multidisciplinary network that conducts cutting-edge fertility preservation research and provides guidance to practitioners interested in providing fertility preservation services. Given their training in both reproduction and the care of pediatric and adolescent females, pediatric and adolescent gynecologists are uniquely poised to fulfill this role for pediatric programs and should be able to discuss the basics of ovarian reserve, gonadal risk, available fertility preservation options, and future implications with patients facing fertility-threatening conditions or treatments.

OOGENESIS AND OVARIAN RESERVE

Counseling patients about the fertility risks of gonadotoxic treatments or conditions, or assessing fertility following gonadotoxic therapy, requires some understanding of oogenesis, ovarian reserve, and the hypothalamic-pituitary-ovarian axis. Maximal oocyte number is achieved *in utero*, with approximately 6–7 million oocytes at 16–20 weeks' gestational age. Oocyte numbers start to decline via atresia and degeneration soon thereafter, with approximately 500,000 to 2,000,000 oocytes remaining at birth; 300,000–500,000 at the time of puberty; and less than 1000 at menopause (Figure 26.1).[10,11] Even in women who are not ovulating, oocytes are continuously being depleted throughout the life span. Gonadal function is important not only for female fertility, but also for the production of sex hormones, important for the maintenance of bone architecture and cardiovascular health. Given that the

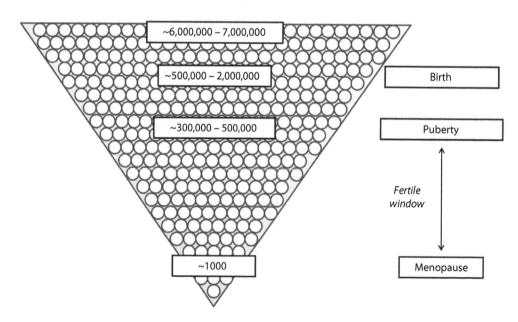

Figure 26.1 Number of remaining oocytes at different reproductive milestones. The fertile window may be shortened in women with a history of gonadotoxic treatments.

number of oocytes is fixed at birth, gonadotoxic therapies or surgical removal of the gonads can have lifelong detrimental effects on both fertility and overall health.

While it is impossible to know exactly how many oocytes are remaining in an individual female at a specific point in time, there are serum and ultrasound markers that can give a general sense of overall ovarian reserve. The ovaries are fairly quiescent until puberty, at which time they fall under the control of the hypothalamic-pituitary-ovarian axis (Figure 26.2), with follicle-stimulating hormone (FSH) secreted at the beginning of each cycle to begin recruitment of a dominant follicle. A cohort of oocytes is recruited every month, but generally only one reaches final maturity and is ovulated, while the rest undergo apoptosis. Once the dominant follicle begins to develop, surrounding granulosa cells secrete estradiol into the circulation, which provides negative feedback to the hypothalamus and pituitary, with a resultant decrease in serum FSH levels (Figure 26.2). As such, serum FSH and estradiol levels must be checked early in the follicular phase (preferably on cycle day 2, 3, or 4) to assess ovarian reserve, with higher FSH levels indicating worse ovarian reserve. Ideal ovarian function is reflected by FSH <10 IU/mL, with

FSH rising above 40 IU/mL in menopause. It is important to draw an estradiol with FSH levels, as negative feedback from increased estradiol levels can drive down the FSH level and provide false reassurance. An elevated estradiol level on cycle day 2, 3, or 4 can also reflect declining ovarian function.

Anti-müllerian hormone (AMH) is produced by the granulosa cells of preantral and antral follicles, which are thought to reflect overall follicular reserve, and is thus another marker of ovarian reserve. Assessing AMH levels is often more practical than FSH/estradiol, as there is minimal fluctuation both within and between cycles, and levels are not as dramatically affected by hormonal treatment, such as birth control pills. AMH rises irregularly during the teen years and peaks in the early 20s, which means serum AMH levels can be difficult to interpret in adolescents.[12] Moreover, AMH levels are often suppressed during chemotherapy,[13] so they are of little utility in patients actively undergoing treatment. Finally, the antral follicles (2–10 mm) can also be assessed directly by ultrasound measurement, but normal ranges have not been established in adolescence.

The majority of the existing literature on fertility after gonadotoxic therapy reports rates of amenorrhea or ovarian failure, not actual fertility. The standard definition of amenorrhea is absence of menses for at least 6 months.[14] Many females become amenorrheic while undergoing gonadotoxic therapy, which can be due to hypothalamic hypogonadism, ovarian failure, or suppression; however, the vast majority of women who will ultimately resume menses will do so within 12 months following last treatment.[15] Unfortunately, even in girls who resume regular menses, ovarian reserve or function may still be significantly damaged, leading to future fertility struggles. Therefore, postpubertal girls who have received gonadotoxic treatment and desire future fertility should be referred to a reproductive specialist who can assess whether posttreatment fertility preservation should occur.

FERTILITY PRESERVATION IN CANCER PATIENTS

Most studies regarding gonadotoxic treatments have been conducted in cancer patients and have shown that female cancer survivors have decreased pregnancy rates and increased rates of infertility, compared to siblings without a cancer history.[16,17] Fertility can be affected by surgical removal of reproductive organs, chemotherapy, or radiation. There is a range in both the timeline and the extent of the effect of nonsurgical gonadotoxic treatments on oocytes, with some girls retaining ovarian function following treatment, but with a shortened reproductive window and earlier age at menopause, and others showing little to no ovarian function after treatment.[18–22] There are publicly available online tools to help providers with risk assessment, but it is important to note that these resources do not take into account differences in baseline characteristics, such as ovarian reserve. Additionally, the risk estimates provided by these resources are for ovarian failure, not necessarily impaired fertility or a shortened reproductive window.

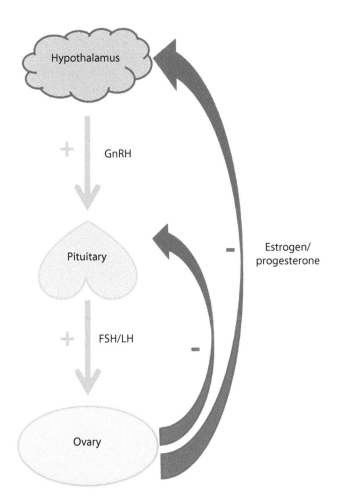

Figure 26.2 Hypothalamic-pituitary-ovarian axis. (FSH, follicle-stimulating hormone; GnRH, gonadotropin-releasing hormone; LH, luteinizing hormone).

Effect of chemotherapy on reproduction

The effect of chemotherapy on ovarian function is dependent on patient age, baseline ovarian reserve, specific chemotherapeutic agent, and cumulative dose (Table 26.1).[23,24] It is not completely understood how chemotherapy leads to oocyte loss, although it is thought to be due to a combination of damage to supporting vasculature and supporting cells, like granulosa cells, resulting in follicular apoptosis and ovarian cortex fibrosis.[25] Alkylating agents, such as cyclophosphamide, procarbazine, and ifosfamide, are particularly damaging to the ovaries,[26] and an online calculator for the "cyclophosphamide equivalent dose" can be used to assess cumulative gonadotoxicity of multiple alkylating agents.[27,28] Heavy metals, such as carboplatin or cisplatin, also may impact female fertility.[29]

Effect of radiation on reproduction

Similar to chemotherapy, the effect of radiation on ovarian tissue is dependent on age, total radiation dose, fractionation schedule, and treatment field.[30] Ovarian insufficiency is reported in greater than 90% of patients who undergo abdominal or pelvic radiation with 20–30 gray (Gy) and total-body irradiation with 15 Gy[31]; however, ovarian reserve may be negatively impacted with doses as low as 2 Gy.[30]

It is important to remember that radiation to the brain can impair the hypothalamic-pituitary-ovarian axis and cause gonadotropin deficiency and amenorrhea, but this does not reflect ovarian insufficiency and can be managed with hormonal interventions.[32] Patients should not undergo fertility preservation procedures or attempt pregnancy during radiation treatment.[33,34] It is also important to counsel patients that radiation to the uterus increases the risk of uterine factor infertility, hypertensive diseases of pregnancy, preterm birth, and miscarriage.[35,36] There are some data to suggest that younger age at the time of radiation, particularly in prepubertal girls, leads to more profound adverse effects on future fertility and pregnancy outcomes.[37] Unfortunately, there have not been any effective methods described to date that could help assess uterine function after radiation to better stratify risk for patients.

Table 26.1 Risk of ovarian failure from commonly used chemotherapy regimens and radiation protocols.

High risk	• Whole abdominal or pelvic radiation doses >6 Gy in adult women • Total-body irradiation (TBI) • Cranial/brain irradiation >40 Gy • CMF, CEF, or CAF × six cycles in women >40 years • Total cyclophosphamide 5 g/m² in women >40 years • Total cyclophosphamide >7.5 g/m² <20 years • Alkylating chemotherapy (e.g., cyclophosphamide, busulfan, melphalan) conditioning for transplant • Any alkylating agent (e.g., cyclophosphamide, ifosfamide, busulfan, BCNU [carmustine], CCNU [lomustine]) + TBI or pelvic radiation • Protocols containing procarbazine: MOPP, MVPP, COPP, ChlVPP, ChlVPP/EVA, BEACOPP, MOPP/ABVD, COPP/ABVD
Intermediate risk	• Abdominal/pelvic radiation • CMF, CEF, or CAF × six cycles in women 30–40 years • Spinal radiation doses >25 Gy CMF, CEF, or CAF × six cycles in women 30–40 years • Bevacizumab (Avastin) • Protocols containing cisplatin • FOLFOX4 • Total cyclophosphamide 5 g/m² in women age 30–40
Low risk	• CMF, CEF, or CAF × six cycles in women <30 years • Nonalkylating chemotherapy: ABVD • Anthracycline + cytarabine
No risk	• Radioactive iodine • MF • Multiagent therapies using vincristine
Unknown risk	• Monoclonal antibodies, e.g., cetuximab (Erbitux) • Tyrosine kinase inhibitors, e.g., erlotinib (Tarceva), imatinib (Gleevec)

Source: From the OncoFertility Consortium (https://savemyfertility.org), with permission.
Abbreviations: ABVD, Adriamycin/bleomycin/vinblastine/dacarbazine; AC, Adriamycin/cyclophosphamide; BEACOPP, bleomycin/etoposide/Adriamycin/cyclophosphamide/Oncovin/procarbazine/prednisone; CAF, cyclophosphamide/Adriamycin (doxorubicin)/fluorouracil; CEF, cyclophosphamide/epirubicin/fluorouracil; ChlVPP, chlorambucil/vinblastine/procarbazine/prednisolone; CHOP, cyclophosphamide/hydroxy-daunomycin/Oncovin/prednisone; COP, cyclophosphamide/Oncovin/prednisone; COPP, cyclophosphamide/Oncovin/procarbazine/prednisone; EVA, etoposide/vinblastine/Adriamycin; MOPP, mechlorethamine/Oncovin (vincristine)/procarbazine/prednisone; MF, methotrexate/5-fluorouracil; MVPP, mechlorethamine/vinblastine/procarbazine/prednisolone.

OTHER FERTILITY-THREATENING CONDITIONS AND TREATMENTS

Young girls with cancer are not the only patients who could benefit from fertility preservation services. Alkylating agents are also used for nononcologic conditions, such as lupus nephritis, vasculitis, and some neurologic disorders, and stem cell transplant might be indicated for conditions such as sickle cell disease. A fertility preservation consult is also indicated for young girls at risk for premature ovarian insufficiency, from conditions such as galactosemia, fragile X syndrome, and mosaic Turner syndrome.[38] The role of fertility preservation is less clear in youth with differences of sex development, although there is recent evidence of potentially viable germ cells at the time of gonadectomy.[39] Another active area of research is whether female-to-male transgender adolescents should be offered fertility preservation procedures prior to transitioning, as the long-term effects of cross-sex hormone therapy with testosterone on future fertility are currently unclear.[40,41] Fertility preservation programs should engage the proper pediatric specialists in order to make sure these patients are offered all options in a timely manner.

OPTIONS FOR FERTILITY PRESERVATION

The different methods of fertility preservation in girls, both established and experimental, are summarized in Table 26.2, and expanded in the next sections.

Medical interventions

Using gonadotropin-releasing hormone agonist (GnRHa) for ovarian suppression during chemotherapy or radiation is still considered experimental. After an initial flare in activity, GnRHa inhibits the pulsatile release of gonadotropins from the anterior pituitary, leading to cessation of ovarian follicle development, similar to prepubertal girls or postmenopausal women. Inhibiting follicular growth makes the developing oocytes and hormone-producing cells of the ovary less transcriptionally active, and therefore, theoretically less sensitive to the gonadotoxic effects of chemotherapy and radiation, potentially protecting future ovarian function.[42] GnRHa may have additional benefits for patients undergoing treatment, most importantly, menstrual suppression in patients with low platelet count.[6] There are ongoing investigations of other medical interventions that may mitigate the effects of chemotherapy and radiation on the ovary, but none that are currently being used clinically (Table 26.3).

Oocyte/embryo cryopreservation

As of 2013, the American Society for Reproductive Medicine (ASRM) declared that oocyte cryopreservation is no longer considered experimental, with fertilization, clinical pregnancy, and live birth rates approximating those achieved with freshly retrieved

Table 26.2 Fertility preservation options for girls.

Method	Considered experimental	Option for prepubertal girls	Approximate time required	Permit natural conception in future	Potential to preserve or restore hormone function	Other considerations
GnRH agonist	Yes	No	<1 day	Yes	Yes	Initial flare in ovarian activity that lasts 7–10 days with unclear effect on ovarian sensitivity to chemotherapy or radiation
Oocyte/embryo cryopreservation	No	No	2 weeks	No	No	May want to consider performing U.S. Food and Drug Administration testing, in case patient needs gestational carrier in the future
Ovarian tissue cryopreservation	Yes	Yes	1 day	Yes	Yes	Concerns about reintroducing malignant cells, especially with hematologic cancers
Ovarian transposition	No	Yes	1 day	Depends on ovarian location	Yes	Does not protect against uterine effects of radiation

Table 26.3 Experimental medical agents that may mitigate the effect of cancer treatment on the ovaries.

Protective agent	Mechanism of action on ovary	Interactions with cytotoxic treatments
GnRH analog	Direct effect on ovary is unclear; suppresses hypothalamic-pituitary-ovarian (HPO) axis, possible ovarian quiescence	No interference with treatment drugs
Imatinib	Inhibit c-Abl kinase apoptosis pathway	May interfere with apoptotic action of chemotherapy drugs
Bone marrow mesenchymal stem cells	Tissue differentiation, angiogenesis, antiapoptosis	May cause chemotherapy drug resistance with Cisplatin
S1P	Inhibit sphingomyelin apoptosis pathway	May interfere with apoptotic action of chemotherapy drugs
Tamoxifen	Antiapoptotic activity; antioxidant activity via IGF-1 axis; possible HPO axis suppression	Adjuvant therapy; no interference with treatment drugs
AS101	Inhibits P13K/PTEN Akt follicle activation pathway; antiapoptosis	No interference with treatment drugs; may have additive/synergistic interaction with treatment drugs
Growth colony-stimulating factor (G-CSF)	Unclear: Possibly angiogenesis; antiapoptosis	No interference with treatment drugs

Source: From the Oncofertility Consortium (http://oncofertility.northwestern.edu/resources/estimating-risk-cancer-therapy), with permission.
Abbreviation: NTD, Nothing to date.

oocytes (Figure 26.3).[7,43] Stimulation for oocyte or embryo cryopreservation should be performed under the supervision of a trained reproductive endocrinology and infertility specialist, preferably who has experience working with pediatric and adolescent patients, in a facility that is comfortable performing anesthesia in adolescents. Centers specializing in fertility preservation should ideally also have specialized mental health providers available to assist patients and their families through this trying time, and if not immediately available, patients should be offered referral.[44] In order to be a candidate for oocyte or embryo cryopreservation, patients must be postpubertal, physically well enough to undergo anesthesia and retrieval, able to delay treatment for at least 2 weeks, and emotionally and physically able to undergo transvaginal monitoring. In postmenarchal females, this method is the most likely to result in subsequent pregnancy and should be offered if ovarian stimulation and oocyte retrieval may safely be performed.[7] Oocyte cryopreservation has been reported in postpubertal but premenarchal girls; however, the outcomes from these cycles remain to be determined, as these patients have not yet attempted conception,[45,46] and this is an ongoing area of research.

For ovarian stimulation, patients administer gonadotropins subcutaneously for an average of 8–12 days, with frequent ovarian monitoring by ultrasound and hormone analysis to assess follicular progress and appropriateness of gonadotropin dose. GnRH antagonist is also initiated once follicles begin developing, to prevent ovulation prior to oocyte retrieval. Once an appropriate number of large follicles (thought to obtain a mature oocyte) are observed by ultrasound, initiation of the ovulation cascade is induced via subcutaneous injection of human chorionic gonadotropin (hCG) or GnRHa. Under conscious sedation, oocytes are generally retrieved transvaginally with ultrasound guidance, although transabdominal retrievals can also be performed, if necessary.

Mature oocytes can be cryopreserved the day of retrieval or fertilized with either partner or donor sperm to create embryos that are cryopreserved in 1–6 days. Given the similarity in efficacy between fresh and frozen oocytes, and because embryos created with a partner's sperm would give that partner legal rights over future disposition of any cryopreserved embryos, cryopreserving oocytes is a better option for most adolescents. Oocytes and embryos are most commonly cryopreserved in an ultrarapid fashion called *vitrification*, which has decreased the damage rate previously seen with traditional slow-freezing, resulting in improved thaw survival and future pregnancy rates.[47,48] Overall pregnancy rates from oocyte cryopreservation are approximately 4.5%–12% per thawed oocyte.[49] As the chance for future pregnancy increases with the number of oocytes retrieved, patients with a lower oocyte yield can be offered back-to-back stimulation cycles to increase the cumulative number of oocytes available for potential fertilization and transfer.[50,51] Patients should also be made aware of the availability of preimplantation genetic diagnosis to potentially screen future embryos for any known genetic predispositions to cancer or other diseases.

A typical oocyte cryopreservation cycle takes approximately 2 weeks (mean 11.5 days, range 9–20 days),[52] and patients can initiate chemotherapy or radiation immediately afterward. Risks associated with an oocyte cryopreservation cycle include development of ovarian hyperstimulation syndrome (OHSS), potential delay in initiation of cancer therapy, surgical risks of the oocyte retrieval procedure, and thromboembolic phenomena.[7] Modified stimulation protocols have subsequently been developed to address and minimize some of these risks. Additionally, "random-start" protocols, in which

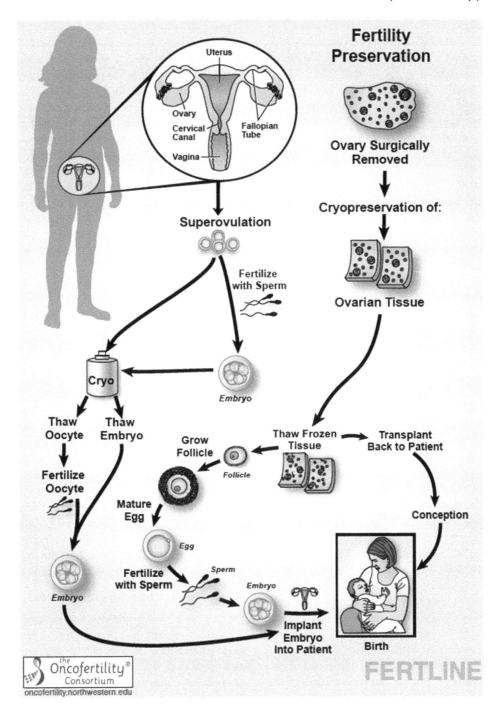

Figure 26.3 Summary of oocyte/embryo cryopreservation versus ovarian tissue cryopreservation (From the Oncofertility Consortium, with permission.)

gonadotropins are initiated as soon as possible irrespective of menstrual phase instead of waiting for menses, have decreased the time frame needed for fertility preservation-related procedures, without compromising oocyte yield or future pregnancy rates.[42,53–55] According to current knowledge, there is no upper limit on the amount of time oocytes or embryos can be cryopreserved without a loss in function. Importantly, the quality and efficacy of oocytes retrieved from postpubertal adolescent girls (prior to any exposure to gonadotoxic treatment) have also recently been brought into question, with some researchers suggesting

the quality may be comparable to women of advanced reproductive age.[56] Research is ongoing on this topic, but patients and their families should be counseled that the quality of oocytes retrieved in adolescence remains to be fully elucidated.

Ovarian tissue cryopreservation

Ovarian tissue cryopreservation (OTC) is currently the only fertility preservation option available to prepubertal girls, and it is also available to postpubertal girls who cannot, or do not want to, delay cancer treatment in order undergo an oocyte cryopreservation cycle (Figure 26.3).[7,57] OTC can also be combined with ovarian stimulation and oocyte cryopreservation to increase overall yield.[58] It is still considered experimental in the United States but is being increasingly used as a fertility preservation option throughout the world. Ovarian tissue cryopreservation theoretically represents an efficient method of preserving thousands of ovarian follicles at one time, as well as provides the potential to return native hormone production once retransplanted.[7,59]

For patients electing OTC, part or all of an ovary is surgically removed, ideally at the time of another procedure requiring anesthesia, such as biopsy or port placement. Surgical techniques include taking care to avoid unnecessary handling of the ovarian cortical region, and to keep the ovary perfused as long as possible, by dividing the ovarian artery last.[60] Once removed, the ovarian tissue is brought to pathology for examination, then the ovarian cortex, where the greatest density of follicles are located,[61] is cut into small strips and cryopreserved via slow-freezing or vitrification. These strips can later be thawed and autotransplanted either orthotopically, into the peritoneum or onto the patient's remaining ovary, or heterotopically in the forearm, abdominal wall, or chest wall. Menstrual cycles have been reported to occur within 4–9 months after transplantation, consistent with the time necessary for follicular growth maturation.[57] Studies have shown survival of transplanted ovarian tissue to range from several months to years, depending on the amount of tissue transplanted and the age and ovarian reserve of the woman when the ovarian tissue was excised, with the longest documented transplant functioning for 7 years.[57] A recent meta-analysis of OTC outcomes suggested the live birth rate may be greater than 35%, and native hormone function greater than 65%.[62] More than 86 births worldwide have been attributed to OTC,[63–65] including from tissue cryopreserved from one peripubertal and one prepubertal patient.[66,67]

A review of OTC surgical outcomes reveals a less than 1% risk of minor complications and no delay of cancer treatment.[68] Risks associated with OTC include the surgical and anesthetic risk involved with laparoscopy or laparotomy for obtaining the tissue and for the subsequent retransplantation. Additionally, the risk of reintroduction of malignancy in the transplanted ovarian tissue is of significant concern, with cancer cells reported in OTC samples from patients with leukemia, breast, gastric, uterine, and cervical cancer.[69–73] To address this concern, research is ongoing as to the safest way to restore fertility and/or ovarian function to patients after OTC.[71,74–77]

In vitro oocyte maturation

Reproductive researchers continue to explore fertility preservation techniques that can both reduce patient risk and minimize treatment delays. One experimental technique, in vitro oocyte maturation (IVM), involves removal of immature oocytes either via transvaginal oocyte retrieval or from surgically resected ovarian tissue, then maturing these oocytes in the laboratory so they can be cryopreserved as mature oocytes or fertilized for embryo cryopreservation. Compared to conventional ovarian stimulation for oocyte cryopreservation, IVM results in less cost and time for patients because it obviates the need for stimulation medications and multiple monitoring visits, in addition to avoiding exposure to large doses of gonadotropins and resultant elevated estradiol levels.[52] Research is also being conducted to advance methods of isolating and maturing oocytes at all stages of development from both fresh and cryopreserved–thawed ovarian tissue.[7] To date, there have not been any live births reported from IVM of immature oocytes obtained at the time of harvesting ovarian tissue for cryopreservation, although this is an area of ongoing investigation, as is cryopreservation of immature oocytes for later IVM.[42,57] Development of techniques to successfully grow and mature oocytes *in vitro* would be particularly pertinent to cancer patients, as it could mitigate the potential risks associated with autotransplantation of cryopreserved ovarian tissue, such as reintroduction of malignant cells and need for multiple surgeries due to shortened graft life.

Ovarian transposition

In patients who require pelvic radiation, the ovaries can be laparoscopically transposed higher in the pelvis to minimize the dose of direct radiation to the ovaries, a technique that has been successfully performed for decades.[78–80] Ovarian transposition often necessitates assisted reproductive technology for future conception, due to the resulting distance of the ovaries from the uterus.[81] Unfortunately, the uterus cannot be moved outside the pelvic radiation field, so patients may still require a gestational carrier for future pregnancies. In patients undergoing radiation at more distant sites from the pelvis, the ovaries and uterus should always be shielded to minimize scatter.

Alternatives to fertility preservation

During any fertility preservation conversation, it is important to discuss alternatives to fertility preservation procedures, specifically doing nothing/accepting risk, receiving donor oocytes or embryos in the future (known or anonymous), or adoption. Due to reports of some adoption agencies expressing unwillingness to work with cancer survivors, the Oncofertility Consortium has compiled a list of "cancer-friendly" adoption agencies (http://oncofertility.northwestern.edu/files/documents/cancer-friendly-adoption-agencies).

CONTRACEPTION DURING AND AFTER GONADOTOXIC TREATMENTS

When patients present to discuss fertility, this is an opportune time to discuss contraception, as pregnancy should be prevented while undergoing chemotherapy and radiation. Since patients with cancer may be in a hypercoagulable state, some oncologists are uncomfortable with estrogen-containing hormonal forms of birth control, because of the associated increased rate of venous thromboembolism.[82] Consideration should be given to placement of a copper or levonorgestrel intrauterine device (IUD), given low failure rates and improved bleeding profiles with the levonorgestrel IUD, which may be especially pertinent in patients with chemotherapy-induced thrombocytopenia.[83] The etonogestrel implant and injectable depot medroxyprogesterone acetate are also alternatives for contraception in this population. Due to the impression that they cannot conceive naturally, cancer survivors are also at increased risk of unplanned pregnancy.[84] Following gonadotoxic treatment, it is important to remember that pregnancies can occur in patients diagnosed with primary ovarian insufficiency, and oral contraceptive pills may not be effective contraception, thought possibly to be due to the extremely high gonadotropin levels overriding the suppressive effects.[85,86]

INTEGRATING FERTILITY PRESERVATION INTO CLINICAL CARE

There are data to suggest that a systematic, multidisciplinary approach to fertility preservation increases both programmatic success and referral rates.[87,88] Fertility preservation teams need to have the proper personnel to be able to provide rapid consultation to potential fertility preservation patients, accurately assess fertility risk, discuss fertility preservation options, and perform fertility preservation procedures. There are publicly available, online tools to assist both caregivers and patients in assessing risk of potentially gonadotoxic therapies and making fertility preservation decisions.[28,89,90] Program development may also need to include education of oncologists and other care providers for patients facing fertility-threatening conditions and treatments, to create awareness of fertility preservation options.[91] Many fertility preservation programs utilize a clinical coordinator or a patient navigator to assist patients during the complex referral and treatment process, and to act as a liaison between the multiple specialties often involved in the patient's care. Additionally, mental health professionals that specialize in both pediatric and fertility care can provide valuable guidance and support for patients and families navigating the fertility preservation process.[92-95] It is also important for centers with a fertility preservation program to either be equipped for long-term storage of harvested tissue or be able to send tissue to such a facility in a timely and cost-effective manner and to have lab personnel with expertise in gamete and tissue handling and cryopreservation. Unfortunately, most fertility preservation procedures are not covered by standard insurance, so access to a financial counselor can also be helpful.[96] Some fertility preservation programs have also chosen to include a reproductive survivorship aspect in their program, where topics such as sexual dysfunction or need for hormone replacement therapy can be addressed.

ETHICAL CONSIDERATIONS

There are many unique ethical considerations pertaining to fertility preservation in pediatric and adolescent girls, and particularly difficult cases may require the involvement of an ethics committee or medical ethicist.[97] Most prominently, most of the patients encountered by the pediatric and adolescent gynecologist will not be of a legal age to consent and will require that both patient and guardian(s) are on the same page regarding fertility preservation procedures, which is sometimes difficult to achieve, particularly with teenagers.[98-102] There is the potential for regret on both the patient's and the parent's side, as well as resentment between them. The existing data suggest that teenagers strongly desire active participation in reproductive conversations and treatment decisions.[103-106] Multiple national and international societies have included statements in their guidelines about fertility preservation, supporting parental/guardian fertility preservation decisions with the child's assent.[5,6,49,107,108] There are also ethical quandaries over disposition of cryopreserved gametes or ovaries in the case of death. Some institutions have handled this by making a blanket policy that oocytes/ovarian tissue will be donated or discarded upon death of the patient, while others leave final disposition up to the patient and guardian.[5,49,109-111] In all pediatric fertility preservation cases, shared decision-making between the parent/guardian, patient, and provider should be pursued as much as possible, as it may help assuage some ethical concerns.[112]

CONCLUSIONS

As survivorship from childhood cancer continues to increase, so has the focus on quality of life after cancer, including fertility. Despite concerns to the contrary, there are no data to suggest that a history of cancer, chemotherapy, or radiation increases the risk for genetic abnormalities, birth defects, or malignancy in the offspring of cancer survivors.[24] Furthermore, there is no evidence that currently used fertility preservation options negatively impact recurrence or survival rates.[24] Patients may not bring up issues surrounding future fertility to their caregivers for multiple reasons, including being overwhelmed by their diagnosis, unaware of risk to fertility, or concerned about potential treatment delays for fertility treatment resulting in poorer outcomes.[6] Pediatric and adolescent gynecologists can play a critical role in educating subspecialists who care for girls facing fertility-threatening conditions or treatments and ensure widespread availability of fertility preservation services so that these families may have the full range of possibilities available to them.

REFERENCES

1. Pui CH, Gajjar AJ, Kane JR, Qaddoumi IA, Pappo AS. Challenging issues in pediatric oncology. *Nat Rev Clin Oncol.* 2011;8(9):540–9.
2. Jemal A, Ward EM, Johnson CJ et al. Annual Report to the Nation on the Status of Cancer, 1975–2014, Featuring Survival. *J Natl Cancer Inst.* 2017;109(9).
3. Phillips SM, Padgett LS, Leisenring WM et al. Survivors of childhood cancer in the United States: Prevalence and burden of morbidity. *Cancer Epidemiol Biomarkers Prev.* 2015;24(4):653–63.

4. Schover LR, Rybicki LA, Martin BA, Bringelsen KA. Having children after cancer. A pilot survey of survivors' attitudes and experiences. *Cancer.* 1999;86(4):697–709.

5. Fallat ME, Hutter J, American Academy of Pediatrics Committee on B, American Academy of Pediatrics Section on HO, American Academy of Pediatrics Section on S. Preservation of fertility in pediatric and adolescent patients with cancer. *Pediatrics.* 2008;121(5):e1461–9.

6. Loren AW, Mangu PB, Beck LN et al. Fertility preservation for patients with cancer: American Society of Clinical Oncology clinical practice guideline update. *J Clin Oncol.* 2013;31(19):2500–10.

7. Practice Committee of American Society for Reproductive M. Fertility preservation in patients undergoing gonadotoxic therapy or gonadectomy: A committee opinion. *Fertil Steril.* 2013;100(5):1214–23.

8. Lewin J, Ma JMZ, Mitchell L et al. The positive effect of a dedicated adolescent and young adult fertility program on the rates of documentation of therapy-associated infertility risk and fertility preservation options. *Support Care Cancer.* 2017;25(6):1915–22.

9. Loren AW, Brazauskas R, Chow EJ et al. Physician perceptions and practice patterns regarding fertility preservation in hematopoietic cell transplant recipients. *Bone Marrow Transplant.* 2013;48(8):1091–7.

10. Baker TG. A quantitative and cytological study of germ cells in human ovaries. *Proc R Soc Lond B Biol Sci.* 1963;158:417–33.

11. Richardson SJ, Senikas V, Nelson JF. Follicular depletion during the menopausal transition: Evidence for accelerated loss and ultimate exhaustion. *J Clin Endocrinol Metab.* 1987;65(6):1231–7.

12. Kelsey TW, Wright P, Nelson SM, Anderson RA, Wallace WH. A validated model of serum anti-mullerian hormone from conception to menopause. *PLOS ONE.* 2011;6(7):e22024.

13. Gupta AA, Lee Chong A, Deveault C et al. Anti-mullerian hormone in female adolescent cancer patients before, during, and after completion of therapy: A pilot feasibility study. *J Pediatr Adolesc Gynecol.* 2016;29(6):599–603.

14. Jacobson MH, Mertens AC, Spencer JB, Manatunga AK, Howards PP. Menses resumption after cancer treatment-induced amenorrhea occurs early or not at all. *Fertil Steril.* 2016;105(3):765–72 e4.

15. Waks AG, Partridge AH. Fertility preservation in patients with breast cancer: Necessity, methods, and safety. *J Natl Compr Canc Netw.* 2016;14(3):355–63.

16. Green DM, Kawashima T, Stovall M et al. Fertility of female survivors of childhood cancer: A report from the childhood cancer survivor study. *J Clin Oncol.* 2009;27(16):2677–85.

17. Barton SE, Najita JS, Ginsburg ES et al. Infertility, infertility treatment, and achievement of pregnancy in female survivors of childhood cancer: A report from the Childhood Cancer Survivor Study cohort. *Lancet Oncol.* 2013;14(9):873–81.

18. Chemaitilly W, Mertens AC, Mitby P et al. Acute ovarian failure in the childhood cancer survivor study. *J Clin Endocrinol Metab.* 2006;91(5):1723–8.

19. Byrne J, Fears TR, Gail MH et al. Early menopause in long-term survivors of cancer during adolescence. *Am J Obstet Gynecol.* 1992;166(3):788–93.

20. Chiarelli AM, Marrett LD, Darlington G. Early menopause and infertility in females after treatment for childhood cancer diagnosed in 1964–1988 in Ontario, Canada. *Am J Epidemiol.* 1999;150(3):245–54.

21. Sklar CA, Mertens AC, Mitby P et al. Premature menopause in survivors of childhood cancer: A report from the childhood cancer survivor study. *J Natl Cancer Inst.* 2006;98(13):890–6.

22. Thomas-Teinturier C, El Fayech C, Oberlin O et al. Age at menopause and its influencing factors in a cohort of survivors of childhood cancer: Earlier but rarely premature. *Hum Reprod.* 2013;28(2):488–95.

23. Demeestere I, Moffa F, Peccatori F, Poirot C, Shalom-Paz E. Multiple approaches for individualized fertility protective therapy in cancer patients. *Obstet Gynecol Int.* 2012;2012:961232.

24. Lee SJ, Schover LR, Partridge AH et al. American Society of Clinical Oncology recommendations on fertility preservation in cancer patients. *J Clin Oncol.* 2006;24(18):2917–31.

25. Meirow D, Biederman H, Anderson RA, Wallace WH. Toxicity of chemotherapy and radiation on female reproduction. *Clin Obstet Gynecol.* 2010;53(4):727–39.

26. Chemaitilly W, Li Z, Krasin MJ et al. Premature ovarian insufficiency in childhood cancer survivors: A report from the St. Jude Lifetime Cohort. *J Clin Endocrinol Metab.* 2017;102(7):2242–50.

27. Green DM, Nolan VG, Goodman PJ et al. The cyclophosphamide equivalent dose as an approach for quantifying alkylating agent exposure: A report from the Childhood Cancer Survivor Study. *Pediatr Blood Cancer.* 2014;61(1):53–67.

28. Northwestern University, The Oncofertility Consortium. Estimating risk: Females. http://oncofertilitynorthwestern.edu/resources/estimating-risk-females. Accessed May 23, 2019.

29. Chow EJ, Stratton KL, Leisenring WM et al. Pregnancy after chemotherapy in male and female survivors of childhood cancer treated between 1970 and 1999: A report from the Childhood Cancer Survivor Study cohort. *Lancet Oncol.* 2016;17(5):567–76.

30. Wallace WH, Thomson AB, Saran F, Kelsey TW. Predicting age of ovarian failure after radiation to a field that includes the ovaries. *Int J Radiat Oncol Biol Phys.* 2005;62(3):738–44.

31. Sanders JE, Hawley J, Levy W et al. Pregnancies following high-dose cyclophosphamide with or

without high-dose busulfan or total-body irradiation and bone marrow transplantation. *Blood.* 1996; 87(7):3045–52.

32. Darzy KH, Shalet SM. Hypopituitarism following radiotherapy revisited. *Endocr Dev.* 2009;15:1–24.

33. Jeruss JS, Woodruff TK. Preservation of fertility in patients with cancer. *N Engl J Med.* 2009;360(9): 902–11.

34. Arnon J, Meirow D, Lewis-Roness H, Ornoy A. Genetic and teratogenic effects of cancer treatments on gametes and embryos. *Hum Reprod Update.* 2001; 7(4):394–403.

35. Anderson C, Engel SM, Mersereau JE et al. Birth outcomes among adolescent and young adult cancer survivors. *JAMA Oncol.* 2017;3(8):1078–84.

36. Reulen RC, Bright CJ, Winter DL et al. Pregnancy and labor complications in female survivors of childhood cancer: The British Childhood Cancer Survivor Study. *J Natl Cancer Inst.* 2017;109(11).

37. Teh WT, Stern C, Chander S, Hickey M. The impact of uterine radiation on subsequent fertility and pregnancy outcomes. *Biomed Res Int.* 2014;2014:482968.

38. Oktay K, Bedoschi G, Berkowitz K et al. Fertility preservation in women with Turner syndrome: A comprehensive review and practical guidelines. *J Pediatr Adolesc Gynecol.* 2016;29(5):409–16.

39. Finlayson C, Fritsch MK, Johnson EK et al. Presence of germ cells in disorders of sex development: Implications for fertility potential and preservation. *J Urol.* 2017;197(3 Pt 2):937–43.

40. Coleman E, Bockting W, Botzer M et al. Standards of care for the health of transsexual, transgender, and gender-nonconforming people, version 7. *Int J Transgend.* 2012;13(4):165–232.

41. Ethics Committee of the American Society for Reproductive Medicine. Access to fertility services by transgender persons: An Ethics Committee opinion. *Fertil Steril.* 104(5):1111–5.

42. Kasum M, von Wolff M, Franulic D et al. Fertility preservation options in breast cancer patients. *Gynecol Endocrinol.* 2015;31(11):846–51.

43. Doyle JO, Richter KS, Lim J, Stillman RJ, Graham JR, Tucker MJ. Successful elective and medically indicated oocyte vitrification and warming for autologous in vitro fertilization, with predicted birth probabilities for fertility preservation according to number of cryopreserved oocytes and age at retrieval. *Fertil Steril.* 2016;105(2):459–66 e2.

44. Lawson AK, Klock SC, Pavone ME, Hirshfeld-Cytron J, Smith KN, Kazer RR. Psychological counseling of female fertility preservation patients. *J Psychosoc Oncol.* 2015;33(4):333–53.

45. Reichman DE, Davis OK, Zaninovic N, Rosenwaks Z, Goldschlag DE. Fertility preservation using controlled ovarian hyperstimulation and oocyte cryopreservation in a premenarcheal female with myelodysplastic syndrome. *Fertil Steril.* 2012;98(5): 1225–8.

46. Oktay K, Bedoschi G. Oocyte cryopreservation for fertility preservation in postpubertal female children at risk for premature ovarian failure due to accelerated follicle loss in Turner syndrome or cancer treatments. *J Pediatr Adolesc Gynecol.* 2014;27(6):342–6.

47. Jadoul P, Kim SS, Committee IP. Fertility considerations in young women with hematological malignancies. *J Assist Reprod Genet.* 2012;29(6):479–87.

48. Rienzi L, Cobo A, Paffoni A et al. Consistent and predictable delivery rates after oocyte vitrification: An observational longitudinal cohort multicentric study. *Hum Reprod.* 2012;27(6):1606–12.

49. Ethics Committee of American Society for Reproductive M. Fertility preservation and reproduction in patients facing gonadotoxic therapies: A committee opinion. *Fertil Steril.* 2013;100(5):1224–31.

50. Turan V, Bedoschi G, Moy F, Oktay K. Safety and feasibility of performing two consecutive ovarian stimulation cycles with the use of letrozole-gonadotropin protocol for fertility preservation in breast cancer patients. *Fertil Steril.* 2013;100(6):1681–5 e1.

51. Kuang Y, Chen Q, Hong Q et al. Double stimulations during the follicular and luteal phases of poor responders in IVF/ICSI programmes (Shanghai protocol). *Reprod Biomed Online.* 2014;29(6):684–91.

52. Reddy J, Oktay K. Ovarian stimulation and fertility preservation with the use of aromatase inhibitors in women with breast cancer. *Fertil Steril.* 2012;98(6): 1363–9.

53. Moravek MB, Confino R, Lawson AK, Smith KN, Klock SC, Pavone ME. Oocyte/embryo utilization rates and disposition decisions in fertility preservation patients. *Reprod Sci.* 2017;24(1 Suppl):102A.

54. Cakmak H, Katz A, Cedars MI, Rosen MP. Effective method for emergency fertility preservation: Random-start controlled ovarian stimulation. *Fertil Steril.* 2013;100(6):1673–80.

55. von Wolff M, Donnez J, Hovatta O et al. Cryopreservation and autotransplantation of human ovarian tissue prior to cytotoxic therapy—A technique in its infancy but already successful in fertility preservation. *Eur J Cancer.* 2009;45(9):1547–53.

56. Duncan FE. Egg quality during the pubertal transition—Is youth all it's cracked up to be? *Front Endocrinol (Lausanne).* 2017;8:226.

57. Practice Committee of American Society for Reproductive Medicine. Ovarian tissue cryopreservation: A committee opinion. *Fertil Steril.* 2014;101(5):1237–43.

58. Dolmans MM, Marotta ML, Pirard C, Donnez J, Donnez O. Ovarian tissue cryopreservation followed by controlled ovarian stimulation and pick-up of mature oocytes does not impair the number or quality of retrieved oocytes. *J Ovarian Res.* 2014;7:80.

59. Hovatta O, Silye R, Krausz T et al. Cryopreservation of human ovarian tissue using dimethylsulphoxide and propanediol-sucrose as cryoprotectants. *Hum Reprod.* 1996;11(6):1268–72.

60. Rowell EE. Optimal technique for laparoscopic oophorectomy for ovarian tissue cryopreservation in pediatric girls. In: Woodruff TK, Gosiengfiao YC, eds. *Pediatric and Adolescent Oncofertility: Best Practices and Emerging Technologies.* Cham, Switzerland: Springer International; 2017:243–9.

61. Edwards RG, Fowler RE, Gore-Langton RE et al. Normal and abnormal follicular growth in mouse, rat and human ovaries. *J Reprod Fertil.* 1977;51(1):237–63.

62. Pacheco F, Oktay K. Current success and efficiency of autologous ovarian transplantation: A meta-analysis. *Reprod Sci.* 2017;24(8):1111–20.

63. Donnez J, Dolmans MM, Pellicer A et al. Restoration of ovarian activity and pregnancy after transplantation of cryopreserved ovarian tissue: A review of 60 cases of reimplantation. *Fertil Steril.* 2013;99(6): 1503–13.

64. Donnez J, Dolmans MM. Ovarian cortex transplantation: 60 reported live births brings the success and worldwide expansion of the technique towards routine clinical practice. *J Assist Reprod Genet.* 2015;32(8):1167–70.

65. Jensen AK, Macklon KT, Fedder J, Ernst E, Humaidan P, Andersen CY. 86 successful births and 9 ongoing pregnancies worldwide in women transplanted with frozen-thawed ovarian tissue: Focus on birth and perinatal outcome in 40 of these children. *J Assist Reprod Genet.* 2017;34(3):325–36.

66. Demeestere I, Simon P, Dedeken L et al. Live birth after autograft of ovarian tissue cryopreserved during childhood. *Hum Reprod.* 2015;30(9):2107–9.

67. Donnelly L. Woman gives birth to baby using ovary frozen in her childhood in "world first." *The Telegraph*; December 14, 2016.

68. Corkum K, Rowell E. Laparoscopic oophorectomy for ovarian tissue cryopreservation in prepubertal and young adolescent females: A review of surgical outcomes. *IPEG's 26th Annual Congress for Endosurgery in Children*, London, England; 2017.

69. Bastings L, Beerendonk CC, Westphal JR et al. Autotransplantation of cryopreserved ovarian tissue in cancer survivors and the risk of reintroducing malignancy: A systematic review. *Hum Reprod Update.* 2013;19(5):483–506.

70. Dolmans MM, Marinescu C, Saussoy P, Van Langendonckt A, Amorim C, Donnez J. Reimplantation of cryopreserved ovarian tissue from patients with acute lymphoblastic leukemia is potentially unsafe. *Blood.* 2010;116(16):2908–14.

71. Laronda MM, Jakus AE, Whelan KA, Wertheim JA, Shah RN, Woodruff TK. Initiation of puberty in mice following decellularized ovary transplant. *Biomaterials.* 2015;50:20–9.

72. Salama M, Woodruff TK. New advances in ovarian autotransplantation to restore fertility in cancer patients. *Cancer Metastasis Rev.* 2015;34(4):807–22.

73. Rosendahl M, Greve T, Andersen CY. The safety of transplanting cryopreserved ovarian tissue in cancer patients: A review of the literature. *J Assist Reprod Genet.* 2013;30(1):11–24.

74. Laronda MM, Rutz AL, Xiao S et al. A bioprosthetic ovary created using 3D printed microporous scaffolds restores ovarian function in sterilized mice. *Nat Commun.* 2017;8:15261.

75. Kniazeva E, Hardy AN, Boukaidi SA, Woodruff TK, Jeruss JS, Shea LD. Primordial follicle transplantation within designer biomaterial grafts produce live births in a mouse infertility model. *Sci Rep.* 2015;5:17709.

76. Laronda MM, Duncan FE, Hornick JE et al. Alginate encapsulation supports the growth and differentiation of human primordial follicles within ovarian cortical tissue. *J Assist Reprod Genet.* 2014;31(8):1013–28.

77. Roth JJ, Jones RE. A single ovary of *Anolis carolinensis* responds more to exogenous gonadotropin if the contralateral ovary is absent. *Gen Comp Endocrinol.* 1992;85(3):486–92.

78. Husseinzadeh N, Nahhas WA, Velkley DE, Whitney CW, Mortel R. The preservation of ovarian function in young women undergoing pelvic radiation therapy. *Gynecol Oncol.* 1984;18(3):373–9.

79. Irtan S, Orbach D, Helfre S, Sarnacki S. Ovarian transposition in prepubescent and adolescent girls with cancer. *Lancet Oncol.* 2013;14(13):e601–8.

80. Farber LA, Ames JW, Rush S, Gal D. Laparoscopic ovarian transposition to preserve ovarian function before pelvic radiation and chemotherapy in a young patient with rectal cancer. *Med Gen Med.* 2005;7(1):66.

81. Morice P, Thiam-Ba R, Castaigne D et al. Fertility results after ovarian transposition for pelvic malignancies treated by external irradiation or brachytherapy. *Hum Reprod.* 1998;13(3):660–3.

82. de Bastos M, Stegeman BH, Rosendaal FR et al. Combined oral contraceptives: Venous thrombosis. *Cochrane Database Syst Rev.* 2014(3):CD010813.

83. Trussell J. Contraceptive failure in the United States. *Contraception.* 2004;70(2):89–96.

84. Murphy D, Klosky JL, Termuhlen A, Sawczyn KK, Quinn GP. The need for reproductive and sexual health discussions with adolescent and young adult cancer patients. *Contraception.* 2013;88(2):215–20.

85. van Kasteren YM, Schoemaker J. Premature ovarian failure: A systematic review on therapeutic interventions to restore ovarian function and achieve pregnancy. *Hum Reprod Update.* 1999;5(5):483–92.

86. Bidet M, Bachelot A, Bissauge E et al. Resumption of ovarian function and pregnancies in 358 patients with premature ovarian failure. *J Clin Endocrinol Metab.* 2011;96(12):3864–72.

87. Ben-Aharon I, Abir R, Perl G et al. Optimizing the process of fertility preservation in pediatric female cancer patients—A multidisciplinary program. *BMC Cancer.* 2016;16:620.

88. Reinecke JD, Kelvin JF, Arvey SR et al. Implementing a systematic approach to meeting patients' cancer and

fertility needs: A review of the Fertile Hope Centers of Excellence program. *J Oncol Pract.* 2012;8(5):303–8.

89. Northwestern University, The Oncofertility Consortium. Oncofertility Decision Tool Web Portal. https://oncofertility.northwestern.edu/resources/oncofertility-decision-tool-web-portal. Accessed May 23, 2019.

90. Cincinnati Children's. Comprehensive Fertility Care and Preservation Program (CFCPP). https://www.cincinnatichildrens.org/service/f/fertility-preservation. Accessed 2018.

91. King L, Quinn GP, Vadaparampil ST et al. Oncology nurses' perceptions of barriers to discussion of fertility preservation with patients with cancer. *Clin J Oncol Nurs.* 2008;12(3):467–76.

92. Logan S, Perz J, Ussher J, Peate M, Anazodo A. Clinician provision of oncofertility support in cancer patients of a reproductive age: A systematic review. *Psychooncology.* 2018;27(3):748–56.

93. Logan S, Perz J, Ussher JM, Peate M, Anazodo A. A systematic review of patient oncofertility support needs in reproductive cancer patients aged 14 to 45 years of age. *Psychooncology.* 2018;27(2):401–9.

94. Ellis SJ, Wakefield CE, McLoone JK, Robertson EG, Cohn RJ. Fertility concerns among child and adolescent cancer survivors and their parents: A qualitative analysis. *J Psychosoc Oncol.* 2016;34(5):347–62.

95. Stein DM, Victorson DE, Choy JT et al. Fertility preservation preferences and perspectives among adult male survivors of pediatric cancer and their parents. *J Adolesc Young Adult Oncol.* 2014;3(2):75–82.

96. Campo-Engelstein L. Consistency in insurance coverage for iatrogenic conditions resulting from cancer treatment including fertility preservation. *J Clin Oncol.* 2010;28(8):1284–6.

97. Dudzinski DM. Ethical issues in fertility preservation for adolescent cancer survivors: Oocyte and ovarian tissue cryopreservation. *J Pediatr Adolesc Gynecol.* 2004;17(2):97–102.

98. English A, Ford CA. The HIPAA privacy rule and adolescents: Legal questions and clinical challenges. *Perspect Sex Reprod Health.* 2004;36(2):80–6.

99. Quinn GP, Knapp C, Murphy D, Sawczyn K, Sender L. Congruence of reproductive concerns among adolescents with cancer and parents: Pilot testing an adapted instrument. *Pediatrics.* 2012; 129(4):e930–6.

100. Klosky JL, Simmons JL, Russell KM et al. Fertility as a priority among at-risk adolescent males newly diagnosed with cancer and their parents. *Support Care Cancer.* 2015;23(2):333–41.

101. Quinn GP, Murphy D, Knapp CA, Christie J, Phares V, Wells KJ. Coping styles of female adolescent cancer patients with potential fertility loss. *J Adolesc Young Adult Oncol.* 2013;2(2):66–71.

102. Crawshaw M. Psychosocial oncofertility issues faced by adolescents and young adults over their lifetime: A review of the research. *Hum Fertil (Camb).* 2013; 16(1):59–63.

103. Quinn GP, Murphy D, Knapp C et al. Who decides? Decision making and fertility preservation in teens with cancer: A review of the literature. *J Adolesc Health.* 2011;49(4):337–46.

104. Bennett SE, Assefi NP. School-based teenage pregnancy prevention programs: A systematic review of randomized controlled trials. *J Adolesc Health.* 2005;36(1):72–81.

105. Zebrack B, Isaacson S. Psychosocial care of adolescent and young adult patients with cancer and survivors. *J Clin Oncol.* 2012;30(11):1221–6.

106. Goossens J, Delbaere I, Van Lancker A, Beeckman D, Verhaeghe S, Van Hecke A. Cancer patients' and professional caregivers' needs, preferences and factors associated with receiving and providing fertility-related information: A mixed-methods systematic review. *Int J Nurs Stud.* 2014;51(2):300–19.

107. Hembree WC, Cohen-Kettenis P, Delemarre-van de Waal HA et al. Endocrine treatment of transsexual persons: An Endocrine Society clinical practice guideline. *J Clin Endocrinol Metab.* 2009;94(9): 3132–54.

108. Deutsch MB, Feldman JL. Updated recommendations from the World Professional Association for Transgender Health Standards of Care. *Am Fam Physician.* 2013;87(2):89–93.

109. Patrizio P, Butts S, Caplan A. Ovarian tissue preservation and future fertility: Emerging technologies and ethical considerations. *J Natl Cancer Inst Monogr.* 2005;(34):107–10.

110. Dolin G, Roberts DE, Rodriguez LM, Woodruff TK. Medical hope, legal pitfalls: Potential legal issues in the emerging field of oncofertility. *Cancer Treat Res.* 2010;156:111–34.

111. Bahadur G. Death and conception. *Hum Reprod.* 2002;17(10):2769–75.

112. Clayman ML, Galvin KM, Arntson P. Shared decision making: Fertility and pediatric cancers. *Cancer Treat Res.* 2007;138:149–60.

Confidential care issues

27

JULIA F. TAYLOR and MARY A. OTT

INTRODUCTION

Providers involved in the care of minor adolescents, especially in areas of sexual and reproductive health, are often recipients of sensitive and private information. Knowing what information to treat confidentially and how to maintain confidentiality can be a challenge. In this chapter, we (1) explain confidentiality, (2) provide ethical and legal justifications for confidential care to minors, (3) identify threats to confidentiality, and (4) discuss effective strategies for providing confidential care to adolescents. We limit the scope of the chapter to adolescents under the age of 18 years, considered legally to be minors, and who typically do not have the legal ability to consent to general health care.

DEFINITION AND EXTENT OF CONFIDENTIALITY

While consent and confidentiality are closely related, they are not synonymous. *Consent* refers to a patient's ability to make a decision after considering the risks, benefits, and alternatives. *Confidentiality*, in contrast, is about the flow and control of health information and potential disclosures of that information to parents or other parties. When health information is confidential, the adolescent is the individual who authorizes disclosure. When health information is not confidential, the parent or legal representative has access to and control over the disclosure of health information. Practically speaking, confidentiality flows from consent. When an adolescent has the right to provide consent for his or her own health care, he or she typically has confidentiality around that health information, although exceptions do exist. However, confidentiality is not limited to minor consent statutes, as described in this chapter.

Confidentiality for minor adolescents is not absolute. It is limited in content and scope, and it is important for providers to know when they can, and cannot, guarantee confidentiality. This sets expectations for both adolescents and parents. Most general health information is not considered confidential. Confidential care, instead, should focus on areas in which adolescents already exercise some autonomy, privacy is important, and the disclosure of sensitive information is imperative to make accurate diagnoses and provide effective treatment. It is generally accepted practice that confidentiality should be maintained when adolescents seek sexual and reproductive health services, such as contraception and treatment for sexually transmitted infections (STIs),[1,2] but providers must understand any legal limitations of minor confidentiality.

If an adolescent discloses an imminent threat of harm to him- or herself or another person, this warrants immediate reporting to authorities. Additionally, providers are mandatory reporters if they have a suspicion of neglect or abuse, including sexual abuse, exploitation, and human trafficking. If a reproductive health condition is life-threatening, such as an ectopic pregnancy in a hemodynamically unstable adolescent, providers can and should break confidentiality.

Potential threats to confidentiality also include state laws that require parental consent or notification for sexual and reproductive health services, such as parental consent laws for abortion and parental notification laws for contraception.[3] While STIs are typically not disclosed to parents because minors may consent to their own care, adolescents should be informed that certain STIs, such as chlamydia, gonorrhea, syphilis, and HIV, may be reported to health departments.

WHY CONFIDENTIALITY IS IMPORTANT

In sexual and reproductive health, public health data show that confidentiality leads to improved quality of care, access, and outcomes. Adolescents provided with confidentiality assurances are more likely to disclose sensitive information to providers.[4] While many providers are uncomfortable asking about sensitive topics such as sexual behavior, when providers do ask about these topics, adolescents are more likely to report that they feel supported by the provider and engaged in their own care.[5] Most of the highly effective forms of contraception are accessed through providers, and data show that adolescents are more likely to access family planning services and less likely to forego care when care is confidential.[6–8] Teens provided with confidential care also have better sexual health outcomes, such as lower rates of teen pregnancy. States that enacted Medicaid family planning waivers allowing confidential care for minors had lower rates of unintended pregnancies.[9] While many providers worry about parent reactions to confidential care, across studies, the majority of parents support confidentiality for minors.[10,11]

ETHICAL JUSTIFICATION FOR CONFIDENTIALITY

Adolescent confidentiality is supported by the ethical principles of respect for persons, beneficence (doing good) and nonmaleficence (not causing harm), and justice.[12] Respect for persons consists of autonomy, or respect for an individual's capacity for self-determination, and support for individuals with limited autonomy. Although minors are not legally considered adults until 18 years of age, the weight of evidence from research on adolescent health-care decision-making suggests that by 12–14 years of age, they have the cognitive capacity to understand a treatment decision, balance risks and benefits, and make a rational, voluntary choice.[13–16] The principle of respect for persons means that we should support an adolescent's emerging autonomy in decision-making, including the adolescent's decision to hold information confidential.

In many instances, the decision to treat information as confidential is the ethically appropriate choice because it benefits or avoids harm for the adolescent. As previously described, adolescents are more likely to disclose sensitive information and seek care if confidentiality is provided, making accurate diagnoses more likely and providing access to necessary sexual and reproductive health services. Confidentiality avoids harm through increased access to reproductive health services.[6-8]

Justice focuses on health disparities and access to care. Adolescents experience a high burden of bacterial STIs and unintended pregnancy.[17,18] Confidential care provides critical access to services to address these disparities. Justice arguments draw from human rights documents. The UN High Commission on Human Rights specifically identifies confidential sexual and reproductive health care for minor adolescents as a basic right and the provision of confidential care an obligation of governments.[19]

LEGAL SUPPORT FOR CONFIDENTIALITY

Legal support for minor confidentiality comes from a variety of sources, including health-care consent laws, federal case law, and federal regulations. Few jurisdictions have laws governing confidentiality. However, in the United States, all 50 states have some type of minor consent laws, and these provide the strongest justification for confidentiality. State minor consent laws provide two types of guidance for adolescents. The first identifies minors who are emancipated, which means that, for the purposes of health-care consent, they should be considered adults. Every state has different laws on emancipation. Groups of minors who may be emancipated depending on state law include married minors, minors who are active duty in the military, pregnant or parenting minors, and minors who have successfully petitioned a court for emancipation.

The second type of guidance identifies specific diagnoses for which all minor adolescents may give consent and, therefore, receive confidential care. All 50 U.S. states and the District of Columbia (DC) allow adolescents to consent to the diagnosis and treatment of STIs.[3] Only 26 states and DC allow all adolescents to consent to contraception; another 20 states allow some minors to consent to contraception.[3] The remaining states are silent, and for these last two groups, providers must look to case law and federal statutes.[20] For an updated state-by-state listing of minor consent laws, see the Guttmacher Institute's state-by-state summary.[3] For more detailed information, see the Center for Adolescent Health and the Law's, *State Minor Consent Laws: A Summary* (3rd ed.).[3,20]

Adolescent confidentiality is additionally supported by case law and federal statutes. A series of court cases has established that minors have constitutional rights, that these constitutional rights include the right to reproductive privacy, and the right to reproductive privacy includes consent and confidentiality around contraceptive use.[21]

Adolescent confidentiality is also supported by federal regulations. Family-planning clinics funded by Title X of the federal Public Health Services Act (42 USC §§300–300a-6 [1970]) are required to provide confidential care to minors, regardless of state law.[21,22] While providers typically consider the Health Insurance Portability and Accountability Act (HIPAA [Pub L No. 104–191, 1996]) a threat to minor adolescent confidentiality, it has important protections built into its 2002 Privacy Rule. According to HIPAA, parents' access to minors' medical records is limited when the minor can consent under state or other laws, when the provider and parent agree that the minor may have confidential care, or at the provider's discretion.[2,20,21] In the last scenario, the provider must clearly document the reasons that confidentiality is clinically necessary.

BEST PRACTICES

Based on these public health data, ethics, and adolescent development, all mainstream professional organizations whose members provide care for adolescents have either their own policy statement or support another organization's policy statement identifying confidential care for adolescents as best practice. These organizations include (but are not limited to) the American Medical Association (AMA),[23] the American Academy of Pediatrics (AAP),[2] the American College of Obstetricians and Gynecologists (ACOG),[24] and the Society for Adolescent Health and Medicine.[1]

THREATS TO CONFIDENTIALITY

Ensuring confidentiality for adolescents requires an awareness of the potential for inadvertent disclosures that can occur before, during, and after clinical care encounters (summarized in Table 27.1). These threats can happen at the level of the provider, the clinic, or the health-care system.

Providers caring for adolescents, especially in the areas of reproductive and sexual health, should be committed to confidentiality as a best practice when caring for adolescents. By understanding the relevant regulations, educating families and office staff, and thoughtfully implementing office-based strategies, clinicians can minimize the threats to confidentiality.

STRATEGIES FOR PROVIDING EFFECTIVE CONFIDENTIAL CARE

Following is a series of recommendations that can help the clinician proactively address confidentiality with patients and parents, avoid inadvertent confidentiality breeches, and manage emerging confidentiality issues in electronic health records (EHRs).

Know the regulations in your state

A working knowledge of relevant state law and institutional policies allows you, as a provider, to feel confident in the limits of confidentiality for adolescents. The Guttmacher Institute maintains an updated index with laws related to reproductive health and organized

Table 27.1 Threats to adolescent confidentiality before, during, and after clinic visits.

Before	During	After
Appointment reminder letters/calls to home	Staff reviews medication list with parent present and includes recent antibiotic for chlamydia infection	After-visit summary includes new prescription of birth control pills
Health portal appointment details (if proxy access available to parents)	Open notes available through health portal (may include sexual history)	Lab results or new problems/diagnoses available via health portal (potentially visible to parents with proxy access)
Front-desk staff checking the patient in confirms reason for appointment: "It says here the appointment was scheduled because you need to be seen before they'll write you another birth control prescription."	Lab orders are associated with diagnoses: sexually transmitted infection testing	Pharmacy calls home number (not patient's cell) when prescription for birth control pills is ready for pick up Explanation of benefits is generated with diagnosis codes of chlamydial infection and contraception surveillance and sent to home address

by state (https:// www.guttmacher.org).[3] The Center for Adolescent Health and the Law (CAHL) provides in-depth analysis and interpretation of each state's relevant consent and confidentiality laws in *State Minor Consent Laws: A Summary* (3rd ed.).[20] A case discussion of confidentiality and adolescent pregnancy can be found in the AMA *Journal of Ethics*.[25] The AAP has a Confidentiality Laws Tip Sheet,[26] and both ACOG and the North American Society for Pediatric and Adolescent Gynecology (NASPAG) have toolkits for making practices youth friendly.[24,26]

Educate patients and parents

Many practices use letters, posters, or confidentiality agreements with adolescents and parents to educate them about confidentiality. In practices that see patients longitudinally, families can be sent a letter when their child reaches 11 or 12 years of age that explains the practice's policies on minor confidentiality and allows parents to anticipate that the adolescent and the provider will spend time alone during visits. NASPAG has created a letter template for practices.[27]

Some providers and clinics use flyers and posters in waiting areas and exam rooms to describe confidentiality policies, educate adolescents and families, and set expectations.[28] Other clinicians provide parents with a letter describing confidentiality policies or ask parents to sign a document acknowledging that they have been informed about and agree with the practice's confidentiality policy. These are not intended to be legal documents, but rather are communication tools to clearly articulate and document expectations about confidentiality for both parents and minor adolescents.

Many clinicians also find it helpful to begin appointments with new adolescent patients using standard language that emphasizes the importance of confidentiality as well as its limits. For example, "We will start off discussing your concerns together as a family, then I will spend some time talking with your adolescent alone before bringing you back in to discuss the final plan. This is how our practice handles all visits with teenagers. If you have

any questions, please let me know." During this conversation, it is important to emphasize that confidentiality allows adolescents to begin taking responsibility for their own health care and provides them with an opportunity to establish a relationship with another trusted adult.

In clinical practice, many providers try to anticipate and address potential parental concerns at the start of the visit. Explaining the purpose of confidentiality, its limits, and that it is a policy applied to all young people is often enough to ease parents' concerns. Sometimes it is helpful to reassure parents that you are not advocating secrecy, and, in fact, you recommend that parents and adolescents talk about difficult topics like sex and relationships.

At an initial visit, it is also important to explain the limits of confidentiality. It is important for the adolescent patient to ensure that he or she understands what services are available in a confidential manner, when disclosure is required, and the possibility of unintended privacy breaches. Following are several examples of how you might address these topics:

- Early on in the appointment, emphasize to minor patients that certain information, dependent on state law, can only be disclosed with their permission.
- If screening for STIs, "Since we are testing for STIs today, I wanted to remind you that these results will be kept confidential, unless the health department requires me to report specific results."
- If prescribing contraceptives, "If you are going to use your health insurance to pay for your prescription, let's think through what might happen if your parents get notified."

Limit unintentional confidentiality breeches at clinic visits

Educating all office staff, including the front desk and nursing staff, about the importance of confidentiality may help limit inadvertent disclosures. Address specific instances in real time if they occur. Many providers have

Table 27.2 Confidentiality-promoting clinic practices.

- When collecting demographic information, ask for the patient's personal cell phone or preferred contact phone number.
- When reviewing demographic information, ask whether or not a message with the clinic's name/phone number can be left.
- Always confirm identity when providing test results by phone. If sending a letter, ask the adolescent if that should be sent home or somewhere else.
- Have staff designate visits as confidential if the adolescent makes the appointment for a sensitive issue.
- Consider a mechanism for patients to receive text or email reminders or to decline reminders about specific appointments.

office guidelines for adolescent visits that highlight the potential for confidentiality breeches at each stage of the clinic visit and ways to prevent them. Example office guidelines to promote adolescent confidentiality are provided in Table 27.2.

Address potential confidentiality breeches associated with the use of electronic health records

The EHRs have the potential to allow adolescents to easily access their own health information and connect with their clinicians, but they also represent a challenge to confidentiality. When designing or selecting a new EHR, clinicians should consider guidance documents from the Society for Adolescent Health and Medicine[29] and the AAP.[30] If an EHR is already in place, clinicians should familiarize themselves with how information is shared across providers, how after-visit summaries (AVSs) are generated, and how electronic health portals are accessed. The AVSs and patient portal represent specific areas where confidentiality is easily breached. Understanding what health information is visible to all EHR users, versus what can be labeled as private or confidential, thereby limiting access, improves your ability to ensure confidentiality. For AVSs, providers should be aware of what information will be printed on an AVS for minor adolescents and whether or not the EHR will designate certain information (medications, diagnoses, appointments, etc.) as private and not to be included on an AVS.

Health portals allow patients (or in some cases parents with proxy access) to view portions of the medical record and directly communicate with clinic staff and providers. Because minors have confidentiality around only certain aspects of care, portal access is complex. There is a compelling argument for parents to have access to a patient portal to schedule their minor adolescent's sports physical or check their diabetes test, etc.; however, parent access to STI testing and treatment information raises significant confidentiality concerns. Some EHRs have multiple levels of access through the portal, and parents can be permitted to access a more limited amount of information. For EHRs that can designate only one level of access, some health-care systems have elected to forgo any type of portal access for minors to prevent breaches of confidentiality. Providers of sexual and reproductive health care for minors need a working knowledge of the information released on minors' health portals and the EHR's policies governing proxy access to portals.

Know the limits of your clinic and health system

As indicated, it is important to know when you are unable to ensure confidentiality for adolescent patients. This is particularly important when disclosure may result in harm to the adolescent. Providers should identify clinics in their area that guarantee confidential care, such as Title X funded family planning clinics and Health Department STI clinics.

In summary, confidentiality of sexual and reproductive health care for minors is essential to providing accurate, ethical, and supportive care, but at times it can be challenging and requires a thoughtful, proactive approach. Table 27.3 provides a summary of available resources to support confidentiality in the clinical care of minor adolescents.

Table 27.3 Resources on adolescent confidentiality.

The Guttmacher Institute	https://www.guttmacher.org
UN High Commission on Human Rights. Committee on the Rights of the Child, General Comment on the implementation of the rights of the child during adolescence	http://www.ohchr.org/EN/pages/home.aspx
Center for Adolescent Health and the Law (CAHL)	http://www.cahl.org/
Understanding Confidentiality and Minor Consent in California: An Adolescent Provider Toolkit	http://www.phi.org/resources/?resource=understanding-confidentiality-and-minor-consent-in-california-an-adolescent-provider-toolkit
American Academy of Pediatrics Confidentiality Laws Tip Sheet	https://www.aap.org/en-us/advocacy-and-policy/aap-health-initiatives/healthy-foster-care-america/Documents/Confidentiality_Laws.pdf
NASPAG. Tools for Clinicians. Adolescent Confidentiality	http://www.naspag.org/page/toolsfortheclinician
Society for Adolescent Health and Medicine. Clinical Care Resources. Confidentiality.	http://www.adolescenthealth.org/Resources/Clinical-Care-Resources/Confidentiality.aspx

REFERENCES

1. Ford C, English A, Sigman G. Confidential health care for adolescents: Position paper for the Society for Adolescent Medicine. *J Adolesc Health*. 2004;35:160–7.
2. Committee on Adolescence. Contraception for adolescents. *Pediatrics*. 2014;134:e1244–56.
3. Guttmacher Institute. An Overview of Minors' Consent Law. State Policies in Brief, 2017. http://www.guttmacher.org/statecenter/spibs/spib_OMCL.pdf. Accessed December 1, 2017.
4. Ford CA, Millstein SG. Delivery of confidentiality assurances to adolescents by primary care physicians. *Arch Pediatr Adolesc Med*. 1997;151:505–9.
5. Brown JD, Wissow LS. Discussion of sensitive health topics with youth during primary care visits: Relationship to youth perceptions of care. *J Adolesc Health*. 2009;44:48–54.
6. Jones RK, Purcell A, Singh S, Finer LB. Adolescents' reports of parental knowledge of adolescents' use of sexual health services and their reactions to mandated parental notification for prescription contraception. *JAMA*. 2005;293:340–8.
7. Klein JD, McNulty M, Flatau CN. Adolescents' access to care: Teenagers' self-reported use of services and perceived access to confidential care. *Arch Pediatr Adolesc Med*. 1998;152(7):676–82.
8. Reddy DM, Fleming R, Swain C. Effect of mandatory parental notification on adolescent girls' use of sexual health care services. *JAMA*. 2002;288:710–4.
9. Yang Z, Gaydos LM. Reasons for and challenges of recent increases in teen birth rates: A study of family planning service policies and demographic changes at the state level. *J Adolesc Health*. 2010;46:517–24.
10. Dempsey AF, Singer DD, Clark SJ, Davis MM. Adolescent preventive health care: What do parents want? *J Pediatric*. 2009;155:689–94 e1.
11. Eisenberg ME, Swain C, Bearinger LH, Sieving RE, Resnick MD. Parental notification laws for minors' access to contraception: What do parents say? *Arch Pediatr Adolesc Med*. 2005;159:120–5.
12. National Commission for the Protection of Human Subjects of Biomedical and Behavioral Research. Belmont report: Ethical principles and guidelines for the protection of human subjects of research. *Fed Regist*. 1979;44:23191–7.
13. Hein IM, De Vries MC, Troost PW, Meynen G, Van Goudoever JB, Lindauer RJ. Informed consent instead of assent is appropriate in children from the age of twelve: Policy implications of new findings on children's competence to consent to clinical research. *BMC Med Ethics*. 2015;16:76.
14. Kilford EJ, Garrett E, Blakemore SJ. The development of social cognition in adolescence: An integrated perspective. *Neurosci Biobehav Rev*. 2016;70:106–20.
15. Nelson LR, Stupiansky NW, Ott MA. The influence of age, health literacy, and affluence on adolescents' capacity to consent to research. *J Empir Res Hum Res Ethics*. 2016;11:115–21.
16. Steinberg L. Does recent research on adolescent brain development inform the mature minor doctrine? *J Med Philos*. 2013;38:256–67.
17. National Data. Washington, D.C.: Power To Decide: The Campaign to Prevent Unplanned Pregnancy, 2017. https://powertodecide.org/what-we-do/information/national-state-data/national. Accessed December 1, 2017.
18. Centers for Disease Control and Prevention. STD Surveillance Report, 2015. https://www.cdc.gov/std/stats15/toc.htm. Accessed December 3, 2016.
19. Adolescent health and development in the context of the Convention on the Rights of the Child CRC/GC/2003/4, 2003.
20. *State Minor Consent Laws: A Summary*. 3rd ed. Chapel Hill, NC: Center for Adolescent Health and the Law; 2010.
21. English A, Ford CA. The HIPAA privacy rule and adolescents: Legal questions and clinical challenges. *Perspect Sex Reprod Health*. 2004;36:80–6.
22. U.S. Department of Health and Human Services OoPA. Clarification regarding "Program Requirements for Title X Family Planning Projects"—Confidential Services to Adolescents, OPA Program Policy Notice 2014-01, 2014. https://www.hhs.gov/opa/sites/default/files/ppn2014-01-001.pdf. Accessed February 1, 2018.
23. American Medical Association. AMA Code of Medical Ethics, Opinion 5.055—Confidential Care for Minors. https://www.ama-assn.org/delivering-care/confidential-health-care-minors. Accessed January 1, 2018.
24. American College of Obstetricians and Gynecologists. *ACOG. Confidentiality in Adolescent Health Care. Toolkit for Teen Care*. Washington, DC: ACOG; 2011.
25. Ott MA. Teen pregnancy and confidentiality. *Virtual Mentor*. 2014;16:884–90.
26. American Academy of Pediatrics. Confidentialty Laws Tip Sheet. https://www.aap.org/en-us/advocacy-and-policy/aap-health-initiatives/healthy-foster-care-america/Documents/Confidentiality_Laws.pdf. Accessed December 1, 2017.
27. North American Society for Pediatric and Adolescent Gynecology. Tools for the Clinician. Updated 2003. http://www.naspag.org/page/toolsfortheclinician. Accessed January 12, 2018.
28. Young A, Shalwitz J, Pollock S, Simmons M. *Sexual Health: An Adolescent Provider Toolkit*. San Francisco, CA: Adolescent Health Working Group; 2003.
29. Society for Adolescent Health and Medicine. Recommendations for electronic health record use for delivery of adolescent health care. *J Adolesc Health*. 2016;54:487–90.
30. Committee on Adolescence, American Academy of Pediatrics. Standards for health information technology to ensure adolescent privacy. *Pediatrics*. 2012;130:987–90.

Family and cultural factors in pediatric gynecology

28

ALLISON B. RATTO

FAMILY AND CULTURAL FACTORS IN PEDIATRIC GYNECOLOGY

Parents have a pervasive influence on the daily lives of children and adolescents, including on their sexual development and behavior. Parents may affect sexual development via the behaviors they model, direct messages about sexuality, and overall parenting and communication styles. One of the principal ways in which parents affect sexual development is as conduits of cultural values, which may be influenced by race/ethnicity, national origin, religious background, and other factors. While parents have a direct interest in the healthy sexual development of their children, parental priorities around sexual behavior and health may differ at times from those of providers or children and adolescents. Understanding the role of families in child and adolescent sexual development and working collaboratively with them is critical to the successful practice of pediatric gynecology.

PARENTING AND SEXUAL DEVELOPMENT

It goes without saying that parents have powerful and lasting impacts on the development and behavior of their children, exerting influence in both direct and indirect ways. Pediatric providers may have complex relationships with parents—while the child or adolescent is the patient, in most cases, it is parents who present the child for treatment and who assume primary responsibility for medical decision-making and treatment implementation. Providers of pediatric and adolescent gynecology (PAGs) face particular challenges in their interactions with parents, as sexual health and development are often highly sensitive topics, which are strongly influenced by parents' values and practices.[1]

Although the primary responsibility of PAGs is to their patients, successful practice in this complex field requires an awareness of parenting practices that promote healthy sexual development for their patients. This begins with an understanding of the challenges that families face in addressing sexuality with their children and adolescents. It is a nearly universal truth that both parents and their children find the topic of sexual development and sexual behavior to be an uncomfortable one to discuss, and thus, they may avoid these conversations.[2,3] Despite public controversy around school-based sexual education, targeted studies of parent opinions indicate that the majority of parents favor comprehensive sex education in schools[4,5] and are also eager for pediatric providers to discuss sexual health topics with their children,[6] perhaps due in part to their own discomfort with these discussions. Studies of

parent-adolescent communication about sexuality indicate that several factors contribute to parental discomfort with discussing sexuality with their children, including concerns about their own lack of knowledge about sexuality, difficulties communicating with their children overall, and concerns about adjusting the topic to their child's developmental level, including fears of encouraging sexual activity.[7-10]

Despite this discomfort, the vast majority of parents report that they have discussed at least some issues related to sexual development with their children, though interestingly, parents often report having had more frequent and comprehensive discussions of sexuality than their children report.[7,10-13] The most frequent topics of parent-child conversations about sexuality include the basic facts of anatomy, puberty, and reproduction; dating relationships; delaying initiation of sexual activity; and (less frequently) the basics of contraception and prevention of sexually transmitted infections (STIs).[2,10,12,13] Rarely discussed topics include masturbation; comprehensive details about sexually transmitted infections and HIV/AIDS; how to obtain access to contraceptives, condoms, and other safer sex materials; and lesbian, gay, bisexual, and transgender (LGBT) issues.[2,10,12,13] As may be evidenced by the most and least frequently discussed topics, parental communication about sexuality tends to have a more negative valence—generally focusing on the risks and consequences of early sexual activity—and often gives less attention to positive aspects of sexuality, such as sexual pleasure and relationship building.[2,7,14] This is particularly true for girls, who receive more communication from their parents about sexuality than boys do, much of it focused on the importance of delaying or avoiding sexual activity and strategies for doing so.[15-18] Mothers also tend to communicate more about sexuality with their children than fathers do, with both daughters and sons.[12,15,18] Generally speaking, parents communicate more about sexuality with older than younger adolescents, though findings generally indicate that these conversations are more effective with preadolescents (i.e., 9- to 12-year-olds), as this increases the likelihood that they will receive relevant information prior to initiating sexual activity and may be more open to their parents' perspectives at earlier ages.[7,13,17]

When parent-child conversations about sexuality do occur, they have the potential to have important effects on child and adolescent sexual behavior. Research has generally supported the idea that adolescents whose parents talk to them directly about sexuality are more likely to have positive sexual outcomes, such as delayed initiation of sexual activity, fewer sexual partners, reduced rates of unplanned pregnancy, and higher usage of contraceptives and STI prevention.[19–22] However, the finding that parent-child communication about sexuality leads to positive sexual outcomes is not considered a conclusive one. There is some evidence that parents communicate more about sexuality with their children when they believe that their child is engaged in sexual activity, meaning that increased parent-child communication is at times correlated with increased sexual activity (rather than decreased or delayed sexual activity).[7,8,22,23] Moreover, the effectiveness of parent-child communication about sexuality is dependent on a number of factors. Timing is one important variable, as previously mentioned—parent-child conversations about sexuality are most likely to be effective when they occur early in development, before initiation of sexual activity.[13] Research has also shown that these conversations are most effective when parents are knowledgeable about sexuality, when communication about sexuality is open and supportive, and when this communication occurs in the context of a generally close, open, and supportive parent-child relationship.[16,21,22,24,25] The overall closeness and quality of the parent-child relationship have also been found to be related to sexual behavior outcomes, with open and supportive mother-daughter relationships that include communication about sexuality being particularly predictive of more positive sexual outcomes.[14,16,21]

The quality of the parent-child relationship is influenced by many factors, but perhaps most strongly by parenting style. Broadly speaking, parenting styles differ widely across families and may be influenced by cultural factors. Psychologists often categorize parenting style into one of three types: *authoritarian*, *permissive*, or *authoritative*[26] (Table 28.1). *Authoritarian* parents often have strict expectations for behavior and are more intrusive and controlling in their children's lives. They tend to be less warm, open, and responsive with their children, placing greater emphasis on achievement, appropriate behavior, and respect for parental authority than on relationships. *Permissive* parents, by contrast, tend to be very nurturing and affectionate, responding immediately to their children's needs. They place few demands on their

children and frequently struggle to set any limits on their children's behavior. They may be overly open with their children, trying to act as their children's "friends," rather than as disciplinarians. *Authoritative* parents set clear rules and consequences for their children's behavior. They have warm, supportive interaction styles, and communicate openly with children about their expectations, while also maintaining appropriate boundaries.

Authoritative parenting is generally described as the most effective style and has been linked to lower rates of engagement in risk behaviors (e.g., related to substance use and sexual health) and better behavioral and health outcomes.[14,27–29] Children of authoritative parents are thought to have more positive outcomes, because this parenting style balances appropriate levels of monitoring and supervision of the child, setting clear expectations for appropriate behavior, and a warm, open approach to communication that allows the child to discuss questions and concerns with the parent.[25,27] Consistent with this broad pattern of findings, children of authoritative parents have been found to have the most positive outcomes in sexual development, including later ages of first sexual experience, higher rates of safer sex behaviors, and decreased likelihood of unplanned and early pregnancy.[16,22,28,29] Because authoritative parenting encompasses a broad set of behaviors, researchers have also worked to understand what aspects of this parenting style are most related to key outcomes. As previously described, supportive and open communication between parents and their children about sexual behavior and other topics is one key factor. Parental monitoring has a somewhat mixed relationship with outcomes—increased monitoring of adolescent behavior is generally linked with delayed initiation of sexual activity and reduced number of sexual partners.[14,16,30,31] However, parents who engage in very high levels of monitoring and control may have a paradoxical effect on behavior and actually increase the likelihood that their children will resist this monitoring and engage in earlier and more risky sexual activity.[14,28,31] Interestingly, the relative effects of monitoring versus openness and support may be moderated by gender, with monitoring being more critical to positive sexual outcomes for boys, and openness and support being the most predictive for girls.[16] A summary of parental factors that relate to sexual outcomes appears in Table 28.2.

Table 28.1 Parenting styles.

- Authoritarian
  - Strict expectations for behavior
  - More intrusive
  - More controlling
  - Emphasize achievement—respect for parental authority
- Permissive
  - Nurturing
  - Affectionate
  - Respond immediately
- Authoritative
  - Set clear rules
  - Consequences for actions

Table 28.2 Parenting factors related to positive sexual health outcomes.

- Direct, informative communication about sexuality
- Having sexuality conversations before initiation of sexual activity
- Authoritative parenting style
- Warm, open communication between parents and adolescents
- Appropriate monitoring of adolescent behavior
- Clearly communicated family values of delaying sexual activity

ENVIRONMENTAL AND CULTURAL INFLUENCES ON SEXUAL DEVELOPMENT

In addition to parenting style and behaviors, other family and environmental factors can also influence adolescent sexual behavior and development. Generally speaking, parental values around sexuality are correlated to adolescent values, such that teens tend to share many of their parents' beliefs about sexuality, though they rarely agree completely.[2,11,31,32] Parents' explicit communication of values around sexual behavior, particularly when parents directly communicate their disapproval of early sexual activity, has been shown to be predictive of adolescents delaying their sexual debut.[2,20,21,31] Values around sexuality are often directly influenced by religious beliefs, with most world religions endorsing the idea that sexual behavior should be restricted to married persons. There are mixed findings regarding the impacts of parental religiosity on communication about sexuality, with some studies finding highly religious parents engage in more communication about sexuality and have more explicit rules about sexual behavior, while others find that religious parents are less open to discussing sexuality and may discuss a smaller range of topics related to sexuality, with most messages focused on negative consequences of sexual behavior.[2,23,32] When parents successfully pass on religious values and identity to their children, however, the findings are fairly consistent that higher rates of adolescent and young adult religiosity are associated with delayed initiation of sexual activity, reduced rates of unplanned pregnancy, and fewer sexual partners.[33–36] Interestingly, virginity pledges (commonly associated with conservative Christians in the United States) are not predictive of delayed sexual initiation or reduced numbers of partners, and may in fact be associated with decreased likelihood of utilizing contraceptives and safer sex practices.[37]

Broader environmental and family factors that may not directly influence sexual beliefs may still impact sexual outcomes and behavior. In general, demographic factors associated with disadvantage, including lower socioeconomic status, living in a disorganized neighborhood, and living in a single-parent home, are linked to higher rates of early sexual activity, unplanned pregnancy, and sexual risk behaviors in adolescents.[22,36,38] It has been suggested that this pattern is due to the decreased monitoring of behavior that often occurs in these households, due to reduced access to resources and increased likelihood of parents working long hours.[22,36] When parents, older siblings, or peers are engaged in risky sexual behaviors, this has also been associated with increased rates of risky sexual behaviors in adolescents.[22,36] Although the idea that lesbian or gay parents would be more likely to have children with more permissive values around sexuality or children who themselves would identify as LGBT has been advanced by some groups who oppose parenting by these individuals, the research has consistently shown that there is no connection between having an LGBT parent and a child's sexual orientation or behavior.[39]

Culture, used here to denote factors related to ethnoracial identity, is another broad and potentially powerful source of influence on sexuality and sexual behavior. As with any discussion of cultural influences, it is important to keep in mind that there is often as much diversity within groups as between them, and thus, we must be cautious never to make assumptions about any individual's particular beliefs or practices based on perceived cultural factors alone. It is also worth noting that in the United States, cultural factors are often strongly confounded by socioeconomic status, which also influences sexual behavior as previously described, making it difficult to know whether observed differences in behavior are due to cultural factors, socioeconomic factors, or the interaction of these.[40] The role of acculturation in development and family processes is also relevant here. Acculturation refers to the process by which values and practices change when two (or more) cultures come into contact; this term is most often used to refer to the changes that occur as immigrants adjust to a new culture.[40] Acculturation is no longer characterized as a unidimensional, unidirectional process, in which an individual moves away from "culture A" and toward "culture B." Rather, it is now understood that acculturation occurs along many different dimensions (e.g., language, cultural knowledge, values, and practices), each of which may progress at different paces, and that individuals may identify to different degrees with different aspects of each culture.[40] Of particular relevance to this chapter is the consistent finding that within immigrant families, children and adolescents experience acculturative forces differently than their parents, with youth tending to identify more strongly with the "new culture" than their parents, which may lead to increased conflicts around values and practices.[40] With these thoughts in mind, a brief overview of cultural differences around sexuality may be helpful to the PAGs, though providers are strongly encouraged to learn more about the sexual values and beliefs of the particular populations and families with whom they work.

Broadly within the United States, sexual attitudes and behaviors have become more permissive over time.[41,42] The most recent data indicate that a majority of U.S. adolescents and adults are accepting of premarital sex, though the overwhelming majority still disapprove of both extramarital sex (i.e., affairs) and adolescent sexual activity.[41,42] Acceptance of sexual activity with same-sex partners and of LGBT individuals and their relationships has also increased substantially over time, with a particular increase since the 1990s.[41] As sexual attitudes have become more permissive over the past several decades, adolescent engagement in sexual activity has also steadily increased, with roughly half of adolescents reporting that they are sexually active.[42,43] Within these broader national trends, there is also some important variability in sexual behaviors, attitudes, and outcomes across ethnoracial groups. Regarding overall risk behaviors, there is a somewhat consistent finding that both African American youth (particularly males) and immigrant youth in the United States are at increased risk for early sexual debut and higher rates of risky sexual behavior.[36,43,44] Findings about the effects of ethnoracial factors on parent-child communication about sexuality are mixed, with some studies finding no differences in frequency of communication, while others find that Asian American parents communicate less about sexuality than other parents, or that African American or Latino parents communicate more about sexuality than other parents.[2,7,10,17,23,31] Research on the ways in which sexual beliefs and values may differ across cultural groups is somewhat limited, given the varied and multifaceted nature of cultural influences on sexual beliefs and practices, but qualitative research, in particular, has provided a window into some of the values and beliefs around sexuality within particular cultural groups.

Caucasian Americans are a varied group, including individuals of Eastern and Western European descent, ethnic Jews, and families who have lived in the United States for several generations. As Caucasians continue to be a slight majority of U.S. society, their beliefs can generally be said to be consistent with the previously discussed broader findings—namely, that there is increased acceptance among Caucasians of premarital (though not adolescent) sexual activity and of LGBT individuals and relationships, particularly relative to other ethnic groups within the United States.[45,46] Religion is often an important factor in influencing sexuality in this group, as previously described, with more religious families tending to hold more conservative views around sexuality. Virginity pledges (as previously discussed briefly) are most common in Caucasian conservative Christians, and discussing their lack of effects on behavior in a culturally sensitive way may be an important role for PAGs to play.[37] Gender roles are increasingly flexible in this group, though many families continue to observe more traditional gender roles, particularly within certain religious groups.[32,47]

African Americans (and indeed, individuals of African descent around the world) have commonly been stereotyped as "hypersexual" and sexually permissive in their values.[48–50] African American women, in particular, have often been sexually objectified, and African American adolescent girls and young women report higher rates of sexual victimization and pressure to engage in sexual activity.[49,51] However, targeted research suggests that while African American youth may engage in higher rates of sexually risky behaviors and initiate sexual activity earlier, African Americans as a group are not more sexually permissive in their attitudes and beliefs than other ethnoracial groups.[41,45,52–54] Following the HIV/AIDS crisis of the 1980s and 1990s, there has been some research to suggest that African American parents engage in more communication around STIs, in particular, with their children, but this finding is not consistent.[2,17,30] Additionally, parents in sub-Saharan Africa (and who subsequently may immigrate to the United States) have generally been found to avoid discussing HIV/AIDS with their children, despite intense public health campaigns across the continent.[3,55] Gender roles are also increasingly flexible in this group,

though that is less true for recent immigrants from the Caribbean and the African continent.[47,48,50]

Latinos in the United States tend to report sexual behaviors and attitudes that are fairly consistent with those of Caucasian Americans.[45,46] However, Latino adolescents tend to receive less communication from their parents about sexuality, despite weighing their parents' opinions more heavily than adolescents from other ethnic groups, and their parents may prefer to communicate about sexuality in more indirect ways.[18,21] They also seem to be at particular risk for unplanned pregnancy relative to other groups.[18] Gender roles tend to be more traditional in this group, with greater flexibility in gender roles among youth relative to their parents, particularly in recent immigrant families.[56] Among U.S. groups, Asian Americans are consistently found to have the most conservative sexual values and beliefs, least comfort with communicating about sexuality, latest ages of sexual debut, and fewest sexual partners.[45,46,57] It has been posited that this pattern is driven by cultural values within Asian societies, which tend to designate sexuality as a taboo subject and outward expressions of sexuality as disruptive to the social order, particularly when they occur outside of marriage.[57] Particularly among recent immigrants, these views of sexuality at times contribute to a perception that routine gynecologic care is inappropriate unless focused specifically on reproductive health, particularly prior to marriage, which in turn contributes to later diagnoses of breast and cervical cancer in Asian American women.[57] Gender roles tend to mirror the findings among Latinos, with Asian Americans generally falling into more traditional roles, particularly among recent immigrants.[47] Like Asian Americans, individuals of Arab and Middle Eastern descent and those from Muslim communities (which are overlapping, though not identical groups) also tend to be highly conservative with regard to sexual behaviors and values. There are often strong values within these communities around restricting sexual activity to marriage, particularly for girls and women, adhering to strict gender roles, and rejecting homosexual relationships.[58,59] Because of these strong beliefs, participation in sexual education that goes beyond teaching basic reproductive facts is often perceived as somewhat threatening to family cultural values, as discussion of safer sex practices is often perceived as condoning premarital sexual activity.[58] Additionally, the existence of intersex conditions may be particularly difficult for these families to cope with, given their strong beliefs around gender roles and the connection of gender to religion.

Much attention has been given in recent years to the practice of female circumcision, also known as female genital mutilation. Female circumcision involves the partial or complete removal of female genitalia—sometimes restricted only to the clitoris, but at times involving much more extensive cutting—for the purposes of protecting a woman's virginity and honor, ensuring suitability for marriage, and symbolizing a girl's passage into adulthood.[60–62] The practice is most often associated with communities in East and Central Africa, but it also exists in other areas, including Indonesia, Malaysia, and parts of the Middle East and North Africa.[62] Although the practice is not actually mandated by Islam and also occurs in some non-Islamic communities, those who observe this practice frequently describe it in Islamic religious terms.[63] Although PAGs will not perform this procedure, as it is not medically necessary and can often result in both physical and psychological harm to the patient,[60-62] they may encounter families who have had the procedure performed elsewhere. It is also important to note that U.S. federal law prohibits female circumcision, as well as the practice of "vacation cutting," whereby a family may travel to another country to have the procedure performed. As legally mandated reporters, PAGs are required to take appropriate steps if they become aware that a family has engaged in this practice.[64] The complexities of caring for a girl or young woman who has undergone this procedure are beyond the scope of this chapter—providers are encouraged to consult the work of Khaja and colleagues[60] and Abdulcadir and colleagues[62] for guides to care and considerations for culturally sensitive practice, as well as guidelines from the American College of Obstetricians and Gynecologists.[65]

RECOMMENDATIONS FOR PRACTICE

As stated at the outset of this chapter, PAGs are faced with the challenge of providing care and communicating about sensitive topics with the patients and families they serve. Providers must balance providing accurate, complete information about sexual development and healthy sexual behavior to both the parent and the patient, with respect for family and cultural values and practices (see Table 28.3). Consistent with the American Academy of Pediatrics' statement on Sexuality Education for Children and Adolescents, providers are encouraged to take an active role in conversations about sexuality with patients and their families, within the context of culturally sensitive and respectful practice.[1] In working with families, PAGs should begin their conversations by asking questions about family values related to sexuality and sexual behavior, to help situate their discussions within a framework that includes and respects these values. Providers should also ask both parents and patients about what conversations families have already had about sexuality, keeping in mind that parents and adolescents may differ in their

Table 28.3 Recommendations for discussing sexuality with families.

---

1. Gather information about family values related to sexuality
2. Ask about prior conversations the family has had
3. Assess family's sexuality knowledge
4. Provide important sexuality information directly to patients with families present, modeling open and direct conversations
5. Share information about effective parenting practices
6. Link families to outside resources

---

reporting of what conversations have occurred.[11] It is also valuable, when possible, to assess both adolescent and parent sexual knowledge, as lack of knowledge of issues related to sexuality is a key barrier to parent comfort and willingness to communicate about sexuality with their child.[8,10] The *Children's Hospital Sexual Education Assessment Survey*[66] provides a structured format for assessing sexual knowledge when possible and useful for providers. Taking the time to gather information about family knowledge and values around sexuality provides a window into the family's comfort with conversations about sexuality and will help PAGs focus their own conversations on the most critical topics related to the patient's health and well-being.

Using this information, PAGs should have direct conversations with both patients and families to provide relevant sexuality education, keeping in mind that families tend to have these conversations too late (i.e., after sexual debut has already occurred)[13] and that families are often eager for medical providers to take an active role in their children's sexual education.[6] Providers can model the types of conversations that parents should reinforce with their children—that is, conversations that are open, direct, and informative. Sharing information about what constitutes normal and healthy sexual development is a particularly appropriate and helpful role for PAGs to play. Providers can also present information about the range of sexual behaviors in which adolescents may engage (e.g., masturbation, kissing, fondling, oral sex, and penetrative intercourse), the risks of engagement in sexual behavior during adolescence, and the steps that adolescents can take to protect themselves from unplanned pregnancies and STIs. By modeling open, fact-based conversations about sexuality with patients and providing parents with education about factors that promote healthy sexual development in children, providers can encourage parenting practices that will benefit their patients. Although it is not the role of the PAGs to act as a parenting coach, it may be appropriate for providers to share information about the ways in which parents can promote positive sexual health outcomes in their children, including monitoring adolescent behavior and whereabouts (without taking a controlling approach), engaging in open and frank conversations with their child about sexuality, clearly communicating their own values and expectations, and providing a warm, supportive family environment.

PAGs will certainly care for patients who identify as lesbian, bisexual, or transgender during the course of their routine practice. Although acceptance of nonheterosexual people and their relationships has increased substantially in the United States over the years, this acceptance is still far from universal.[41] Children and adolescents who identify as LGBT continue to be at significantly increased risk for mood and anxiety disorders, as well as for high-risk behaviors such as running away, self-harm, and suicidality.[67] This is particularly true for LGBT youth from ethnic minority backgrounds and those who experience family rejection due to their LGBT identity.[67-69] For this reason, it is vital that providers emphasize with families the importance of unconditional acceptance of these children and their identities. Attempts to change a child's sexual orientation or gender identity increase the risk of psychological distress and high-risk behaviors and thus must be strongly discouraged. Providers are encouraged to emphasize the importance of acceptance of the child and his or her identity as vital to the child's physical and emotional well-being.

Finally, while PAGs are important resources and sources of support to families as they work to promote their children's sexual health, families will also benefit from outside resources. Providers are encouraged to familiarize themselves with helpful websites, books, and other resources that parents can use to educate their children about sexuality and encourage healthy sexual behavior. Many such resources are freely available through nonprofit organizations (e.g., Planned Parenthood). Providers may also wish to consider linking families with structured programs that have been shown to improve parent-child communication about sexuality and increase the likelihood of positive sexual outcomes.[19,70,71] By working in supportive and culturally sensitive ways with families, PAGs can support healthy sexual development and positive outcomes for their patients.

REFERENCES

1. American Academy of Pediatrics. Sexuality education for children and adolescents. *Pediatrics.* 2001;108(2):498–502.
2. Diiorio C, Pluhar E, Belcher L. Parent-child communication about sexuality: A review of the literature from 1980 to 2002. *J HIVAIDS Prev Educ Adolesc Child.* 2003;5(3–4):7–32.
3. Namisi FS, Flisher AJ, Overland S et al. Sociodemographic variations in communication on sexuality and HIV/AIDS with parents, family members and teachers among in-school adolescents: A multi-site study in Tanzania and South Africa. *Scand J Public Health.* 2009;37(Suppl 2):65–74.
4. Ito KE, Gizlice Z, Owen-O'Dowd J, Foust E, Leone PA, Miller WC. Parent opinion of sexuality education in a state with mandated abstinence education: Does policy match parental preference? *J Adolesc Health.* 2006;39(5):634–41.
5. Eisenberg ME, Bernat DH, Bearinger LH, Resnick MD. Support for comprehensive sexuality education: Perspectives from parents of school-age youth. *J Adolesc Health.* 2008;42(4):352–9.
6. Thomas D, Flaherty E, Binns H. Parent expectations and comfort with discussion of normal childhood sexuality and sexual abuse prevention during office visits. *Ambul Pediatr.* 4:232–6.
7. Byers ES, Sears HA, Weaver AD. Parents' reports of sexual communication with children in kindergarten to grade 8. *J Marriage Fam.* 2008;70(1):86–96.
8. Miller KS, Fasula AM, Dittus P, Wiegand RE, Wyckoff SC, McNair L. Barriers and facilitators to maternal communication with preadolescents about age-relevant sexual topics. *AIDS Behav.* 2009;13(2):365–74.
9. Jaccard J, Dodge T, Dittus P. Parent-adolescent communication about sex and birth control: A conceptual framework. *New Dir Child Adolesc Dev.* 2002;2002(97):9–42.
10. Jerman P, Constantine NA. Demographic and psychological predictors of parent–adolescent communication about sex: A representative statewide analysis. *J Youth Adolesc.* 2010;39(10):1164–74.
11. Jaccard J, Dittus PJ, Gordon VV. Parent-adolescent congruency in reports of adolescent sexual behavior and in communications about sexual behavior. *Child Dev.* 1998;69(1):247–61.
12. Wyckoff SC, Miller KS, Forehand R et al. Patterns of sexuality communication between preadolescents and their mothers and fathers. *J Child Fam Stud.* 2008;17(5):649–62.
13. Beckett MK, Elliott MN, Martino S et al. Timing of parent and child communication about sexuality relative to children's sexual behaviors. *Pediatrics.* 2010;125(1):34–42.
14. de Graaf H, Vanwesenbeeck I, Woertman L, Meeus W. Parenting and adolescents' sexual development in western societies: A literature review. *Eur Psychol.* 2011;16(1):21–31.
15. Wilson EK, Koo HP. Mothers, fathers, sons, and daughters: Gender differences in factors associated with parent-child communication about sexual topics. *Reprod Health.* 2010;7(1):31.
16. Kincaid C, Jones DJ, Sterrett E, McKee L. A review of parenting and adolescent sexual behavior: The moderating role of gender. *Clin Psychol Rev.* 2012;32(3):177–88.
17. Tobey J, Hillman SB, Anagurthi C, Somers CL. Demographic differences in adolescents' sexual attitudes and behaviors, parent communication about sex, and school sex education. *Electron J Hum Sex.* 2011;14(3):1–2.
18. Raffaelli M, Green S. Parent-adolescent communication about sex: Retrospective reports by Latino college students. *J Marriage Fam.* 2003;65(2):474–81.
19. Wight D, Fullerton D. A review of interventions with parents to promote the sexual health of their children. *J Adolesc Health.* 2013;52(1):4–27.
20. Lehr ST, DiIorio C, Dudley WN, Lipana JA. The relationship between parent-adolescent communication and safer sex behaviors in college students. *J Fam Nurs.* 2000;6(2):180–96.
21. Romo LF, Lefkowitz ES, Sigman M, Au TK. A longitudinal study of maternal messages about dating and sexuality and their influence on Latino adolescents. *J Adolesc Health.* 2002;31(1):59–69.
22. Miller BC. Family influences on adolescent sexual and contraceptive behavior. *J Sex Res.* 2002;39(1):22–6.
23. Swain C, Ackerman L, Ackerman M. The influence of individual characteristics and contraceptive beliefs on parent-teen sexual communications: A structural model. *J Adolesc Health.* 2006;38(6):753.e9–753.e18.

24. Somers CL, Vollmar WL. Parent-adolescent relationships and adolescent sexuality: Closeness, communication, and comfort among diverse US adolescent samples. *Soc Behav Personal.* 2006;34(4):451–60.

25. Pluhar EI, Kuriloff P. What really matters in family communication about sexuality? A qualitative analysis of affect and style among African American mothers and adolescent daughters. *Sex Educ.* 2004;4(3):303–21.

26. Baumrind D. Child care practices anteceding three patterns of preschool behavior. *Genet Psychol Mongraphs.* 1967;75(1):43–88.

27. Baumrind D. The influence of parenting style on adolescent competence and substance use. *J Early Adolesc.* 1991;11(1):56–95.

28. DeVore ER, Ginsburg KR. The protective effects of good parenting on adolescents. *Curr Opin Pediatr.* 2005;17(4):460–5.

29. Huebner AJ, Howell LW. Examining the relationship between adolescent sexual risk-taking and perceptions of monitoring, communication, and parenting styles. *J Adolesc Health.* 2003;33(2):71–8.

30. DiClemente RJ, Wingood GM, Crosby R, Cobb BK, Harrington K, Davies SL. Parent-adolescent communication and sexual risk behaviors among African American adolescent females. *J Pediatr.* 2001;139(3):407–12.

31. Bersamin M, Todd M, Fisher DA, Hill DL, Grube JW, Walker S. Parenting practices and adolescent sexual behavior: A longitudinal study. *J Marriage Fam.* 2008;70(1):97–112.

32. Regnerus MD. Talking about sex: Religion and patterns of parent-child communication about sex and contraception. *Sociol Q.* 46:79–105.

33. Sinha JW, Cnaan RA, Gelles RJ. Adolescent risk behaviors and religion: Findings from a national study. *J Adolesc.* 2007;30(2):231–49.

34. Simons LG, Burt CH, Peterson FR. The effect of religion on risky sexual behavior among college students. *Deviant Behav.* 2009;30(5):467–85.

35. Landor A, Simons LG, Simons RL, Brody GH, Gibbons FX. The role of religiosity in the relationship between parents, peers, and adolescent risky sexual behavior. *J Youth Adolesc.* 2011;40(3):296–309.

36. Zimmer-Gembeck MJ, Helfand M. Ten years of longitudinal research on U.S. adolescent sexual behavior: Developmental correlates of sexual intercourse, and the importance of age, gender and ethnic background. *Dev Rev.* 2008;28(2):153–224.

37. Rosenbaum JE. Patient teenagers? A comparison of the sexual behavior of virginity pledgers and matched nonpledgers. *Pediatrics.* 2009;123(1):e110–20.

38. Browning CR, Burrington LA, Leventhal T, Brooks-Gunn J. Neighborhood structural inequality, collective efficacy, and sexual risk behavior among urban youth. *J Health Soc Behav.* 2008;49(3):269–85.

39. Tasker F. Lesbian mothers, gay fathers, and their children: A review. *J Dev Behav Pediatr.* 2005;26(3):224–40.

40. Atkinson DR. *Counseling American Minorities.* 6th ed. New York, NY: McGraw-Hill; 2004.

41. Twenge J, Sherman R, Wells B. Changes in American adults' sexual behavior and attitudes, 1972–2012. *Arch Sex Behav.* 2015;44(8):2273–85.

42. Wells B, Twenge J. Changes in young people's sexual behavior and attitudes, 1943–1999: A cross-temporal meta-analysis. *Rev Gen Psychol.* 2005;9(3):249–61.

43. Eaton D, Kann L, Kinchen S et al. Youth risk behavior surveillance—United States, 2005. *MMWR.* 2006;55(S05):1–108.

44. Hussey JM, Hallfors DD, Waller MW, Iritani BJ, Halpern CT, Bauer DJ. Sexual behavior and drug use among Asian and Latino adolescents: Association with immigrant status. *J Immigr Minor Health.* 2007;9(2):85–94.

45. Ahrold TK, Meston CM. Ethnic differences in sexual attitudes of U.S. College students: Gender, acculturation, and religiosity factors. *Arch Sex Behav.* 2010;39(1):190–202.

46. Meston CM, Ahrold T. Ethnic, gender, and acculturation influences on sexual behaviors. *Arch Sex Behav.* 2010;39(1):179–89.

47. Lennon S, Rudd N, Sloan B, Sook Kim J. Attitudes toward gender roles, self-esteem, and body image: Application of a model. *Cloth Text Res J.* 1999;17(4):191–202.

48. Kempadoo K. Caribbean sexuality—Mapping the field. *Caribb Rev Gend Stud.* 2008;(3).

49. Williams JK. African-American sexuality and HIV/AIDS: Recommendations for future research. *J Natl Med Assoc.* 2008;100(1):44.

50. Epprecht M. The making of "African Sexuality": Early sources, current debates. *Hist Compass.* 2010;8(8):768–79.

51. Townsend TG, Thomas AJ, Neilands TB, Jackson TR. I'm no Jezebel; I am young, gifted, and black: Identity, sexuality, and black girls. *Psychol Women Q.* 2010;34(3):273–85.

52. Owen JJ, Rhoades GK, Stanley SM, Fincham FD. "Hooking up" among college students: Demographic and psychosocial correlates. *Arch Sex Behav.* 2010;39(3):653–63.

53. Cuffee JJ, Hallfors DD, Waller MW. Racial and gender differences in adolescent sexual attitudes and longitudinal associations with coital debut. *J Adolesc Health Off Publ Soc Adolesc Med.* 2007;41(1):19–26.

54. Hipwell AE, Keenan K, Loeber R, Battista D. Early predictors of sexually intimate behaviors in an urban sample of young girls. *Dev Psychol.* 2010;46(2):366–78.

55. Bastien S, Kajula LJ, Muhwezi WW. A review of studies of parent-child communication about sexuality and HIV/AIDS in sub-Saharan Africa. *Reprod Health.* 2011;8(1):25.

56. Raffaelli M, Ontai LL. Gender socialization in Latino/a families: Results from two retrospective studies. *Sex Roles.* 2004;50(5/6):287–99.

57. Okazaki S. Influences of culture on Asian Americans' sexuality. *J Sex Res.* 2002;39(1):34–41.
58. Orgocka A. Perceptions of communication and education about sexuality among Muslim immigrant girls in the US. *Sex Educ.* 2004;4(3):255–71.
59. Smerecnik C, Schaalma H, Gerjo K, Meijer S, Poelman J. An exploratory study of Muslim adolescents' views on sexuality: Implications for sex education and prevention. *BMC Public Health.* 2010;10(1):533.
60. Khaja K, Lay K, Boys S. Female circumcision: Toward an inclusive practice of care. *Health Care Women Int.* 2010;31(8):686–99.
61. Public Policy Advisory Network on Female Genital Surgeries in Africa. Seven things to know about female genital surgeries in Africa. *Hastings Cent Rep.* 2012.
62. Abdulcadir J, Margairaz C, Boulvain M, Irion O. Care of women with female genital mutilation/cutting. *Swiss Med Wkly.* 2011;140(w13137).
63. Osten-Sacken T von der, Uwer T. Is female genital mutilation an Islamic problem? *Middle East Q.* 2007;Winter 2007:29–36.
64. Female Genital Mutilation. 18 U.S. Code § 116.
65. Female genital Mutilation. College Statement of Policy. American College of Obstetricians and Gynecologists. Washington, DC. April 2019. https://www.acog.org/-/media/Statements-of-Policy/Public/98FemaleGenitalMutilationREV.pdf?dmc=1&ts=20190517T1615326105. Accessed May 17, 2019.
66. Kumar M, Lim R, Langford C, Seabrook J, Speechley K, Lynch T. Sexual knowledge of Canadian adolescents after completion of high school sexual education requirements. *Paediatr Child Health.* 2013;18(2):74–80.
67. Mustanski BS, Garofalo R, Emerson EM. Mental health disorders, psychological distress, and suicidality in a diverse sample of lesbian, gay, bisexual, and transgender youths. *Am J Public Health.* 2010;100(12):2426–32.
68. Balsam KF, Huang B, Fieland KC, Simoni JM, Walters KL. Culture, trauma, and wellness: A comparison of heterosexual and lesbian, gay, bisexual, and two-spirit Native Americans. *Cultur Divers Ethnic Minor Psychol.* 2004;10(3):287–301.
69. Ryan C, Huebner D, Diaz R, Sanchez J. Family rejection as a predictor of negative health outcomes in white and Latino lesbian, gay, and bisexual young adults. *Pediatrics.* 2009;123(1):346–52.
70. Klein JD, Sabaratnam P, Pazos B, Auerbach MM, Havens CG, Brach MJ. Evaluation of the parents as primary sexuality educators program. *J Adolesc Health.* 2005;37(3):S94–9.
71. Schuster MA, Corona R, Elliott MN et al. Evaluation of Talking Parents, Healthy Teens, a new worksite based parenting programme to promote parent-adolescent communication about sexual health: Randomised controlled trial. *BMJ.* 2008;337:a308.

Health-care transition

29

ARIEL WHITE and LISA TUCHMAN

INTRODUCTION

Transition is the normal, healthy process of moving from adolescence to adulthood.[1,2] Transition is not a one-time event but rather a normal developmental process that occurs throughout adolescence.[1] Adolescents and young adults go through transition in multiple facets of their lives, including health, school, employment, and social transitions, though timing may vary depending on the unique characteristics of the individual adolescent.[1-3] While the transfer of care from pediatric to adult health care may happen at different times depending on individual needs, developmentally appropriate transition support in all of these developmental domains should be integrated into clinical care for all youth.[4] Lack of communication with patients regarding expectations during health-care transition may lead to poor health outcomes, particularly for youth with chronic conditions.[5] Without good physical and mental health support, other life transitions may be derailed, which puts youth at a social and economic disadvantage as they become adults.[1] It is the responsibility of the health-care provider not only to address medical needs, but to help patients stay as healthy as possible, thrive in their adult lives, and find their place in the world. When a child is born, there are many resources mobilized around that child. As that child nears adulthood, the goal should be to integrate the child into the community to contribute his or her fullest potential such that needed resources are minimized and contribution is maximized.

The ideal process of health-care transition is intentionally changing the model of health-care delivery from pediatric care to adult care in a way that is developmentally appropriate for the individual patient.[1,2] This process often leads to a patient graduating from a pediatric-care setting and transferring to an adult health-care practice or setting. However, transition from a pediatric model to an adult model of care can also occur within the patients' already established medical home.[4] This is especially true in the Family Practice or Internal Medicine/Pediatric clinic setting, where patients may be cared for from birth. The developmental approach and expectations change as the patient ages, while the health-care setting does not. For example, shared decision-making and approach to confidentiality change as a youth becomes more developmentally mature. Health-care transition can incorporate both the process of modifying the provider approach to the patient as well as the transfer of care to an adult-oriented health-care provider, as appropriate.[4] Regardless of practice setting, transition readiness should increase over time. Transition readiness is the process of acquiring behaviors that support self-care, health-care decision-making, and self-advocacy. Transition readiness is

influenced by a complex interaction of factors including the youth's own cognitive maturity and/or development, type and complexity of physical and mental health issues, health system and insurance supports and barriers, and family resources. In the case of an adolescent transitioning from a pediatric to an adult practice setting, the provider should be periodically assessing transition readiness and providing support for areas where patients need extra help (Figures 29.1 and 29.2). There are many transition assessment tools available.[6] Some are disease or condition specific, and some are appropriate for all adolescents. It is important to recognize that transfer to an adult practice setting can happen before optimal transition readiness occurs. In this case, adult practices accepting young adult patients should be prepared.[7] This includes having a practice policy in place that addresses privacy and confidentiality and establishing a process for welcoming young adults into the practice, including a description of available services. It may also be helpful to provide young adult–friendly online or written information about the practice and offer a "get-acquainted" appointment. At the first visit, the adult provider should address any concerns that the young adult has about transferring to an adult approach to care and use the opportunity to clarify the process of shared decision-making, privacy and consent, access to information, adherence to care, and preferred methods of communication, including attending to health literacy needs.

The process of health-care transition includes health-care practice-, patient-, and family-based elements to facilitate a safe, efficient, and organized transfer of care.[2] The goal is to promote lifelong function and healthy habits, as well as to foster connection between the youth and the health-care system. There are many differences between adult versus pediatric models of health care that need to be considered when helping youth and families anticipate expectations in the adult-oriented health setting. While a pediatric-care model involves close care coordination and allocation of supportive resources by the health-care team, an adult-care model expects patients to take responsibility for their own care and seek out resources proactively. Additionally, the pediatric-care model tends to be more future oriented, while adult care focuses on optimizing the present. Other differences include tolerance of nonadherence, higher levels of pain tolerance, and different approaches to palliative care in the adult health-care model. Youth have identified benefits to receiving care in adult health settings, including better efficiency, providers speaking more directly to them than to their parents, and addressing reproductive health issues more thoroughly.[8] Finally, adult patients are responsible for covering the cost and logistics of their health care,

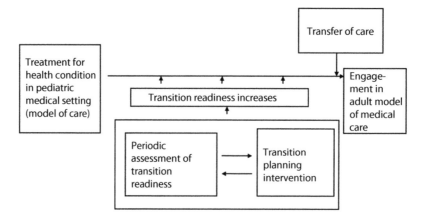

Figure 29.1 Conceptual model of transition process (to adult model of care). (From Tuchman LK et al. *Pediatrics.* 2010;125[3]:566–73, with permission.)

while youth are often covered on their parents' insurance, and are expected to take ownership of their health by transporting themselves to appointments on time and requesting treatment information and results.

A successful transition becomes particularly important when working with a patient with special health-care needs. An individual with special health-care needs is defined as someone with or at higher risk for developing a chronic health condition (physical, developmental, behavioral, or emotional) and who requires health services beyond what is required by children generally.[9,10] Therefore, youth with special heath-care needs encompass a heterogeneous population with conditions ranging from chronic illnesses, such as diabetes, cystic fibrosis, and sickle cell disease, to individuals with developmental disabilities or mental illness. Due to medical advances, nearly half a million children with special health-care needs are reaching adulthood annually in the United States.[2,10] Healthy People 2020 reports that in 2005–2006, 41.2% of youth with special health-care needs had a health-care provider discuss transition with them. The report sets a goal of a 10% increase in transition discussions, or 45.3%, between providers and youth with special health-care needs by 2020.[8] A 2013 analysis of the National Survey of Children with Special Health Care Needs found that there has not been significant improvement in discussion of transition with this patient population since 2005–2006. While providers encouraged youth to take ownership of their health, they

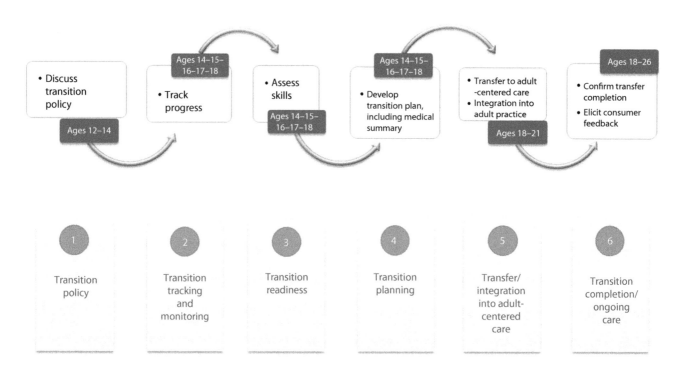

Figure 29.2 Six core elements of transition: Preparing for pediatric to adult health-care transition. (From Got Transition, Washington, DC, with permission.)

failed to discuss moving to an adult provider or navigating the insurance process.[11] Goals of transition should be tailored to the abilities of the patient. Youth with chronic illness may be able to navigate the adult health-care system with or without assistance or may have a severe condition that warrants more careful planning and communication between health-care teams and families.[2] Coordination of an organized, well-planned transition by the pediatric and adult medical teams improves patient heath status and access to care, as well as family perception of quality of care.[12] Patients with mental illness may have a more difficult time transitioning and, therefore, may require extra support during this time. Youth with chronic physical health conditions are at an increased risk of psychiatric comorbidity that may impact the transition process.[13]

In 2011, the American Academy of Pediatrics (AAP), the American Academy of Family Physicians (AAFP), and the American College of Physicians (ACP) released a Clinical Report recommending a formalized transition process for all youth.[2] This report provides an algorithm for health-care transition starting in early adolescence and continuing until young adulthood.[2] Despite widespread support for coordinated transition, data indicate that transition programs are not well implemented at the health system level.[14] In a 2016 study surveying 209 adolescents from 16 to 22 years old with special health-care needs, 64% of participants reported that they had never discussed transition to adult care with their pediatric provider.[15] This trend was also observed in a study of 139 hospitalized youth ages 15–21 years, which showed that less than 40% of participants had discussed transition or taking personal responsibility for their health.[16] Without a well-coordinated transition, adult providers may feel poorly prepared to care for young adults with chronic conditions, which may lead to gaps in care and subsequent poor health outcomes.[2] The 2011 Clinical Report was updated in 2016 to better define the infrastructure, education and payment models that need further development in order to improve transition readiness and success.[17]

ELEMENTS OF SUCCESSFUL TRANSITION TO AN ADULT MEDICAL HOME

As a child grows into a young adult, the first step in transition is to add preventative screening questions and counseling appropriate for the patient's stage of life, ideally in the absence of a parent, into regular visits. In general, the provider should start to incorporate time with the adolescent alone during ambulatory visits around the time of puberty. This approach may be modified in the case of a patient with developmental delay who is not able to participate or cannot tolerate an interview alone. During the confidential interview, the provider should use a screening tool or mnemonic such as SHADESS (strengths, school, home, activities, drugs/substance use, emotions/eating/depression, sexuality, safety) to guide developmentally appropriate questions about home life, activities, education and school performance, future plans, family, peer relationships, sexuality, body image, drug use, and safety.[18]

Through the course of this interview, the provider should focus on the patient's strengths to help develop rapport and assess patient resilience.[18] These questions allow the provider to provide preventative counseling and help the patient anticipate transition. In addition to focusing on strengths, the SHADESS assessment differs from the more traditional HEEADSS (home, education, employment, activities, drugs, sexuality, suicide) in that it places school before home, as home environment can be more sensitive for some youth, and screens for a broader range of emotions.[18] If time constraints do not allow for a full assessment, a brief psychosocial screen can be used. If this screen uncovers concerns, further evaluation is warranted.[18] While confidential screening and discussion of SHADESS can begin in adolescence, the AAP, AAFP, and ACP Clinical Report recommends definitive health-care transfer to a new provider or to an adult model of care ideally between the ages of 18 and 21 years.[2] This recommendation is supported by the American College of Obstetricians and Gynecologists Committee Opinion on transition of young adults, which recommends a preventative health-care visit for women between the ages of 18 and 26 years to conduct preventative screening and assess barriers to transition to adult care.[19]

In 2011, after the release of the Clinical Report by the AAP, AAFP, and ACP on transition, "Got Transition," a national resource center, published. The Six Core Elements of Transition to help guide ambulatory clinics to develop a clear transition policy that incorporates a protocol for planning and implementing a smooth transition[13,20] (Figure 29.3). Discussion of transition policy should begin when the patient is between 12 and 14 years. Progress should be tracked by the provider throughout adolescence, with special attention paid to transition readiness and life skills development. Transition readiness can help lead development of an individualized transition plan and eventual transfer of care. Relevant documents should be collected and transferred with the patient. After transfer of care, the transferring provider should follow up, ideally within 3–6 months, to confirm successful completion of transfer with the patient and/or accepting provider. This policy should be communicated clearly with patients and families and be readily available in the form of posters, brochures, and/or web-based information. When beginning and facilitating transition, the provider should aim to normalize the process, address patient and family anxiety, and help youth develop skills to facilitate change.[20] Ultimately, the patient and the family should guide the transition process.[3] The provider should encourage promotion of developmentally appropriate independence and empower the youth to take more control over their health-care decision-making.[2] There are also Six Core Element guidelines for accepting a young adult into an adult-oriented practice (Figure 29.4). The adult practice can anticipate many of the needs of these young adults as they are transferred into their practice. This includes discussing a transition policy that includes confidentiality, expectations around visits, and family involvement. It is also recommended to have

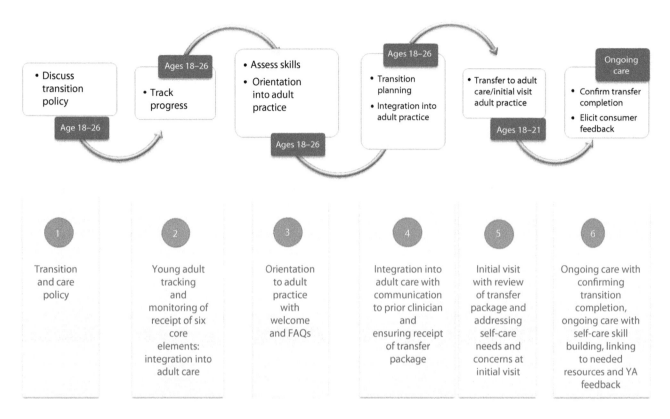

Figure 29.3 Six core elements of transition: Integrating young adults into your adult practice. (From Got Transition, Washington, DC, with permission.)

a system to keep track of youth entering an adult practice and assess integration and engagement and identify areas of additional support needed. Most youth and families will appreciate an orientation to the adult practice with a warm welcome. Prior to the first visit, communication with the transferring provider and ensuring receipt of pertinent medical records facilitates being prepared and anticipates needs of the new patient. At the initial visit with the adult provider, addressing self-care needs and concerns sets the stage for expectations and adds a potential extra level of support needed. Ongoing care can continue to support self-care skill building, linking to needed resources with the prior provider available as a resource as needed.

Ideally, providers should start preparing patients and their families for eventual transition at 12 years of age or younger by discussing the clinic transition process and identifying special health-care needs that may affect transition. Transition planning should formally begin by age 14 and should be well established by 16–17 years of age.[2,20] Ideally, transition should be addressed at every encounter.[19] If the patient is moving to a new medical home, a list of area providers who are interested and available to see young adults should be provided.[2] If a patient is transferring providers, a visit to the planned adult medical home can be considered in the year prior to transition.[2,20] At 18 years old or earlier, if developmentally appropriate, a full adult model of care should be implemented even if there is no change of provider.[2] Any concerns the patient has about transitioning to an

adult-care model should be addressed. If the patient is changing providers, a summary letter to the new provider, as well as transfer package, including assessment of transition readiness by current provider, medical summary and plan of care with transition goals and any pending actions, emergency care plan, and legal documents, should be prepared to move with the patient to his or her new medical home.[20] Adult providers should be communicating with the pediatrician as needed to make sure care continues smoothly and should assist the patient in finding adult subspecialty providers if needed.[20]

For a patient with chronic health-care needs, transition planning may be more comprehensive. Transition of patients with complex care needs should include the development of a formal care plan to be communicated to future providers, as well as coordination with case management and subspecialty providers.[2,20] A written plan should be started at age 14 and updated annually.[1] Insurance and guardianship planning, as appropriate, should start early to prevent gaps in care.[21-24]

Transition readiness varies for each individual patient. While the 2011 AAP, AAFP, and ACP Clinical Reports regarding transition identifies age ranges to start and implement transition plans, the provider should allow the patient and, as appropriate, the patient's family to guide the timeline of transition and decide when they are ready to move to an adult provider.[3] This recommendation is further emphasized in the 2016 updated Clinical Report.[17] The physician must also take the individual physical and

Please fill out this form to help us see what you already know about your health and how to use health care and the areas that you need to learn more about. If you need help completing this form, please ask your parent/caregiver.

Date:

Name: Date of Birth:

Transition Importance and Confidence   *On a scale of 0 to 10, please circle the number that best describes how you feel right now.*

How important is it to you to prepare for/change to an adult doctor before age 22?

0 (not)	1	2	3	4	5	6	7	8	9	10 (very)

How confident do you feel about your ability to prepare for/change to an adult doctor?

0 (not)	1	2	3	4	5	6	7	8	9	10 (very)

My Health   *Please check the box that applies to you right now.*

	Yes, I know this	I need to learn	Someone needs to do this... Who?
I know my medical needs.	☐	☐	☐
I can explain my medical needs to others.	☐	☐	☐
I know my symptoms including ones that I quickly need to see a doctor for.	☐	☐	☐
I know what to do in case I have a medical emergency.	☐	☐	☐
I know my own medicines, what they are for, and when I need to take them.	☐	☐	☐
I know my allergies to medicines and medicines I should not take.	☐	☐	☐
I carry important health information with me every day (e.g. insurance card, allergies, medications, emergency contact information, medical summary).	☐	☐	☐
I understand how health care privacy changes at age 18 when legally an adult.	☐	☐	☐
I can explain to others how my customs and beliefs affect my health care decisions and medical treatment.	☐	☐	☐

Using Health Care

I know or I can find my doctor's phone number.	☐	☐	☐
I make my own doctor appointments.	☐	☐	☐
Before a visit, I think about questions to ask.	☐	☐	☐
I have a way to get to my doctor's office.	☐	☐	☐
I know to show up 15 minutes before the visit to check in.	☐	☐	☐
I know where to go to get medical care when the doctor's office is closed.	☐	☐	☐
I have a file at home for my medical information.	☐	☐	☐
I have a copy of my current plan of care.	☐	☐	☐
I know how to fill out medical forms.	☐	☐	☐
I know how to get referrals to other providers.	☐	☐	☐
I know where my pharmacy is and how to refill my medicines.	☐	☐	☐
I know where to get blood work or x-rays if my doctor orders them.	☐	☐	☐
I have a plan so I can keep my health insurance after 18 or older.	☐	☐	☐
My family and I have discussed my ability to make my own health care decisions at age 18.	☐	☐	☐

Figure 29.4 Six core elements of health-care transition: Sample transition readiness assessment for youth. (From Got Transition, Washington, DC, with permission.)

psychosocial needs of the patient into consideration and modify their transition timeline as appropriate.[3]

Research looking at predictive measures of transition success, defined as a smooth transfer of care without gaps, is limited. While multiple tools to measure transition readiness are available; none have predictive validity for transition success.[25] However, these tools may assist in the clinical setting as teams develop transition protocols and may help maximize the likelihood of successful transition by identifying where youth may need extra support. For example, the American College of Physicians published a transition tool set for providers to use for patients with physical and/or developmental disabilities, as well as for specific chronic illnesses, such as sickle cell disease, congenital heart disease, and diabetes, broken down by subspecialty.[26] This toolkit contains disease-/condition-specific tools developed by internal medicine subspecialties to assist physicians in transitioning young adults with chronic diseases/conditions into adult-care settings. Included in the tool set is a readiness assessment and clinical summary templates to be completed by the referring provider and a self-care assessment to be filled out by the accepting provider to help assess gaps in medical knowledge or skill, as well as any additional issues that need to be addressed by the new medical team.[26] Instruments available assess patients' understanding of their medical conditions and ability to take responsibility for their care (take their medicines, keep appointments, etc.), as well as quantify patients' perceptions of importance to have ownership of their health-care decision-making.[26] Competency for self-care, issues of guardianship, insurance, and eligibility of services should also be addressed as part of the transition process for youth with special health-care needs.[1,21,22]

In a 2016 update to the 2011 Clinical Report, authors highlight the importance of developing infrastructure such as care coordination, lists of patient resources, and communication adult subspecialty providers able to care for young adults to better facilitate the transition process. Focus on building this infrastructure in adult facilities is particularly essential, as adult practices are more likely to lack this support than their pediatric counterparts. The updated report also highlights the need for education focusing on young adult heath, care of chronic conditions of pediatric onset, and transition readiness for medical providers and trainees. Educating patients and families about medical transition, as well as process of obtaining guardianship or power of attorney as needed, is also important. As transition programs grow, payment mechanisms to compensate clinicians for providing care and counseling around transition will need to be developed. Finally, the updated Report calls for continued research to further characterize best practices for facilitating transition and assessing transition outcomes.[17]

BARRIERS TO TRANSITION

Despite the importance of organized, continuous, and patient-centered transition to an adult medical home, analyzing the success of transition programs is difficult. Individual clinics and patients have unique needs and challenges, and evidence-based models for what defines a successful transition are lacking. Potential barriers to successful transition may include clinic issues such as visit time constraints, inadequate reimbursement, or deficit of adult providers with experience managing chronic disease of childhood into adulthood.[27,28] Patients with chronic illness who are not stable or require frequent hospitalizations are poor candidates for transition due to their acute illness. Barriers may also include patient discomfort with the adult health-care model, hesitancy to let go of pediatric providers with whom they have developed therapeutic relationships, or issues of adherence with medications and follow-up, which may indicate that the patient is having difficulty managing his or her health care on his or her own without the support of the pediatric-care model.[24] Patient readiness assessments have been developed, but

none have shown predictive validity for successful transition outcome.[6] More research is needed to develop transition readiness assessments that are able to consistently predict successful transition.

Patient race and socioeconomic status may also affect whether or not patients receive adequate transition counseling. The 2005 National Survey of Children with Special Health Care Needs found significant differences in transition counseling provided to racial and ethnic minority patients.[29] The survey asked parents or guardians of youth with special health-care needs ages 12–17 if they had received counseling from their child's provider about transition, adult versus pediatric care, insurance eligibility, and youth self-responsibility. While 56.7% of non-Hispanic white participants stated they had received this counseling, only 28.7% of black youth and 26.3% of Hispanic youth received this service, indicating that minority youth may be at higher risk of poor health outcomes due to lack of adequate transition counseling.[29]

While important guidelines and best practices for transition have been clearly outlined, proof of the effectiveness of these guidelines has not been extensively studied. One framework for assessing the success of transition is the "Triple Aim," a model developed by the Institute for Health Care Improvement to analyze the impact of the medical home model of care.[30,31] It was also adopted by the Department of Health and Human Services in the 2011 National Strategy for Quality Improvement in Health Care after the passage of the Affordable Care Act as a model for improving health-care access and quality.[32] The Triple Aim highlights three major goals of a successful transition: (1) improve experience of the individual patient with the health-care system; (2) improve the health of populations; and (3) reduce the cost per capita of health care.[33]

Evidence is lacking with regard to how best to build a transition program that meets the goals laid out in the Triple Aim model. Inconsistency in measuring outcomes makes it difficult to compare populations of youth.[33] Most current evidence examines only one of three Triple Aim goals and focuses on transition for youth with a specific illness; therefore, it is not generalizable. Implementing structured programs and processes is associated with improvement in population health, consumer experience, reported adherence, and service utilization.[34] Studies looking at cost of transition interventions have been inconclusive.[32] Outcome data are still lacking, given transition processes vary greatly depending on the individual being transitioned and his or her specific health profile. More research is needed to fully understand best practices for building a transition plan that remains generalizable while maximizing individual patient success.

YOUTH IN FOSTER CARE

Youth in foster care and young adults who have recently aged out of foster care often have complex health-care needs due to the adverse effects of neglect or abuse in childhood, as well as lack of consistent social and emotional support.[35] Youth who have been in foster care have higher rates of physical illness as well as increased incidence of mental health needs.[35] Furthermore, once adolescents age out of the foster care system, they are at further risk for poor health outcomes due to lack of social resources, such as housing, help managing insurance, and employment.[36] Therefore, health may suffer due to lack of access to and/or ability to afford appropriate services and medications.[36] Finally, youth who have experienced the foster care system have often been in multiple foster homes and have not experienced consistent relationships with adults during their youth.[37] Therefore, building a trusting relationship between the patient and provider is especially important when working with youth who have been in foster care. A smooth transition to an adult medical home with providers who have experience with the unique health needs of this population is particularly important in developing a strong partnership between the patient and the health-care system.[37]

CONCLUSION

All youth will go through transition in multiple aspects of their lives as they become adults, including in health care. Because of medical advances, almost all youth will reach adulthood and require adult-oriented health care. Providers should have a structured process to guide a smooth transition to an adult-care model to avoid gaps in care. Careful planning is especially important for youth with chronic conditions, mental illness, or other social determinants that put them at risk for health disparities. Many resources and best practice guidelines are available to guide practitioners to facilitate successful transition, which have been shown to impact quality of care and engagement. However, more research is needed to better understand how implementing these practices will affect health outcomes.

REFERENCES

1. Shaw TM, DeLast DE. Transition of adolescent to young adulthood for vulnerable populations. *Pediatr Rev.* 2010;31(12):497–505.
2. American Academy of Pediatrics, American Academy of Family Medicine, American College of Physicians et al. Clinical report: Supporting the health care transition from adolescence to adulthood in the medical home. *Pediatrics.* 2011;128(1):182–209.
3. Age limit of pediatrics. American Academy of Pediatrics policy statement. *Pediatrics.* 2017;140(3):1–3.
4. Tuchman LK, Schwartz LA, Sawicki GS et al. Cystic fibrosis and transition to adult medical care. *Pediatrics.* 2010;125(3):566–73.
5. Tepper V, Stefanie Z, Ryscavage P. HIV healthcare transition outcomes among youth in North America and Europe: A review. *JIAS.* 2017;20(3):60–70.
6. Schwarz LA, Daniel LC, Brumly LD, Barakat LP, Wesley KM, Tuchman LK. Measures of readiness to transition to adult health care for youth with chronic physical health conditions: A systematic review and recommendations for measuring testing and development. *J Pediatr Psychol.* 2014;39(6):588–601.

7. Got Transition. Integrating young adults into adult health care. Six core elements of heath care transition 2.0. https://www.gottransition.org/resourceGet.cfm?id=220. Accessed June 3, 2019.
8. Tuchman LK, Slap GB, Britto MT. Transition to adult care: Experiences and expectations of adolescents with a chronic illness. *Child Care Health Dev.* 2008;34(5):557–63.
9. McPherson M, Arango P, Fox H et al. A new definition of children with special health care needs. *Pediatrics.* 1998;102:137–40.
10. McPheeters M, Davis AM, Taylor JL et al. Agency for Healthcare Research and Quality. Effective Health Care Program Technical Brief Number 15. Transition care for children with special health needs; 2014.
11. McManus MA, Pollack LR, Cooley WC et al. Current status of transition preparation among youth with special health care needs in the United States. *Pediatrics.* 2013;131(6):1090–7.
12. Lemke M, Kappel R, McCarter R, D'Angelo L, Tuchman LK. Perceptions of health care transition care coordination in patients with chronic illness. *Pediatrics.* 2018;141(5):e20173168.
13. McManus M, White P. Transition to adult health care services for young adults with chronic medical illness and psychiatric comorbidity. *Child Adolesc Psychiatr Clin N Am.* 2017;26(2):367–80.
14. Sawicki GS, Garvey KC, Toomey SL et al. Transition to adult care among Medicaid-insured adolescents. *Pediatrics.* 2017;140(1):e20162768.
15. Syverson EP, McCarter R, He J et al. Adolescents' perceptions of transition importance, readiness, and likelihood of future success. *Clinical Pediatrics.* 2016;55(11):1020–5.
16. Dwyer-Matzky K, Blatt A, Asselin B, Wood DL. Lack of preparedness for pediatric to adult-oriented health care transition in hospitalized adolescents and young adults. *Acad Pediatr.* 2018;18(1):102–10.
17. White PH, Cooley WC. Transition Report Authoring Group, American Academy of Pediatrics, American Academy of Family Physicians, American College of Physicians. Supporting the health care transition from adolescence to adulthood in the medical home. *Pediatrics.* 2018;42(5):1–20.
18. Ginsburg KR. The SSHADESS Screen: A strength based psychosocial assessment. In Ginsburg KR, Sara B, Kinsman SB, eds. *Reaching Teens: Strength-Based Communication Strategies to Build Resilience and Support Healthy Adolescent Development.* Elk Grove Village, IL: American Academy of Pediatrics; 2014:139–43.
19. The transition from pediatric to adult health care: preventive care for young women aged 18–26 years. Committee Opinion No. 626. American College of Obstetricians and Gynecologists. *Obstet Gynecol* 2015; 125:752–4.
20. Got Transition. The six core elements of health care transition. http://www.gottransition.org/resources/index.cfm##six. Accessed June 3, 2019.

21. Okumura MJ, Hersh AO, Hilton JF et al. Change in health status and access to care in young adults with special health care needs: Results from the 2007 national survey of adult transition and health. *J Adolesc Health*. 2013;52:413–8.

22. Harden AP, Hackell JM, Committee of Practice and Ambulatory Medicine. American Academy of Pediatrics Policy Statement: Age limit of pediatrics. *Pediatrics*. 2017;140(3):1–3.

23. Bloom SR, Kuhlthau K, Van Cleave J et al. Health care transition for youth with special health care needs. *J Adolescent Health*. 2012;51:213–9.

24. Dowshen N, D'Angelo L. Health care transition for youth living with HIV/AIDs. *Pediatrics*. 2011;128(4):762–70.

25. Schwartz LA, Daniel LC, Brumley LD et al. Measures of readiness to transition to adult health care for youth with chronic physical conditions: A systemic review and recommendations for measurement testing and development. *J Pediatr Psychol*. 2104;39(6):588–601.

26. Pediatric to Adult Care Transition Initiative. The American College of Physicians. https://www.acponline.org/clinical-information/high-value-care/resources-for-clinicians/pediatric-to-adult-care-transitions-initiative

27. AAP Department of Research. Research update: Survey: Transition services lacking for teens with special needs. *AAP News*. 2009;30(11).

28. Peter NG, Forke C, Ginsburg KR et al. Transition from pediatric to adult care: Internists' perspective. *Pediatrics*. 2009;123(2):417–23.

29. Lotstein DS, Kuo AA, Strickland B et al. The transition to adult health care for youth with special health care needs: Do racial and ethnic disparities exist? *Pediatrics* 2010; 126(Suppl 3): S129–36.

30. Berwick DM, Nolan W, Whittington J. The triple aim: Care, health, and cost. *Health Aff (Millwood)*. 2008;27(3):759–69.

31. Peikes D, Zutshi A, Genervo J et al. *Early Evidence on the Patient-Centered Medical Home*. Princeton, NJ: Mathematica Policy Research; 2012.

32. US Department of Health and Human Services. *Report to Congress National Strategy for Quality Improvement in Health Care*. Rockville, MD: AHRQ; March 2011.

33. Prior M, McManus M, White P et al. Measuring the "triple aim" in transition care: A systematic review. *Pediatrics*. 2014;134(6):e1648–61.

34. Gabriel P, McManus M, Rogers K et al. Outcome evidence for structured pediatric to adult health care transition interventions: A systemic review. *J Pediatr*. 2017;118:263–9.

35. Ahrens KR, Garrison MM, Courtney ME. Health outcomes in young adults from foster care and economically diverse backgrounds. *Pediatrics*. 2014;134(6):1067–74.

36. Collins JL. Integrative review: Delivery of healthcare services to adolescents and young adults during and after foster care. *J Pediatr Nurs*. 2016;31:653–66.

37. Lopez P, Allen PJ. Addressing the health needs of adolescents transitioning out of foster care. *Pediatr Nurs*. 2007;33(4):345–55.

Legal considerations in pediatric and adolescent obstetrics and gynecology

30

STEVEN R. SMITH

INTRODUCTION

Health-care providers caring for the gynecologic and obstetric needs of adolescents and young adults face some of the thorniest legal issues in all of medicine. (We use the common legal word "minors" to refer to such patients.) With minor patients, gynecologic practice often involves difficult emotional, controversial, and unresolved questions of our society. The law reflects both the passion and ambiguity of these questions.[1]

Despite the complexity of the legal issues involved in treating minor patients, it is critical that clinicians understand the basic rights of their patients, parents, and others associated with care. This chapter discusses questions of consent to treatment, child abuse, and other required reporting. It also considers the conflicting obligations gynecologists have, both to minor patients and their parents, and, in some cases, to society. Legal issues related to confidentiality will be considered in less detail because of the specific consideration of that subject and an extensive list of resources in Chapter 27.

What is the law

One reason that discussing the law affecting minors and health care is complicated is that there is no such thing as "The Law." This is true for several reasons. First, state law has traditionally governed the regulation of medical care, the definition of the legal rights of minors, and the relationships between parents and minors. State law still plays the dominant role in defining and regulating the provision of medical care to minors, although federal law has become increasingly important. Laws in areas of adolescent rights and health care vary somewhat among the states. There are many common points in legal principles from one state to another—and we particularly focus on areas of common agreement. In some important ways, however, the differences among states can be quite significant—an example is the rules related to minors receiving abortion services.[2]

A second reason for the complexity in the law is the federal system in America. The federal government has legal authority that usually (but not always) trumps state law. The Constitution of the United States limits what states can do, an example being the limitation on the ability of states to prohibit abortion[3] or same-sex marriage.[4] The federal government, however, is also subject to constitutional limitations, so not every effort to control what states do is successful, as was the case when the federal government sought to require states to expand Medicaid as part of the Affordable Care Act.[5]

The third thing that makes it difficult to know what the law "is," is the multiplicity of sources of law, at the federal, state, and local levels. There are constitutions, statutes (or ordinances) passed by legislative bodies, regulations of various sorts adopted by administrative agencies, and decisions of courts throughout the country. Often the work of these bodies is ambiguous, inconsistent, or collectively does not address a legal question. And (except for the constitutions) these sources of law are changing frequently. It is sometimes not at all clear what the law actually is. This is, for example, sometimes because of ambiguity in the language of statutes or regulations and sometimes because it is not clear how various parts of the law (regulations and court decisions, for instance) will interact. For these reasons, the "practice of law" (like the practice of medicine) is often not an exact science but one involving judgment.

Federal statutes have directly or indirectly (notably through federal funding requirements) increasingly influenced medical practice.[7] Federal court decisions regarding the constitutional rights of minors are examples of federal rules that have generally changed the law affecting the rights of adolescents. While this trend is clear, state laws are still dominant in many areas of health care.

THE FUNDAMENTAL RIGHTS OF CHILDREN AND PARENTS

General rules of parents and children

Under traditional common law, children were virtually the property of their parents and were completely subject to parental decisions, direction, and discipline.[6] Throughout much of the last hundred years, however, the concept of parental ownership and control of children increasingly has weakened.[7] As a matter of statutory and constitutional law, parents still have wide latitude in raising their children.[77] However, minors have increasingly been recognized as separate legal entities with their own rights and interests.[8] As a result, the relative authority of parents and their children, especially older adolescent children, in making medical decisions is in flux and often uncertain.[9]

Children traditionally have been protected from their own immature judgment by their limited ability both to enter into contracts (except for necessities) and to consent to medical care (except under very limited circumstances).[10] The law generally considered minors to be incapable of making binding legal decisions until the age of majority. State law defines the age of majority, and most states now use 18 for general decision-making capacity.[11]

Emancipated minors and mature minors

There have been some well-recognized exceptions to minors' inability to make legally binding decisions. The most common is the "emancipated minors" rule.[12] Emancipated minors may make legally binding decisions, because they are viewed as formally free of the control and responsibility of their parents. This is usually as a result of marriage, military service, or (in some states) economic independence coupled with parental approval.[13] Most states also have recognized that "mature minors" may make legally binding decisions.[14] The concept of the mature minor generally refers to those who are able to understand and make complex decisions even though they have not reached the age of majority.[15]

Legal trends in recent decades

The legal tendency during the last three decades, consistent with studies of the decision-making ability of older minors, has been to give minors the legal authority to make legally binding decisions at an earlier age.[16] This is not an uninterrupted trend, however, and in some places the trend has been reversed for a while, leading to somewhat expanded parental control over fundamental decisions for adolescents under 18.[17] Special rules also have been applied to substance abuse treatment—generally allowing expanding authority for minors to seek treatment for substance abuse.[18]

An especially helpful state-by-state review of minor's consent laws is contained as part of the Guttmacher Institute website. It has specific consent reports dealing with minors' access to contraception, abortion, sexually transmitted infections (STIs) care, and prenatal care. It also has a comprehensive report covering all of these topics.[19] These reports are updated frequently.

THE LAW OF INFORMED CONSENT

Medical care may ordinarily be provided only if the patient (or someone legally authorized to act for the patient—a parent, for example) has given consent.[20] Consent to treatment is part of the general right of autonomy, the right of all adults to decide for themselves what will be done to their bodies. When the treatment is important or risky—surgery or invasive testing, for example—the patient must be informed of the risks and benefits and of alternative treatments and their consequences. That is, the patient must give "informed consent"[21] (Table 30.1).

Although informed consent is a general requirement of medical treatment, there are a few, limited exceptions—the most important being the "emergency exception." Emergency care generally can be provided to minors without parental consent, and lifesaving care may be undertaken on the intervention of state social service agencies or courts.[22]

Parents must generally consent to treatment for their unemancipated children. Some modifications of these general rules have been recognized, however, for adolescent obstetric and gynecologic care.[23] These have been made by statute in some states and by federal court decisions.[24] Virtually all states allow adolescents to consent to some kinds of gynecologic care, most often for treatment for STIs and commonly (but not universally) for pregnancy and contraception.[25] Several states, as part of the increased concern over child abuse, expressly allow the victims of abuse to consent to treatment for the sequela of abuse. Other changes in federal and state law have permitted adolescents to seek treatment without parental consent for drug or alcohol dependence. Many states have limited the scope of these minor consent laws so that they do not apply to abortion.[26]

By way of examples of the variations of state laws regarding kinds of care and consent, all states (and DC) allow minors to consent to STI services. Twenty-six states (and DC) allow all minors (who are at least 12 years old) to consent to contraceptive services, while 20 allow only some categories of minors to consent, and four states have no law on the subject. Most restrictive are the laws regarding consent to abortion. Two states (and DC) allow minors to consent to abortion services; 21 states require the consent of at least one parent, but some other states have notification provisions to be discussed subsequently. In addition, six states have parental involvement statutes (involving minors seeking abortion) that have been enjoined by the courts, and five other states have no policy or case law on the subject.[19] These laws also raise complex confidentiality-notification issues, as we discuss.

Most often the consent questions arise in the context of whether a minor may consent to treatment without the

Table 30.1 The general principles of informed consent.

Element of informed consent	Nature of the obligation
Nature of the proposed "procedure" (may include other intervention)	The practitioner provides an overview of the procedure that is proposed in ways the patient (or the patient's surrogate) can understand. This may include a procedure or an intervention such as pharmaceuticals.
Risks and benefits	The significant risks are generally measured by a combination of the probability of an event happening and how serious the consequences would be (loss of the use of a limb versus a rash, for example). This element is usually the most likely to cause difficulties and deserves careful attention.
Alternatives	The viable alternatives to the proposed treatment should be discussed with the patient.
Consequences of doing nothing	Where rejection of a proposed procedure (or an alternative) carries a risk of harm, that risk should be explained.

Table 30.2 Permutations of consent/involvement.

	Consents	Refuses consent	Not involved/ does not decide
AA	AA agrees	AA refuses	AA cannot or will not decide
Mother	AA and mother agree	AA and mother refuse	AA and mother cannot or will decide
Father	AA, mother, and father agree	AA, mother, and father refuse	AA, mother, and father cannot or will not decide

additional consent of her parents.[27] In some cases, it is even more complicated. For example, may treatment be provided over the minor's objection?[78] The complexity that can occur with consent to the treatment of adolescents is illustrated in the example of Patient AA, a 16-year-old, who is brought to the office by her mother for a complaint that ordinarily would call for a gynecologic examination. In the examining room, AA tells the nurse she does not want the exam, essentially refusing the examination to which her mother has given consent. There are several permutations of consent/involvement that can occur, as illustrated in Table 30.2.

To make this case even more complex, the parents of AA could disagree about the desirability of her receiving the examination.

In this case where the father is not involved, at least three legal issues face the health-care provider: (1) whether AA can withdraw the consent that her mother gave, (2) whether the provider can or must tell the mother about this, and (3) whether the provider physician has additional "informed consent" obligations. In light of AA's age, absent a meaningful medical issue requiring the examination, it is likely that she can refuse this examination, but her mother should be informed of the refusal. Furthermore, the provider will have the additional obligation of informed consent to tell AA of the health risks of refusing the examination. If, for example, an STI is a possibility, AA must be informed of the risks of not being tested or leaving the disease untreated.[22]

It is also important to note that although consent is a legal requirement, it also presents excellent opportunities for communication with patients and their parents. For example, the provider may want to consider why AA does not want the examination and what medical importance that may have. Furthermore, it is an opportunity to discuss the continuing importance of such examinations.

REPORTING ABUSE AND NEGLECT

All states require that physicians report child abuse or neglect. The statutes vary somewhat from state to state, but they usually have broad definitions of reportable events. Often "known" or "suspected" abuse or neglect must be reported. Abuse includes physical, sexual, or emotional abuse.[28] Sexual abuse usually includes sexual assault or molestation, sexual exploitation, and human trafficking or prostitution.[29]

Child abuse reporting statutes are mandatory. Failure to report known or suspected abuse, neglect, or sexual exploitation is a criminal offense in most states and may also give rise to civil liability. States generally provide immunity, however, against liability for those who in good faith report cases of suspected child abuse.[30]

Difficult questions of reporting arise when a patient seeks medical attention but has probably been abused. Consider a 12-year-old patient who is pregnant. Almost by definition, she has been the subject of statutory rape (sexual contact with someone under the age of legally recognized consent).[31] Theoretically, this might trigger the reporting requirement, but a provider (or the provider's attorney) can determine the necessity of reporting only by carefully examining the state statutes and related regulations and court decisions.[32]

Every health-care organization and practitioner should have in place a routine system for reporting known or suspected abuse.

LAWS REGARDING DISCLOSURE AND CONFIDENTIALITY

Patient confidentiality is among the most important and enduring values of medicine.[33] Maintaining confidentiality is an ordinary part of the physician–patient relationship. The law provides substantial protection of that value through physician licensing, potential malpractice liability, state and federal regulations, the Health Insurance Portability and Accountability Act (HIPAA) and the Health Information Technology for Economic and Clinical Health (HITECH) Act.[34] Chapter 27 explains these concepts in detail, so here we only highlight select legal issues.

Special problems regarding disclosure to parents are common in treating minors and are worth emphasizing.[79] As a general rule of thumb, absent a statute requiring disclosure, if a minor can legally consent to a medical procedure or may receive it without the consent of parents, parents usually do not have the right to have the minor's health information. (Like all rules of thumb, this one is generally, but not universally, true.) In addition, if the parent has agreed to confidentiality between the doctor and child, the parent has probably given up the right to access the information.[35] Both HIV testing and the more recent human papillomavirus vaccination have demonstrated the risks of breaches of confidentiality to important medical treatment for minors.[36]

The terms "disclosure" or "provide information" to parents may have several meanings. The first question is whether disclosure is "permissive" or "mandated." A permissive statute makes it clear that in some circumstances (e.g., "in the best interest of the minor"),[37] the health-care provider *may*, but is not required to, provide the information to the parents or others. If it is "mandated," then the provider must provide the information to the parents, absent a specific exception in the statute or one created by regulation or the courts.

A second basic disclosure question is whether it is "reactive" or "proactive." Reactive means that should the parents contact the physician and request information, it must be provided. Proactive means that the physician must reach out to the parent(s) with the information. Proactive is required, for example, where the rule says that "as part of providing this service, the parents must be notified." Some states, as we see, have such a requirement for abortion services.

Having an understanding of the disclosure laws regarding the services provided is essential for any provider. Several principles can help in the everyday application of the laws:

- It is important that minor patients (and to the extent possible, their families) have a clear understanding of, and reasonable expectations concerning, the protection of confidentiality during the course of treatment.[38] The minor patient especially should know ahead of time how confidential her medical information will be. Where it is practical, families should have a sense of the physician's intention. For example, compare, "In my medical practice I have found that the confidentiality of patients is important to successful treatment, so my policy has been to avoid disclosing patient information, except where required by the ethical principles, the law, or good medical practice," with, "In my practice, I feel that the family is an integral part of all treatment, so I generally share with the family all of the information about treatment, except where prohibited by the law or extraordinary circumstances." Those create very different expectations.[39]
- Where the treatment involves issues of sexuality or substance abuse, an understanding of the limits of confidentiality is especially important.
- The initial presumption should be against disclosure without careful thought. It is possible to disclose information later but impossible to "undisclose" things.
- It is important to find out who really has the right to information. Minors seeking treatment may come from single-parent homes in which one parent may not have custody rights. In such cases, that parent probably does not have a right to the medical information about his or her child, and it may be a violation of the law to provide the information.[13]
- The possibility of parental abuse warrants caution in some cases. If the disclosure would harm the child, it is almost never required. But if abuse is found or suspected, it probably has to be reported to a state agency.
- Electronic health records pose additional problems of maintaining confidentiality—a topic covered extensively in Chapter 27.[40]
- The disclosure of a minor's information to parents, or to a state abuse reporting agency, is not a waiver of confidentiality. It is a limited disclosure only. The minor, and her family, retains an interest in the privacy of the information, and the physician has the obligation to continue to protect the general confidentiality of the patient's information.

SPECIAL LEGAL ISSUES IN OBSTETRICS AND GYNECOLOGY CARE FOR MINORS

Sexually transmitted infections

Patient BB (age 15) arrives in your office seeking treatment for an STI and asking for assurance of complete confidentiality. All states permit physicians to provide treatment for the STI and to give related advice with the minor's consent (not the parents'). Eighteen states allow, *but do not require*, a physician to provide parental notification if such notification is in the best interest of the minor. Physicians must remember, however, that *informed* consent is still required and must include reasonable information about the benefits and risks of the proposed treatment and about alternatives.[41]

Confidentiality cannot be absolute, however. States require physicians to make a report to the state about the diagnosis of STIs by informing the department of health of basic information about the disease. The reports generally are mandatory. In addition, questions regarding reimbursement for the treatment (including pharmaceuticals) will likely require the release of pertinent information. This may be a special concern where a claim is made through the parents' insurance.

Contraception

During the office visit, BB also asks for contraceptives—again asking for confidentiality. Whether you can provide for contraceptives, and do so without any parental notification, depends on the state.[42,43] A few states limit the right of minors to consent to contraceptive services (e.g., to those married, or previously pregnant).[44] In addition to state law, there is a constitutional right of adolescents involved. In *Carey v. Population Services*, the U.S. Supreme Court held that the right of privacy includes the right of minors to have access to some contraceptives.[45] It struck down a New York statute that limited access by minors younger than 16, holding that a state cannot completely prohibit the use or availability of nonprescription contraceptives to minors. Thus, even in states without a specific statute allowing minors to consent to contraceptive services, there is some constitutional protection for obtaining the services.

Sterilization

Unlike contraception, permanent sterilization of competent minors is disfavored, and ordinarily a minor (or even her parents) would not be able to consent to it without a strong health justification. Sterilization is sometimes sought because minors with a serious intellectual disability are unable to understand their own sexuality and the consequences of sexual contacts. They would be unable to care for any children they might bear.[46] There is, of course, a very sad history of the use of eugenic sterilization in the United States. For good reason, therefore, courts currently permit sterilization only in very limited cases after a process to determine that such a step is justified. Courts are reluctant to remove the fundamental right to procreation and are concerned about the potential for abuse.

Pregnancy

Most states expressly allow minors to consent to prenatal care, and almost all, by implication, probably allow such consent.[47] In a few states, parents of the soon-to-be mother may be notified, but that is generally not required.[48]

Abortion

It probably comes as no surprise that abortion is a legal and political tempest.[49] As we noted earlier, two states and DC allow minors to consent to abortion. Among the 37 states that require parental involvement, 26 require parental consent, and the other 11 require parental notification.[50] It is clear that state statutes are not the end of the story.

The Supreme Court has required that states recognize the right of minors to have some access to abortion services.[51] In *Planned Parenthood v. Danforth*, the Supreme Court held that the right of privacy to decide to have an abortion extends to minors. A state, therefore, does not have the constitutional authority to delegate to parents the decision of a "competent and mature minor" to have an abortion.[52] The Court held unconstitutional an ordinance that provided that all minors younger than 15 years old were too immature to make abortion decisions,[53] but in *Planned Parenthood Association of Kansas City v. Ashcroft*, the Court upheld a state statute requiring all minors to obtain either parental or judicial consent for an abortion.[54] In a judicial bypass process, a minor goes to state court to seek permission (without parental consent) to have an abortion.[55] These courts are *required* to give consent to the abortion if the minor is mature enough to make the decision or if the abortion is in her best interest.

The judicial bypass exception is so complicated that it is unlikely that most minors would be able to negotiate it by themselves. In some areas of the country, there are organizations that will assist adolescents with the bypass procedures, and minor patients may know of these from their friends. Physicians treating minors who may need or want to have an abortion, however, should determine whether a parental consent or notification statute exists and whether they are permitted to assist the minor in completing the bypass.[56] Several studies suggest that courts overwhelmingly approve abortions when application is made through the bypass process, but the adolescent patient is likely to need assistance in going through the court process.[57,58]

In terms of informed consent, the Supreme Court has upheld state laws that require graphic informed consent.[59] This includes information about the development of the fetus. A number of states have adopted such laws.[60]

The Court has held that states may regulate aspects of abortion but may not do so in a way that "unduly burdens" the right to have an abortion. Applying this principle, in 2016 the Court struck down Texas laws requiring medical facilities and arrangements that did not in fact meaningfully contribute to the safety of abortions.[61]

Most states require parental notification, and about half the states require parental consent (in both cases subject to a judicial bypass).[50] In *Ohio v. Center for Reproductive Health*[62] and *Hodgson v. Minnesota*,[63] the Court held that a state may constitutionally require the notification of one or even both parents when a minor seeks an abortion as long as the state also provides for a "judicial bypass." In jurisdictions requiring parental notification for certain types of obstetric and gynecologic care, the practitioner

should inform minors at the beginning of treatment of this reporting requirement. This is another area where significant changes may occur in the future, so particularly careful monitoring of changes in federal, state, and local law is important.

Abortion is fraught with political, religious, and social concerns that play out in the laws. The statutes change frequently, and in some states there are ongoing cat and mouse struggles between state lawmakers and federal courts. This all makes for a very difficult legal landscape for practitioners (Table 30.3).

RESEARCH INVOLVING CHILDREN

Special legal and ethical issues arise when children are engaged in research studies. This section briefly reviews a few issues, primarily federal regulations. In addition, a number of states have laws directly or indirectly regulating research involving children. At the end of this section, we note some legal issues involving "near research." "Children" is used in this section (rather than "minors"), because that is the term used in the federal regulations. The definition of children essentially looks to the state law of consent. That is, a child in the federal regulations is someone who is not of legal age to consent to the procedures involved in the research.[65]

Federal law defines research broadly—as "a systematic investigation...designed to develop or contribute to generalizable knowledge."[66] Almost any research funded by the federal government is subject to regulation under the "Common Rule" regarding human subjects, established by the Department of Health and Human Services (HHS).[67] In addition, many foundations, other sponsors, publishers, and institutions (universities and teaching hospitals) require that research comply with the same rules. The U.S. Food and Drug Administration has similar rules regarding research related to pharmaceuticals and devices.[68] The Common Rule was under review for several years. In January 2019, revisions to the rule (known as the "Common Rule 2018") became effective.[80] In addition to the regulations regarding the use of children as research subjects (discussed next), the Common Rule has specific regulations regarding the use of pregnant women, human fetuses, and neonates in research.[81]

Any practitioner who is involved in a research project should contact the sponsor, principal investigators, and institutions in which the research will be done to determine that the research has been approved by the Institutional Review Board (IRB), what the obligations of the practitioner will be in protecting the child and her parents, the rules regarding obtaining consent and assent, and the procedures involved in reporting adverse events. There may be potential professional and legal problems in undertaking unapproved research. Seeking "forgiveness rather than permission" is not a good strategy when using children in research. The institution's IRB staff can be invaluable in advising researchers and answering questions. Because children are a vulnerable population, their participation in research can be especially complex.[69]

Table 30.3 Summary of the legal principles.

Legal principle	Explanation
The law varies from state to state and may change quickly.	The result is that definitive and permanent answers about treating pediatric and adolescent patients (minors) are usually not possible.
Diagnosis and treatment can be undertaken only with consent.	For minors, parents ordinarily have the legal authority to give consent to treatment. Where minors have the right to consent themselves, the rules of *informed* consent still apply.
"Informed consent" requires that the patient or decision-maker be given sufficient information on which to base a sensible decision.	This generally includes a description of the treatment or procedure proposed, its costs and benefits, alternatives, and the consequences of refusing treatment. The informed consent process is an excellent opportunity for communication with patients.
There are exceptions to parental consent rules for some minors or for some kinds of health care.	"Emancipated minors" may generally make decisions for themselves.[64] "Mature minors" in most states may make certain basic decisions for treatment related to pregnancy, contraception (not including sterilization), sexually transmitted diseases, and the like.
Where there is disagreement between a minor patient and parents regarding care, or between parents of a minor patient, the law in practice often becomes murky.	Where the life or health of a minor is at stake, the bias should be toward providing emergency or necessary treatment. A health-care provider should be prepared for these disagreements by establishing (generally with the assistance of an attorney) good practices for dealing with the problem when it arises.
Physicians have a general obligation to protect patient confidentiality.	Parents generally, but not always, have a right to information about their minor children. State and federal laws, including the Health Insurance Portability and Accountability Act, are further limiting the release of confidential medical information. Where there is doubt about the propriety of releasing information to parents, it is generally better to be conservative under the theory that it is difficult to retract information improperly released.
Many states have laws permitting providers to withhold some kinds of sensitive information from parents.	This information generally includes information about sexually transmitted infections, contraception, and pregnancy. These rules vary from state to state, however.
Laws regarding consent to abortions and parental notification are complex.	It is common for states to require parental consent or a "judicial bypass" for a minor to obtain an abortion. Parental notification laws (regarding abortion) are common, but there may well be judicially described exceptions to these laws.
All states require the reporting of child abuse.	There can be legal consequences for failure to report, including civil liability and even criminal liability. In addition, there may be licensing consequences. Such liability is uncommon but possible. It is essential to know what the reporting requirements are and to have a system to ensure that reports are actually made.

Table 30.4 is an overview of the mix of risks, direct benefits to the child, importance to generalized knowledge, and permission–assent that are contained in the federal regulations regarding children.

In addition, in each of these categories, the research must provide for the following:

1. Permission of the parent or guardian for the child to participate.
2. "Assent" of the child (meaning that if capable, the child must express a willingness to participate).[74]

Valuable additional guidance regarding adolescents in research and when parental permission may be waived is available from the American College of Obstetricians and Gynecologists.[75]

In addition to the regulation of formal research, "near research" (new techniques and approaches that are innovative but not in standard or common use) also may raise legal issues. If these do not involve pharmaceuticals or devices, they are often not regulated. They may be used but require caution and generally a special informed consent that calls attention to the option of standard (versus the innovative, nonstandard) care.[76]

PRACTICAL ADVICE

By way of conclusion, there are several practical tips that those treating pediatric and adolescent patients should consider to avoid unnecessary problems and complications:

- Establish an ongoing relationship with an attorney you trust. Ask the attorney to help you understand the legal requirements in your state, and seek help establishing procedures and practices that will help you comply with legal requirements. Do not hesitate to contact the attorney as questions or problems arise in practice.
- Have annual "checkups." (You should take the advice you give patients.) Your attorney should help you do

Table 30.4 Federal regulations associated with research in children.

Risk	Direct benefits to the child	Review required	Other considerations
1. Minimal risk[70]	None required	May be approved by the Institutional Review Board (IRB)	
2. Minor increase in risk over "minimal risk"; intervention is similar to those inherent in everyday medical situations[71]	None required, but likely to yield generalizable knowledge about the child's disorder that is vital to understanding the condition generally	May be approved by the IRB	Risk is justified by benefits to the subjects, and the risk–benefit ratio is at least as favorable as alternative approaches
3. Greater than minimal risk[72]	Direct benefit to the child must exist	May be approved by the IRB	Likely to yield "generalizable knowledge" about the child's condition, which is vitally important
4. Greater than minimal risk[73]	No direct benefit to the child	Must first be approved by the IRB and then submitted to the Department of Health and Human Services (HHS) for additional review	Reasonable opportunity to understand "serious problem" affecting children; research will be conducted with sound ethical principles

an annual review of your practice to make adjustments that respond to changes in the law.

- Understand the elements of informed consent in your state and who may give consent to what procedures involving minors.
- Understand the limits and obligations of confidentiality. Have a plan regarding disclosure to parents that meets the legal requirements and is consistent with HIPAA.
- Discuss confidentiality issues with patients, especially adolescent patients. They should generally understand the limits of confidentiality. Consider making agreements with parents regarding confidentiality, so that they agree in appropriate cases that you will not disclose information to them (parents can agree to give up the right to information).
- Take *informed* consent seriously. Use it as a way of communicating important information with patients and parents.
- If you are involved with abortions or sterilizations, be very clear on the legal requirements of your state.
- Have a system in place to report abuse and neglect.
- Maintain good records. Keep them honestly and accurately.

It is ultimately important to remember that the law is not a series of random rules. Rather, with all of its faults, it is an effort by society to implement the most important values and goals of society. Inevitably, there are conflicting values and compromises that produce changing and imperfect rules. Physicians, in cooperation with attorneys when needed, can work sensibly through these rules. The two professions, when they work together over time, can also improve the law to make it a better vehicle for achieving important values.

REFERENCES

1. Mutcherson KM. Whose body is it anyway? An updated model of healthcare decision-making rights for adolescents. *Cornell J Law Public Policy.* 2004–2005;14:251–325.
2. Vukadinovich DM. Minors' rights to consent to treatment: Navigating the complexity of state laws. *J Health Law.* 2004;37:667–91.
3. *Roe v. Wade,* 410 U.S. 113, 1973.
4. *Obergefell v. Hodges,* 576 U.S., 2015.
5. *National Federation of Independent Business v. Sebelius,* 567 U.S. 519, 2012.
6. Diaz A, Neal WP, Nucci AT et al. Legal and ethical issues facing adolescent health care professionals. *Mt Sinai J Med.* 2004;71:181–5.
7. Hill BJ. Constituting children's bodily integrity. *Duke LJ.* 2015;64:1295–362.
8. Rosato J. What are the implications of Roper's dilemma for adolescent health law symposium: Adolescents in society: Their evolving legal status: Essay. *JL & Pol'y.* 2011 2012;20:167–90.
9. Ewald LS. Medical decision making for children: An analysis of competing interests. *St Louis Univ Law J.* 1982;25:689–733.
10. Boldt Richard C., Henry LM. Medical decision making by and on behalf of adolescents: Reconsidering first principles. *J Health Care L & Pol'y.* 2012;15:37–73.
11. Newman A. Adolescent consent to routine medical and surgical treatment: A proposal to simplify the law of teenage medical decision-making. *J Leg Med.* 2001;22:501–32.
12. Lane S, Kohlenberg E. Emancipated minors: Health policy and implications for nursing. *J Pediatr Nurs.*

2012;27(5):533–48. https://www.pediatricnursing.org/article/S0882-5963(11)00540-9/pdf.

13. Cohen LT, Millock PJ, Asheld BA, Lane B. Minor patients: Consent to treatment and access to medical records. *J Am Coll Radiol*. 2015;12(8):788–90.

14. Benston S. Not of minor consequence: Medical decision-making autonomy and the mature minor doctrine. *Indiana Health Law Rev*. 2016;13(1):1–6.

15. Partridge BC. The decisional capacity of the adolescent: An introduction to a critical reconsideration of the doctrine of the mature minor. *J Med Philos*. 2013;38(3):249–55.

16. Harris LJ. Teen health care decisions: How maturity and social policy affect four hard cases. In: *Studies in Law, Politics, and Society*. Vol. 72. Bingley, UK: Emerald Publishing; 2017:185–217. https://doi.org/10.1108/S1059-433720170000072006

17. Austin AW. Medical decisions and children: How much voice should children have in their medical care. *Arizona Law Rev*. 2007;49:143–69.

18. Boldt RC. Legal issues with respect to treatment for substance misuse and mental illness roundtable on adolescent decision making. *J Health Care L & Pol'y*. 2012;15:75–116.

19. Guttmacher Institute. *An Overview of Minors' Consent Law*. New York, NY: Guttmacher Institute; 2017. https://www.guttmacher.org/state-policy/explore/overview-minors-consent-law. Accessed October 3, 2017.

20. *Schloendorff v. Society of New York Hospital*, 105 N.E. 92, N.Y. 1914.

21. Katz AL, Webb SA, Committee on Bioethics. Informed consent in decision-making in pediatric practice. *Pediatrics*. 2016;138:e20161485. http://pediatrics.aappublications.org/content/early/2016/07/21/peds.2016-1485. Accessed October 4, 2017.

22. Rozovsky PA. *Consent to Treatment: A Practical Guide*. 4th ed. Boston, MA: Little, Brown; 2007.

23. English A. Reproductive health services for adolescents: Critical legal issues. *Adolesc Gynecol*. 2000;27:195–211.

24. Fanaroff JM, Committee on Medical Liability and Risk Management. Consent by proxy for nonurgent pediatric care. *Pediatrics*. 2017;139(2);e20163911. http://pediatrics.aappublications.org/content/early/2017/01/19/peds.2016-3911. Accessed October 4, 2017.

25. Tillett J. Adolescents and informed consent: Ethical and legal issues. *J Perinat Neonatal Nurs*. 2005;19(2):112–21.

26. Phillis N. When sixteen ain't so sweet: Rethinking the regulation of adolescent sexuality. *Mich J Gender & L*. 2010–2011;17:271–314.

27. Alderson P, Sutcliffe K, Curtis K. Children's competence to consent to medical treatment. *Hastings Cent Rep*. 2006;36(6):25–34.

28. Fox J. In the courts: A balancing act: The protection of child abuse victims and the rights of a defendant. *Child Legal Rts J*. 2015;35(3):250–2.

29. Chaffee T, English A. Sex trafficking of adolescents and young adults in the United States: Healthcare provider's role. *Curr Opin Obstet Gynecol*. 2015;27(5):339–44.

30. Culhane JG. Duty per se: Reading child abuse statutes to create a common law duty in favor of victims. *Widener Law Rev*. 2013;19(1):73–92. http://search.ebscohost.com/login.aspx?direct=true&db=lft&AN=87778739&site=ehost-live. Accessed October 1, 2017.

31. Cocca CE. *Jailbait: The Politics of Statutory Rape Laws in the United States*. Albany, NY: State University of New York Press; 2004.

32. Horton O. Mind the gap: Theorizing asymmetry between parental involvement and statutory rape laws notes. *Yale JL & Feminism*. 2016–2017;28:171–210.

33. Smith SR. Medical and psychotherapy privileges and confidentiality: On giving with one hand and removing with the other. *Ky Law J*. 1987;75:473–557.

34. U.S. Department of Health and Human Services. The HIPAA Privacy Rule; 2015. https://www.hhs.gov/hipaa/for-professionals/privacy/index.html. Accessed October 4, 2017.

35. Cullitan CM. Please don't tell my mom—A minor's right to informational privacy. *JL & Educ*. 2011;40:417–60.

36. Jackson S, Hafemeister TI. Impact of parental consent and notification policies on the decisions of adolescents to be tested for HIV. *J Adolesc Health*. 2001;29:81–93.

37. Cohen IG. Beyond best interests. *Minn L Rev*. 2011–2012;96:1187–274.

38. Ford CA, Millstein SG. Delivery of confidentiality assurances to adolescents by primary care physicians. *Arch Pediatr Adolesc Med*. 1997;151:505–9.

39. Blasdell J. Ramifications for parental involvement laws for minors seeking abortion services. *J Gender Social Policy Law*. 2002;10:287–304.

40. Spooner SA. Protecting privacy in the child health EHR. In: *Pediatric Biomedical Informatics*. Singapore: Springer; 2016:27–36. (Translational Bioinformatics.) https://link.springer.com/chapter/10.1007/978-981-10-1104-7_2. Accessed September 30, 2017.

41. Tillett J. Legal issues in adolescent care. *Nurse Practitioner*. 2011;36(9):8–9. http://journals.lww.com/tnpj/Citation/2011/09000/Legal_issues_in_adolescent_care.3.aspx. Accessed September 30, 2017.

42. Jones RK, Boonstra H. Confidential reproductive health services for minors: The potential impact of mandated parental involvement for contraception. *Perspect Sex Reprod Health*. 2004;36:182–91.

43. Mulchahey KM. Practical approaches to prescribing contraception in the office setting. *Adolesc Med Clin*. 2005;16:665–74.

44. Guttmacher Institute. *Minors' Access to Contraceptive Services*. New York, NY: Guttmacher Institute; 2016. https://www.guttmacher.org/state-policy/explore/minors-access-contraceptive-services. Accessed October 4, 2017.

45. *Carey v. Population Services*, 431 US 678, 1977.
46. Dickema DS. Involuntary sterilization of persons with mental retardation: An ethical analysis. *Ment Retard Dev Disabil Res Rev*. 2003;9:21–6.
47. Mason JK. *Medico-Legal Aspects of Reproduction and Parenthood*. 2nd ed. New York, NY: Routledge; 2017:448.
48. Manian M. Minors, parents, and minor parents. *Mo L Rev*. 2016;81:127–204.
49. Butler JD, Walbert DF. *Abortion, Medicine, and the Law*. Martinsville, IN: Fideli Publishing; 2011:793.
50. Guttmacher Institute. *Parental Involvement in Minors' Abortions*. New York, NY: Guttmacher Institute; 2016. https://www.guttmacher.org/state-policy/explore/parental-involvement-minors-abortions. Accessed October 4, 2017.
51. Guggenheim M. Minor rights: The adolescent abortion cases. *Hofstra Law Rev*. 2001–2002;30:3.
52. *Planned Parenthood v. Danforth*, 428 U.S. 52, 1976.
53. *City of Akron v. Akron Center for Reproductive Health*, 462 U.S. 416, 1983.
54. *Planned Parenthood of Kansas City v. Ashcroft*, 462 US 476, 1983.
55. Bridges KM. An anthropological meditation on ex parte anonymous—A judicial bypass procedure for an adolescent's abortion. *California Law Rev*. 2006;94:215–42.
56. Council on Ethical and Judicial Affairs, American Medical Association. Mandatory parents: Consent to abortion. *JAMA*. 1993;269:82–6.
57. Treadwell L. Informal closing of the bypass: Minors' petitions to bypass parental consent for abortion in an age of increasing judicial recusals. *Hastings Law J*. 2007;58:869–90.
58. Vanderwalker I. Abortion and informed consent: How biased counseling laws mandate violations of medical ethics. *Mich J Gender & L*. 2012 2013;19:1–70.
59. *Planned Parenthood of Southeastern Pennsylvania v. Casey*, 505 U.S. 833, 1992.
60. Adler NE. Ozer EJ, Tschann J. Abortion among adolescents. *Am Psychol*. 2003;58:211–17.
61. *Whole Woman's Health v. Hellerstedt*, 579 U.S., 2016.
62. *Ohio v. Akron Center for Reproductive Health*, 497 U.S. 502, 1990.
63. *Hodgson v. Minnesota*, 497 U.S. 417, 1990.
64. Kolaitis IN, Frader JE. Informed consent: Pediatric patients, adolescents, and emancipated minors. In: *Ethical Issues in Anesthesiology and Surgery*. Basel, Switzerland: Springer International; 2015:1–6.
65. 45 CRF §46.402(a).
66. 45 CFR §46.102(d).
67. 45 CFR §46.
68. 21 CFR §50 Subpart D.
69. Field MJ, Behrman RE, Children I of M (US) C on CRI. *Understanding and Agreeing to Children's Participation in Clinical Research*. Washington, DC: National Academies Press; 2004. https://www.ncbi.nlm.nih.gov/books/NBK25560/. Accessed March 6, 2018.
70. 45 CFR §46.404.
71. 45 CFR §46.406.
72. 45 CFR §46.405.
73. 45 CFR §46.407.
74. Grady C, Wiener L, Abdoler E et al. Assent in research: The voices of adolescents. *J Adolesc Health*. 2014;54(5):515–20.
75. Guidelines for adolescent health research. Committee Opinion No. 665. American College of Obstetricians and Gynecologists. *Obstet Gynecol*. 2016;127:e183–6.
76. Sawicki NN. Choosing Malpractice: A New Narrative for Limiting Physician Liability. *SSRN*. https://papers.ssrn.com/sol3/papers.cfm?abstract_id=3037986. Accessed March 6, 2018.
77. Alderson P. Children's consent and the zone of parental discretion. *Clinical Ethics*. 2017;12(2):55–62.
78. Lang A, Paquette ET. Involving minors in medical decision making: Understanding ethical issues in assent and refusal of care by minors. *Semin Neurol*. 2018;38(5):533–38.
79. Alderman EM. Confidentiality in pediatric and adolescent gynecology: When we can, when we can't, and when we're challenged. *J PediatrAdol Gynec*. 2017;30(2):176–83.
80. U.S. Department of Health & Human Services, Office for Human Research Protections, Revised Common Rule; https://www.hhs.gov/ohrp/regulations-and-policy/regulations/finalized-revisions-common-rule/index.html (accessed April 19, 2019).
81. 45 CRF §§401-409, Part D, https://www.ecfr.gov/cgi-bin/retrieveECFR?gp=&SID=83cd09e1c0f5c6937cd9d7513160fc3f&pitd=20180719&n=pt45.1.46&r=PART&ty=HTML#sp45.1.46.b (accessed April 23, 2019).

Appendix 1: Additional video resources

Video A1.1	Vaginoscopy and hysteroscope *Mary Ann Jamieson and Amanda Black*	https://youtu.be/gHr8ldqQysM
Video A1.2	Laparoscopic gonadectomy *Sari Kives*	https://youtu.be/ez6hyyxMmtQ
Video A1.3	Laparoscopic management of ovarian torsion *Sari Kives*	https://youtu.be/PI7GdxNLCQA
Video A1.4	Vaginoscopy *Sari Kives*	https://youtu.be/Du9OsHcU1K4
Video A1.5	Lysis of labial adhesions *Elizabeth Quint*	https://youtu.be/rWug22WYitk
Video A1.6	Laparoscopic presacral neurectomy *Linda Yang and Suketu Mansuria*	https://youtu.be/2yUJIMRTK4A

Appendix 2: Establishing a pediatric and adolescent gynecology clinical and educational program

JOSEPH S. SANFILIPPO, EDUARDO LARA-TORRE, and VERONICA GOMEZ-LOBO

BACKGROUND

As pediatric and adolescent gynecology (PAG) is an important aspect of the health of youth, training requirements and licensing examinations for obstetrics and gynecology, pediatrics and adolescent medicine in North America have included PAG for many decades. More recently, the American Board of Obstetrics and Gynecology has further recognized the importance of this field through the introduction of PAG subject articles in the annual Maintenance of Certification (MOC) process as well as a special certification known as Focused Practice in PAG, introduced in October 2018 with its first written examination. Unfortunately, many hospitals and training programs do not have access to experts in the field. In recognition of the importance of providing this service, we provide an approach on establishing a clinical, educational, and academic program in PAG.

ESTABLISHING A PEDIATRIC AND ADOLESCENT GYNECOLOGY SERVICE

Many hospitals and departments are recognizing the importance of PAG, as noted by the number of sites that are recruiting experts in the field through the North American Society for Pediatric and Adolescent Gynecology (NASPAG).* Many sites provide PAG care through a gynecologist, pediatrician, family medicine provider, or adolescent medicine provider who develops an interest in addressing this sector of health care. These individuals can greatly increase their knowledge of the field through attendance at a NASPAG Annual Clinical and Research Meeting as well as through reading NASPAG's educational guidelines. Many of the current experts of the field have begun their programs in this manner. As the field has grown, it is important that the program can provide care or referral for care for the many subjects included in this textbook (Table A2.1).

RESIDENT EDUCATION IN PEDIATRIC AND ADOLESCENT GYNECOLOGY SERVICE

Learning objectives from the Council on Resident Education in Obstetrics and Gynecology in the United States, the American Board of Pediatrics, and the Royal College of Physicians and Surgeons of Canada include

requirements that educational programs train their physicians in PAG subjects.[1] Trainees, however, report receiving little training in this area.[1] In response to this need, the NASPAG Resident Education Committee has published a short[2,†] and a long curriculum[‡] to assist programs in educating their residents in our field. Dissemination of this curriculum through pediatrics, obstetrics and gynecology, and family practice residents was evaluated and noted improved self-evaluation of PAG knowledge in residents in all three fields.[3]

FELLOWSHIP EDUCATION

A number of 13 training programs in PAG[§] and 26 training programs in adolescent medicine.[¶] As Adolescent Medicine Programs have been established for a longer time and are accredited by the Accreditation Council for Graduate Medical Education (ACGME), educational requirements and structure have been well established. The PAG fellowships have been coordinating through NASPAG and currently have established educational guidelines.[**]

RESEARCH IN PEDIATRIC AND ADOLESCENT GYNECOLOGY

As PAG clinical and training programs are established, the need for evidence-based care has grown and requires research in this important field. In May 2016, the Gynecologic Health and Disease Branch (GHDB) of the Eunice Kennedy Shriver National Institute of Child Health and Human Development (NICHD) held a Scientific Vision Meeting. The cross-cutting theme of this meeting was "the need to stimulate study of the adolescent period in relation to the development of gynecologic conditions." In response to this recommendation, GHDB has worked with the Fertility and Infertility Branch to craft several Funding Opportunity Announcements.[††] Furthermore, in recognition that children and adolescents may respond differently

---

* https://www.naspag.org/general/custom.asp?page=jobsinpag; January 2019

† https://www.jpagonline.org/article/S1083-3188(17)30513-2/pdf
‡ https://www.naspag.org/page/EducatorTools
§ https://www.naspag.org/general/custom.asp?page=PAGFellowship
¶ https://www.adolescenthealth.org/getattachment/Training-and-CME/Fellowships-Training/Training-Opportunities-in-Adolescent-Medicine_2019-(3).pdf.aspx?lang=en-US
** See "Educational Goals and Training Objectives" on the Additional Resources tab at https://www.crcpress.com/Sanfilippos-Textbook-of-Pediatric-and-Adolescent-Gynecology-Second-Edition/Sanfilippo-Lara-Torre-Gomez-Lobo/p/book/9781138551572
†† https://www.nichd.nih.gov/about/org/der/branches/ghdb/programs

Table A2.1   Components of a Pediatric and Adolescent Gynecology Program.

Program components	Who can provide	Comments

Comprehensive adolescent care:
  Confidential services
  Contraception
  Prevention and treatment of sexually transmitted infections
  Puberty and menstruation counseling
  Sexuality counseling
  Care of disabled adolescents
	Adolescent Medicine, Gynecology, Pediatrics, Family Practice	May identify a Title X provider in the community for confidential contraceptive administration
		Social work support is ideal

Adolescent pregnancy management	Obstetrics, Family Medicine	Special program for adolescent pregnancy can provide resources for risk reduction, parenting, etc.

Endocrine conditions:
  Abnormal puberty
  Obesity
  PCOS
  Nutrition and eating disorders
	Adolescent Medicine, Gynecology, Endocrinology	Multidisciplinary care can greatly enhance diagnosis and care

Medical management of:
  Pelvic pain
  Heavy menstrual bleeding
	Gynecology, Adolescent Medicine	Collaboration with a comprehensive pain team will enhance care

Surgical and medical management of:
  Genital injuries
  Pelvic masses
  Congenital anomalies
	Gynecology, Pediatric Surgery, Pediatric Urology	

Transgender care	Adolescent Medicine, Endocrinology, Gynecology and Mental Health-Care Provider	Multidisciplinary care is required
Disorders of sex development	Endocrinology, Urology, Gynecology, Genetics, Mental Health-Care Provider	Multidisciplinary care is required
Dermatology and vulvar conditions	Gynecology, Dermatology, Pediatrics	
Fertility preservation	Gynecology, Urology, Oncology, Adolescent Medicine, Endocrinology, Reproductive Endocrinology	Develop a referral program ideally with a patient navigator for options not available such as sperm and oocyte cryopreservation
Child abuse	Child Abuse Pediatrician, Gynecology, Adolescent Medicine, Sexual Assault Nurse Examiner (SANE)	Encourage local jurisdiction to have a SANE program with a board-certified abuse expert

to medications, the Best Pharmaceuticals for Children Act (BPCA) was signed into law in 2002 to promote pharmaceutical studies in pediatric populations.[3] Children and adolescents, however, continue to be underrepresented in pharmaceutical research, which may be in part related to the federal regulations 45 C.F.R. § 46 and federal and state laws that affect research with minors. Given the importance of including children and adolescents in research, the American College of Obstetricians and Gynecologists as well as the Society for Adolescent Medicine have provided guidelines regarding these regulations.[4,5]

CONCLUSIONS

As the field of PAG continues to grow and develop, institutions will need to develop clinical, educational, and academic programs in PAG. There are many resources available to providers interested in the field, including

this textbook, the *Journal of Pediatric and Adolescent Gynecology*,* and many others that may be found on NASPAG's web page.†

REFERENCES

1. Wheeler C, Browner-Elhanan KJ, Evans Y, Fleming N, Huguelet PS, Karjane NW, Loveless M, Talib HJ, Kaul P. Creation and dissemination of a multispecialty graduate medical education curriculum in pediatric and adolescent gynecology: The North American Society for Pediatric and Adolescent Gynecology Resident Education Committee Experiences. *J Pediatr Adolesc Gynecol.* 2018;31:3–6.

* https://www.jpagonline.org
† https://www.naspag.org

2. Huguelet PS, ChelvaKumar G, Conner L et al. Improving resident knowledge in pediatric and adolescent gynecology: An evaluation of the North American Society for Pediatric and Adolescent Gynecology Short Curriculum. *J Pediatr Adolesc Gynecol*. 2018;31:356–61.

3. Bonny AE, Lange HL, Gomez-Lobo V. Hormonal contraceptive agents: A need for pediatric-specific studies. *Pediatrics*. 2015;135:4–6.

4. Guidelines for adolescent health research. Committee Opinion No. 665. American College of Obstetricians and Gynecologists. *Obstet Gynecol*. 2016;127:e183–6.

5. Santelli JS, Smith Rogers A, Rosenfeld WD et al. Guidelines for adolescent health research. A position paper of the Society for Adolescent Medicine. Society for Adolescent Medicine. *J Adolesc Health*. 2003;33:396–409.

Index

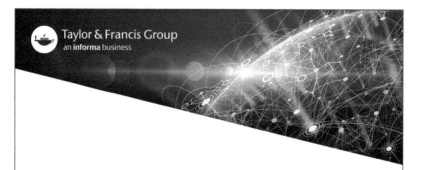

Accessing the E-book edition

Using the VitalSource® ebook

Access to the VitalBook™ ebook accompanying this book is via VitalSource® Bookshelf – an ebook reader which allows you to make and share notes and highlights on your ebooks and search across all of the ebooks that you hold on your VitalSource Bookshelf. You can access the ebook online or offline on your smartphone, tablet or PC/Mac and your notes and highlights will automatically stay in sync no matter where you make them.

1. **Create a VitalSource Bookshelf account at** *https://online.vitalsource.com/user/new* or log into your existing account if you already have one.

2. **Redeem the code provided in the panel below to get online access to the ebook.** Log in to Bookshelf and select **Redeem** at the top right of the screen. Enter the redemption code shown on the scratch-off panel below in the **Redeem Code** pop-up and press **Redeem**. Once the code has been redeemed your ebook will download and appear in your library.

No returns if this code has been revealed.

DOWNLOAD AND READ OFFLINE

To use your ebook offline, download BookShelf to your PC, Mac, iOS device, Android device or Kindle Fire, and log in to your Bookshelf account to access your ebook:

On your PC/Mac

Go to *https://support.vitalsource.com/hc/en-us* and follow the instructions to download the free **VitalSource Bookshelf** app to your PC or Mac and log into your Bookshelf account.

On your iPhone/iPod Touch/iPad

Download the free **VitalSource Bookshelf** App available via the iTunes App Store and log into your Bookshelf account. You can find more information at *https://support. vitalsource.com/hc/en-us/categories/200134217-Bookshelf-for-iOS*

On your Android™ smartphone or tablet

Download the free **VitalSource Bookshelf** App available via Google Play and log into your Bookshelf account. You can find more information at *https://support.vitalsource.com/ hc/en-us/categories/200139976-Bookshelf-for-Android-and-Kindle-Fire*

On your Kindle Fire

Download the free **VitalSource Bookshelf** App available from Amazon and log into your Bookshelf account. You can find more information at *https://support.vitalsource.com/ hc/en-us/categories/200139976-Bookshelf-for-Android-and-Kindle-Fire*

N.B. The code in the scratch-off panel can only be used once. When you have created a Bookshelf account and redeemed the code you will be able to access the ebook online or offline on your smartphone, tablet or PC/Mac.

SUPPORT

If you have any questions about downloading Bookshelf, creating your account, or accessing and using your ebook edition, please visit *http://support.vitalsource.com/*

9 781032 240046